CURRENT PSYCHOTHERAPIES

CURRENT PSYCHOTHERAPIES
NINTH EDITION

Editors

Raymond J. Corsini
Danny Wedding

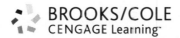

BROOKS/COLE
CENGAGE Learning™

Australia • Brazil • Japan • Korea • Mexico • Singapore • Spain • United Kingdom • United States

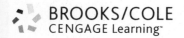

BROOKS/COLE
CENGAGE Learning™

Current Psychotherapies: Ninth Edition
Raymond J. Corsini and Danny Wedding

Publisher/Executive Editor: Linda Schreiber

Acquisitions Editor: Seth Dobrin

Assistant Editor: Nicolas Albert

Editorial Assistant: Rachel McDonald

Media Editor: Dennis Fitzgerald

Marketing Manager: Trent Whatcott

Marketing Assistant: Darlene Macanan

Marketing Communications Manager:
    Tami Strang

Content Project Management:
    Pre-Press PMG

Creative Director: Rob Hugel

Art Director: Caryl Gorska

Print Buyer: Rebecca Cross

Rights Acquisitions Account Manager, Text:
    Bob Kauser, Roberta Broyer

Rights Acquisitions Account Manager,
    Image: Leitha Etheridge-Sims

Production Service: Pre-Press PMG

Photo Researcher: Pre-Press PMG

Copy Editor: Pre-Press PMG

Cover Designer: Gia Giasullo, Studio

Cover Image: Dave Cutler / Getty Images

Compositor: Pre-Press PMG

For product information and technology assistance, contact us at
Cengage Learning Customer & Sales Support, 1-800-354-9706.

For permission to use material from this text or product,
submit all requests online at **www.cengage.com/permissions**.
Further permissions questions can be e-mailed to
permissionrequest@cengage.com.

Library of Congress Control Number: 2009942932

ISBN-13: 978-0-495-90336-9

ISBN-10: 0-495-90336-1

Brooks/Cole
20 Davis Drive
Belmont, CA 94002-3098
USA

Cengage Learning is a leading provider of customized learning solutions with office locations around the globe, including Singapore, the United Kingdom, Australia, Mexico, Brazil, and Japan. Locate your local office at **www.cengage.com/global**.

Cengage Learning products are represented in Canada by Nelson Education, Ltd.

To learn more about Brooks/Cole, visit **www.cengage.com/brookscole**

Purchase any of our products at your local college store or at our preferred online store **www.CengageBrain.com.**

Printed in the United States of America
1 2 3 4 5 6 7 13 12 11 10

In memory of Raymond J. Corsini (1914–2008)

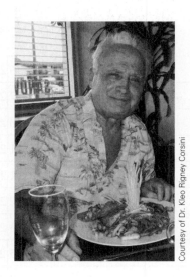

CORE STRUCTURE

	Psychoanalysis	Adlerian	Analytical	Client-Centered	Rational Emotive	Behavior	Cognitive	Existential	Gestalt	Interpersonal	Family	Contemplative	Integrative	Multicultural
Overview **Page**	15	67	113	148	196	235	276	310	342	383	417	454	502	536
Basic Concepts	16	67	113	148	197	236	276	311	343	383	417	454	503	537
Other Systems	19	70	115	152	200	240	278	—	343	386	422	457	505	542
History	22	75	117	154	201	242	280	314	348	387	423	462	507	543
Precursors	22	75	117	154	201	242	280	314	348	387	423	462	507	543
Beginnings	22	76	118	155	202	243	280	314	349	389	424	462	507	544
Current Status	27	77	119	157	203	244	281	316	350	390	426	464	508	546
Personality	30	78	120	158	205	245	283	317	351	391	429	465	510	548
Theory of Personality	30	78	120	158	205	245	283	317	351	391	429	466	510	548
Variety of Concepts	33	81	123	161	209	247	285	318	354	393	430	471	511	—
Psychotherapy	37	82	125	163	211	249	290	322	359	394	433	473	512	549
Theory of Psychotherapy	37	82	125	163	211	249	290	322	359	394	433	473	512	549
Process of Psychotherapy	41	84	127	166	213	251	292	323	362	395	435	476	516	550
Mechanisms of Psychotherapy	45	90	129	167	220	256	295	330	364	402	439	479	519	553
Applications	49	93	131	170	221	258	295	333	366	404	441	481	520	555
Who Can We Help?	49	93	131	170	221	258	295	333	366	404	441	481	520	555
Treatment	51	94	132	174	222	264	296	333	367	404	441	485	521	556
Evidence	54	97	136	176	225	265	300	335	370	405	444	490	522	559
Psychotherapy in a Multicultural World	57	99	138	182	225	267	301	336	375	408	446	493	524	560
Case Example	58	99	139	183	229	267	301	337	376	411	447	494	526	560
Summary	61	105	142	190	231	270	304	339	378	413	449	495	531	563
Annotated Bibliography	62	106	144	190	232	271	306	340	379	413	450	498	532	564
Case Readings	63	107	145	191	233	271	306	340	380	414	450	498	532	564
References	63	107	145	191	233	272	306	341	380	414	451	498	533	564

CONTENTS

CONTRIBUTORS

Jacob Arlow, MD
Deceased

Aaron T. Beck, MD
University Professor of Psychiatry,
University of Pennsylvania,
Philadelphia, Pennsylvania

Larry E. Beutler, PhD
William McInnes Distinguished Professor
of Psychology
Director, National Center for the
Psychology of Terrorism
Pacific Graduate School of Psychology
Palo Alto, California

Raymond J. Corsini, PhD
Deceased

Lillian Comas-Diaz, PhD
Transcultural Mental Health Institute
Washington, DC

Claire Douglas, PhD
Private Practice,
Training and Supervisory Analyst
C. G. Jung Institute of Los Angeles
Malibu, California

Frank Dumont, EdD
Professor Emeritus
McGill University
Montreal, Canada

Albert Ellis, PhD
Deceased

Erica Goldenberg Pelavin, LCSW, PhD
Private Practice

Herbert Goldenberg, PhD
Deceased

Irene Goldenberg, EdD
Professor of Psychiatry, University of
California-Los Angeles, Los Angeles,
California

Lynne Jacobs, PhD
Private Practice, Gestalt Therapy
Institute of the Pacific, Los Angeles,
California

Ruthellen Josselson, PhD
School of Psychology
Fielding Graduate University
Baltimore, Maryland

Ellen Luborsky, PhD
Private Practice, New York, New York

Michael P. Maniacci, PsyD
Clinical Psychologist and Consultant in
Private Practice, Chicago, Illinois

Harold H. Mosak, PhD
Distinguished Service Professor of
Clinical Psychology, Adler School of
Professional Psychology, Chicago,
Illinois

John Norcross, PhD
Professor of Psychology & Distinguished
University Fellow, University of Scranton,
Scranton, Pennsylvania

Maureen O'Reilly-Landry, PhD
Private Practice, New York, New York

Ken Pope, PhD
Private Practice, Norwalk, Connecticut

Nathanial J. Raskin, PhD
Emeritus Professor of Psychiatry and
Behavioral Sciences, Northwestern
University Medical School, Chicago, Illinois

Carl Rogers, PhD
Deceased

Helen Verdeli, PhD
Assistant Professor of Clinical Psychology
Teachers College
Columbia University
New York, New York

Roger Walsh, MD, PhD
Professor of Psychiatry, Philosophy,
and Anthropology, University of
California-Irvine, Irvine, California

Danny Wedding, PhD, MPH
Professor of Psychiatry and Director,
Missouri Institute of Mental Health,
St. Louis, Missouri

Marjorie Weishaar, PhD
Clinical Professor of Psychiatry and
Human Behavior, Brown University
Providence, Rhode Island

Myrna Weissman, PhD
Professor of Epidemiology in Psychiatry
Department of Psychiatry
Columbia University
New York, New York

G. Terence Wilson, PhD
Oscar K. Buros Professor of
Psychology, Rutgers University,
Piscataway, New Jersey

Marge Witty, PhD
Professor of Clinical Psychology,
Illinois School of Professional Psychology,
Argosy University, Chicago, Illinois

Irvin D. Yalom, MD
Professor Emeritus of Psychiatry
Stanford University
Palo Alto, California

Gary Yontef, PhD
Private Practice, Gestalt Therapy Institute
of the Pacific, Santa Monica, California

ACKNOWLEDGMENTS

Every book is shaped and refined by the comments of those readers who take time to provide feedback. This book is no different, and we have benefited from the suggestions of literally hundreds of our students, colleagues, and friends. We have been particularly vigilant about getting feedback from those professors who use *Current Psychotherapies* as a text, and their comments help shape each new edition. The following individuals were especially helpful in preparing the ninth edition, and we genuinely appreciate their contributions: Martin Antony, Adam Blatner, Bernard Beitman, James Bray, Kleo Corsini, Barbara Cubic, Vicki Eichhorn, Connie Evashwick, Debbie Joffe Ellis, Frank Farley, Ken Freedland, James Hennessy, Jessica Kohout, Annie Kim, Judy Kuriansky, Carla Leeson, Marsha Linehan, Anthony Marsella, Lisa Marty, Richard Nelson-Jones, John Norcross, Chris Pearce, Lauralyn Perkins, Stephanie Silbey, Sombat Tapanya, and Bob Woody. In addition, I appreciate numerous suggestions from colleagues in the Society of Clinical Psychology (Division 12 of the American Psychological Association).

In addition, we'd like to acknowledge the following reviewers of the ninth edition: Vergel L. Lattimore, PhD, Methodist Theological School in Ohio; Harry Pitsikalis, York College; Raluca Gaher, University of South Dakota; Joy Burnham, University of Alabama; Dr. Cherrye G. Watts, Central Michigan University; Stephanie Porterfield, PhD, University of Oklahoma; Holly Orcutt, Northern Illinois University; Mary Ann Goodwyn, Louisiana Tech University; Carl Jylland-Halverson, University of Saint Francis; Victor Wiesner, Sam Houston State University; Timothy S. Hartshorne, Central Michigan University; La Pearl Logan Winfrey, Wright State University; Sherryl M. McGuire, University of Oklahoma; Noah Shapiro, New York University; Benjamin R. Tong, PhD, California Institute of Integral Studies; Matthew Miller, Rowan University; Mary M. Livingston, Louisiana Tech University; George M. Wawrykow, PhD, ABPP, Prairie View A&M University; and Roger L. Johnson, Dallas Baptist University.

PREFACE

The ninth edition of *Current Psychotherapies* reflects our commitment to maintaining the currency alluded to in the book's title, and the text in its entirety provides a comprehensive overview of the state of the art of psychotherapy. The book was first published in 1973, and since that time it has been used by more than a million students and translated in more than a dozen languages. One reviewer recently refered to the text as "venerable."

New chapters on Interpersonal Psychotherapy and Multicultural Psychotherapy have been added to the latest edition. A previous chapter on Multimodal Psychotherapy has been eliminated to keep the book to a reasonable length; however, this chapter is still available on the *Current Psychotherapies* Web site. Dr. Irvin Yalom has returned to *Current Psychotherapies* and has contributed a new chapter on Existential Psychotherapy coauthored by Ruthellen Josselson; a previous excellent chapter on Existential Psychotherapy, written by Ed Mendelowitz and Kirk Schneider, is still available on the book's Web site. In addition, anyone interested can watch an interview of Dr. Raymond J. Corsini at this site by simply clicking on "Corsini videos"

All other chapters in the book have been updated or totally rewritten. A new author has been added for the chapter on Family Therapy. All chapters have been revised to include up-to-date references and the most current psychotherapy research available. Each chapter describing a particular approach to psychotherapy examines the evidence base supporting that particular theory, and I have asked each contributor to share his or her ideas about the current controversy regarding the importance—and limitations—of evidence-based practice. In addition, all of the core chapters now address the very important topic of multiculturalism, and I'm delighted to add a separate chapter on Multicultural Psychotherapy to the new editon.

In a preface to an earlier edition, Raymond J. Corsini described six features of *Current Psychotherapies* that have helped ensure the book's utility and popularity. These core principles guided the development of the ninth edition.

1. *The chapters in this book describe the most important systems in the current practice of psychotherapy.* Because psychotherapy is constantly evolving, deciding what to put into new editions and what to take out demands a great deal of research. The opinions of professors were central in shaping the changes we have made. Before each new edition, professors who have taught from the book at least 2 years are asked what they would want in the next edition and what they no longer want in the current one. Their diverse opinions helped us decide what changes to make.

2. *The most competent available authors are recruited.* Newly established systems are described by their founders; older systems are covered by those best qualified to describe them.

3. *This book is highly disciplined.* Each author follows an outline in which the various sections are limited in length and structure. The purpose of this feature is to make it as convenient as possible to compare the systems by reading the book "horizontally" (from section to section across the various systems), as well as in the usual "vertical" manner (from chapter to chapter). The major sections of each chapter include an overview of the system being described, its history, a discussion of the theory of personality that shaped the therapy, a detailed discussion of how psychotherapy using the system is actually practiced, and

an explanation of the various applications of the approach being described. In addition, each of the therapies described is accompanied by a case study illustrating the techniques and methods associated with the therapy. Students interested in more detailed case examples can read this book's companion volume, *Case Studies in Psychotherapy* (Wedding & Corsini, 2011). Those students who want to understand psychotherapy in depth will benefit from reading both *Current Psychotherapies* and *Case Studies in Psychotherapy.*

4. Current Psychotherapies *is carefully edited.* Every section is examined to make certain that its contents are appropriate and clear. In the long history of this text, only one chapter was ever accepted in its first draft. Some chapters have been returned to their original authors as many as four times before finally being accepted.

5. *Chapters are as concise as they can possibly be and still cover the systems completely.* We have received consistent feedback that the chapters in *Current Psychotherapies* need to be clear, succinct, and direct. We have taken this feedback seriously, and every sentence in each new edition is carefully edited to ensure that the information provided is not redundant or superfluous.

6. *The glossary for each new edition is updated and expanded.* One way for students to begin any chapter would be to read the relevant entries in the glossary, thereby generating a mind-set that will facilitate understanding the various systems. Personality theorists tend to invent new words when no existing word suffices. This clarifies their ideas, but it also makes understanding their chapter more difficult. A careful study of the glossary will reward the reader.

Ray Corsini died on November 8, 2008. He was a master Adlerian therapist, the best of my teachers and a cherished friend. This edition of *Current Psychotherapies* is dedicated to his memory.

Danny Wedding
danny.wedding@mimh.edu

1 | INTRODUCTION TO 21ST-CENTURY PSYCHOTHERAPIES

Frank Dumont

Other men are lenses through which we read our own minds.
Ralph Waldo Emerson (1850)

Psychotherapy, as far as it leads to substantial behavior change, appears to achieve its effect through changes in gene expression at the neuronal level.
Eric Kandel (1996)

EVOLUTION OF THIS SCIENCE

This book surveys a diverse set of effective psychotherapies. Each represents a vision of the Human as well as a set of distinct treatment procedures for addressing the emotional distress and the accompanying behavioral and cognitive problems that drive people to seek help. As one reviews the evolution of this textbook through nine editions and the theories of personality development that underpin each of the therapeutic modalities treated within it, it's evident that these modalities have an increasingly short half-life. Entire schools of psychotherapy have undergone dramatic change, some more rapidly than others—and some have virtually disappeared (e.g., Transactional Analysis). The editors of this book continue to showcase several therapies that have their origins in the early 20th century, but they do this because these earlier therapies have evolved to reflect changes in the science of developmental psychology and have continually improved their clinical effectiveness. Therapies of more recent vintage have been added, which, although built on strong historical foundations, would strike even psychotherapists of the 1960s and 1970s as novel if not strange. In any event, to understand where we are heading, we need to know where psychotherapy started and how it has changed. The following section addresses this matter.

Historical Foundations of Psychotherapy

From the origins of recorded history, humans have sought means to remedy the mental disorders that have afflicted them. Some of these remedies were (and continue to be) patently unscientific, if not ineffective, such as the ceremonial healing rituals found in shamanistic societies. Pre-Christian, temple-like *asklepeia* and other retreat centers of the eastern Mediterranean region, using religio-philosophical lectures, meditation, and simple rest, competed with secular medicine to assuage if not remedy psychological disorders. This latter stream of psycho-physiological treatment, in which Hippocrates worked, was surprisingly scientific. Hellenist physicians, through their empirical studies, understood that the brain was not only the seat of knowledge and learning but also the source of depression, delirium, and madness. Indeed, he wrote, "Men ought to know that from nothing else but the brain come joys, delights, laughter and sports, and sorrows, griefs, despondency, and lamentations . . . and by the same organ we become mad and delirious, and fears and terrors assail us . . . all things we endure from the brain when it is not healthy" (5th c. B.C.E., quoted by Stanley Finger, 2001, p. 13). Hippocrates himself insisted that his students address illnesses by natural means. He repudiated the popular notion that such illnesses as seizures were "divine" and should be treated by appealing to and placating gods. Although the Hippocratic tradition endured uninterruptedly to the time of his renowned disciple Galen, who lived six centuries later, psychotherapy in its present guise did not clearly emerge until the 18th century.

The Unconscious

The reader will find that the construct *unconscious* plays a salient role in certain chapters of this volume, especially those that have a psychodynamic character, but it was also a key construct in the psychotherapies that emerged in the 19th century. The scientific study of the unconscious is commonly thought to have started with the renowned polymath Gottfried Wilhelm Leibniz (1646–1716). Leibniz studied the role of subliminal perceptions in our daily life (and, incidentally, coined the term "dynamic" to describe the forces operative in unconscious mentation). His investigations of the unconscious were continued by Johann Friedrich Herbart (1776–1841), who attempted to mathematicize the dynamics describing the passage of memories to and from the conscious and the unconscious. Herbart suggested that ideas struggle with one another for access to consciousness as dissonant ideas repel one another and associated ideas help pull each other into consciousness (or drag each other down into unconsciousness). Leibniz and Herbart are examples of 17th- and 18th-century scientists who attributed significance to an understanding of the unconscious in their work (Whyte, 1960).

Mesmer and Schopenhauer. Two of the most influential and creative thinkers in the early 19th century were Franz Anton Mesmer (1734–1815) and Arthur Schopenhauer (1788–1860). Their impact can be seen in the psychiatric literature that evolved into the full-fledged systems of Pierre Janet, Sigmund Freud, Alfred Adler, and Carl Gustav Jung. Thomas Mann (a Nobel laureate in literature) stated that in reading Freud, he had an eerie feeling that he was actually reading Schopenhauer (1788–1860) translated into a later idiom (Ellenberger, 1970, p. 209).

Mesmer and his disciple the Marquis de Puységur, regarded as the pioneers of hypnotherapy, effectively discredited the exorcist tradition that had dominated pre-Enlightenment Europe (Leahey, 2000, pp. 216–218). That there were many quaint and unsubstantiated hypotheses in the Mesmerian system does not diminish the fact that the notion of rapport between therapist and patient, the influence of the unconscious in shaping behavior, the personal qualities of the therapist, spontaneous remission of disorders, hypnotic somnambulism, the selective function of unconscious memory, importance of patients' confidence in treatment procedures, and other common factors in our current therapeutics armory can be traced back to this period in European history.

Three distinct streams of investigation into how the mind works emerged in the 19th century. The contributors to these three streams were (a) systematic, lab-bench empiricists, (b) philosophers of nature, and (c) clinician–researchers. A multitude of psychotherapies were spun out from these investigations.

Psychotherapy-related Science in the 19th Century

The Natural-Science Empiricists

Some of the greatest scientists of the 19th century, such as Gustav T. Fechner (1801–1887) and Herman von Helmholtz (1821–1894), conducted seminal research in the area of cognitive science. Fechner's work tapped into and overlapped with the investigations of Herbart. Fechner began with the distinction between the theaters of the waking and sleeping states—and especially the dream state. That the unconscious existed as a realm of the mind was evident even to the untutored farm laborer. Anyone who had ever struggled to recall a memory—and succeeded—knew that he or she retained knowledge that was not always readily accessible. This knowledge had to reside somewhere. In the late 1850s, Fechner, in his psychophysics experiments, attempted to measure the intensity of psychic stimulation needed for ideas to cross the threshold from the unconscious to full awareness, as well as the intensity of the resultant perception. Fechner's studies reverberated throughout Europe, and the reader may unknowingly resonate to his findings not only in Freud's writings (Freud quoted him in several of his works) and the chapters of this book but also in those of myriad other contemporary theorists and practitioners, most notably the Gestaltists and (Milton H.) Ericksonians.

Helmholtz, another experimentalist, "discovered the phenomenon of 'unconscious inference'," which he perceived "as a kind of instantaneous and unconscious reconstruction of what our past taught us about the object" (Ellenberger, 1970, p. 313). Wilhelm Griesinger, Joannes von Müller, and many other such experimentalists and brain scientists dominated the academic scene of Vienna, Heidelberg, Leipzig, and other German-language universities and institutes, making many contributions that infused the work of later psychodynamicists.

The spirit and approach of these lab-based scientists resounded throughout Europe and in large part constituted what became known there as the *somatiker* (organicist) tradition. Several of Freud's mentors, such as Ernst Brücke (1819–1892) and Theodor Meynert (1833–1892), were organicists. Although the organicists worked feverishly throughout the century to find solutions to psychiatric disorders, Emil Kraepelin on the cusp of the 20th century finally conceded defeat, admitting that 50 years of hard bench work had given medicine few tools for curing psychiatric disorders (Shorter, 1997, pp. 103, 328). He turned his attention to classifying diseases, meticulously describing them, schematizing their course, and establishing benchmarks for prognosis. This provided an opportunity for the *psychiker* (those who were convinced that only a psychological approach to mental illness would prove effective) to gain prominence. The work of all the brass-instrument methodologists and empiricist dream scholars still pales in significance by comparison with the influence of the psycho-philosophical writers of the first half of the 19th century.

The Psychologist—Philosophers

The philosophers of nature had a much greater, long-term influence on the development of the psychotherapies described in the following chapters of this book than did laboratory-based scientists. These philosophers can be historically situated in the same school of thought that nurtured Schiller and Goethe. They were Romantics in the philosophical sense, firmly rooted in nature, beauty, homeland, sentiment, the life of the mind, and of course, the mind at its most enigmatic: the unconscious. Arthur Schopenhauer, Carl Gustav Carus, and Eduard von Hartmann were among the most notable of this group.

Carl Gustav Carus (1789–1869), though largely unread today, can justifiably be singled out in a book on psychotherapy because he developed one of the most sophisticated schemas that exist for the unconscious (see Ellenberger, 1970, pp. 202–210). Carus speculated that there are several levels to the unconscious. When humans interact, all levels of the unconscious as well as the conscious interact. To extrapolate to the clinic, when patient and therapist are at work, the conscious of each speaks to the unconscious as well as to the conscious of the other. But further, the unconscious of each speaks to the conscious as well as the to unconscious of the other. Needless to emphasize, both are communicating with each other in paravocal, nonverbal, organic, and affective modes of which both participants are largely unaware. In this perspective, *both* the therapist and the patient engage, willfully or not, in transference and countertransference (see Dumont & Fitzpatrick, 2001). Nonlinear messages are systemically (often simultaneously) sent in all directions. What Carus taught us is that transference occurs at an unconscious level.

Before Carus, Schopenhauer (1819) published "The World as Will and Idea." This masterpiece of the Western canon, once it caught on, provided ideational grist for generations of psychological researchers who followed. It inspired those psychologists who were children of the Philosophy of Nature and had embraced (or resigned themselves to) nonbiological methods for curing the fashionable disorders of the day—even those disorders that today would be classified as (DSM) Axis I disorders. Schopenhauer's book was in large part a treatise on human sexuality and the realm of the unconscious. His principal argument was that we are driven by blind, irrational forces of which we are largely unaware and that we know things that we are unaware that we know. His irrationalist and pansexual view of human behavior and mentation was deterministic and also pessimistic (see Ellenberger's [1970] analysis, pp. 208–210). Schopenhauer's thoughts influenced the psychology of many later thinkers, not least Friedrich Nietzsche and Sigmund Freud.

The tracts of Schopenhauer and Carus set the epistemological stage for von Hartmann's and Nietzsche's influential writings on our tacit cognitions, which they believed drove the daily, unreflective behavior of people. In Nietzsche's view, humans lie to themselves even more than they do to each other. What we consciously are thinking is "a more or less fantastic commentary on an unconscious, perhaps unknowable, but felt text" (cited in Ellenberger, 1970, p. 273). He developed notions of self-deception, sublimation, repression, conscience, and neurotic guilt. Cynic *par excellence* Nietzsche averred that every complaint is an accusation and every admission of a behavioral fault or characterological flaw is a subterfuge to conceal more serious personal failures. In brief, he unmasked many of the defense mechanisms that humans employ to embellish their persona and self-image. Nietzsche, in his unsystematic and aphoristic way, cast a long shadow over the personology and psychotherapies of the 20th century.

The Clinician–Researchers

In the nascent clinical psychology of the 19th century, a great number of gifted clinicians made discoveries and innovations in their clinical practice that had implications for psychotherapy generally and for the development of theories of personality as well. Some were humble practitioners like the celebrated hypnotherapist Ambroise Liébault, others great scholars like Moritz Benedikt (1835–1920), whose work in criminology, psychiatry, and neurology won the admiration of Jean-Martin Charcot. Benedikt developed the useful concept of seeking out and clinically purging "pathogenic secrets," a practice that Jung later made an essential element of his analytic psychotherapy. Théodore Flournoy, Josef Breuer, Auguste Forel, Eugen Bleuler, Paul Dubois (greatly admired by Raymond Corsini), Sigmund Freud, Pierre Janet, Adolf Meyer, Carl Gustav Jung, and Alfred Adler all made signal contributions to the science of psychotherapy. Though many of their contributions have outlived their usefulness, the many offshoots of their findings and systems can be traced in clinical psychotherapy and in other psychological disciplines.

A corollary of the notion that psychotherapies are in constant evolution is the recognition that clinicians have often perpetuated the strategies and techniques they learned in their graduate professional programs, dated though they may have become, rather than learning and developing important new principles and procedures through their professional practice and diligent reading of the literature in their specialty. Remaining at a fixed stage of one's continually evolving profession is not a desirable outcome of training, for, to paraphrase an aphorism from sport psychology, practice makes permanent but not necessarily perfect. Improving our performance of an outdated or largely flawed technique is not a clinical desideratum.

Chapters 2 through 15 of this volume represent scientifically recognized advances over what preceded them. Like all current and major psychotherapies, they have all emerged to a greater or lesser degree from the historical matrix described above. Even the contemplative therapies described in chapter 13 have their roots not only in the ancient traditions of the Middle and Far East but also in those of the Near East and the *asklepeia* of Hellenic Greece.

THE IMPACT OF THE BIOLOGICAL SCIENCES ON PSYCHOTHERAPY

When patients[1] learn new ideas, whether true or false, whether in the clinic or in the course of daily life, concomitant alterations of the brain occur (see, e.g., LeDoux's [2002], *Synaptic Self*). Every encounter with our environment causes a change within us and in our neural functioning. Moreover, education implies permanence. Once skills and ideas are truly learned and lodged in permanent storage, it is difficult if not

---

[1] Throughout this chapter we have used the term *patient,* which etymologically implies *suffering* and characterizes most people who seek therapy. It is a derivative of a Latin verb that means to endure a painful situation. In the 8th edition of this book, Ray Corsini noted the discipline-specific connotations of patient and *client*, the former for medical contexts and the latter for his private practice.

impossible to unlearn them. Given the solution to a puzzle, taught the secret of cracking a safe, or having developed the skill of riding a bicycle, one cannot unlearn that knowledge. Neuronal decay and lesions can, of course, undo memory and occur to a certain extent in aging and, catastrophically, in strokes, illness, or violent accidents. The task of the therapist in most cases is to help the patient fashion *alternative* and future memories, supported by newly learned motivational schemas.

Klaus Grawe (2007), in his important book *Neuropsychotherapy: How the Neurosciences Inform Effective Psychotherapy,* noted that "Psychotherapy, as far as it leads to substantial behavior change, appears to achieve its effect through changes in gene expression at the neuronal level" (p. 3, citing Kandel, 1996, p. 711). Further embedding patients in their dysfunctional past by prodding them to ruminate about that past does not erase their painful memories nor their penchant for dwelling on these memories. Nor does it teach them more adaptive patterns of behavior. Therapists teach patients how to avoid dysfunctional, harmful behavioral routines and maladaptive habits. Effective therapists also help their clients develop alternative skills (social, interpersonal, self-disciplinary, and technical) that will advance their well-being and that of others with whom they interact. The neurosciences have demonstrated that neuronal restructuring, which occurs in all learning processes, enables the adaptive changes in affect, behavior, and mentation that are the core objectives of psychotherapy (cf. Dumont, 2009; 2010).

A neurological perspective on psychotherapy does not exclude attention to changing clients' environment or introducing constructive environmental stimuli into their lives. On the contrary, even minor novelties in clients' lifestyle can have enormous consequences in the way they perceive and experience themselves. We now know that effective therapists and their clients can optimize desirable outcomes by epigenetically triggering the expression of *immediate-early genes* (IEGs) through exposure to nurturant social events (Güntürkün, 2006). (*Epigenetics* refers to the expression of certain genes that results from their activation by specific but common environmental events.) Culture generally and one's immediate family specifically function as genetic enablers. Such epigenetic effects can operate for better or for worse, depending on the quality of the experiences. In brief, it is the complex bio-cultural matrix of the organic *and* the environmental that co-construct our way of being and our potential for growth (Baltes, Reuter-Lorenz, & Rösler, 2006).

ORGANICISTS AND DYNAMICISTS: CLASHING STANDPOINTS

Readers will immediately recognize the potential for cultural confrontations in these propositions. However, our view is that confrontation is neither necessary nor useful. The ancient animosity between the *somatiker* and the *psychiker,* the psychopharmacological organicists and psychodynamicists, the behavioral geneticists and the cognitive-behaviorists can be resolved through a systemic integration of the many variables that are at play at any moment. Indeed, such integration is necessary. To ignore organic *or* environmental variables in one's treatment of one's clientele is to neglect essential aspects of the whole person, and to treat all affective disorders as if there were no organicity in the causal skein of variables that brought them about is an ancient error.

One example of this error is ignoring patients' medication histories. Kenneth Pope and Danny Wedding (2010) discuss the danger inherent in neglecting to monitor patients who are taking psychotropic medication. Patients need to be pharmacologically guided and their experiences between sessions closely monitored. Medicating patients for psychological purposes requires preset clinical objectives and conscientious ongoing assessment of progress. Grawe (2007) stated:

> From a neuroscientific perspective, psychopharmacological therapy that is not coordinated with a simultaneous, targeted alteration of the person's experiences cannot be justified. The widespread practice of prescribing psychoactive medication without assuming responsibility for the patient's concurrent experience is, from a neuroscientific view, equally irresponsible. . . . The use of pharmacotherapy alone—in the absence of the professional and competent structuring of the treated patient's life experience—is not justifiable . . . (pp. 5–6)

Nurture is profoundly shaped by nature. Similarly, aspects of our nature (that is, our genetic inheritance) are epigenetically expressed for better or for worse by the kinds of experiences to which we are subjected throughout our life. This explains in part why, among identical twins, one can become severely diabetic while the other does not. In this perspective, therapists become responsible to some degree for both the natural and nurturant components of the patients' lives that come under their purview.

Evolutionary Biology and Behavioral Genetics

Neuroscience is not the sole biological research domain whose findings will have implications for psychotherapy. Evolutionary psychology will likely further clarify many of the temperamental traits that therapists need to understand to be effective. Steven Pinker (2002) has extensively documented the principle that all humans share the same, unique nature. If we exclude anomalous genetic mutations, the normative stance of all clinicians treating a patient is that they are dealing with an organism struck from the same genetic template as themselves.

Evolutionary psychology is closely related to the field of behavioral genetics, another discipline that will have an impact on the therapeutic modalities that clinicians of the future will assuredly develop. This discipline will shine a focused light on the lawfulness that governs the human genome and the biopsychosocial regularities that occur in the course of one's life. There are more regularities, that is, universal behavioral traits, than we have traditionally imagined (see Brown, 1991). While accepting the parameters established by our genetic inheritance and the regularities our genes prescribe for our human interactions and life course, clinicians will still need to treat the idiosyncratic dysfunctions their patients reveal to them. Moreover, as suggested above, psychotherapy will involve monitoring the situational variables and events that can trigger the expression of latent genes. Finally, the related fields of molecular genetic analysis, cognitive neuropsychology, and social cognitive neuroscience, which are advancing at an impressive rate, will inevitably infiltrate our porous integrationist models of helping.

CULTURAL FACTORS AND PSYCHOTHERAPY

Demographics

In this 9th edition of *Current Psychotherapies,* a new chapter is dedicated to current approaches to multicultural psychotherapy. This initiative is not simply a reflection of the self-evident importance of cultural factors in counseling and psychotherapy that have been developing in recent decades. It is also a reflection of the changing demographic character of the planet, the human tides that are swirling about the previously distant continents of the globe, the tightening communicational network of masses of people engaged in commerce, armed conflict, research, diplomacy, and higher education, and the internationalization of professional psychological counseling. Although chapters on Jungian psychotherapy (Chapter 4), existential psychotherapy (Chapter 9), and, most notably, contemplative psychotherapies (Chapter 13) have dealt heretofore with the ethno-cultural variables implicated in the treatment of diverse ethnic populations, a new chapter (Chapter 15) will be dedicated exclusively to this approach.

The complexities involved in multicultural counseling are incomparably greater than those involved in conducting therapy in a homogeneous culture where each member of the therapeutic dyad springs from the same ethno-cultural background. Where the patient and the therapist are solidly grounded in different traditional cultures, it matters if the "authority" figure is a member, say, of a minority, nondominant culture or the dominant, majority culture. In marital counseling, the difficulties multiply like fractals if the couple seeking help is biracial. In this case, the matrix of interactive variables becomes even more complex if the therapist/counselor *unknowingly* identifies with one spouse rather than the other. Gender by culture permutations add another layer of systemic interactions. And of course it is not enough to simply acknowledge one's differentness. Counselors are never fully aware of how different they are from the clients sitting across from or beside them for the simple reason that they are never fully conscious of the dynamics driving their own reactions to the client's socially conditioned sensitivities. Much of therapists' mentation operates beyond awareness, for their own cognitive and affective structures are intermeshed in the invisible, bottomless depths of their unconscious.

Cantonese speakers counseling Cantonese speakers in Hong Kong face a different set of parameters and challenges than Hispanic counselors in San Diego counseling other Hispanics. The philosophical and socio-economic differences that characterize members of the same society will determine the suitability of nonindigenous psychotherapies that are most congenial to both of them. But within homogeneous non-Caucasian populations, there is the same constellation of contingencies that confront Euro-American peoples. Job stresses, finances, physical illness, personal history, family dynamics, personological variables of genetic and environmental origin, even the weather will all affect what happens between a therapist and a client.

Language and Metaphor

Language, behavioral mannerisms, local and national poetry, metaphor, and myth are the instruments that shape the structures of our mind (see, for example, Lakoff & Johnson [1980] in *Metaphors We Live By*). Popular metaphors permeate all aspects of human thought. They ultimately shape a nation's culture and collective personality. Those who are not familiar with these elements of their clients' culture will find it difficult to enter the labyrinthine recesses where their ancestral and self-made daemons (some benevolent, some hurtful) reside.

All therapists have clinical stories they can tell of mistakes they have made by the innocent use of a metaphor, a careless juxtaposing of questions, a refusal of a courtesy, or insensitivity to a taboo of their client's culture. Painfully, their former friends and patients have left, never to return, with hardly a word of explanation. For this reason, it has often been proposed that psychotherapies need to be indigenized. Rather than exporting Euro-American psychotherapies, say, to China, some would encourage Chinese healers to develop psychotherapies that reflect *their* philosophies, values, social objectives, and religious convictions. Yang (1997, 1999), for example, has suggested that Chinese counselors can more easily help resolve the paradoxes and dilemmas that characterize Chinese village, family, and personal life than non-Chinese can. Likewise, Hoshmand (2005, p. 3) avers that "indigenous culture provides native ways of knowing what is salient and congruent with the local ethos and what are credible ways of addressing human problems," a view supported by Marsella and Yamada (2000). Similarly,

Cross and Markus (1999) note that "the articulation of a truly universal understanding of human nature and personality . . . requires the development of theories of behavior *originating* in the indigenous psychologies of Asian, Latin American, African, and other non-Western societies" (p. 381).

The complex issues that we have alluded to here will be more fully addressed in Chapter 15.

NEGOTIATING FAULT LINES IN THE EBT TERRAIN

Division 12 (1995) of the American Psychological Association (APA) established a Task Force on Promotion and Dissemination of Psychological Procedures to grapple with the issues of empirically based treatments (EBTs). Since then there has been a flood of research conducted to demonstrate the scientific validity of those therapies their partisans espouse. As in earlier editions of *Current Psychotherapies,* the contributors to this book have wrestled with this issue. There are a number of serious fault lines in the terrain defining this debate, and although they have all been addressed by the professions serving the mental health needs of society, they still constitute threats to clinical credibility.

Psychotherapy: An Art or a Science

Patients typically work in session with one therapist for 50 minutes a week but are exposed for the rest of the week to innumerable contingencies outside the clinic that can confound their fine-tuned plans and firmest resolve. Many of these contingencies are unforeseen and beyond their control. Paul Meehl (1978) called these random events *context-dependent stochastologicals* (pp. 812–814); they are a tangle of variables internal and external to the person that intertwine with job stresses, financial concerns, troubled children, angry spouses or in-laws, difficult colleagues, bad weather, life-threatening illness, dubious insurance claims, and the forgotten baggage of personal history and past defeats. Each patient has a unique set of such variables, but to make the situation even more complicated, they are often afflicted by a number of distinct disorders. This comorbidity complicates the categorization of disordered patients for purposes of validating therapy for them (Beutler & Baker, 1998). For many practitioners and onlookers, the science of prognosticating outcomes in psychotherapy inspires as much confidence as predictions of stock market fluctuations. There is simply too much opacity in the universe of variables, known and unknown, to make confident prognoses.

Spontaneity and Intuition: "Throw-Ins"

Readers of the chapters of this book will be faced with clients who present complex puzzles to them, each client manifesting varying degrees of anxiety, coping skills, and emotional stability—and often with no clear idea what their treatment will consist of nor how effective this expensive service likely will be. Long before clinical interns enter that arena, they will need to have made some multilayered existential choices: whether (or not) to become artisanal therapists, manual-based "craftsmen," or complex humanistic variants between these two extremes. Yalom (1980) wrote about a cooking course he once took with an Armenian chef. She could not speak English, nor could Yalom or other students speak Armenian. The students learned by watching, like so many Inuit children. Besides noting the main ingredients, Yalom observed that as the pots and skillets were shuffled from counter to stove, a variety of spices were tossed in—a pinch of this and a pinch of that. "I am convinced," he wrote, "those surreptitious throw-ins made all the difference" (p. 3). He likened this process to psychotherapy. Often unknown to therapists, it's their unscripted "throw-ins" that can make all the difference.

AN UNUSUAL EXAMPLE OF PSYCHOTHERAPY

A Corsini "Throw-in"

About 50 years ago, when I was working as a psychologist at Auburn Prison in New York, I participated in what I believe was the most successful and elegant psychotherapy I have ever done. One day an inmate, who had made an appointment, came into my office. He was a fairly attractive man in his early 30s. I pointed to a chair, he sat down, and I waited to find out what he wanted. The conversation went something like this (P = Prisoner; C = Corsini):

P: I am leaving on parole Thursday.
C: Yes?
P: I did not want to leave until I thanked you for what you had done for me.
C: What was that?
P: When I left your office about two years ago, I felt like I was walking on air. When I went into the prison yard, everything looked different, even the air smelled different. I was a new person. Instead of going over to the group I usually hung out with—they were a bunch of thieves—I went over to another group of square Johns [prison jargon for noncriminal types]. I changed from a cushy job in the kitchen to the machine shop, where I could learn a trade. I started going to the prison high school and I now have a high school diploma. I took a correspondence course in drafting and I have a drafting job when I leave Thursday. I started back to church even though I had given up my religion many years ago. I started writing to my family and they have come up to see me and they remember you in their prayers. I now have hope. I know who and what I am. I know I will succeed in life. I plan to go to college. You have freed me. I used to think you bug doctors [prison slang for psychologists and psychiatrists] were for the birds, but now I know better. Thanks for changing my life.

I listened to this tale in wonderment, because to the best of my knowledge I had never spoken with him. I looked at his folder and the only notation there was that I had given him an IQ test about two years before. "Are you sure it was me?" I finally said. "I am not a psychotherapist, and I have no memory of ever having spoken to you. What you are reporting is the sort of personality and behavior change that takes many years to accomplish—and I certainly haven't done anything of the kind."

"It was you, all right," he replied with great conviction, "and I will never forget what you said to me. It changed my life."

"What was that?" I asked.

"You told me I had a high IQ," he replied.

With one sentence of five words I had (inadvertently) changed this person's life.

Let us try to understand this event. If you are clever enough to understand why this man changed so drastically as a result of hearing these five words, "You have a high IQ," my guess is that you have the capacity to be a good therapist.

I asked him why this sentence about his IQ had such a profound effect, and I learned that up to the time that he heard these five words, he had always thought of himself as stupid and crazy—terms that had been applied to him many times by his family, teachers, and friends. In school, he had always received poor grades, which confirmed his belief in his mental subnormality. His friends did not approve of the way he thought and called him crazy. And so he was convinced that he was both an ament (low intelligence) and a dement (insane). But when I said, "You have a high IQ," he had an "aha!" experience that explained everything. In a flash, he understood why he could solve crossword puzzles better than any of his friends. He now knew why he read long novels rather than comic books, why he preferred to play chess rather than checkers, why he liked symphonies as well as jazz. With great and sudden intensity, he realized through my five words that he was really normal and bright and not crazy or stupid. He had experienced an abreaction that ordinarily would take months. No wonder he had felt as if he were walking on air when he left my office two years before!

His interpretation of my five words generated a complete change of self-concept—and consequently a change in both his behavior and his feelings about himself and others.

In short, I had performed psychotherapy in a completely innocent and informal way. Even though . . . there was no agreement between us, no theory, and no intention of changing him—the five-word comment had a most pronounced effect, and so it was psychotherapy.

MANUALIZATION OF TREATMENT

Spontaneous, unplanned throw-ins are hardly a basis for a *science* of psychotherapy. Doing psychotherapy in this manner makes it more like a craft, or at its pinnacle—as Yalom and Josselson do it—an art. Even repeatedly demonstrating that one can improve client well-being and achieve therapeutic objectives by a manualized series of interventions does not explain *how* the variables have caused the outcome. Intensive research has been conducted in the last decade precisely to identify the mechanisms that are bringing about change. Although ambitious programs of process research, as distinguished from outcome research, are being conducted (see, e.g., Norcross & Goldfried, 2005), these causal links and their nature are not yet fully understood. Such understanding will only surface when we have a mature neuroscience that can describe the mechanisms involved. This problem is obviated for those who are only seeking manualized approaches to therapy, that is, sets of sequential, algorithmized steps for proceeding through phases of therapy (see Prochaska, Norcross, & DiClemente, 1995, for one cogent model).

There are several practical advantages to manualized psychotherapy. Engineering therapy in the guise of an architecture of stages or building blocks makes sense pedagogically. One proceeds from the known to the unknown and untried in a methodical, stepwise fashion, clearly specifying layered objectives and mobilizing the personal, social, and institutional resources that are so useful—and so often necessary. These processes through which the patient can be guided are amenable to various configurations. The chapters of this book (2 through 15) have been structured in such a way that the enterprising student can design a manual for each using the elements as they are presented.

OBSTACLES TO A SCIENCE OF PSYCHOTHERAPY

The sheer number of potent client and personological variables that must be considered when computing the outcome variance of a procedure dwarfs the influence of the technique. Citing numerous studies, Michael Mahoney wrote in 1991 "the *person* of the therapist is at least eight times more influential than his or her theoretical orientation and/or use of specific therapeutic techniques" (p. 346). Norcross and Beutler (2008) stated that there are "tens of thousands of potential permutations and combinations of patient, therapist, treatment, and setting variables that could contribute" to improving treatment decisions (p. 491). They noted the earlier studies of Beutler and colleagues in which the latter conducted various analyses of these multitudinous variables with a sample of depressed patients. They reduced "tens of thousands" to a manageable number, trusting that the loss of specificity in their constructs would not overshadow the utility of their generic approach. This is analogous to the task undertaken by Allport and Odbert (1936) and several generations of trait psychologists who followed them, who reduced 18,000 personality descriptors to a handful of core personality factors using the factor analytic techniques developed largely by Raymond B. Cattell.

The immensity of the task dawns on us when we consider the hundreds of other DSM disorders that call for varied treatments on the one hand and Meehl's innumerable random events on the other. The complex and changing context of our patients' daily lives is like a headwind that keeps pushing us back toward Yalom's kitchen and the critical importance of "throw-ins."

SOURCES OF HOPE

The pursuit of *what* works is more important to a pragmatic species like *homo sapiens* than the pursuit of *why* it works. This is especially true of psychotherapy, which is an applied and very practical science. Like wave and particle theories in the physics of light, art and science in psychotherapy are not incompatible paradigms. Both are valid, and elements of both appear in every clinical session. As unanticipated material comes to light, all clinicians to one degree or another rely on intuitive inspiration and creative imagination in deciding what to do next in therapy.

Some therapies, such as behavioral and cognitive therapies, are more amenable to manualization than others such as existential psychotherapy but ought not to be preferred simply for that reason. On the other hand, the manualization of therapies must not be caricatured simply as a cookbook approach to treating disorders. The variables and the random events that continually pop up in a patient's life and complicate therapists' best-thought-out plans require adjustment and compromise. Therapeutic judgment and creativity are always called into play. Pursuing the mirage of a blueprint that unfolds seamlessly from start to finish entails a loss of therapists' time and effectiveness and drains patients' emotional and financial resources. There is room in evidence-based therapies and manualized therapies for the poetry, spirituality, spontaneity, sentiment, free will, even the mystery and romance of human self-discovery and growth that both patients and humanistically inclined therapists crave. There should be no tension between getting better and *feeling* better. In fact, like butter in the batter, affect and reason are as inseparable here as elsewhere.

INDUSTRIALIZING PSYCHOTHERAPY

Although pastoral counseling and faith-based therapeutic procedures are still widely practiced in North America, and indeed globally, secular, science-based approaches to treating mental disorders have become normative. As psychotherapy has gained recognition as a health discipline, a growing chorus of voices (of both patients and mental heath services professionals) has clamored for insurance programs to reimburse mental health costs. The establishment of managed health care (MHC) is a business issue and perhaps of little interest to students who wish to commit their careers to helping people, but the reality is that students will need to ensure that they can run a solvent enterprise after they graduate, even if it is a humble independent practice. Like it or not, therapists are quickly drawn into a web of institutional requirements that will secure not only the safety of the public they serve but their own livelihood as well.

The industrialization of all health professions, whether it be counseling, social work, psychiatry, clinical psychology, neuropsychology, school psychology, or psychometrics has "been the linchpin of the development and use of empirically based clinical practice guidelines" (Hayes, 1998, p. 27). Readers may recoil from these institutional realities, but they are well advised to generate their personal therapeutic models during their studies and training such that they meet the demands of the accreditation, licensure, insurance, and medical organizations that will facilitate the growth and solvency of their practice.

Epilogue to This Chapter

In the previous edition of this book, Ray Corsini (2008) wrote,

> I believe that if one is to go into the fields of counseling and psychotherapy, then the best theory and methodology to use must be one's own. The reader will not be either successful or happy using a method not suited to her or his own personality. Truly successful therapists adopt or develop a theory and methodology congruent with their own personality . . . In reading these accounts, in addition to attempting to determine which school of psychotherapy seems most sensible, the reader should also attempt to find one that fits his or her philosophy of life, one whose theoretical underpinnings seem most valid, and one with a method of operation that appears most appealing in use. (p. 13)

A final value of this book lies in the greater self-understanding that may be gained by close reading. This book about psychotherapies may be psychotherapeutic for the reader. Close reading vertically (chapter by chapter) and then horizontally (section by section) may well lead to personal growth as well as to better understanding of current psychotherapies.

These counsels from a great therapist and scholar are a fitting conclusion to this chapter.

Valedictory

Some readers of previous editions of this book will note that this is the first time that Ray Corsini has not been the sole author of this introductory chapter. Ray died November 8, 2008, in Honolulu at the age of 94. He left those of us who survive him bereft of one of the most creative, loyal, challenging, and inspiring colleagues we've had the privilege of knowing and working with. Danny Wedding, Ray's co-editor of *Current Psychotherapies,* and all those, including me, who have had the privilege of working with Ray over the years, bid him a fond farewell and wish him well in this journey.

REFERENCES

Allport, G. W., & Odbert, H. S. (1936). Trait-names: A psycho-lexical study. *Psychological Monographs, 47,* (1, Whole No. 211).

Baltes, P. B., Reuter-Lorenz, P. A., & Rösler, F. (2006). Prologue: Biocultural co-constructivism as a theoretical metascript. In P. B. Baltes, P. A. Reuter-Lorenz, & F. Rösler (Eds.), *Lifespan development and the brain: The perspective of biocultural co-constructivism* (pp. 3–39). Cambridge, UK: Cambridge University Press.

Beutler, L. E., & Baker, M. (1998). The movement toward empirical validation: At what level should we analyze, and who are the consumers? In K. S. Dobson & K. D. Craig (Eds.), *Empirically supported therapies: Best practice in professional psychology* (pp. 43–65). Thousand Oaks, CA: Sage.

Brown, D. E. (1991). *Human universals.* New York: McGraw-Hill.

Corsini, R. J. (2008). Introduction. In R. J. Corsini & D. Wedding (Eds.), *Current psychotherapies* (8th ed., pp. 1–14). Belmont, CA: Brooks/Cole, Thomson Learning.

Cross, S. E., & Markus, H. R. (1999). The cultural constitution of personality. In L. A. Pervin & O. P. John (Eds.), *Handbook of personality* (pp. 378–396). New York: Guilford.

Dumont, F. (2009). Rehearsal, confession, and confabulation: Psychotherapy and the synaptic self. *Journal of Contemporary Psychotherapy, 39*(1), 33–40.

Dumont, F. (2010). *A history of personality psychology: Theory, science, and research from Hellenism to the twenty-first century.* Cambridge, UK: Cambridge University Press.

Dumont, F., & Fitzpatrick, M. (2001). The real relationship: Schemas, stereotypes, and personal history. *Psychotherapy: Theory, Practice, Research, and Training, 38,* 12–20.

Ellenberger, H. F. (1970). *The discovery of the unconscious: The history and evolution of dynamic psychiatry.* New York: Basic Books.

Finger, S. (2001). *Origins of neuroscience: A history of explorations into brain function.* Oxford: Oxford University Press.

Grawe, K. (2007). *Neuropsychotherapy: How the neurosciences inform effective psychotherapy.* Mahwah, NJ: Erlbaum.

Güntürkün, O. (2006). Letters on nature and nurture. In P. B. Baltes, P. A. Reuter-Lorenz, & F. Rösler (Eds.), *Lifespan development and the brain: The perspective of biocultural co-constructivism* (pp. 379–397). Cambridge, UK: Cambridge University Press.

Hayes, S. C. (1998). Scientific practice guidelines in a political, economic, and professional context. In K. S. Dobson & K. D. Craig (Eds.), *Empirically supported therapies: Best practice in professional psychology* (pp. 26–42). Thousand Oaks, CA: Sage.

Hoshmand, L. T. (2005). Thinking through culture. In L. T. Hoshmand (Ed.), *Culture, psychotherapy, and counseling: Critical and integrative perspectives* (pp. 1–24). Thousand Oaks, CA: Sage.

Lakoff, G., & Johnson, M. (1980). *Metaphors we live by.* Chicago: University of Chicago Press.

Leahey, T. H. (2000). *A history of psychology: Main currents in psychological thought* (5th ed.). Upper Saddle River, NJ: Prentice Hall.

LeDoux, J. (2002). *Synaptic self: How our brains become who we are.* New York: Viking/Penguin.

Mahoney, M. (1991). *Human change processes: The scientific foundations of psychotherapy.* New York: Basic Books.

Marsella, A. J., & Yamada, A. M. (2000). Culture and mental health: An introduction and overview of foundations, concepts, and issues. In I. Cuellar, & F. A. Paniagua (Eds.), *Handbook of multicultural mental health: Assessment and treatment of culturally diverse populations* (pp. 3–24). New York: Academic Press.

Meehl, P. (1978). Theoretical risks and tabular asterisks: Sir Karl, Sir Ronald, and the slow progress of soft psychology. *Journal of Consulting and Clinical Psychology, 46,* 806–834.

Norcross, J. C., & Beutler, L. E. (2008). Integrative psychotherapies. In R. J. Corsini & D. Wedding, *Current psychotherapies* (pp. 481–511). Belmont CA: Brooks/Cole, Thomson Learning.

Norcross, J. C., & Goldfried, M. R. (Eds.) (2005). *Handbook of psychotherapy integration* (2nd ed.). New York: Oxford University Press.

Pinker, S. (2002). *The blank slate: The modern denial of human nature.* New York: Viking.

Pope, K. S., & Wedding, D. (2011). Contemporary challenges and controversies. In R. J. Corsini & D. Wedding (Eds.), *Current psychotherapies* (9th ed., pp. 568–603). Belmont, CA: Brooks/Cole.

Prochaska, J. O., Norcross, J. C., & DiClemente, C. C. (1995). Stages of change: Prescriptive guidelines. In G. P. Koocher, J. C. Norcross, & S. S. Hill (Eds.), *Psychologists' desk reference* (pp. 226–231). New York: Oxford University Press.

Schopenhauer, A. (1819/1969). *The world as will and representation* (Trans. E. F. J. Payne). Toronto: General Publishing.

Shorter, E. (1997). *A history of psychiatry: From the era of the asylum to the age of Prozac.* New York: Wiley.

Task Force on Promotion and Dissemination of Psychological Procedures. (1995). Training in and dissemination of empirically validated psychological treatments. *Clinical Psychologist, 48,* 3–23.

Whyte, L. L. (1960). *The unconscious before Freud.* New York: Basic Books.

Yalom, I. D. (1980). *Existential psychotherapy.* New York: Basic Books.

Yang, K. S. (1997). Indigenizing Westernized Chinese psychology. In M. H. Bond (Ed.), *Working at the interface of cultures: Eighteen lies in social science* (pp. 62–76). New York: Routledge.

Yang, K. S. (1999). Towards an indigenous Chinese psychology: A selective review of methodological, theoretical, and empirical accomplishments. *Chinese Journal of Psychology, 41*(2), 181–211.

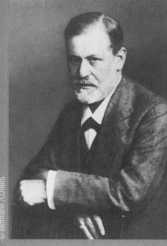

Sigmund Freud, 1856–1939

2 | PSYCHOANALYSIS

Ellen B. Luborsky, Maureen O'Reilly-Landry, and Jacob A. Arlow

OVERVIEW

"It doesn't add up."

How could a seemingly nice person abuse a child? Why would someone not show up at her own wedding, one she'd planned for a year? How could a child from a great neighborhood with fine schools and an intact family never develop any ambition?

The next time you wonder, give credit where credit is due. Over one hundred years ago, Sigmund Freud pronounced that the surface, or manifest, level of life is but the topsoil of mental activity. Much of it happens at an unconscious level. Symptoms and problem behavior begin to make sense when the deeper levels are understood.

Psychoanalysis, a system of treatment as well as a way to understand human behavior, has given rise to discoveries and controversies that are actively with us today. It has seeped into the language ("Was that a Freudian slip?") and made an impact on our thinking.

Consider your reaction to the questions raised at the beginning of the chapter. Did you wonder whether the abuser had himself been abused? (Repetition of an early experience not consciously remembered.) Did you suspect that the woman who never showed up at her wedding had mixed feelings she couldn't face? (Inner conflict, with warded off emotional experience.) Did you think that the student without ambition had more issues than meet the eye? (The surface story functioning as a cover for, or defense against, inner emotional experience.)

Psychoanalytic thinking has evolved over the last century, so that classical and modern psychoanalytic approaches now coexist. It has spawned different forms of psychotherapy, with psychodynamic psychotherapy being its most direct descendant. According to Rangell (1973), most of the widely practiced forms of psychotherapy are based on some element of psychoanalytic theory or technique.

Psychoanalysis has affected fields that range from child development to philosophy to feminist theory. It has inspired thinkers and therapists who disagree with Freud's premises to come up with methods of their own. Whether because it is rejected, adapted, or accepted, Freud's legacy is still with us.

The purpose of this chapter is to better understand psychoanalysis, particularly those concepts that have had staying power. Freud's own concepts evolved over the course of his lifetime, and they continue to do so. Controversy and change have accompanied psychoanalysis since it began. The tests of time and of research have highlighted some ideas and discredited others. Both the clinical and the empirical evidence for the usefulness of psychoanalytic thinking will be explored.

The goals of this chapter are

- To present the central psychoanalytic concepts
- To examine the ways in which those concepts have evolved
- To demystify the language and principles of psychoanalysis
- To look at the treatment methods that have emerged from a psychoanalytic perspective
- To consider different applications of psychodynamic ideas
- To examine research evidence for psychoanalytically oriented treatment
- To give examples of how psychodynamic ideas can be used in psychotherapy

Basic Concepts

You have been trained to find an anatomical basis for the functions of the organism and their disorders, to explain them chemically and view them biologically. But no portion of your interest has been directed to the psychical life, in which, after all, the achievement of this marvelously complex organism reaches its peak. (Freud, 1916, p. 20)

Psychoanalysis seeks to understand human behavior through an investigation of inner experience, and to treat psychological problems through a clinical application of that understanding. Consequently, the central tenets include both theoretical concepts and clinical methods.

Basic Theoretical Concepts

The Unconscious

The division of the psychical into what is conscious and what is unconscious is the fundamental premise of psychoanalysis. (Freud, 1923, p. 15)

The *unconscious* consists of states of mind that are outside awareness. They include both emotional and cognitive processes, along with forms of memory that affect the patient's reactions and behavior. Although the concept of the unconscious mind predates psychoanalysis, Freud's unique contribution was to discover how the concept could be used to understand and inform the treatment of psychological problems.

The scientific status of the unconscious has been in question since the concept was proposed. Recent discoveries of neuroscience offer some support for the influence of mental processes that are outside conscious awareness.

Psychodynamics

Our purpose is not merely to describe and classify the phenomena, but to conceive of them as brought about by the play of forces in the mind. . . . We are endeavoring to attain a *dynamic concept* of mental phenomena. (Freud, 1917, p. 60)

Psychodynamics is the "play [that is, the interplay] of forces of the mind." The concept of *inner conflict* is a prime example of psychodynamics at work. The term *inner* or *intrapsychic conflict* refers to conflict between parts of the self that hold opposing perceptions or emotions, one or more of which is out of awareness. This may result either in problematic behavior or in symptoms. For example, a patient may express the conviction that he loves his wife and would never do anything to hurt her, while having affairs outside of the marriage. He may be *acting out* feelings that conflict with his consciously held beliefs. Or a patient may get a headache whenever Monday comes. The symptom may express a conflict between the part of her that knows she must go back to work and the part that dreads doing so.

Symptoms in psychodynamic theory are often seen as an expression of inner conflict. Whereas in the medical or diagnostic model a symptom is a sign of a disorder, here a symptom is a clue, expressed through the language of behavior, to the patient's core conflicts. Decoding its meaning in the course of treatment allows the feelings once expressed through the symptom to be expressed in less harmful ways. The *symptom-context method* is a clinical-research method that aids in that process.

Psychodynamic Psychotherapy. Psychotherapies that follow in a psychoanalytic tradition are referred to as psychodynamic treatments. They retain the central *dynamic* principles of psychoanalysis but do not make use of the *metapsychology*, or formal theories of the structure of the mind. Even Freud came to the conclusion that metapsychological hypotheses are "not the bottom, but the top of the whole structure [of science] and they can be replaced and discarded without damaging it" (Freud, 1915b. p. 77).

Dynamic psychotherapy evolved from psychoanalysis to fill the need for a form of treatment that was not so lengthy and involved. Whereas psychoanalysis is typically conducted three to five times a week, with the patient lying down, dynamic psychotherapy usually takes place once or twice a week, with the patient sitting up. *Supportive-expressive (SE)* psychotherapy is a current form of dynamic treatment that incorporates clinical-research methods.

Defenses

The term "defense". . . is the earliest representative of the dynamic standpoint in psychoanalytic theory. (Freud, A., 1966, p. 42)

Defense mechanisms are automatic forms of response to situations that arouse unconscious fears or the anticipation of "psychic danger." Examples of common defenses include *avoidance* and *denial*. These both function as "ways around" situations that bring up thoughts or emotions that the patient cannot tolerate. Effective defenses are essential for healthy functioning because they render painful and potentially overwhelming feelings manageable. However, they often cause problems in real life, because they tend to obscure or distort reality. For example, a student who spends all of her time online instead of studying for exams may be using the defense of avoidance to counteract the intense anxiety she would feel if she opened up the semester's untouched work. Other defenses will be discussed in the next sections of this chapter.

Transference.   *Transference,* Freud's cornerstone concept, refers to the transfer of feelings originally experienced in an early relationship to other important people in a person's present environment. They form a pattern that affects the patient's attitudes toward new people and situations, shaping the present through a "template" from the past.

> Each individual, through the combined operation of his innate disposition and the influences brought to bear on him during his early years, has acquired a specific method of his own in the conduct of his erotic life. This produces a stereotype plate [or template], or several such, which is constantly repeated . . . in the course of a person's life. (Freud, 1912, pp. 99–100)

In psychoanalysis, the analysis of the transference is fundamental to the treatment. The patient's transference to the analyst enables them both to see its operating force and to work on separating reality from memories and expectations. The transference contains patterns from the past that may be remembered through actions or through repetition of the past, rather than through recollection; " . . . the patient does not say that he remembers that he used to be defiant and critical toward his parents' authority; instead he behaves that way to the doctor" (Freud, 1914, p. 150).

Transference has been investigated through clinical research on the Core Conflictual Relationship Theme (CCRT) method. This research, which both clarifies and validates the concept, will be explored later in this chapter.

Countertransference refers to the therapist's reactions to the patient. As the counterpart to the transference, it refers to the therapist's reactions to a patient that may be linked to personal issues the therapist needs to resolve. Countertransference has been used recently to evaluate whether the therapist's reactions may be responses to the patient's emotions or to nonverbal communications from the patient.

Basic Clinical Concepts

Free Association.   "Say what comes to mind" is a typical beginning to any psychoanalytic treatment. Unlike other forms of treatment, psychoanalysis invites all thoughts, dreams, daydreams, and fantasies into the treatment. Psychoanalysts believe that the expression of unedited thoughts will bring richer material about the inner workings of the mind. The less edited the material, the more likely that it will contain clues to parts of the self that may previously have been expressed through symptoms. Free association also gives the patient a chance to hear himself.

Therapeutic Listening.   Freud recommended maintaining a state of "evenly hovering attention" to what the patient says. That means that the analyst does not seize on one topic or another but, rather, listens to all the levels of the communication at once. That includes what the patient is literally saying, what kinds of emotions she conveys, and the analyst's reactions while listening. This form of listening is at the foundation of the analytic method, since it allows a full hearing of the patient. A second kind of therapeutic listening occurs when the analyst develops a sense of the patient's patterns—those that may form the transference as well as those that link symptoms with their meanings.

Therapeutic Responding.   *Interpretation* is the fundamental form of responding in traditional psychoanalysis. It involves sharing an understanding of a central theme of the patient, often a facet of the transference. Interpretations are intended to help a patient come to terms with conflicts that may have been driving his behavior or symptoms, offered when the analyst senses that the patient is ready to grapple with them.

The interpretation of dreams has a special place in psychoanalytic treatment. "The interpretation of dreams is the royal road to a knowledge of the unconscious activities of the mind" (Freud, 1932, p. 608). Freud believed that the *manifest content,* or surface story, of dreams could be decoded to reach the deeper, *latent content.* Ways to understand the language of the dream will be explored in the next section.

Empathy as a form of therapeutic responding has received increasing attention since the second half of the twentieth century. Empathic responding means attuning to the patient's feeling states and conveying a sense of emotional understanding. Research now links the therapist's empathy with the outcome of the treatment.

The Therapeutic Alliance.   The *therapeutic* or *working alliance* is the partnership between the patient and therapist forged around working together in the treatment. Greenson (1967) clarified the difference between the working alliance and the transference and emphasized the importance of the alliance to the treatment. Current research confirms that a positive *helping alliance* is one of the factors that is consistently associated with a good outcome in psychotherapy.

Other Systems

Psychoanalysis serves as both the grandfather and the current relative to many forms of psychotherapeutic practice. Some other systems and theorists (notably Jung and Adler) branched off from psychoanalysis during Freud's lifetime. Others began as later adaptations and either remained under the "analytic umbrella," as did dynamic psychotherapy, or highlighted an essential difference, as did Carl Rogers.

A number of distinct, but still essentially psychoanalytic, theories have emerged since Freud's time. These include classical psychoanalysis, ego psychology, interpersonal psychoanalysis, object relations and other relational perspectives, and self-psychology. Although psychoanalysis as a system of thought comprises many theories, three basic ideas are common to all and provide a framework for comparison with other systems of psychology: the role of the unconscious, the phenomenon of transference, and the relevance of past experiences to present personality and symptoms.

The Unconscious Mind

The first central concept that distinguishes psychoanalysis from many other systems of psychology is a belief in the importance of the unconscious in understanding the human psyche. Other systems of psychology that acknowledge the significance of the human unconscious are, understandably, those developed by theorists who studied directly with Freud. Most notable among these is Carl Jung. Jung retained Freud's belief in the unconscious but saw it as consisting of two important aspects. In addition to the type of personal unconscious that Freud described, Jungian analysts believe in a *collective unconscious.* The collective unconscious is made up of archetypal images, or symbolic representations of universal themes of human existence that are present in all cultures, as opposed to the more personal Freudian unconscious. Similar to psychoanalysis, neurosis in Jungian analysis results when one is excessively cut off from the contents of the unconscious and the meaning of the archetypes, which can be understood through various methods, including dream analysis. Jung brought in aspects of mysticism and spirituality that were rejected or ignored by earlier psychoanalysts but which are now beginning to receive attention from modern psychoanalysts, particularly those with an interest in meditation and Eastern religions.

Adler, another of Freud's students, departed from the belief in the unconscious as part of an intrapsychic system based on repression of drives, but he continued to believe that people know more about themselves than they actually understand.

The Existentialists are also concerned with the unconscious. Like psychoanalysts, they believe that people experience internal unconscious conflicts and that these are excluded from conscious awareness but still exert an influence on behavior, thoughts, and feelings. For them, it is anxiety about basic existential fears such as death, isolation, and meaninglessness that is being defended against.

Gestalt therapy was also an outgrowth of psychoanalysis but departed from it in radical ways, not only in eschewing much of its basic theory, but also by developing very structured and active therapeutic techniques. Despite these substantial differences, Fritz Perls held on to a belief in the therapeutic value of bringing what is unconscious into consciousness. Similarly, Moreno's Psychodrama, by enacting problematic interpersonal situations, helps a patient get in touch with and express feelings she may not have realized she had. Alvin Mahrer's experiential psychotherapy also differs from psychoanalysis in a wide variety of ways. Mahrer regards unconscious material as unique to each individual and believes it represents one of many aspects of a deeper potential for experiencing life. Finally, certain schools of family therapy deal with the ways in which members unconsciously play out particular roles in relation to each other.

The "depth psychologies," those that acknowledge that deeper underlying processes and experiences have significant effects on human behavior, contrast sharply with behavioral and cognitive approaches. Such therapies, which include behavior therapy, rational emotive behavior therapy (REBT), cognitive and cognitive-behavior therapy (CBT), and multimodal therapy, are all rooted in learning theory. In these systems, the undesired symptom, behavior, or thought is understood as having been learned and reinforced by environmental events. These models do not look for meaning beyond observed behavior or conscious experience, and behavioral observation and self-report are their primary methods of assessment.

Some therapies derived from these models have demonstrated effectiveness in treating problems such as phobias and other well-defined anxiety disorders, as well as certain symptoms of major depression. Thus, they have made a valuable contribution to the alleviation of psychological suffering. However, many difficulties for which adults seek psychotherapy are not so readily delineated and categorized. A woman may seek psychological treatment, for example, because she is unable to maintain a close and satisfying relationship, or because she experiences a sense of malaise for which she has no explanation. Further, even with well-defined symptoms, when "treatment-resistant" cases occur, these systems offer no conceptual tools for looking beyond the observable to understand what might have gone wrong.

The Transference

A second idea common to psychoanalytic therapies is the transference. Freud was the first to recognize the therapeutic value of transference phenomena, in which the patient comes to experience others, the analyst in particular, in ways that are colored by his early experiences with important people in his life. Countertransference, or the response of the analyst to the patient and his transference, is also utilized in various ways in psychoanalysis. Most contemporary psychoanalysts regard countertransference as useful clinical information about the patient, including the types of feelings he might evoke in others. Attention to transference and countertransference reflects interest both in the unconscious and in the importance of childhood experiences and early relationships. Jungian analysts and contemporary psychoanalysts work actively with the transference and countertransference, reflecting a move within both orientations toward recognizing the mutual influence between patient and therapist.

Gestalt, Adlerian, and Client-centered (Rogerian) therapists have less confidence in the therapeutic value of transference. They place greater value on actively cultivating a positive relationship with the client by maintaining a stance that is visibly empathic, supportive and non-judgmental and attempting to bypass any negative transference phenomena. Being empathic and non-judgmental are also highly valued by psychoanalysts, but they remain open to the expression of both positive and negative feelings about the therapist and attempt to understand and interpret either. They believe that understanding these feelings is important if deep and lasting therapeutic change is to occur.

In REBT, the therapist attempts to eradicate transference phenomena at the outset by demonstrating that the client's feelings are based on irrational, maladaptive wishes. Behaviorally and cognitively oriented therapists attempt to enhance the working alliance, but transference is not part of their theories. Their more active stance, in which homework assignments are routinely given and explicit instructions are provided about how to change thoughts and behavior, establishes the therapist as an authority figure, a role that is utilized to encourage compliance.

The Role of Childhood Experiences

A third characteristic shared by psychoanalytically oriented clinicians is a belief that childhood experiences influence personality development, current relationships, and emotional vulnerabilities. Many contemporary psychoanalysts incorporate research findings demonstrating the long-term impact of the quality of a child's early attachment, childhood trauma, early experiences of loss, and other related areas into their thinking about personality development. Any system for which transference is an important concept is necessarily one that recognizes this past-present relationship. Jungian analysts work actively with transference material and are similar to psychoanalysts in their view that aspects of early formative relationships affect the analytic relationship, affording the patient an opportunity to work through these feelings and move beyond their negative impact.

Although Ellis does not use the term *transference,* he acknowledges that transferential thoughts and feelings toward the therapist might arise but regards them as little more than irrational beliefs. Rather than examine and attempt to understand them, he points out their unrealistic nature and applies his very systematic REBT procedure with the intention of eradicating them.

In psychodrama, early past experiences are thought to have an impact on one's current situation, and these are explicitly role-played in an effort to rework and replace the psychologically harmful experiences with more positive ones. Rogerians and existentialists are concerned with the therapeutic relationship, but past experiences do not figure prominently in their thinking.

For systems greatly influenced by learning theory, such as cognitive, behavioral, and cognitive-behavioral therapies, as well as multimodal therapy, the past is significant only in terms of the direct antecedents to the dysfunctional behavior. This major difference from the analytic perspectives may limit the types of psychological problems that the systems that rely on learning theory are able to address.

Common Factors

Various approaches to psychotherapy differ in what they see as fundamental to the process. Dynamic psychotherapies differ from behavioral forms of treatment in their understanding of the origins of psychological problems, as well as in aspects of technique.

Although the differences among forms of therapy are frequently highlighted in writings about treatment, they also share important fundamentals. Establishing a working alliance is important in all forms of treatment, whether it is made explicit, as in psychodynamic theory, or not. So is the frame, or structure, of the treatment and the establishment of treatment goals. The role of common factors will be further explored in the Evidence section of this chapter.

HISTORY

Precursors

Psychoanalysis, as originated by Sigmund Freud (1856–1939), represented an integration of the major European intellectual movements of his time. This was a period of unprecedented advance in the physical and biological sciences. The crucial issue of the day was Darwin's theory of evolution. Originally, Freud had intended to pursue a career as a biological research scientist, and in keeping with this goal, he became affiliated with the Physiological Institute in Vienna, headed by Ernst Brücke. Brücke was a follower of Helmholtz and was part of the group of biologists who attempted to explain biological phenomena solely in terms of physics and chemistry. It is not surprising, therefore, that models borrowed from physics and chemistry, as well as the theory of evolution, recur regularly throughout Freud's writings, particularly in his early psychological works.

Freud came to psychoanalysis by way of neurology. During his formative years, great strides were being made in neurophysiology and neuropathology. This was also the time when psychology separated from philosophy and began to emerge as an independent science. Freud was interested in both fields. He knew the works of the "association" school of psychologists (Herbart, von Humboldt, and Wundt), and he had been impressed by the way Gustav Fechner applied concepts of physics to problems of psychological research.

In the mid-nineteenth century, there was great interest in states of split consciousness. The French neuropsychiatrists had taken the lead in studying conditions such as somnambulism, multiple personalities, fugue states, and hysteria. Hypnotism was one of the principal methods used in studying these conditions. The use of the couch, with the patient lying down, began with the practice of hypnosis. The leading figures in this field of investigation were Jean Martin Charcot, Pierre Janet, Hippolyte Bernheim, and Ambrose August Liebault. Freud worked with several of them and was particularly influenced by Charcot.

Beginnings

Freud made frequent revisions in his theories and practice as new and challenging findings came to his attention. In the section that follows, special emphasis will be placed on the links between Freud's clinical findings and the consequent reformulations of his theories. These writings serve as nodal points in the history of the evolution of his theories: *Studies on Hysteria, The Interpretation of Dreams, Three Essays on Sexuality, On Narcissism,* the metapsychology papers, *Beyond the Pleasure Principle* (the Dual Instinct Theory), and *The Ego and the Id* (the Structural Theory).

Studies on Hysteria (1895)

The early history of psychoanalysis begins with hypnotism. Josef Breuer, a prominent Viennese physician, told Freud of his experience using hypnosis. When he placed the patient in a hypnotic trance and encouraged her to relate what was oppressing her mind at the moment, she would frequently tell of some highly emotional event in her life. While awake, the patient was completely unaware of the "traumatic" event or of its connection with her disability, but after relating it under hypnosis, the patient was cured of her disability. The report made a deep impression on Freud, and it was partly in pursuit of the therapeutic potential of hypnosis that he undertook studies first with Charcot in Paris and later with Bernheim and Liébault at Nancy, France.

When Freud returned to Vienna, he used Breuer's procedures on other patients and was able to confirm the validity of Breuer's findings. The two then established a working relationship that culminated in *Studies on Hysteria.* Freud and Breuer noted that recalling the traumatic event alone was not sufficient to effect a cure. The discharge of the appropriate amount of emotion was also necessary. Anna O., a patient whom Breuer cured in this way, referred to the treatment as "the talking cure."

The task of treatment, they concluded, was to achieve *catharsis* of the undischarged affect connected with the painful traumatic experience. The concept of a repressed trauma was fundamental in Freud's conceptualization of hysteria, which led him, in an aphoristic way, to say that hysterics suffer mainly from reminiscences.

Breuer and Freud differed on how the painful memories in hysteria had been rendered unconscious. Breuer's explanation was a "physiological" one, in keeping with theories of psychoneuroses current at that time. In contrast, Freud favored a psychological theory. The traumatic events were forgotten or excluded from consciousness precisely because the individual sought to defend herself from the painful emotions that accompany recollection of repressed memories. That the mind tends to pursue pleasure and avoid pain became one of the basic principles of Freud's subsequent psychological theory.

Breuer refused to continue this line of research, but Freud continued to work independently. Meanwhile, Freud learned from his clinical experience that not all patients could be hypnotized and that many others did not seem to go into a trance deep enough to produce significant results. He began using suggestion, by placing his hand on the patients' foreheads and insisting that they attempt to recall the repressed traumatic event. This method was linked to an experiment he had witnessed while working with Bernheim. In his *Autobiographical Study* (1925, p. 8), Freud described the incident:

> When the subject awoke from the state of somnambulism, he seemed to have lost all memory of what had happened while he was in that state, but Bernheim maintained that the memory was present all the same; and if he insisted upon the subject remembering, if he asseverated that the subject knew it all and had only to say it, and if at the same time he laid his hand on the subject's forehead, then the forgotten memories began to return, hesitatingly at first, but eventually in a flood and with complete clarity.

Accordingly, Freud abandoned hypnosis in favor of a new technique of forced associations. However, Elisabeth von R, the first patient whom Freud treated by "waking suggestion," apparently rebuked Freud for interrupting her flow of thoughts. Freud took her response seriously, and the method of "free association" began to emerge.

Clinical Experience and Evolving Technique.   The responses of Freud's patients to his procedures made for modification in his technique as well as in his thinking. Not only did he attend to Elizabeth van R's response to his "forced" questions, but he also began to notice that she actively refused certain questions. This observation prompted his thinking about *resistance,* or a force of "not wanting to know" in the patient. That furthered his emerging use of free association, where the task was to bring the resistances to the fore, rather than trying to circumvent them.

This technical innovation coincided with another interest that pervaded Freud's thought at the time. He had found that two elements were characteristic of the forgotten traumatic events to which he had been able to trace the hysterical symptoms. In the first place, the incidents invariably proved to be sexual in nature. Second, in searching for the pathogenic situations in which the repression of sexuality had set in, Freud was carried further and further back into the patient's life, reaching ultimately into the earliest years of childhood. Freud first concluded that the patients he observed had all been seduced by an older person. In his further investigation, Freud realized that this was not always true, and he began to develop his theory of childhood sexuality, eventually coming to believe in the importance of childhood fantasies about sexuality.

Following the same principle of learning from patients, dynamic therapists who work with the survivors of childhood sexual abuse have reopened the topic of abuse and its aftermath in patients' lives (Davies & Frawley, 1994). Thus, in the century that has followed Freud, attention has returned to actual abuse, along with the possibilities of complex, interwoven symbolic material.

The Interpretation of Dreams (1900)

The second phase of Freud's discoveries concerned a solution to the riddle of the dream. *Dreams* and *symptoms,* Freud came to realize, had a similar structure. He saw both as products of a compromise between two sets of conflicting forces in the mind—between unconscious wishes and the repressive activity of the rest of the mind. In effecting this compromise, an inner censor disguised and distorted the representation of the unconscious wishes. This process makes dreams and symptoms seem unintelligible, but Freud's descriptions of the mechanisms of representation in the dream gave way to the understanding of dreams and their symbols.

The Interpretation of Dreams was the place where Freud first described the *Oedipus complex,* an unconscious sexual desire in a child, especially a male child, for the parent of the opposite sex, usually accompanied by hostility to the parent of the same sex, as well as guilt over this wish to vanquish that parent. The development of that theory coincided with Freud's own self analysis. Although the Oedipus complex continues to have an important place in classical psychoanalytic theory, more recent approaches that emphasize early attachment rather than childhood sexuality do not give it the same credence.

The Structure of Mind.   In the concluding chapter of *The Interpretation of Dreams,* Freud attempted to elaborate a theory of the human mind that would encompass dreaming, psychopathology, and normal functioning. The central principle of this theory is that mental life represents a fundamental conflict between the conscious and unconscious parts of the mind. The unconscious parts of the mind contain the biological, instinctual sexual drives, impulsively pressing for discharge. Opposed to these elements are forces that are either conscious or readily available to consciousness, functioning at a logical, realistic, and adaptive level.

Because the fundamental principle of this conceptualization of mental functioning concerned the depth or "layer" of an idea in relation to consciousness, this theory was called the *topographic theory.* According to this theory, the mind could be divided into three systems: *consciousness,* resulting from perception of outer stimuli as well as inner mental functioning; the *preconscious,* consisting of those mental contents accessible to awareness once attention is directed toward them; and finally the *unconscious,* comprising the primitive, instinctual wishes.

The concepts developed in *The Interpretation of Dreams*—unconscious conflict, infantile sexuality, and the Oedipus complex—enabled Freud to attain new insights into the psychology of religion, art, character formation, mythology, and literature. These ideas were published in *The Psychopathology of Everyday Life* (1901), *Jokes and Their*

Relationship to the Unconscious (1905a), *Three Essays on Sexuality* (1905b), and *Totem and Taboo* (1913).

Libido Theory.   Freud conceived of mental activity as representative of two sets of drives: Libidinal drives seek gratification and are ultimately related to preservation of the species; these are opposed by the ego drive, which seeks to preserve the existence of the individual by curbing the biological drives, when necessary. The term *libido* refers to sexual energies, although they have different meanings and manifestations at different ages.

Freud proposed a developmental sequence of the libidinal drives. The *oral phase* extends from birth to about the middle of the second year. One of the earliest analysts, Karl Abraham (1924), observed that people whose oral needs were excessively frustrated turned out to be pessimists, whereas those whose oral desires had been gratified tended to be more optimistic. The oral phase is followed by the *anal phase.* A child may react to frustrations during that phase by becoming stubborn or contrary. Through *reaction formation* the child may overcome the impulse to soil by becoming meticulously clean, excessively punctual, and quite parsimonious in handling possessions.

Somewhat later (ages 3 1/2 to 6), the child enters the *phallic phase.* In this stage, children become curious about sexual differences and the origin of life, and they may fashion their own answers to these important questions. They enjoy a sense of power and can idealize others. By this time, complex fantasies, including Oedipal fantasies, have begun to form in the mind of the child.

Today's child may still come home from nursery school saying he wants to marry his teacher. Freud's theories have allowed the culture to be relaxed about such statements, and the vast differences in the meaning of such feelings to a child and to an adult are better understood.

These early psychosexual phases are followed by a period of *latency,* from the age of 6 to the onset of puberty. Then, under the influence of the biological changes of puberty, a period of turbulence and readjustment sets in, and when development is healthy, this period culminates in the achievement of adequate mastery over drives, leading to adaptation, sexual and moral identity, and attachment to significant others.

On Narcissism (1914)

The next phase in the development of Freud's concepts focused on his investigation into the psychology of the psychoses, group formation, and love—for one's self, one's children, and significant others. He found that some individuals led lives dominated by the pursuit of self-esteem and grandiosity. These same factors seemed to operate in the relationship of an individual to the person with whom he or she was in love. The beloved was aggrandized and endowed with superlative qualities, and separation from the beloved was seen as a catastrophic blow to self-esteem. These observations on narcissism remain relevant to more recent attention to the narcissistic personality disorder.

The Ego and the Id (1923)

Having recognized that in the course of psychic conflict, conscience may operate at conscious and/or unconscious levels, and that even the methods by which the mind protects itself from anxiety may be unconscious, Freud reformulated his theory in terms of a structural organization of the mind. Mental functions were grouped according to the role they played in conflict. Freud named the three major subdivisions the ego, the id, and the superego.

The *ego* orients the individual toward the external world and serves as a mediator between one's external and internal worlds. The *id* represents the organization of the instinctual pressures on the mind, basically the sexual and aggressive impulses. The *superego* is a split-off portion of the ego, a residue of the early history of the individual's moral training and a precipitate of the most important childhood identifications and ideal aspirations. Under ordinary circumstances, there is no sharp demarcation among these three major components of the mind. Intrapsychic conflict, however, highlights the differences and demarcations between them.

One of the major functions of the ego is to protect the mind from internal dangers and from the threat of a breakthrough into consciousness of unacceptable conflict-laden impulses. The difference between mental health and mental illness depends on how well the ego can succeed in this responsibility. In his monograph *Inhibitions, Symptoms and Anxiety* (1926), Freud pointed out that the key to the problem is the appearance of anxiety, perhaps the most common symptom of neurosis. Anxiety serves as a warning signal, alerting the ego to the danger of overwhelming anxiety or panic that may supervene if a repressed, unconscious wish emerges into consciousness. Once warned, the ego may utilize any of a wide array of defenses. This new view had far-reaching implications for both the theory and the practice of psychoanalysis.

Beyond Freud

Psychoanalysis has gone through many changes since Freud. The earlier defections by Adler and Jung have already been noted, but a serious split began within psychoanalysis even during Freud's lifetime. This grew out of the teaching and the influence of Melanie Klein in London, which eventually spawned what is known as the British school of psychoanalysis. Klein emphasized the importance of primitive fantasies of loss (the *depressive position*) and persecution (the *paranoid position*) in the pathogenesis of mental illness. Melanie Klein's influence is preeminent in England, many parts of Europe, and South America.

When Nazi persecution forced many of the outstanding European analysts to migrate to this country, the United States became, for a time, the world center of psychoanalysis. The leading figures in this movement were Heinz Hartmann, Ernest Kris, and Rudolph Loewenstein. These three collaborators tried to establish psychoanalysis as a general psychology. They did so by extending Hartmann's concepts of the adaptive function of the ego (Hartmann, 1939) and clarifying fundamental working hypotheses concerning the development of the psyche (Hartmann & Kris, 1945). Hartmann, in particular, emphasized the role of the transformation of the basic instinctual drives in a set of metapsychological propositions that have been largely abandoned in recent years. Closely related to the work of Hartmann, Kris, and Loewenstein were the efforts of Anna Freud, derived from studies of long-term child development. Her book *The Ego and the Mechanisms of Defense* became a classic.

For a while, issues concerning the development of the sense of self and personal identity were most prominent in the psychoanalytic literature. These were the focal point of works by D. W. Winnicott and John Bowlby in England and Edith Jacobson and Margaret Mahler in the United States. All of these studies underlined the importance of the child's early attachment to the mother and the emergence of the self as an independent entity.

Whereas Mahler emphasized the emergence of a sense of self through a process of separation and individuation, Winnicott emphasized the continuing influence of the psychological experience of the young child, where representations of the external world take the form of *transitional phenomena*. Winnicott's concept of the *transitional object* can be seen to this day, whenever a child carries around a teddy bear or baby blanket. These objects serve as concrete ways for the child to maintain a connection between herself and her attachments.

Current Status

Most people associate psychoanalysis with classical Freudian theory and techniques, without realizing how much the field has changed. As a result, psychoanalysis and psychodynamic therapies have been criticized for being irrelevant to today's culture, for being appropriate only to an elite group of highly educated patients, and for not being based on empirical findings. This view, however, is inaccurate. Psychoanalysis is a continually evolving field that has been revised and altered by psychoanalytic theorists and clinicians ever since its origin. This evolution began with Freud himself, who often rethought and substantially revised his own ideas.

Changing Clinical Concepts

In the century that has passed since Freud, psychoanalysts have developed different branches of psychoanalysis, including ego psychology, interpersonal theory, self-psychology, and various relational theories. In fact, there are so many differing theories that Wallerstein (1988) spoke of the need to recognize many psychoanalyses instead of just one. Perhaps the most significant differences within the field today concern the nature of the analyst's view of the treatment situation. The issue is often drawn in terms of whether psychoanalysis is a one-person or a two-person psychology. A "one-person" psychology focuses exclusively on the mental reactions of the patient, whereas a "two-person" psychology considers the treatment as emerging from the interaction between two individuals. The *relational* viewpoint takes the "two-person" perspective and emphasizes the mutuality within the therapeutic relationship (Aron, 1996).

A related issue is the question of the "blank screen." In classical analytic theory, the analyst was thought of as a "blank screen" onto which the patient might project his transference. In order to facilitate this process, the patient lies on the couch with the analyst behind her, out of sight. However, current thinkers have pointed out that "the blank screen is not blank." In other words, patients have reactions to an analyst who says very little and is out of sight, just as they have reactions to one who is visible and interactive.

The Interpersonal school of psychoanalysis, which began with Harry Stack Sullivan, introduced a view of the analyst as an active participant as well as observer in the therapeutic relationship. Sullivan believed that an individual cannot be meaningfully understood outside of her interpersonal and social context. He described a process of *selective inattention,* a variation on the concept of the unconscious, in which a person will actively exclude from awareness certain anxiety-producing aspects of her interpersonal experiences (Sullivan, 1953). Because she is missing this information, she may construct a distorted view of the world. He advocated conducting a *detailed inquiry* of troubled relationships in order to bring to light those aspects of which the patient has been unaware.

For interpersonalists the patient's feelings about the therapist may be reactions to the analyst's actual behavior and not merely manifestations of transference (Sullivan, 1954). A contemporary interpersonal analyst will attempt to be aware of the ways in which he may be contributing to the patient's view of him. But he will also try to notice his own experience during the session, attempting to recognize when he has been "transformed" by reacting to some aspect of the patient. Exploration of the therapist's reactions may then shed light on the nature of the patient's relationships in the rest of her life (Levenson, 1972). The analyst's own experience of the patient now becomes an invaluable source of clinical information.

This emphasis on the patient's real interaction with the analyst was a radical departure from the less involved stance of the classical analyst. It has led some analysts to let the patient sit up and look at them and to take a more interactive role in the treatment. The interpersonal view has strongly influenced many relational perspectives.

Psychodynamic Psychotherapy

Psychodynamic psychotherapy is the most commonly practiced form of psychoanalytic treatment. It is less intensive than psychoanalysis, and sessions are held one or two times each week; the patient is sitting up and facing the therapist. Training in psychodynamic therapy is offered in many psychology, psychiatry, and social work programs and can be conducted without formal advanced training at a psychoanalytic institute. Modifications in technique have enabled psychoanalytic concepts to be applied to new populations and settings. In supportive-expressive (SE) psychotherapy, the balance of supportive and expressive elements is calibrated to meet the needs of the patient. The level of psychological health or sickness of the patient is among the factors that help the therapist determine the appropriate balance of the treatment.

Incorporating Research and New Ideas

In recent years, psychoanalysts have incorporated ideas from other fields. Empirical findings from research literature in sexual trauma (Alpert, 1995), cognitive psychology (Bucci, 1997), mother-infant interactions (Beebe & Lachmann, 2002), attachment (Lyons-Ruth, 2003) and other areas have been integrated into psychoanalytic thinking. Ideas from feminist theory (Benjamin, 1988) have also informed and enriched the field of psychoanalysis. Nobel laureate Eric Kandel (2005) has examined psychoanalytic concepts through the lens of neuroscience, and Schore (2003) has brought together developmental, psychological, and neurological research findings to significantly advance this new field of neuropsychoanalysis. Schore suggests that much of what occurs in psychotherapy is a function of right-brain, or non-verbal and non-linear activity, which clearly suggests that the value of the talking cure goes beyond the actual talking itself. Finally, despite frequently voiced perceptions to the contrary, research on psychodynamic therapies and psychoanalytic concepts is actively pursued, with positive results. That research will be reviewed in the Evidence section of this chapter.

Psychodynamic Diagnostic Manual

In 2006, the first *Psychodynamic Diagnostic Manual (PDM)* was published. The PDM is a psychodynamic alternative to the *Diagnostic and Statistical Manual (DSM)*, which is currently used for making psychiatric diagnoses (American Psychiatric Association, 2000). The *DSM* was conceived as a means for researchers and clinicians to have a common language for communicating about psychiatric disorders. It lists observable symptoms and characteristics for each diagnostic category but provides no conceptual framework for organizing the information.

In contrast, the *PDM* is based on a psychodynamic model of human functioning and integrates up-to-date information from the empirical literature on cognitive psychology, trauma, and attachment. For example, psychoanalytic research has revealed two distinct types of depression; one results from an overly self-critical personality, while the other stems from fears of abandonment and loss (Blatt, 2005).

Whereas the *DSM* emphasizes what is observable, the *PDM* describes the subjective experience of people who exhibit particular symptoms. For example, the subjective experience of anxiety is different for one who is neurotic ("I can't stand the fear; I need comfort"), one who is borderline ("My sense of self was hollow, like I didn't have a self"), and one who is psychotic ("They have been blowing poison gas through the keyhole. It's destroying me and obliterating my thoughts").

The *PDM* represents an extremely significant effort to provide a conceptual framework that meaningfully organizes what is known about the complexity of human psychological functioning.

Psychoanalytic Training

When psychoanalytic training began in this country, it was offered exclusively to physicians, but this is no longer the case. Today, admission to most psychoanalytic institutes requires that one first earn a Ph.D. or Psy.D. in clinical psychology or successfully complete a psychiatry residency. Institutes vary in their admission policies for clinical practitioners in social work. Whereas advanced training to be a psychoanalyst is extensive, training in psychoanalytic or psychodynamic psychotherapy is part of many graduate programs in psychology, psychiatry, or social work.

Psychoanalytic training generally consists of at least four years of course work, accompanied by closely supervised treatment of psychoanalytic patients who are in treatment at least three (and most often four to five) times per week for several years. A candidate is also required to undergo a personal analysis conducted by a senior psychoanalyst. This is an important part of the training; it provides an opportunity for candidates to learn firsthand what being an analytic patient, or *analysand,* is like and to observe a senior psychoanalyst at work. Even more important, a practicing psychoanalyst needs to know himself or herself well, since the work is deeply personal, and one's own emotional vulnerabilities and conflicts must be confronted and worked through if one is to be truly helpful to one's patients. For these reasons, some graduate programs recommend that students enter a personal psychoanalysis or psychoanalytically oriented therapy themselves.

Psychoanalytic Organizations

Much has changed in the organizational structure of psychoanalysis in recent years. The American Psychoanalytic Association (APsaA), founded in 1911, remains the largest of psychoanalytic societies in the United States, with 42 affiliate societies and 29 professional training programs. APsaA is part of the International Psychoanalytical Association, the largest worldwide psychoanalytic organization. The American Psychological Association's Division of Psychoanalysis lists 92 psychoanalytic training programs. Whereas many institutes have evolved from a Freudian framework, others, such as the William Alanson White Institute, have an interpersonal/relational orientation. The New York University Postdoctoral Program houses a range of theoretical orientations and encourages an exchange of ideas between them. Both the American Psychological Association (Division 39, Psychoanalysis) and the American Academy of Psychoanalysis are good resources for further information.

Psychoanalytic Journals

Because so many theoretical orientations and professional disciplines now represent psychoanalysis, there are simply too many psychoanalytic journals to list them here. They include *The International Journal of Psychoanalysis, American Journal of Psychoanalysis, Contemporary Psychoanalysis* (interpersonal), *Psychoanalytic Dialogues* (relational), and *The International Journal of Psychoanalytic Self Psychology,* to name a few of the more popular ones reflecting the range of orientations. There are also journals on specific topics, such as *Gender and Psychoanalysis.*

PERSONALITY

Theory of Personality

Personality evolves out of the interaction between biological factors and the vicissitudes of experience. That interaction is influenced not only by the nature of the life events but also by the ways those experiences are absorbed and handled. Likewise, overall mood and attitudes toward life are affected by early experiences. "Basic mood" begins to develop during the first year of life, and "confident expectancy" is a mood state that can emerge after a happy first year in which the baby's needs are met.

Problems in early life may become embedded in personality through fixation or regression, hidden through defense mechanisms, or embodied through *enactment*. In *fixation,* aspects of the child's personality get stuck at the developmental moment in which a traumatic event or unresolved conflict occurred. For example, a young adult never leaves home, in spite of pressures from those around him to move out and move on. His parents were "always gone" when he was a child, leaving him with an array of nannies, and he became fixated on the home as a form of family connection. In *regression*, the child reverts to earlier forms of behavior in response to stress. Many parents are familiar with this phenomenon, since the birth of a baby typically causes the older sibling to regress. This is usually a temporary event, but in some cases a regression has more lasting effects. *Enactment* is a form of "action memory," in which memories of sequences of troublesome experience are replayed in action. A common example comes when parents find themselves disciplining a child in just the way their parents did, even though they thought they would do it differently.

Defense Mechanisms

Psychological defense mechanisms play a pivotal role in the structure of personality. The concept of a psychological defense had its beginning in Freud's writings, but it was his daughter Anna Freud who developed the concept. Whereas Freud paid a good deal of attention to the conflict between id and superego, Anna Freud brought the ego to the fore, delineating specific ego defenses and their important role in the development of the psyche. She observed in her clinical work with adults and children that there are specific types of defenses and that people tend to use them with some consistency. For example, one person might utilize her thinking ability to keep threatening feelings at bay by speaking about them in emotionally detached and abstract terms (*intellectualization),* whereas another might express unacceptable desires symbolically through a bodily symptom (*conversion* or *somatization*).

In many people, defenses are activated by stress, but they may have a full range of other ways of responding. Other people have what Wilhelm Reich (1949) called character armor, in which their defenses pervade how they act and respond. Even positive traits can serve as defenses. Anna Freud gives the example of a matchmaker who used altruism as a defense. All her energies went into other people's love lives, but she avoided experiencing her own needs and did not have a personal life of her own.

The ego psychologists, following Anna Freud's focus on the ego's defenses, shifted the focus to the ways people adapt to reality and showed how defensive style shapes their experience of themselves, others, and the world in general. For example, those with more histrionic personality styles tend to be impressionistic and intuitive, whereas those who are more obsessional are likely to be focused, goal-oriented, and conscientious (Shapiro, 1965).

Otto Kernberg (1975) investigated the character structure of patients in the "borderline" spectrum, so called because it was first considered as the area between neurosis and psychosis. Borderline patients tend to use certain pathological defense mechanisms. The most common are *projection* (projecting one's own feelings onto another person) and *splitting* (seeing some people as all good and others as all bad, or alternately idealizing and devaluing the same person). Lyons-Ruth (2003) has shown how this type of personality structure may develop through certain forms of interaction between mothers and young children.

The types of defenses a person employs have implications for later mental and physical health. Vaillant (1977, 2002) conducted a large longitudinal study, in which he followed Harvard students from graduation until old age. He showed that the use of more mature defenses, such as sublimation (channeling one's impulses into positive, culturally desirable activities) and humor, as opposed to those that are less mature and pathological, such as projection, is highly predictive of both physical and mental health later in life.

Knowledge of the defensive and personality style of patients has useful clinical implications, as well. McWilliams (1994) has formulated very useful ways of assessing and treating people seeking psychoanalytic psychotherapy, based on their personality style and structure. For treating post-traumatic stress disorder and other stress-related problems, Horowitz (2001) delineated different treatment approaches found to be most effective, based on the particular defensive style.

Culture and Development

Erik Erikson, one of Freud's students, drew on his background in developmental psychology and anthropology, expanding Freud's theory of psychosexual development to include the effects of culture and society on psychological growth. Erikson (1963) postulated eight stages of psychosocial development from infancy to old age, in contrast to Freud's five stages of psychosexual development, which ended with childhood.

Each of Erikson's stages was based on a specific psychosocial conflict or crisis. The resolution of each crisis is associated with a particular psychosocial outcome that shapes the way the individual relates to other people and to society.

Erikson wrote a great deal about the ways in which our sense of identity develops throughout the life cycle, and he is best known for his formulation of the "identity crisis" of adolescence (Erikson, 1950). The period from 12 to 18 years (characterized in terms of the tension between identity and role confusion) is one in which an adolescent struggles to figure out who he is as a person in relation to his family, peers, and society. He then brings this sense of himself, however secure or confused, to his efforts to establish healthy and satisfying love relationships, which is the challenge of the next stage, in which the major psychosocial issue to be confronted is that of intimacy versus isolation.

Freud also believed that culture plays an important role in personality development, and for him, the superego is an internalization of the moral codes of family and society. However, Erikson believed that society's impact extends beyond its moral authority, and he placed great importance on the continual interaction between the person, culture, and family.

Early Relationships

Margaret Mahler saw the first three years of life as an unfolding process of *separation-individuation* (Mahler, Pine, & Bergman, 1975). She believed that the mother-infant relationship began with a state of oneness that she termed *symbiosis*. From there, the child gradually separates and forms her own sense of identity. In order to do so, she *internalizes* the relationship with the mother, giving her the ability to experience a feeling of connection with her mother as she develops her own autonomy. Disturbances in the process give rise to lasting conflicts, with anxiety around separation and problems in establishing a secure identity.

Mahler's concept of symbiosis has been disproved by child development research, but the idea that the child internalizes the relationship with the mother is consistent with attachment theory on "inner working models" of relationships (Bowlby, 1988).

Over time, many psychoanalysts have moved toward orientations that place greater emphasis on the social and relational aspects of psychological functioning. Freud initially hypothesized that people are motivated by a quest for pleasure and gratification of certain basic drives, such that specific people become significant to a child because they satisfy his basic biological needs. A mother becomes important to a baby because she feeds him when he is hungry and thus becomes associated with the child's own gratification and pleasure. From the relational perspective, on the other hand, the primary motivation is the desire to be in a relationship with another person (Greenberg & Mitchell, 1983).

Object Relations

Fairbairn (1954) and others developed an idea that has come to be known as *object relations theory*. (He used the word *object* to mean a person who has great emotional significance to the child, having retained the term from Freud's earlier descriptions of caregiving adults as being "the objects of the drives," or those toward whom the drives are directed.) Fairbairn worked with abused children and observed that they remained extremely attached to parents who had severely abused them, suggesting they were looking to their parents for more than mere pleasure through need gratification. What is more, these children later sought out relationships characterized by the same abusive pattern as the earlier relationship.

Object relations theory concludes that human emotional life and relationships center around the unconscious mental images we hold of our earliest and most intense relationships, or *internalized object representations*. In order to avoid the terror of loss and abandonment, a child (or adult) will do whatever she can to maintain her connection to her early love objects. She might do so by seeking out others to whom she can relate in ways that match her internalized images of those who comprised her early emotional life; in this way, she recaptures the soothing feeling of connectedness. Object relations theory has helped psychoanalysts to understand better why people find themselves in relationships that appear to be maladaptive and self-destructive. It has been applied to a wide range of populations and situations and has provided particular insights into more serious and therapeutically challenging types of disturbances, such as borderline and narcissistic personalities (Kernberg, 1975). It has also led to a variety of other relational perspectives (Mitchell, 1988).

Numerous other psychoanalysts further elaborated on the early mother-infant relationship as it relates to personality development. One of these was Donald Winnicott (1965), who trained as a pediatrician before becoming a psychoanalyst. Winnicott (1965) believed that healthy emotional development requires a *good-enough mother* who provides a *holding environment* for her child with her consistent, loving presence. From this experience, the baby emerges with a sense of security and the ability to soothe herself during periods of stress and anxiety.

Self-Psychology

Heinz Kohut (1977) took a new look at a group of narcissistic patients for whom other formulations did not appear to apply. His was interested in those who presented with a chronic state of emptiness, a lack of inner vitality, and an unstable sense of themselves and their self-worth, which was frequently masked by a more grandiose or expansive presentation. Kohut observed that these patients often reported a lack of "mirroring" experiences in their childhoods, such that they failed to receive support and admiration for what Kohut regarded as "healthy narcissism."

Young children frequently demand attention from adults by showing off and exaggerating their own power and abilities. A very young child might run around shouting, "Look at me, I'm the fastest runner in the world!" The parents of Kohut's patients, rather than mirroring the child's joy, typically responded with a lack of warmth and often with criticism or ridicule. Many of his patients also lacked an adult figure to safely idealize, something Kohut regarded as crucial to healthy development. In this self-psychological model, narcissistic disturbances result from environmental deficiencies rather than biological drives or psychological conflict.

Kohut found that psychoanalytic interpretations did not help narcissistic patients. Instead, he proposed offering empathy, mirroring, and support for positive self-esteem. In a well-known case of "Mr. Z," he used his empathic approach to reanalyze a patient who had not done well with traditional analytic techniques (Kohut, 1979).

Attachment and Personality Development

Psychodynamic theory and attachment theory have arrived at congruent views of personality development. Both regard early relationships as formative in the development of the child's emotional well-being and sense of self, and decades of attachment research supports this (Bowlby, 1969; 1988; Main, Kaplan, & Cassidy, 1985). Psychoanalysts are increasingly integrating these findings into their thinking. Lyons-Ruth (1991), for example, has proposed that Margaret Mahler's concept of *separation-individuation* be renamed "attachment-individuation." She points out that the child first develops an attachment to the parent and then *individuates* internalizing this relationship. Fonagy (2002) has demonstrated that the ability to *mentalize,* or mentally represent internal psychological states, develops from a secure early attachment relationship and is related to the later ability to regulate emotions and calm oneself during times of stress and anxiety. The intersection between attachment research and psychodynamic concepts continues to offer the potential for fresh thinking and discoveries.

Variety of Concepts

Defense Mechanisms

Freud first described defenses as the ego's struggle against painful or unendurable ideas or affects (Freud, 1894). He later shifted to using the word *repression* for that purpose, but the concept of defense returned in his later writings, and it has had staying power in the practice of psychodynamic forms of treatment.

Repression came to refer to the process of removing a painful memory or feeling from consciousness, whereas *defenses* came to mean the varied ways in which the ego keeps itself protected from painful thoughts and feelings, especially those experienced as dangerous. The danger often has less to do with active danger in the current world and more to do with a sense of "felt danger." The "felt danger" may have its origins in early, sometimes traumatic experience. For example, a child who was adopted from a Russian orphanage at two years of age reacts to new people with ease. But he wriggles away from his adoptive mother. He has developed a defense that is easy to decode, since we know its history. He seems on the surface as if he is at ease with adults, but he defends against getting close, since he knows too well that people leave. Without such an obvious trail of documented history, patients discover their own "trail" in treatment, as a way to begin to undo early defenses.

The analysis of defense starts with noticing the defenses in operation. After becoming aware of their function, the patient can gradually look at the once intolerable content behind them. The therapist needs to respect that the content behind the "fence" of the defense may be difficult to tolerate and may even be part of a trail of memories to what was once a very painful experience. Here are some examples of prominent defenses:

In *projection,* the patient attributes unacceptable impulses or feelings of his own to another person (or agency). Angry, controlling, sexual, or jealous feelings are frequently projected onto others. Projection is the major mechanism of paranoia.

Obsessional thinking and *compulsive rituals* are defenses against unacceptable thoughts or unbearable feelings. Rather than allowing the individual to feel worried about the potential consequence of an aggressive thought, or overwhelmed by an anxiety-provoking one, obsessional thinking shifts the focus to small details that can be cognitively controlled. Compulsive rituals have a similar function, reducing anxiety through behavior.

Denial is the refusal to accept external reality when it is too threatening, and may involve "the reversal of real facts into their opposites" (A. Freud, 1966, p. 93). Young children exhibit harmless denial when they use the "magical thinking" of childhood, but it becomes a serious problem if this defense mechanism survives beyond childhood. It is frequently associated with alcohol or drug dependence, where acknowledging the related problems would mean facing the addiction.

Avoidance is a much more common mechanism than denial. It involves withdrawing from the experience of "psychic pain" or anxiety. However, in doing so, the patient also avoids the entire situation that caused the perception of emotional pain.

Primary and Secondary Process Thinking

Primary process thinking is nonlogical thinking. It is the language of the dream, of creative processes, and of the unconscious. The connections between thoughts have to do with images, memories, and emotion, rather than rational thinking. *Secondary process* thinking is logical, verbal thinking. These modes of thinking have been linked to the different modes of processing of the left and right hemispheres of the brain (Erdelyi, 1985).

Dream Interpretation

Freud considered the dream to be "the royal road to the unconscious" and *The Interpretation of Dreams* to be his greatest achievement. He believed that to understand his theory of dreams is to understand psychoanalysis.

Following the method Freud developed to interpret dreams, the dreamer holds the key to its meanings. Unlike Jungian analysis, psychoanalytic dream interpretation does not tend to attach preset meanings to dream symbols. Instead, the dreamer's associations, or thoughts about each dream image, serve as clues to understanding the dream. When the dreamer comes up with associations to the dream elements, they offer links between the dream image and its meaning to the dreamer.

The *manifest content* of the dream is the overt dream story, and the *latent content* consists of its underlying meanings. *Day residue,* or images that come from events of the day, may make their way into the dream. The interpretation of the dream emerges by listening to the dream and the dreamer's associations to elements of it, while seeking the deep thematic links between them. Understanding the language of the dream gives the analyst the ability to make sense out of what might sound like nonsense to others.

Although some aspects of Freud's thoughts on dreaming (such as the idea that the dream is the guardian of sleep) have not withstood the test of science, his insights into the language of the dream still open doors to the "royal road." The language of the dream consists of the use of nonlogical forms of expression, including condensation, [personal] symbolism, allusions, and displacement.

Here is an example of some of these mechanisms at work in a dream:

DREAM: "I dreamt about a flower. I was the flower and I was the picker."

BACKGROUND: The patient, a young woman of 20, had recently had an abortion. Her first thought about the flower was that it was a daisy. Her association to a daisy was "he loves me, he loves me not," which made her think of her boyfriend (an allusion), who would not commit to their relationship. Then she thought of picking off the petals. This was a symbolic reference to the abortion, as "taking off" the flower. When asked for her association to picking the flower, her eyes became misty with tears. The dream condensed her feelings and thoughts about the abortion into one moving image.

Freud believed that these mechanisms disguised hidden wishes and that interpreting the dream reversed the censorship created through these forms of disguise. Psychodynamic therapists now are likely to consider the dream as a symbolic representation of whatever is essential to the patient, in dream language. Whether the dream is considered as a product of censorship or as a different form of processing during sleep, understanding the language of dreams can still take the dreamer down the royal road to personal discovery.

Clinical-Research Concepts

Psychotherapy researchers have developed methods that allow for the study of psychotherapy process and outcome. The methods highlighted here have both clinical and research uses. Their clinical use is as procedures in the practice of supportive-expressive (SE) psychotherapy. They may also be used in other forms of treatment.

The Core Conflictual Relationship Theme Method (CCRT). The CCRT is a method to examine the inner workings of the patient's relationship patterns. It serves as an operational version of the transference (Luborsky & Luborsky, 2006). The therapist listens for repeating patterns in the stories the patient tells about encounters with others ("relationship episodes"), including responses to the therapist. The pattern is termed *conflictual* because the responses are most often at odds with what the patient really wants for himself.

Each CCRT pattern is composed of these three elements:

1. The wish (W), either stated or implied
2. The response of others, either real or anticipated (RO)
3. The response of self (RS)

Common wishes include the wishes to be loved, to be respected, and to be accepted. Here are some examples of CCRT material as it appears in session:

CCRT Example 1

P: I am getting behind in my work. It's driving me crazy. Every time she passes by my desk it gets so dragged out that I have no time to myself. If this keeps up, my manager is going to get wind of it.

W (implied): To be respected

RO: Takes over; doesn't consider patient's needs

RS: Feels trapped

CCRT Example 2

P: (Stares blankly for a few minutes, and then speaks) Nothing much to say (in a monotone). Rob is in L.A., and there is no point calling. He is much too busy meeting this one and that one to want to talk.

W (implied): To be cared for

RO (anticipated): Indifference, not caring

RS: Give up, get depressed

The CCRT is not decoded by one example alone. It comprises repeating episodes that bring the conflictual theme to light. The wish (W), response of other (RO), and response of self (RS) can be thought of as three strands of a rope that have become intertwined. The first task of the CCRT method is to notice the strands at work. That starts the action of the second aspect of the method, which involves disentangling the strands so that new forms of responses can begin. In fact, research suggests that is just what happens in successful SE psychotherapy. The patient's wishes remain the same, but the responses of others and self show some change (Luborsky & Crits-Christoph, 1998). In other words, the patient still wants what he wants for himself, but he no longer has such negative expectations of others or so many self-defeating responses from himself.

The Symptom–Context Method.   The Symptom-Context method offers a way to decode the meanings of symptoms that can be used both in clinical and research situations. Instead of considering the symptom as having a life of its own, this method provides a way to examine why the symptom emerges.

Just as clinicians look for the "triggers" for depression or problems of abrupt onset, the Symptom-Context method looks at the "material" surrounding the symptom—that is, the emotional and verbal responses of the patient. When this approach is used as a research method, the researcher blocks off the segment of the session before and after the appearance of the symptom (its nodal point). That segment is compared to other, non-symptom segments of the same length (its control nodal point).

In treatment, the Symptom-Context method gives the patient and therapist a way to make sense out of what was once a mysterious, disturbing event. Its power begins to diminish once the context gives clues to its meaning. This is particularly useful for patients with anxiety disorders, PTSD, or stress-related physical symptoms.

An Example of the Symptom-Context Method

P: In the car coming over here, I started getting a headache. . . . I think it was because of what we've been talking about. You know, him. . . . And my sister wants me to drive her all the way to Staten Island to visit him.

Context: The patient has been talking about her father, who singled her out for berating during her childhood. She has been working on the issue in therapy long enough to suspect that the headache is a manifestation of the conflict in her head, between the pressure to see her father, and her anger against him.

The Helping Alliance Methods.   The Helping Alliance is the partnership between the patient and the therapist around the work of the treatment. In clinical writings, it has been referred to as the therapeutic, or working, alliance. The Helping Alliance methods include scales and questionnaires designed to be used in research to track the state of the Helping Alliance.

Two kinds of Helping Alliance were found through factor analysis of clinical research material. The first kind, called Helping Alliance 1, is an alliance in which the patient feels that the therapist is there to help her. In other words, she feels that the therapist is doing his job and is on her side. The second kind, Helping Alliance 2, is an alliance in which the patient feels like a partner in the therapy process. He sees working together as a way to move his recovery forward. Both forms of alliance are linked with a successful treatment outcome in psychotherapy research.

In SE psychotherapy, two different therapeutic tools are important in the development of the Helping Alliance. The first is the therapist's empathy for the patient's experience. Research shows that a strong Helping Alliance early in the treatment is linked to the therapist's empathy, both of which are predictors of a good outcome for the therapy. The second is the process of examining problems that occur within the treatment, acknowledging anything that the therapist may have done that has bothered the patient, and setting about to clarify the problem. That is referred to as *rupture and repair,* a process that initial research suggests is beneficial to the treatment (Safrin et al., 2001).

PSYCHOTHERAPY

Theory of Psychotherapy

As a form of therapy, psychoanalysis brings the "whole person" to the couch, including his problems, stresses, memories, dreams, fantasies, and feelings, in order to discover the inner sources of his problems. The psychoanalytic process begins as the patient opens up, so that previously unknown parts of the self can be owned and recognized.

During the patient's free associations, the analyst starts to hear patterns in the midst of the stories the patient tells and begins to pick up the emotional "hot spots" in the patient's life. At the same time, the patient may begin to convey his difficulties through the ways he reacts to the analyst. The convergence of these streams of information forms the basis of the transference. This gives the analyst and patient a chance to work on repeating patterns while they are active in the treatment. The analyst also listens for sources of inner conflict that may be linked to symptoms or life problems. Change comes through the process of reworking old patterns so that the patient can become freer to respond in new ways.

The therapeutic relationship itself is the other central change agent. Greenson (1967) and Zetzel (1970) pointed out how an alliance between therapist and patient is beneficial to the treatment. Whereas in psychoanalysis the treatment relationship develops through the intensity of the treatment, in psychodynamic psychotherapy a strong working alliance is actively encouraged. Current psychoanalytic thinking emphasizes the importance of the emotional communication between patient and therapist as a way to gain information and create connection.

Change in Psychodynamic Psychotherapy

What makes for change in dynamic psychotherapy? The theories about what matters in treatment have their origins in the central principles of psychoanalysis. Change is seen as a gradual process of (1) opening up to self-discovery, (2) discovering patterns of relating and perceiving that stand in the way of current functioning, (3) finding ways to disentangle the influences of the past from the present, and (4) finding new ways to cope. The first (1) objective is achieved through free association on the part of the patient and the "evenly hovering" attention of the analyst. The next (2) objective refers to the analysis of the transference or, in SE psychotherapy, the examination of the CCRT. The third (3) objective involves the gradual discovery of the sources of pain, through memories and through the unwelcome reminders that may come via symptoms and behavior in relationships. The final phase (4) is achieved by working through the changes from the preceding steps and developing an increasing ability to use the working alliance with the therapist as a backdrop for a new sense of emotional competence.

Psychoanalysis and Psychodynamic Treatment

Although psychoanalysis is the subject of a vast amount of writing, psychodynamic treatment is more frequently used in practice. Psychodynamic treatment began in order to shorten and simplify the lengthy process of psychoanalysis. It remains popular for the same practical reasons. Supportive-expressive (SE) psychotherapy was developed in order to add clarity to the clinical process. It works from central dynamic principles and includes the use of clinical-research methods in the treatment.

Gains in psychoanalysis and in dynamic psychotherapy derive from two sources: the therapeutic relationship and the exploration of the patient's problems. In supportive-expressive (SE) psychotherapy, the relationship and the structure of the treatment serve as the basis for the supportive aspect of the treatment. Exploration of the patient's problems, using the CCRT and the Symptom-Context methods as tools, constitutes the expressive aspect.

Table 2.1 illustrates the ways in which the psychoanalytic principles emerge in treatment. The term *psychodynamic psychotherapies* here refers to both psychoanalysis and dynamic psychotherapy, since both make use of the same fundamentals in their treatments.

The Purpose of the Psychoanalytic Method

Why make the unconscious conscious? Why talk about the past? The psychoanalytic stereotype is that of patients spending dozens of years of talking to the ceiling and getting nowhere. Aimless analysis may sometimes occur, but that is not the intent of the method, nor is it likely in a well-conducted treatment. Let's look at the theoretical

TABLE 2.1   **Application of Psychoanalytic Principles to Treatment**

Psychoanalytic Principle	Psychodynamic Psychotherapies	SE Psychotherapy
Allow a positive regard for the analyst as a base for the treatment.	Develop a working alliance.	Apply Helping Alliance methods.
Understand the transference. Unconscious conflict results in symptoms.	Analyze the transference. Explore conflicts that may be connected to symptoms.	Apply CCRT methods. Apply Symptom-Context method.

reasons for the psychoanalytic method. (The psychodynamic and clinical-research methods applicable to each of these points are given in parentheses.)

1. *To uncover the inner problems that had been disguised as symptoms.* Just as replacing a garden hose does not solve a problem in water quality, in psychodynamic psychotherapies, the goal is to resolve the problem at its source. In order to understand the meanings expressed in the symptom, the treatment allows in all kinds of material that might at first appear to be random and unrelated. The thematic and emotional links become apparent only after enough "emotional data" have been collected. An "emotional understanding" of the meaning and function of the symptom should prevent *symptom substitution,* in which a different symptom emerges that expresses the same inner problem, and should help reduce the likelihood that the same symptom will continue to recur. {Expressive work; Symptom-Context method.}

2. *To become integrated.* In intrapsychic, or internal, conflict, the parts of the self are at odds with each other. For example, one part may hold the belief in high achievement, while the other part may feel burdened and resentful of work. In conflict, one part sabotages the other, as in the student who never makes it to class. In "working through the conflict" the student may come to know the part of himself that feels resentful and may give that part a chance to speak in session, rather than through behavior. The next task is to find solutions in life that work for both parts of the self. That may take the form of no longer holding on to old feelings that carried pain or frustration, so that what once was at impasse becomes possible. Or it might take the form of a different kind of adaptation, as in the student who decides to spend a semester in Alaska instead of in class. {Free association; working through; CCRT}

3. *To uncover the sources of past pain that may be embedded in the present, causing ripples, or at times whirlpools, of the past in the present.* Perhaps the most powerful reason to take the time to consider what may lie behind symptoms and problems in living is the power of the past to find its way into the present. Selma Fraiberg (1987) tells poignant stories of her work with mothers who had been neglected or abused themselves as children. Their own babies began life in a form of repetition of that neglect, because the mothers could not respond to their babies' cries. Through her work with the mothers and their memories, Fraiberg and her colleagues helped two generations at once, separating the past from the present by first allowing past pain to be understood and then focusing on the present, new baby. An except from the one of these cases, "Ghosts in the Nursery," is included in Case Studies in Psychotherapy, the companion book to this text. {Early memories; therapist's empathy; Symptom-Context method}

4. *To discover what stands in the way of taking appropriate actions for the self.* Even the best plans sometimes go nowhere because other forces within the patient stand in her way. For example, a patient spent several sessions outlining her plan to apply to business school and then develop her own business. But she then canceled her next session and did not return the therapist's phone calls. When she finally showed up, weeks later, she and the therapist discovered that she had expected the therapist to hold her to a plan she was not ready to follow. In fact, the people who would have been behind her plan were not even there. They were her parents as she remembered them from childhood, always planning for her, especially her mother. The therapeutic work needed to back up, and take a look at the transference, so that the patient could become free to make her own choices. The CCRT offered them a way to examine the anticipated responses of others (RO) as well as her own response (RS). {Transference; CCRT}

The sources of change in dynamic treatment are summarized in Table 2.2.

TABLE 2.2   **Sources of Change in Dynamic Treatment**

Theoretical Principle	Treatment Process	Clinical Method	Clinical-Research Method	Goal
Unconscious conflict causes symptoms or problems in living.	Uncover inner sources of conflict; pt gives voice to parts of the self.	Pt: free association T: open listening	CCRT (for conflict) Symptom-Context (for symptom's meaning)	Decode symptom; find new resolution to inner conflict.
Transference causes problems in current relationships.	Uncover the workings of the transference.	Attend to the transference to the analyst and others.	CCRT method	Disentangle old expectancies from current attitudes.
Early problems resurface in later functioning.	Examine the transformation of past problems into new forms.	Listen for early memories and notice ways current stresses may trigger them.	Symptom-Context method (for the role of stresses in triggering old issues)	Give a new ear to old pain so that it no longer causes acute stress; disentangle the past and the present.
The therapeutic relationship serves as the foundation of treatment.	Forge a treatment relationship that builds trust.	Empathy, along with examination of problems as they occur	Helping Alliance methods; rupture and repair	Build a treatment alliance that gives the patient a sense that someone is "there for him."

The Purpose of Free Association

The reason for encouraging free association, rather than structuring the treatment around specific problems, is that neither the patient nor the therapist knows where the keys to the patient's problems will come from until they find them. That is because powerful aspects of the patient's inner life have been operating without his full awareness. As he gradually allows more of himself to be known, both to himself and to the therapist, the patient can begin to take charge of a "fuller self." New potential emerges once he gets in touch with sources of conflict that were previously operating in the language of symptoms. "Free speech" is the first step.

EXAMPLE

A patient who has just turned 30 finds that he loses interest in every woman he dates after 3 months. He tried "holding his nose" and staying, but that did not change his feelings. His current girlfriend suggested therapy.

P: So, tell me what is wrong with me. I mean, could it be that I just haven't met the drop-dead gorgeous girl who deserves me? Just kidding. Mia says I'm scared of rejection. I don't know about that.

The patient is backing into his own feelings by talking about his girlfriend's ideas first. The therapist is listening, her first job in the treatment. She knows better than to jump in too quickly with any answer to the patient's problems. Instead, she is interested in beginning a process where the patient gets in touch with himself. Her two tasks, developing a Helping Alliance and starting the exploratory work, are beginning together.

Psychoanalytic Variations

Although the fundamentals of the theory of psychotherapy are shared by most therapists working in a psychodynamic tradition, the emphasis on one element or another varies considerably. For example, classical psychoanalysts focus most on the exploratory work, with the analysis of the transference as the crux of the work. Self-psychologists focus on the nature of the therapeutic relationship, using empathy, rather than understanding, as a prime tool. Relational analysts focus on what gets conveyed through the relationship forged between patient and analyst. The diversity in viewpoints makes a refreshing change from the early days of psychoanalysis (Orfanos, 2006).

However, underneath the differences, a common set of principles continues to operate. In addition to the fundamentals mentioned above, there is the importance of individual differences and the view of the treatment as an opportunity to help the patient rediscover himself. The patient's unique story is the topic of the treatment, with its previously hidden parts as sources of both pain and potential. The dynamics to understand are not a theory to fit to the patient. Instead, they are principles that can guide the therapist's ways of understanding the patient, once enough clinical material has emerged.

Process of Psychotherapy

Psychoanalytically oriented psychotherapy is an unfolding interpersonal process aimed at both discovery and recovery. It is shaped by the personality and problems of the patient, the nature of the therapeutic relationship, and the pathway discovered by patient and therapist as most fitting for the patient. It moves through a series of stages that do not have a time line, except in time-limited versions of dynamic treatment. Instead, the stages are paced by the process and progress of the treatment.

Phases of Dynamic Psychotherapy

Just like a book, the phases of dynamic psychotherapy can be divided in three: the beginning, or *opening phase;* the middle, which consists of the major work of the treatment, including *working through* the basic themes; and the end, commonly called the *termination phase.* Whereas the beginning and the end are defined by their place in the treatment, the middle phase is defined more by the nature of the processes and progress that take place. Consequently, the opening and termination phases will be discussed here as such, and the work of the treatment will be described in terms of the elements that go into the treatment.

The Opening Phase.   The opening phase begins before the door opens. What made the patient decide to come into treatment at this time? How hard was it to make the decision? Has she ever been in treatment before? How "bad off" is she? Are there symptoms that might be dangerous to her well-being? Does she have clear goals, or is she "here because she's here"? The therapist will be interested in all of these questions, but he will not want to bombard the patient with them. He will want to set a tone and a pace that allow the patient to begin to get comfortable being in therapy and telling her story.

Psychoanalysis and dynamic psychotherapy differ in certain respects during the first phase. A notable difference is that analysts typically wait for the patient to tell her story, rather than asking many questions. Whether or not questions are explicitly posed, the therapist will want to understand

- Why the patient is seeking treatment at this time
- What kinds of triggers to the current problems seem to be present
- How troubled the patient appears to be (psychological health-sickness)

The therapist takes cues from the patient right from the start. Thus some patients will be able to talk over their reasons for coming into treatment in an organized way, whereas others convey their reasons by their level of distress and difficulty talking. The therapy begins where the patient is.

The introductory phase typically lasts for several sessions. Some therapists use the first three sessions to get an initial sense of the patient and her problems and to go over treatment goals together. Others begin without a formal procedure, trusting that the process will unfold organically. In SE psychotherapy, some form of evaluation, however informal, takes place during the first several sessions. The therapist seeks to get a sense of the patient's psychological well-being in order to consider what form of treatment will be in her best interest. Related decisions include the frequency of the treatment, as well as the balance of supportive and expressive elements. If the initial assessment raises concerns about psychotic process, drug abuse, or severe depression, it also is the responsibility of the therapist to refer the patient for a psychiatric evaluation. Psychological testing may be used to better understand a patient's cognitive and psychological problems.

The practical arrangements of the treatment need to be made during the introductory phase. Those include establishing the frequency of the sessions, agreeing on the fee, and communicating any policies the therapist has regarding missed or canceled appointments.

In psychoanalysis, particularly classical analysis, the patient moves from sitting up to lying on the couch either after a few sessions or when she is ready. In dynamic psychotherapy, the patient remains sitting up, facing the therapist. Psychoanalysis typically takes place three to five times a week, whereas psychotherapy sessions typically occur either once or twice a week. This reflects a difference in the process between the two forms of treatment. In psychoanalysis, the patient goes through what has been called a *transference neurosis*. That is, she replays her core relationship problems in the analysis, and they are resolved by working through their action in the treatment. Frequent sessions intensify that process. In dynamic psychotherapy, work on the transference also takes place, but it is less likely to be replayed in the same way. The CCRT offers a tool for uncovering its action in SE psychotherapy.

The Helping Alliance begins in the opening phase, through the partnership forged between patient and therapist around beginning the treatment. An early positive Helping Alliance correlates with positive results in treatment, according to psychotherapy research studies. This does not mean that a therapy is doomed if the patient starts with mistrust and misgivings, but it does mean that forging a good connection is an auspicious start.

The Elements of the Treatment

The two central elements of the treatment are the therapeutic relationship and the exploration of the patient's problems. The balance of these two elements varies by the form of dynamic treatment being practiced and, more important, by the needs of the patient. In SE psychotherapy, the amount of supportiveness and the amount of expressiveness are tailored to the needs and pathology of the patient. In other words, a patient who is more psychologically fragile will need more support from the therapist than one who functions well in daily life. Some patients respond more to the empathy and the feeling of connection; others respond more to the quest for self-discovery that happens through expressive work. The guide to the right balance of these elements is the patient.

The Supportive Relationship.   In SE psychotherapy, the supportive relationship includes all elements of the therapeutic relationship that offer sources of human connection and structural support to the patient. These elements include the Helping Alliance, the therapist's empathy, the structure of the treatment contract, and attention to the realities of the patient's life. Although many people think of "support" as a lesser element, something either to avoid or to fall back on when nothing else works, empirical studies link support with a positive outcome of the treatment (Orlinsky, Graw, & Parks, 1994).

In all dynamic treatments, the therapeutic relationship is considered a source of the therapeutic action. The therapist's empathy sets the stage for connection. "One begins to empathize with the patient as soon as one goes to open the door, even before seeing him" (Greenson, 1978, p. 158). Empathy connects the therapist and patient to a level of the patient's experience that may not be expressed in words. Since patients often come to therapy when they find themselves in the midst of different kinds of negative emotion, it is encouraging for them to find that the therapist can get the "feel" of their lives.

EXAMPLE

P sits in her chair in a way that makes her look as if the chair is her skin. She is not moving. The therapist sits very still, finding that she has quieted herself to be in tune with the patient's slow rhythm. Time passes. The therapist watches the patient's face.

P: Tomorrow is another day.
T: (Nods)
P: You don't know what it's like to get up in the morning, look around the room, and see . . . (She begins to get teary.)
T: (Hands her the tissues)
P: Thanks.
T: (Nods)

The patient is trying to come to terms with the end of her marriage. There are no words the therapist can offer her right now that are as useful as her presence. The patient needs someone to *be with* her feelings.

The Expressive Work

The expressive work is a gradual process of making sense of the patient's problems, in the context of the whole person. Before forming any hypotheses about the problems, the therapist needs to deepen her sense of the patient by tuning her ear to listen for all the levels of communication that take place. Freud called this "evenly hovering attention"; instead of preselecting what matters, the therapist listens to everything the patient brings. Luborsky & Luborsky (2006) refer to this process as *open listening,* and Rubin (1996) likens this form of listening to Buddhist meditation, in which the focus is not the content but a state of being.

Meanwhile, the patient is asked to "say what comes to mind," a suggestion that different patients use in different ways. Some want to begin at the beginning and start with their memories and earlier problems. Some begin with today—with whatever events and thoughts come to mind. Some stay problem focused and select those situations that cause stress. In that way the treatment belongs to the patient, and he is shaping it as his own by the nature of the concerns he brings.

It is not only what the patient says that helps the therapist develop an understanding of the patient, but also how he conveys himself. That includes his tone of voice, *affect* (emotional tone), and behavior. Many current analysts consider their countertransference reactions as possible sources of information as well.

EXAMPLE

P: (In a bland voice) So I went to Washington, spent the day collecting the data that I needed, and made the train back that night.

T: (T is silently wondering why this patient bores him. There is nothing wrong with what he is saying. Most patients give an account of the details of their daily life. He has been coming to treatment for three months, so he must be getting something out of it.)

P: Marjorie was there . . . (He falls silent.)

T: (Marjorie . . . She was the one who broke up with him last year. Maybe she is key to live feelings.) What was it like to see her again?

P: You remembered.

T: A surprise?

P: Yes. People don't.

T: That must bother you.

P: Not really. I'm used to it.

T: How did you get so used to it?

P: (Winces, the first show of real affect the therapist has seen in a long time.)

T: (No longer feeling bored, and suspecting that his reaction is related to the patient's CCRT pattern) There may be good reasons why you got used to it. It would be rather frustrating to keep expecting people to remember what you have to say, if they never do.

P: I'd say so. (His body posture relaxes ever so slightly.)

T: (The therapist is glad to have found a way to understand the patient's bland way of presenting himself. He did not want to mention it directly, feeling fairly certain that the patient would be insulted if he did. He realizes that his own worry about being rude had stopped him from looking more closely at the issue. He then begins to consider the patient's CCRT pattern.)

The therapist's countertransference response had let him know that something active had been missing. He took advantage of an opening in the patient's discourse to get to a "live issue." That allowed him to consider the patient's CCRT. In this case it would be

W: (Wish) [implied and deeply buried] To be recognized, remembered

RO: (Response of others) [anticipated] Not recognized, not remembered

RS: (Response of self) No emotional reaction, no affect

The therapist could also consider the patient's bland presentation as a defense against affect. The defense against the pain he would feel if he let in the disappointing response of others had become a defense against all feeling.

Deepening the Exploration

The expressive work deepens through the gradual emergence of patterns in the patient's problems. That includes patterns in relationships and in handling stresses and emotions. Unlike symptom-focused treatments, dynamic treatments start with the premise that any information can be useful in that process of discovery. Just as in mining for gold in a muddy stream, you don't know where the nuggets are until you find them.

In the middle phase of treatment, the patient and therapist gain a deeper understanding of what forces make for problems in the patient's life. That takes place by an examination of problems in relationships, through the understanding of the transference or CCRT pattern. The patient's emotions begin to make sense as their connections to her past and present life become clear. The emergence of symptoms takes on new meaning once the links to the patient's inner conflicts are understood. The Symptom-Context method can help in that process.

By the later phase of the exploratory work, the patient has gained understanding of the past patterns in her life and is no longer experiencing inner conflict that stops her from functioning. She may continue to *work through* the remaining ways in which old patterns may surface, as she gets ready to figure out new ways to cope. With some patients that happens as a natural outgrowth of the process of the therapy. Others make active efforts to develop new coping strategies, now that their energies are no longer tied up in past patterns and conflicts. In this phase of the work, the patient may notice herself "freed up" in situations that used to be impossible for her to handle.

The Termination Phase

The end of the treatment comes when it comes. The best ending is an ending of the need for treatment, when the patient is engaged with her life in ways that feel positive, without the initial symptoms and turmoil that brought her to treatment in the first place. She should also have mastery of her core themes, so that she no longer falls back into the same problems once she has finished treatment. She should have developed new ways to cope, so that she feels that she can handle her life.

In reality, people "get off the train" of treatment at different points. Some end due to symptom relief, some end due to difficulties in the treatment, or some stay until the deeper issues are resolved. Of course, there is really no such thing as being finished, if "finished" means having no problems and having complete confidence, but an end to a psychoanalytically based treatment should mean that the patient knows herself better, accepts herself and her feelings, and is not frightened of what she will find or feel if she really tunes into herself. She should instead be in a place, psychically, where the old demons have been tamed and no longer "spook" her in the present, and she is ready to move on.

Termination is not as simple as setting a date to conclude treatment. It is a process instead, and considerable feeling comes up in ending therapy. Patients have typically become attached to their analysts, and there are many feelings about letting that person go. Old conflicts and symptoms may resurface as an expression of anxiety about stopping. However, these experiences should be brief and the patient should be able to get them back under control if she is really ready to end. It is important during this phase to explore any fantasies the patient has about how things will be after the analysis is over. That gives the patient and analyst a chance to share the patient's hopes and fears, as well as to give the patient greater confidence going forward. An "open door" policy is often useful as an ending stance. That means the therapy is a place the patient can return to if she ever has the need. In the meantime (which could be forever), she takes it with her.

Mechanisms of Psychotherapy

If someone listened through the walls to a psychodynamic treatment session, he would not be hearing "mechanisms." Instead, he would hear someone talking about his life, telling anecdotes, memories, feelings, and fears. He would hear the therapist's responses to those concerns—sometimes to the content, sometimes to the feelings, often to both. But those exchanges contain the treatment mechanisms, since the essential mechanism of psychotherapy is an interpersonal process. The two central elements of the treatment, the therapeutic relationship and the exploratory work, both contribute to their workings.

The Therapeutic Relationship

The Helping Alliance is pivotal to the therapeutic relationship. It is the partnership between therapist and patient around the work of the treatment. Some patients experience that alliance as going to a therapist who gives them help (Helping Alliance 1), whereas others experience it more as a partnership between patient and therapist (Helping Alliance 2). Research links both forms with a good outcome for the treatment, provided it is a positive alliance, or one that the patient feels offers help.

The Helping Alliance can be enhanced by the therapist's efforts to keep the channels of communication clear. This means actively listening to the patient so that she feels the therapist is a partner in sharing her real concerns. It also means noticing if problems occur in the alliance and seeking to address them.

A process of *rupture and repair* can benefit the alliance if misunderstandings or negative reactions have occurred. This process consists of talking over what may have been problematic for the patient, acknowledging any real difficulties that arose, and accepting the patient's feelings about whatever went wrong. Being able to look at a mishap without brushing it away or overreacting can serve as a useful experience for the patient. Safran & Muran (1996) found it actually to be beneficial to the treatment outcome, especially for patients with negative expectations of relationships.

EXAMPLE

P: (P cancelled the last session. She arrives at this one just on time, and sits down.) So.

T: (Waits. She notes that the patient is focused on the arm of the chair and looks annoyed.)

P: Nothing much to report. Work is busy. What else is new? A lot has happened, I guess.

T: (Wondering why she is so evasive, and whether something might be bothering her about the therapy. Since she canceled the last session, there could be a reason for both.) You haven't been here in a few weeks, is that right?

P: (Shrugs)

T: So I imagine a lot has happened that you haven't talked about here.

P: As if that matters.

T: I get the feeling I am pretty useless in your life right now.

P: (Shrugs again)

T: But I do remember just a few weeks ago you talking about some really important things. I wonder what happened in between? I must have done something, or said something, that made it feel different here.

P: Done something.

T: OK, what did I do?

It turned out that what the therapist did was to take a phone call during the patient's session, something she ordinarily never does, but she had been worried about her own child, who was home sick. The therapist acknowledged that she had taken the call. She wondered if that felt to the patient like she was no longer interested in her. After hearing the patient's feelings, the therapist apologized for causing the patient to feel that she wasn't interested in her: "The last place you need to feel that is here." After several sessions of work on this rupture, repair began. The incident ended up helping the treatment, because the patient said that she had figured she would have quit therapy until the therapist admitted her mistake. It also led them to work on the patient's transference expectations, through CCRT work on her negative expectations of others and her own defensive responses. And it led the therapist to reflect on the narrow bridge between her personal and professional lives.

As we noted earlier, the therapist's empathy is another crucial aspect of the therapeutic relationship. Understanding the affect states that the patient goes through makes the partnership deeper. "Most experienced psychoanalysts will agree that in order to do effective psychotherapy, knowledge of psychoanalytic theory and an intellectual understanding of the patient are not sufficient. In order to help, one has to know a patient differently—emotionally" (Greenson, 1978, p. 147).

The Exploratory Work

The exploratory, or expressive, work of the treatment is made up of the human process of dialogue in a protected place. It is protected from intrusions by the "saving of the hour" for the patient. It is protected from the ears of others by the practice of confidentiality. And it is protected from having any agenda other than the patient's well-being by the nature of the therapeutic contract. The patient's part of the process in the expressive work is to "say what comes to mind." The therapist's part is a sequence of listening and responding, which gradually yields an understanding of the sources of the patient's problems. In psychoanalysis, the analyst's interpretations of the transference are pivotal.

Transference and the CCRT

The transference is the cornerstone concept of psychoanalysis. It reflects the deep patterning of old experiences in relationships as they emerge in current life. Just as if someone had made footprints in the woods and started looking for a path in the dark, people find themselves retracing their patterns of relating and responding without realizing it. It is not so easy to illuminate an unfamiliar path and walk a new way. Old paths wind through the shadows of habit and history. The analysis of the transference provides the lantern.

Even though volumes have been written about the transference and its role in psychoanalysis, its inner workings may still seem mysterious. The Core Conflictual Relationship Theme method (CCRT) demystifies the concept by describing the different elements of the process. Each CCRT pattern is made up of repeated episodes, consisting of the patient's wishes (W), responses from others, either real or anticipated (RO), and responses from the self (RS). People tend to have either one or several central patterns, just as Freud described when he first came up with the concept of the transference. In fact, Luborsky & Crits-Christoph (1998) found that the CCRT corresponded to the central defining characteristics that Freud gave for the transference pattern. Thus the CCRT is an operational version of the transference.

In understanding the patient's CCRT, the therapist looks for the "convergence of spheres." That term refers to the commonality in the CCRT themes in each of three fundamental areas of the patient's life: his current relationships, his past relationships, and the therapeutic relationship. Both the current and the past relationships are central relationships, typically with family members from the past and either family members or others who are close to the patient in the present.

As the patient and therapist notice the ways in which this pattern intrudes into the present, they become able to begin changing its impact. In clinical practice, it is important not to overload the patient with interpretations. For this reason, the therapist usually brings up one sphere at a time, an area related to the topic the patient has been talking about. As the treatment progresses, the patient may be ready to notice links between the spheres, once the pattern has become evident.

EXAMPLE

P: I wished I could have walked out of the meeting, but I was stuck. You know how bad it would have looked if I had gotten out of my chair and knocked it over? (Laughs) Anyway, I was good and I sat there till I saw someone else move his chair. The only problem is how am I going to stand this job, with all of their meetings?

T: How are you going to stand that stuck, trapped feeling?

P: Exactly. Oh, now that you say that, I remember I felt that way in the last job. When is it going to be over?

T: When will there be a job that isn't a trap?

P: Will you find me one? (Laughs)

T: Let's take a look at what makes you feel trapped. Maybe we can figure it out that way.

In this sequence, the patient is actively aware of his feeling state and realizes that there is some pattern to it. The therapist picks up the patient's signs of readiness to look at this pattern in the context of the job sphere, since that is the patient's current focus. In supervision, his supervisor points out that the patient could develop those same feelings about the therapy. After all, he is stuck in a room, sitting in a chair, having a meeting. The therapist decides to remember that possibility and to keep his ears open to see if that theme becomes active in the treatment.

Symptoms and the Symptom–Context Method

When a symptom appears in the course of the treatment, it gives the patient and therapist an opportunity to investigate its meaning. By taking a look at its context, they can begin to decode the symptom and find out what is making it erupt. The symptom can be thought of as a language for forces that are out of the patient's awareness, often an inner conflict. The context gives hints to what it might mean. The context includes not only the events in the patient's life but also his feelings about them. In a therapy session, the material the patient has just been talking about is the immediate context.

This method has a number of clinical uses. In instances of "momentary forgetting," in which the patient suddenly forgets what he is talking about, paying attention to the context helps the patient and therapist discover whether there was something emotionally disruptive that could have prompted the lapse of memory. A different kind of clinical use comes into play with patients whose symptoms are intrusive and frightening, as in anxiety disorders and post-traumatic stress disorder. Understanding the meaning of the symptom makes it less frightening, and the translation into words can begin to shift its form.

EXAMPLE

P: It's happening again. . . . My throat feels like it's closing up. (The patient had just been talking about early sexual abuse.)

T: What do you think about that?

P: (in a rasping voice) What he did to me. (Referring to a form of sexual abuse that involved her throat.) I can't talk.

This patient has been in treatment long enough that she can readily use the Symptom-Context method to understand her symptoms. She reached that point through the gradual discovery that situations that triggered feelings or memories of the abuse also caused bodily symptoms.

Transformation

The goal of the expressive work is a kind of personal transformation. By gaining an understanding of parts of the self that were previously at odds or out of awareness, the patient can work out new ways of handling her needs and her feelings. This is a gradual process. As the patient gains self-understanding, she becomes more aware of the ways she has "been in her own way." She can begin to shift her expectations toward more positive ones and can find ways to go toward what she really wants, instead of defending herself against her fears. The maladaptive defense mechanisms that were operating before become less powerful. As described earlier in this chapter, research on the CCRT suggests this is the course of events in successful treatment. Patients keep wishing for the same things they always wanted for themselves, but their negative patterns of responses from others and self undergo change.

APPLICATIONS

Who Can We Help?

Psychoanalysis functions both as a form of psychotherapy and as a conceptual system to understand how people function psychologically. As a form of treatment, psychoanalytic therapies are particularly well suited for the many patients who have what Sullivan termed "problems in living," which include difficulties with work and love. Often, people present with generalized patterns of behavior that interfere with their conscious goals for happiness and success. Such difficulties are usually complex and lack an obvious cause, and a psychoanalytic approach helps discern the causes, often by tracing them to an unconscious conflict or relational pattern. A man, for example, might repeatedly fall in love with and marry the same kind of woman, although he knows from previous experience that these relationships will end disastrously. Or perhaps a woman unconsciously arranges her life so that any success at work will be followed by an even greater failure.

Stress and Distress

People with various symptoms of stress or distress, including depression, anxiety, or hypomania, are also well suited for a dynamic approach. A dynamic therapist attempts to understand a symptom in the context of the whole person. She takes into account biological and personality predispositions, past history, current circumstances, and unconscious and cultural meaning. A woman suffering from post-partum depression, for example, may have a genetic vulnerability, hormonal fluctuations, and stress and sleep deprivation, all of which contribute to a biological susceptibility to depression. A psychodynamic therapist would help her to explore the personal meaning of having her own baby to care for, looking at both her past and her present circumstances. Through this process, she may recognize the unconscious anxiety she has about her own unmet wish to be nurtured, which had been interfering with her ability to make an emotional connection with her baby. Once she has worked these feelings through, she will be able to form a positive bond with her child and to have more children without becoming depressed.

Psychoanalytic treatments are beneficial for those who would like to gain a deeper understanding of their problems. Those in the mental health professions often wish for a high level of insight and self-knowledge, in order to be better able to help others with their difficulties. Because it can get at issues that are unconscious, psychoanalysis can also be quite helpful to people who feel generally troubled but do not know why.

Personality Disorders

Psychoanalytic treatment is probably the treatment of choice for personality problems and disorders. This is because psychoanalysts have developed sound theories and techniques to understand and treat them, whereas many other schools of psychotherapy have not. Such disorders are difficult to treat because, as the name suggests, they involve problems that pervade the patient's personality, rather than a specific symptom or condition. Personality disorders call for intensive, long-term treatment to address these issues at a deep level, including work on the patient's defenses and underlying feelings.

Range of Applications

As a system for thinking about people and their problems, a psychodynamic model has a wide range of applications. Understanding the patient's personality structure helps the therapist decide which types of therapeutic interventions are likely to be most effective. The Psychodynamic Diagnostic Manual (PDM) (2006), a psychodynamically based system of classification of psychological difficulties, can be used in that process. Projective psychological tests can sometimes provide information about personality structure, areas of potential conflict, or the presence of a thought disorder.

In supportive-expressive (SE) psychotherapy, the therapist balances two basic elements of the treatment, the supportive relationship and the expressive work, in order to meet the needs of the patient. In that way the therapist is able to tailor the treatment to the level of the patient's pathology.

Psychoanalysis is now useful for many who might have at one time been deemed untreatable or "unanalyzable." Variations of psychoanalysis are currently being used to understand and effect change with a much wider spectrum of people and situations than ever before. Object relations theory, in particular, has widened enormously the scope of treatable conditions, making psychoanalysis useful for many more people and situations. Kernberg (1975), for example, has established an object relations approach to working with patients with personality disorders in the narcissistic and borderline spectrum.

Psychoanalytic formulations have been used to elucidate the dynamics of life in the inner city and their effect on psychological treatment (Altman, 2009). A relational approach has been found to be especially useful for people suffering from the long-term effects of chronic relational trauma, such as physical, emotional, or sexual abuse (Davies & Frawley, 1994). Other psychodynamic approaches to therapy have also been used to address the particular issues of gay men and lesbians, as well as older adults and the chronically medically ill (Greenberg, 2009).

Child and Family Treatment

Problems with a family can be addressed in various ways using a psychodynamic approach. A psychoanalytic perspective informs certain schools of family therapy, such as object relations couples therapy (Scharff & Scharff, 1997) and has been utilized in an integrative way by combining individual and family/couples approaches (Gerson, 2009; Wachtel & Wachtel, 1986). When couples or families work to discover the sources of their problems together, they often find that some of those problems have come about as a result of their own personal histories, conflicts, and vulnerabilities. Understanding those patterns together provides an opportunity to shift the present interactions away from the past paradigms.

Play therapy is an application of dynamic concepts for children, based on Melanie Klein's concept that play is for children what free association is for adults. Such therapy gives the patient an uncensored opportunity to play out issues and express feelings in a way that causes no harm. Symbolic play allows children to express themes that might feel threatening in words. Parents can be thrown out the window, children can take over the house, animals can fight battles, and no one really gets hurt. Working with parents to help them with their relationships with their children can involve the application of dynamic theory. Either with the parents alone or with the parents and child together, the therapist can help separate the current parenting relationship from those in the parents' past. The work of Selma Fraiberg, excerpted in the *Case Studies in Psychotherapy* volume, gives an unparalleled example of that kind of work.

Combinations of Treatments

Like other forms of psychotherapy, dynamic therapies may be combined with the use of medication for symptoms that are too severe to respond to psychotherapy alone. That is often the case in a major depression or other major mood disorder. Medication does not replace psychotherapy, and the two together are often more effective than either one alone. Understanding the meaning of symptoms and the psychological function they might serve is still an important task. Some dynamically oriented therapists combine tools such as relaxation and breathing techniques for addressing the immediate symptoms and the Symptom-Context method for understanding their meaning.

Treatment

Freud compared writing about psychoanalysis to explaining the game of chess. It is easy to formulate the rules of the game, to describe the opening phases, and to discuss what has to be done to bring a chess game to a close. But what happens in between is subject to infinite variation. The same is true of psychoanalysis. Since every patient (and every therapist) is different, no two treatments are alike. Even so, dynamic treatments have inherent operating principles and treatment techniques that are not immediately visible but are nevertheless at work. The following case fragment illustrates how they intermingle.

Example

P: I have something I have been meaning to bring up . . . Night . . . (Pt's voice is soft, and the therapist listens closely. After several minutes the patient starts again.) Katie made the soccer team. (Her voice is bright now.) Which is great, except for all the driving. The amount of miles I have put on that car . . .

T: (T is wondering, what happened to what she had been meaning to bring up? It seemed that the patient had abruptly shifted gears. She notices the pun in her thinking and decides to ask about exactly that.) You know, I am still wondering about what you started the session with. It seemed like you shifted gears, just like the car.

P: (Smiles) I have an automatic. But you're right. So what was I avoiding? (The patient has been in treatment long enough to know that avoiding has reasons.) Well, you're going to think, "She's a fat pig" if I tell you.

T: If I'm going to think that you're a fat pig, I can see why you stopped talking.

P: Well, maybe you won't, but I do. . . . OK, here's the thing. Jon (her husband) goes to bed early. He goes upstairs at 9:00, because he's up at 5 to catch the train. And there I am. I just got the kids to bed, with the whole night in front of me. I keep telling you I want time to myself, but there it is, and what do I do?

T: What do you do?

P: Nothing. Clean the kitchen counters. Leave the TV low, so I don't bother anyone. OK here it is. Eat. (Patient looks embarrassed.) I ate an entire package of Oreos last night. The whole package so I could throw the wrapping away and no one would know the difference.

T: That must have been hard to talk about.

P: Not as bad as I thought.

T: And you must be wondering what I think.

P: Well I really don't think you would judge me, but . . . I mean, who wouldn't? Why would anyone do something so stupid? I mean, I am trying to lose weight. Good reason not to eat that garbage. I should work on my writing if I ever want to get anything published. Good reason not to waste my time. I have no time to myself during the day and finally the kids are in bed and Jon's up there too. You'd think I'd be happy about it.

T: It sounds like you are really mad at yourself.

P: I am.

T: And that you figure I would judge you too. It's hard to get to the "why's" if you and I are both sitting in judgment, but I bet there are feelings hidden under there.

P: (Nods) Lonely.

T: (With empathy) Lonely.

P: (Looks at T, and then back out the window) Even though the house is full, it's empty. . . . Yeah, OK, I'm trying to fill it up, but you can't fill it with Oreos. (Looks at T, and they both smile.) . . . Is my time up?

T: Actually, we have 10 minutes left.

P: Oh, that's so strange. I was sure it was over.

T: Well, I wonder if there was something about what we just talked over that made you feel like I'd be ready to get rid of you.

P: You mean, having feelings?

T: Having feelings like . . .

P: Lonely, mad that I get left with everything.

T: And get left?

P: Yeah, that. (Her eyes start to tear.) When I married Jon I thought I was done with that. He is solid.

T: But he goes to bed and leaves you, and gets up early and does it all over again.

P: (Nods) And now are we out of time?

This session gave the patient some relief. She told the therapist that she finally began writing again. But a month later the Oreos have returned.

P: I started doing it again—eating. I was doing better with it, and then this last week, I got back in my old habit, you know, the night thing.

T: I wonder if anything went on this week that might have been difficult?

P: No. Good things actually. Katie got into a summer program we wanted her to do. Jon got offered a promotion at work. Got to buy some champagne.

T: And your life?

P: Yeah, that is my life. Me and my Oreos. (Looks the therapist in the eye.) You know when I was a kid, it was the same thing. When I came home from school, no one was there, but there was always food.

T: What did you have to eat then?

P: There'd always be something. Look in the refrigerator, look in the cupboard. Something. But I wished we'd have something really good.

T: Like Oreos, by any chance?

P: Now I'm throwing them away. My friend Andrea had all that junk in her lunch, and I wished I could have it too.

In this sequence the symptom is *multidetermined.* As the session unfolds, more links between the patient's feelings, present and past, and the symptom come to light. That kind of layering is itself a psychoanalytic principle. As more layers of related feelings collect, they add to the pull of the symptom.

The next thing to notice is the *sequence* of the session. The patient's emotional themes link her most spontaneous comments together. For example, just after she reveals emotionally laden material, she figures the session will be over. The sense that the session will be over comes from an inner theme, not from a realistic sense of time. Talking about her feeling of being left triggered the fear that she would be left by the therapist (by ending the session). Her response in this case was to become anxious. In the home sequences that she reports, she covers over the feeling by eating.

The therapist is quick to note evasions in the patient's process. They could be thought of as a form of defense. Since the patient and therapist have worked with each other for 9 months, they have an easy rapport. The patient has also already learned through previous examples that she may be avoiding things with which she doesn't feel comfortable. The patient and therapist functioned as partners in this exchange, discovering what is really behind changing the subject. Their Helping Alliance helped the patient trust the therapist when dealing with a topic that was embarrassing to reveal. So did the therapist's *analysis of the defense.* When she made a joke about the car changing gears, she was also pointing out the patient's method of defense against difficult feelings. When she commented that "no wonder" the patient wouldn't talk about eating if the therapist would think she was a "fat pig," she was pointing out one of the functions of the defense.

A CCRT pattern is suggested, through the convergence of the responses described from her childhood, in the present with her husband, and with the therapist. The possible CCRT pattern looks like this:

W: (implied) To be close

RO: Leaves, does not stay close

RS: Eats, fills the space with a substitute; avoids feeling (in the early part of the session, she tends to avoid feelings, whereas later she becomes anxious instead. This is actually a sign of improvement since the anxiety is really underneath the avoidance and use of food).

The Symptom-Context method is at work when the patient and therapist examine the context for overeating. It gives them clues to the patient's feeling state. Another technique that the therapist follows is responding to the patient's affect. She slows down the dialogue and makes time for empathy with the patient's feeling state.

The potential for change is suggested by the patient's positive response to the session and in her greater ease in moving into the material the second time. More work will be needed in order to better understand the patient's feelings and their history. But what we have here is simply a fragment of a treatment, and it represents a good start.

The Psychoanalytic Situation

Shame, fear, pride, political correctness, social conformity—these are among the forces that stand in the way of the patient acknowledging her own truth. The *psychoanalytic situation,* in which nothing is the wrong thing to say, gradually undoes those layers of inhibition. "The special conditions of the psychoanalytic situation are designed to promote the optimal unfolding of the patient's unconscious subjective life" (Rubin, 1996, p. 24).

As the analyst listens to all the layers of the patient's experience, the patient begins to do the same. Logic, consistency, and the other person's approval are not the goals of psychoanalytic discourse. It has its own logic, where the heart and the unconscious mind intermingle with the waking, rational self. As the patient comes to accept the varied parts of herself, a greater flexibility emerges.

As the transference is worked through, the patient may find that he can relate to others in new ways. The transference can be understood as a form of memory in which repetition in action replaces recollection of events. Once memory's voice is heard, its power to keep a patient repeating the same pathways weakens. Analysis of the transference helps the patient distinguish fantasy from reality, past from present. Analysis of transference helps the patient understand how he may have misperceived or misinterpreted. In place of the automatic ways in which he responded before, the patient becomes able to evaluate impulses and anxieties, rather than either acting on them or covering them over. Ironically, after making room in his consciousness for the illogical and irrational parts of the self, the patient is ready to make decisions on a more mature and realistic level.

Evidence

People often think of psychoanalysis as a "dinosaur" among psychotherapeutic treatments, with a few stray fossils around and no science that could bring it back to life. That happens to be untrue. Not only is psychoanalysis actively practiced in a variety of forms, but there has been ongoing psychodynamic research for decades. Research supports the efficacy of dynamic treatment and specifically supports the workings of its cornerstone principles. Although clinical research does not suggest that dynamic treatment yields more consistent success than other forms of psychotherapy, it does confirm its effectiveness, and studies of its working mechanisms confirm its most fundamental methods.

Psychotherapy Research

Psychotherapy research often focuses on which form of therapy has the best outcomes, compared to other forms. Researchers who have an *allegiance* to one particular form of treatment often obtain results that support their favored approach. However, when psychotherapy studies are combined into meta-analyses, the results are different. Large-scale meta-analyses that aggregate data come up with two findings. The first, often ignored, may be more important than the second.

The first finding is that psychotherapy works. Two thirds to three quarters of patients in psychotherapy get better, a very high rate of success (Lambert & Bergin, 1994). The finding that good "talk therapy" helps the majority of patients is often overlooked in the wake of all the attention given to psychotropic medication. Supportive-expressive, or dynamic, psychotherapy is one of the forms of therapy that attain this level of success.

The second finding is that no one form of therapy consistently outperforms the others. Differences that are too small to be statistically significant are the norm, especially when the studies are corrected for the effects of the researchers' allegiance (Luborsky et al., 1999). This has been called the "Dodo bird finding" after a story in *Alice and Wonderland.* In that story, the Dodo bird gives prizes to everyone who participated in a race, declaring that "everyone has won, and all shall have prizes."

Why is it that everyone gets a prize, when each runner really thinks he should be the winner? The most likely reason is that well-performed psychotherapies share some fundamental factors. Prominent among them is the Helping Alliance. Dynamic psychotherapies highlight the importance of the alliance between patient and therapist, and other treatments rely on the partnership between client and therapist, even if it is not described as an aspect of technique. Whether explicit or implicit, the Helping Alliance is key in moving the treatment forward. Research also reveals that the therapist's empathy is also linked with positive treatment outcomes. Empathy is another aspect of psychodynamic technique that may be present in other forms of treatment, whether explicitly or not.

Other shared characteristics include the structure and frame of the treatment and an explanatory system that the patient gradually masters. That does not mean there are no meaningful differences between forms of treatment. There are important differences, as you will see as you read the chapters of this book. However, meta-analyses suggest that the differences do not overpower the effect of psychotherapy itself. The Dodo bird's prize goes to those general ("g") factors that all good treatments share.

Evidence-Based Practice

In order to gather clearer evidence on the effectiveness of different treatments, researchers have begun to establish *empirically supported therapies* (ESTs). By establishing precise guidelines for the treatment and for the type of disorder being treated, researchers intend to bring more objectivity to the studies comparing psychotherapies. However, pitfalls arise in relating the results of this approach to real life. Most ESTs are brief treatments, using specified techniques for specific disorders, with subjects whose problems fit with the criteria for that disorder alone. This makes for a clean research design, but in real life, people frequently have commingled problems, and those people are not eligible for the studies (Westen, Novotny, & Thompson-Brenner, 2004).

The other real-life difference comes from the way psychotherapies are practiced. Whereas in studies of ESTs, the treatments follow "pure culture" methods, in reality good therapists adapt their treatment to the individual patient. In supportive-expressive therapy, that adjustment takes the form of balancing the supportive and expressive elements in accordance with the needs of the patient. Thomson-Brenner and Weston (described in Westen et al., 2004) found that therapists of different orientations tended to alter the degree of their activity in session, depending on the needs of the patient. Dynamic therapists reported using more structuring techniques (techniques associated with CBT) when dealing with emotionally constricted patients. And CBT therapists reported using interventions that explored relationship patterns (techniques associated with dynamic therapists) with emotionally deregulated clients. This means that in real life, the differences between forms of treatment are not always as clean as the differences suggested by EST research.

Effective Psychotherapy

Seligman (1995) considered the question of the real-world effects of psychotherapy in a simple way. He polled actual patients for their impressions on a variety of factors. One of these factors was length of treatment. The patients said they found longer treatments more effective than brief ones.

This type of research is not the whole answer either, as Seligman would be quick to agree. However, this approach provides another way to look at psychotherapy using research that is relevant and meaningful.

Dynamic psychotherapies aim to treat the whole person and the patterns of his problems. When specific symptoms alone are studied, the important forces in dynamic treatment may be overlooked. Dynamic concepts and methods are supported by research evidence, which has been found through different kinds of studies.

Evidence for Psychodynamic Concepts and Methods

The Transference.   Evidence on the key psychoanalytic concept, the transference, has accumulated through research on the Core Conflictual Relationship Theme (CCRT) method (Luborsky & Crits-Christoph, 1998; Luborsky & Luborsky, 2006). The CCRT is an operational version of the transference that allows it to be studied in research on the process of psychotherapy. Here are some of the findings:

- The same CCRT pattern can be found in patients' narratives about different people.
- There is a parallel between the CCRT pattern with the therapist and with others.
- Interpretations of the CCRT are beneficial to the treatment when they clarify the habitual responses of self (RS) and other (RO).

The Unconscious Mind.   Research in neuroscience has given the concept of unconscious processes scientific support through the study of implicit and explicit memory. The term *explicit memory* refers to the conscious retrieval of information, whereas *implicit memory* refers to memory that does not come to mind but is demonstrated through behavior (Westen, 1999). Implicit memory would be the kind of memory linked to transference patterns that are demonstrated through behavior in new relationships. Another form of memory, *associative memory,* links a network of things by their similarities. That process is akin to one tracked in dynamic inquiry into unconscious meanings, such as when the therapist follows the train of thought by its nonlogical, emotional links.

Schore has studied the role of early relationships in early brain development. He notes that the processing of emotional understanding of the right hemisphere precedes verbal understanding. Schore hypothesizes that "the implicit self-system of the right brain that evolves in preverbal stages of development represents the biological substrate of the dynamic unconscious" (Schore, 2005, pp. 830–831).

Finding Meaning in Symptoms.   The meanings of a symptom can be found through the Symptom-Context method, which tracks the connection of a symptom to its context (Luborsky, 1998; Luborsky & Luborsky, 2006). The researcher compares samples of material from psychotherapy that contain a psychological symptom with samples of material that do not. This method has yielded three notable findings:

- The symptom emerges after a state of helplessness.
- Feelings of hopelessness, lack of control, and helplessness are linked to symptoms.
- The context for a symptom is significantly different from the context for a nonsymptom.

The Role of the Past in the Present.   The belief that past relationship problems persist into the present is basic to psychoanalysis. Attachment research on the intergenerational transmission of attachment patterns (Main, Kaplan, & Cassidy, 1985) validates that hypothesis. Attachment researchers have also validated Bowlby's concept that "inner working models" of relationships develop through attachment experience and affect the child's sense of security and functioning in relationships.

Sprinters and Runners

What would happen if someone decided to discover which were better, sprinters or long-distance runners? One of each type might be stopped after a quarter of a mile and tested for their heart rate and how rapidly they covered the distance. Would the winner really be the winner, or simply the one who best fit the research design? In order to study the effectiveness of psychotherapy, it is worth keeping in mind both the complexity of real people and their problems *and* the natural differences among forms of treatment. The performance of psychodynamic therapies, like that of the long-distance runner, may be best measured over time.

Research suggests that symptom relief may be achieved through several "well-performing" therapies. But psychoanalysis was never about symptom relief alone. Patients go into all forms of treatment because of symptoms that are troubling them, and they should get relief from those symptoms. But dynamic psychotherapies offer something else as well: a changed sense of self that is no longer stuck in old patterns.

Psychotherapy in a Multicultural World

Culture infuses all of our assumptions, and when considering theories of psychotherapy, it is all too easy to forget that both theorists and their patients are affected by culture. There is no such thing as culture-free thinking, any more than there is word-free language. Even within a culture, the name of a culture may not tell the whole story because of different subcultures that may be present. One person's experience may involve multiple experiences across different cultures and continents. Another's cultural story may be a hybrid of differing beliefs and backgrounds within the same family. The potential for misunderstanding multiplies when a patient and therapist make assumptions about each other based on cultural fragments or stereotypes.

How can the search for understanding still take place? How can a patient and analyst navigate a shared journey when they may not even know which ways they diverge or which assumptions they do not share? Altman (2009) refers to culture as the third force in the consulting room, proposing that if the analyst and patient are already working in a two-person psychology, issues of race, class, and culture create a third and critical element in the relationship.

Cultural Assumptions of Psychoanalysis

In the early days of psychoanalysis, questions of cultural differences were not considered important. On the contrary, Freud sought to create a psychology that applied to a "universal man" (Davidson, 1988). Did his own cultural assumptions limit his theories? Rendon (1993) wrote, " . . . psychoanalysis has been ethnocentric. It has been practiced mostly by and for certain ethnic groups and sectors of society" (p. 120). That bias has been challenged by feminist writers (Benjamin, 1988; Chodorow, 1989). Chodorow (1999) analyzed the ways that personal beliefs about culture and gender, along with unconscious fantasies, influence subjective experience. Altman (2009) considers the ways race and class influence the developing self while challenging the assumptions often ascribed to "blackness" and "whiteness." Leary (1995) points out that race and ethnicity are frequently taboo topics, all too often left unexplored.

While anthropologists criticized Freud's *Totem & Taboo* for its obsolete assumptions after it was published in 1918, anthropology and psychoanalysis have since cross-fertilized each other, with anthropologists delving into life histories and autobiography and psychoanalysts taking culture into account when studying differences in personality structure among non-Occidental individuals (Wittkower & Dubreuil, 1976).

Research on Cultural Differences and Psychoanalytic Concepts

The mid to late 20th century brought collaboration between psychoanalysts and anthropologists, which led to a mingling of theories and perspectives (Mead, 1957). Utilizing data from the Human Relations Area Files (HRAF), a collection of all known ethnographic data, psychological anthropologists (Whiting & Child, 1953; Whiting & Whiting, 1975) studied Freudian theory across cultures, showing the influence of early socialization experiences on personality development. Herdt and Stoller (1990), an anthropologist and a psychoanalyst, respectively, studied gender identity and eroticism cross-culturally.

Tori and Bilmes (2002) studied psychological defenses in Thailand in order to see whether this concept was only relevant in Western countries. These investigators found evidence that the Thai population studied utilized ego-defense mechanisms, although there were differences in which defenses were most common there as compared to the United States. However, despite these differences, the fundamental concept still proved useful in understanding how individuals in different cultures cope with emotions.

Differences in Nonverbal Behavior

Differences in the interpretation of nonverbal behavior can lead to misunderstanding in treatment. While direct eye contact typically connotes honesty and connection to most people in the United States, it has different meanings in other cultures. For example, in Asian cultures, looking away may be a signal of respect to someone of a higher status (Galanti, 2004). Likewise, the psychoanalytic use of the couch and expectations about speaking your mind may mean very different things in different cultures. Cultural differences add a layer of meaning to the basic structure of a treatment.

The Psychoanalytic Method and Cultural Meanings

The psychoanalytic method of inquiry can be used to uncover some of the ways divergent cultural influences may influence both patient and treatment, including the complex effects of dislocation and adaptation to another culture. ". . . In our pluralistic society, conflict and symptomatology are often the products of two or three generational disparities in cultural values" (Davidson, 1998, p. 88).

Recent writings on treatment with patients from diverging backgrounds identify the ways that experiences of loss and dislocation may be hidden in a patient's problems, along with the value of working that through.

Immigration from one country to another is a complex and multifaceted psychosocial process with significant and lasting effects on an individual's identity. Leaving one's country involves profound losses. Often one has to give up familiar food, native music, unquestioned social customs, and even one's language. The new country offers strange-tasting food, new songs, different political concerns, unfamiliar language, obscure festivals, unknown heroes, psychically unearned history, and a visually unfamiliar landscape. However, alongside the various losses is a renewed opportunity for psychic growth and alteration. (Akhtar, 1995, p. 1051)

Cultural differences can alert the analyst to areas that need to be explored in therapy.

CASE EXAMPLE

This case example illustrates the application of a classical psychoanalytic approach to a pivotal session in the treatment. The same session would be handled somewhat differently by therapists representing other psychoanalytic perspectives. In order to clarify some of the differences, the case description will be followed by the view of a relational analyst and the view informed by the use of the CCRT.

A Psychoanalytic Session

The patient was a middle-aged businessman whose marriage had been marked by repeated strife and quarrels. His sexual potency had been tenuous. At times he suffered from premature ejaculation. At the beginning of one session, he began to complain about having to return to treatment after a long holiday weekend. He said, "I'm not so sure I'm glad to be back in treatment even though I didn't enjoy my visit to my parents. I feel I just have to be free." He then continued with a description of his visit home, which he said had been depressing. His mother was bossy, aggressive, manipulative, as always. He felt sorry for his father. At least in the summertime, the father could retreat to the garden and work with the flowers, but the mother watched over him like a hawk. "She has such a sharp tongue and a cruel mouth. Each time I see my father he seems to be getting smaller and smaller; pretty soon he will disappear and there will be nothing left of him. She does that to people. I always feel that she is hovering over me ready to swoop down on me. She has me intimidated just like my wife."

The patient continued, "I was furious this morning. When I came to get my car, I found that someone had parked in a way that hemmed it in. It took a long time and lots of work to get my car out. I was very anxious, and perspiration was pouring down the back of my neck.

"I feel restrained by the city. I need the open fresh air; I have to stretch my legs. I'm sorry I gave up the house I had in the country. I have to get away from this city. I really can't afford to buy another house now, but at least I'll feel better if I look for one.

"If only business were better, I could maneuver more easily. I hate the feeling of being stuck in an office from 9 until 5. My friend Bob had the right idea—he arranged for early retirement. Now he's free to come and go as he pleases. He travels, he has no boss, no board of directors to answer to. I love my work but it imposes too many restrictions on me. I can't help it, I'm ambitious. What can I do?"

At this point, the therapist called to the patient's attention the fact that throughout the material, in many different ways, the patient was describing how he feared confinement, that he had a sense of being trapped.

The patient responded, "I do get symptoms of claustrophobia from time to time. They're mild, just a slight anxiety. I begin to feel perspiration at the back of my neck. It happens when the elevator stops between floors or when a train gets stuck between stations. I begin to worry about how I'll get out."

The fact that he suffered from claustrophobia was a new finding in the analysis. The analyst noted to himself that the patient felt claustrophobic about the analysis. The conditions of the analytic situation imposed by the analyst were experienced by the patient as confining. In addition, the analyst noted, again to himself, these ideas were coupled with the idea of being threatened and controlled by his mother.

The patient continued, "You know, I have the same feeling about starting an affair with Mrs. X. She wants to and I guess I want to also. Getting involved is easy. It's getting uninvolved that concerns me. How do you get out of an affair once you're in it?"

In this material, the patient associates being trapped in a confined space with being trapped in the analysis and with being trapped in an affair with a woman.

The patient continued, "I'm really chicken. It's a wonder I was ever able to have relations at all or get married. No wonder I didn't have intercourse until I was in my twenties. My mother was always after me, 'Be careful about getting involved with girls; they'll get you in trouble. They'll be after you for your money. If you have sex with them, you can pick up a disease. Be careful when you go to public toilets; you can get an infection,' etc. She made it all sound dangerous. You can get hurt from this; you can get hurt from that. It reminds me of the time I saw two dogs having intercourse. They were stuck together and couldn't separate—the male dog was yelping and screaming in pain.

I don't even know how old I was then, maybe 5 or 6 or perhaps 7, but I was definitely a child and I was frightened."

At this point, the analyst suggest that the patient's fear of being trapped in an enclosed space is the conscious derivative of an unconscious fantasy in which he imagines that if he enters the woman's body with his penis, it will get stuck; he will not be able to extricate it; he may lose it. The criteria he used in making this interpretation are the sequential arrangement of the material, the repetition of the same or analogous themes, and the convergence of the different elements into one common hypothesis that encompasses the data—namely, an unconscious fantasy of danger to the penis once it enters a woman's body. The goal of this interpretation is to move toward what must have been an unconscious fantasy of childhood, that of having relations with his mother, and a concomitant fear, growing out of the threatening nature of her personality, that in any attempt to enter her she would swoop down upon him. In this case, there was a threat of danger associated with these wishes—namely, a fantasy that within the woman's body there lurked a representation of the rival father who would destroy the little boy or his penis as it entered the enclosure of the mother's body.

As the therapist helped him become aware of the persistent effects of these unconscious childhood conflicts, the patient would gain some insight into the causes of his impotence and his stormy relations with women, particularly his wife, as well as his inhibited personal and professional interactions with men. To this patient, having to keep a definite set of appointments with the analyst, having his car hemmed in between two other cars, being responsible to authorities, and getting stuck in elevators or in trains were all experienced as dangerous situations that evoked anxiety. Consciously, he experienced restrictions by rules and confinement within certain spaces. Unconsciously, he was thinking in terms of experiencing his penis inextricably trapped inside a woman's body. This is the essence of the neurotic process: persistent unconscious fantasies of childhood impose a mental set that results in selective and idiosyncratic interpretations of events.

Drive Theory versus Relational Theory

The analyst in this case (Jacob Arlow) looks through the lens of drive theory. He sees the patient's problems as having originated in the psychosexual anxieties of Oedipal conflict. The patient's repressed sexual and aggressive impulses are behind his symptoms. Rather than succumb to these urges, he develops a symptom, claustrophobia, to represent the conflict symbolically, enabling him to simultaneously repress and express the impulse. This analyst sees his role as an objective observer who interprets the patient's experience in order to make conscious what had previously been unconscious. In so doing, he works within a "one-person model," offering insights that give the patient a deep-level understanding of his problems.

A relational analyst would see the same material as an intersection of reality with long-standing relational patterns. She would be more likely to focus her responses on the ways the relationship patterns were activated in the present, by spending time on the patient's feelings about the treatment. For example, when the patient talked about not wanting to come back to analysis after the weekend, she would have inquired about those feelings, "shining a flashlight" on what the patient was experiencing with her. She would have had an interest in the patient's early relationships as memories to explore, using them to understand the patient's past and current feelings, rather than interpreting them in accordance with Oedipal theory. She would have tried to "get a feel" for the patient's early world by empathizing with what was frustrating in his early experiences.

She would be working from a two-person model, in which she is participant as well as observer. Her focus would be on the patient's relationships, past and present.

Looking Through the Lens of the CCRT

In looking at the session through the lens of the CCRT, the *convergence of spheres* becomes apparent. The patient describes the same themes in his relationship with his mother, his work, the analyst, and his wife. That convergence makes it a good time for the patient and analyst to look at the pattern. The fact that the theme is reflected in the session itself means that the patient's feelings about the analyst need to be further explored. Considering the session in that way makes it seem to be a pivotal session, just as it did to the treating analyst. However, what seems pivotal is the convergence of the CCRT pattern, not the Oedipal material.

The CCRT pattern conveyed by this patient would be

W: (Implied) To be free, independent

RO: Controlling; trapping

RS: Get angry; get anxious; get impotent

The patient's perception of the mother as controlling seems like an important driving force in his conflictual pattern. The patient's symptoms, impotence and claustrophobia, both seem to be expressions of the CCRT pattern. The patient's impotence appears to be linked to his perception of (female) others as controlling, and while his own response is to feel angry and trapped. The patient's claustrophobia also seems symbolically related to his CCRT pattern, since the symptom involves the fear of being trapped. The Symptom-Context method could be used to determine the context of that symptom, including feelings, thoughts, and events that precede it.

We noted, when we traced themes in this psychoanalytic session, that for this patient, having to keep a definite set of appointments with the analyst, having his car hemmed in between two other cars, being responsible to authorities, and getting stuck in elevators or in trains were all experienced as dangerous situations that evoked anxiety. Whether seen through the lens of classical or relational analysis, or through the CCRT, the pattern in the transference is key in the process. The differing techniques use different language and approaches to help the patient come to terms with its impact.

SUMMARY

Psychoanalysis began as a way to explain and treat human behavior that did not follow the laws of logic. What made people remain in states of psychic pain, with physical symptoms that had no apparent cause? From his early use of hypnotic techniques with patients who were then called hysterics, Freud began to develop a way to treat the conditions of psychic distress. Both his theories and technique evolved along with his clinical experience. As he discovered that psychological cures were often not as simple as recovering memories and regaining health, he noticed resistances within his patients that he began to explore. Theories of defense and of inner conflict as a source of symptoms evolved from there. He postulated an unconscious mind as the keeper of early patterns of relating, otherwise known as the transference.

Since Freud, psychoanalytic ideas and forms of treatment have continued to evolve in different ways. In the century since his early discoveries, they have been alternately challenged, followed, rejected, and expanded. The classical psychoanalytic tradition has stayed the closest to Freud's original ideas, whereas other theorists and practitioners have made changes in focus and technique. These include the ego psychologists, self-psychologists, the object relations school, and the current interpersonal and relational analysts. Psychoanalytic concepts have been evaluated through clinical research, through methods that give operational status to their inner workings, notably the CCRT and the Symptom-Context method.

Psychodynamic treatments make use of two basic elements of cure: the therapeutic relationship and exploratory work. Varied forms of treatment have evolved from the psychoanalytic core. They include both forms of psychoanalysis and dynamic psychotherapy, including supportive-expressive (SE) psychotherapy, which expands the range of patients who can be treated through a dynamic approach. Pivotal to all the forms of treatment are the fundamental psychodynamic beliefs in the power of old patterns of relationships to "trip the system" of current relationships, and the power of unconscious aspects of the self to appear in the form of symptoms.

One of Freud's seminal contributions to the history of psychology was his insight that there is more to us as human beings than what is on the surface, and that we can hide things about ourselves, even from ourselves. That is as true today as it was a century ago. Psychodynamic treatment continues to offer a way for patients to make sense of their own behavior and develop a clearer personal path. Psychoanalytic thinking continues to evolve by engaging in new ideas and clinical research. But perhaps most important of all, it is enriched by the source that sparked its origins: the patient.

ANNOTATED BIBLIOGRAPHY

The following books are recommended for those who want to learn more about psychoanalysis as theory and practice.

Freud, A. (1966). *The ego and the mechanisms of defense. The writings of Anna Freud* (Vol. 2). New York: International Universities Press. [Originally published in 1936.]
Anna Freud has one of the finest and clearest writing styles in psychoanalysis. *The Ego and the Mechanisms of Defense* is an established classic for its lucidity in portraying the theoretical implications of the structural theory and its application to problems of technique. In a relatively small volume, the author offers a definitive presentation of the psychoanalytic concept of conflict, the functioning of the anxiety signal, and the many ways in which the ego attempts to establish defenses. The sections on the origin of the superego, identity, and the transformations in adolescence present a clear picture of how the child becomes an adult.

Freud, S. (1915–1917). *Introductory lectures on psychoanalysis.* London: Hogarth Press.
These lectures make up Volumes 15 and 16 of *The Complete Psychological Works of Sigmund Freud.* The books are based on a set of lectures Freud gave at the University of Vienna. His lectures are a model of lucidity, clarity, and organization. Introducing a new and complicated field of knowledge, Freud develops his thesis step by step, beginning with simple, acceptable, common-sense concepts, and advancing his argument consistently until the new and startling ideas that he was to place before his audience seemed like the inevitable and logical consequences of each individual's own reflection. *Introductory Lectures on Psychoanalysis* offers the easiest and most direct approach to the understanding of psychoanalysis.

Greenberg, J. R., & Mitchell, S. A. (1983). *Object relations in psychoanalytic theory.* Cambridge, MA: Harvard University Press.

This landmark book contrasts drive theory and the relational model, in terms of theory and history. The latter paradigm follows from the British object relations theorists who believe that an innate need to maintain relationships is what motivates human behavior and that early relational patterns remain active throughout life.

Greenson, R. (1967). *The technique and practice of psychoanalysis.* New York: International Universities Press.
This book offers a clearly written introduction to psychoanalytic theory and technique. The psychoanalytic essentials of free association, the transference, and resistance are explained, as is the working alliance. The author gives clinical examples that demonstrate the psychoanalytic method and describes the "skills required of a psychoanalyst." Greenson has a rare capacity to make complex concepts clear.

Luborsky, L. & Luborsky, E. (2006). *Research and psychotherapy: The vital link.* Lanham, MD: Jason Aronson.
This book does three things. It brings clinical experience and research together in one volume, showing how the two can enrich each other. It introduces Luborsky's innovative methods, which can be used both in the practice of psychotherapy and as research tools. Finally, it offers a clear, stepwise introduction to the practice of supportive-expressive (SE) psychotherapy, a form of psychodynamic therapy.

McWilliams, N. (2005). *Psychoanalytic psychotherapy: A practitioner's guide.* New York: Guilford.
The third of a trilogy, this volume builds on McWilliams's previous books on psychoanalytic diagnosis and case formulations. She discusses in a sophisticated but accessible way the essential aspects of psychodynamic therapy.

CASE READINGS

Arlow, J. A. (1976). Communication and character: A clinical study of a man raised by deaf-mute parents. *Psychoanalytic Study of the Child, 31,* 139–163.

The adaptive capacities of the individual, even under difficult environmental circumstances, are illustrated in this well-documented case of a person raised by deaf-mute parents. In many respects, overcoming real hardships and conquering shame contributed to the character development of this person.

Fraiberg, S. (1987) Ghosts in the nursery: A psychoanalytic approach to problems with impaired infant-mother relationships. In L. Fraiberg (Ed.), *Selected Writings of Selma Fraiberg* (pp. 100–136). Columbus, OH: Ohio State University Press.

Selma Fraiberg takes the psychoanalytic concept of the role of the past in the present into the lives of neglected infants. The mothers in these case studies could not respond to their own babies until Fraiberg and her colleagues responded to their own, previously forgotten memories of being neglected themselves. That opened up the potential for the mothers to hear their own real babies. Fraiberg offers a moving account of the ways two generations can be helped at once.

Freud, S. (1963). The rat man. In S. Freud, *Three case histories.* New York: Crowell-Collier.

The case of the "rat man" was a landmark in Freud's developing theory of psychoanalysis. In precise, clinical reporting, Freud outlined the role of the primary process, magical thinking, ambivalence, and anal fixation in the structure of an obsessive-compulsive neurosis. Although in his later writings Freud expanded his clinical theory and metapsychology, this case report is a prime example of how Freud used clinical observation to develop his ideas and shed light on previously obscure problems.

Grossmark, R. (2009). The case of Pamela. *Psychoanalytic Dialogues, 19(1),* 22–30. [Reprinted in D. Wedding and R. J. Corsini (Eds.). (2010). *Case studies in psychotherapy* (6th ed.). Belmont, CA: Brooks/Cole.]

A vivid rendering of a psychoanalytic treatment conducted from a relational perspective. A woman unconsciously reenacts her traumatic experiences in her relationship with her analyst, who uses his own countertransference to better understand his patient's inner world.

Winnicott, D. W. (1972). Fragment of an analysis. In P. L. Giovacchini, *Tactics and technique in psychoanalytic therapy* (pp. 455–493). New York: Science House.

Winnicott's approach to psychoanalytic theory and practice represented an important turning point in psychoanalysis. This case report illustrates his special approach, which emphasizes the influence of interpersonal interactions and feelings. Winnicott's technical precepts have had a strong and lasting effect on psychoanalytic practice.

REFERENCES

Abraham, K. (1924). The influence of oral eroticism on character formation. In *Selected papers of Karl Abraham, Vol. 1* (pp. 393–496). London: Hogarth Press.

Akhtar, S. (1995) A third individuation: Immigration, identity, and the psychoanalytic process. *Journal of the American Psychoanalytic Association 43,* 1051–1084. Alpert, J. (1995) Sexual abuse recalled: Treating trauma in the era of the recovered memory debate. New York: Jason, Aronson.

Altman, N. (2009). *The analyst in the inner city: Race, culture and class through a psychoanalytic lens* (2nd ed.). New York: Routledge.

American Psychiatric Association. (2000). *Diagnostic and statistical manual of mental disorders, 4th ed., Text revision (DSM–IV–TR).* Washington, DC: American Psychiatric Association.

Ansbacher, H., & Ansbacher, R. (Eds.). (1956). *The individual psychology of Alfred Adler.* New York: Basic Books.

Arlow, J. A. (1963). Conflict, regression and symptom formation. *International Journal of Psychoanalysis, 44,* 12–22.

Arlow, J. A. (1969). Unconscious fantasy and disturbances of conscious experience. *Psychoanalytic Quarterly, 38,* 28.

Arlow, J. A., & Brenner, C. (1988). The future of psychoanalysis. *Psychoanalytic Quarterly, 57,* 1–14.

Aron, L. (1996). *A meeting of minds: Mutuality in psychoanalysis.* Hillsdale, NJ: Analytic Press.

Beebe, B., & Lachmann, F. (2002). *Infant research and adult treatment: Co-constructing interactions.* Hillsdale, NJ: Analytic Press.

Benjamin, J. (1988). *The bonds of love: Psychoanalysis, feminism, and the problem of domination.* New York: Pantheon.

Berenfeld, S. (1944). Freud's earliest theories and the school of Helmholtz. *Psychoanalytic Quarterly 13,* 341–362.

Beres, D., & Arlow, J. A. (1974). Fantasy and identification in empathy. *Psychoanalytic Quarterly, 43,* 4–25.

Blatt, S. J. (2005). *Experience of depression: Theoretical, clinical, and research perspectives.* Washington, DC: American Psychological Association.

Bodnar, S. (2004). Remember where you come from: Dissociative process in multicultural individuals. *Psychoanalytic Dialogues, 14,* 581–603.

Bowlby, J. (1969). *Attachment and loss: Vol. 1. Attachment.* New York: Basic Books.

Bowlby, J. (1988). *A secure base: Clinical applications of attachment theory.* London: Routledge.

Brenner, C. (1982). *The mind in conflict.* New York: International Universities Press.

Breuer, J., & Freud, S. (1895). *Studies on hysteria.* Standard edition of the complete psychological works of Freud, Vol. 2. London: Hogarth Press.

Bucci, W. (1997). *Psychoanalysis and cognitive science: A multiple code theory.* New York: Guilford Press.

Chodorow, N. J. (1989). *Feminism and psychoanalytic theory.* New Haven: Yale University Press.

Chodorow, NJ. (1999). *Personal meaning in psychoanalysis, gender, and culture.* New Haven: Yale University Press.

Davies, J., & Frawley, M. (1994) *Treating the adult survivor of childhood sexual abuse: A psychoanalytic perspective.* New York: Basic Books.

Davidson, L. (1988). Culture and psychoanalysis—From marginality to pluralism. *Contemporary Psychoanalysis, 24,* 74–90.

Drescher, J., D'Ercole, A. & Schoenberg. (2003). *Psychotherapy with gay men and lesbians: Contemporary dynamic approaches.* New York: Haworth Press.

Ellis, A. (1994). *Reason and emotion in psychotherapy, revised.* Secaucus, NJ: Citadel.

Erdelyi, M. (1985). *Psychoanalysis: Freud's cognitive psychology.* New York: W.H. Freeman.

Erikson, E (1950). *Childhood and society* (2nd ed.). New York: Norton.

Erikson, E. (1968). *Identity, youth and crisis.* New York: Norton.

Fairbairn, W. R. D. (1954). *An object relations theory of the personality.* New York: Basic Books.

Fenichel, O. (1945). *The psychoanalytic theory of neurosis.* New York: Norton.

Fonagy, P., Gergely, G., Jurist, E. L. & Target, M. (2002). *Affect regulation, mentalization and the development of the self.* New York: Other Press.

Fraiberg, S. (1987) Ghosts in the nursery: A psychoanalytic approach to problems with impaired infant-mother relationships. In L. Fraiberg (Ed.), *Selected Writings of Selma Fraiberg* (pp. 100–136). Columbus, OH: Ohio State University Press.

Freud, A. (1966). *The ego and the mechanisms of defense.* New York: International Universities Press.

Freud, S.[1] (1894). *The neuropsychoses of defense.* (Standard Edition, Vol. 3.)

Freud, S. (1895). *Studies on hysteria.* (Standard Edition, Vol. 2.)

Freud, S. (1900). *The interpretation of dreams.* (Standard Edition, Vol. 4.)

Freud, S. (1901). *The psychopathology of everyday life.* (Standard Edition, Vol. 6.)

Freud, S. (1905b). *Three essays on sexuality.* (Standard Edition, Vol. 7.)

Freud, S. (1911). *Formulations regarding the two principles of mental functioning.* (Standard Edition, Vol. 12.)

Freud, S. (1913). *Totem and taboo.* (Standard Edition, Vol. 13.)

Freud, S. (1914b). *On narcissism: An introduction.* (Standard Edition, Vol. 14.)

Freud, S. (1915a). *Repression.* (Standard Edition, Vol. 14.)

Freud, S. (1915b). *The unconscious.* (Standard Edition, Vol. 14.)

Freud, S. (1923). *The ego and the id.* (Standard Edition, Vol. 19.)

Freud, S. (1926). *Inhibitions, symptoms and anxiety.* (Standard Edition, Vol. 20.)

Fromm, E. (1955). *The sane society.* New York: Holt, Rinehart and Winston.

Fromm-Reichmann, F. (1950). *Principles of intensive psychotherapy.* Chicago: University of Chicago Press.

Galanti, G. (2004). *Caring for patients from different cultures.* Philadelphia, PA: University of Pennsylvania Press.

Gerson, MJ (2009). *The embedded self: A psychoanalytic guide to family therapy* (2nd ed.). Hillside, NJ: Routledge.

Gill, M. N. (1987). The analyst as participant. *Psychoanalytic Inquiry, 7,* 249.

Goldberg, A. (1998). Self-psychology since Kohut. *Psychoanalytic Quarterly, 67,* 240–255.

Greenacre, P. (1956). Re-evaluation of the process of working through. *International Journal of Psychoanalysis, 37,* 439–444.

Greenberg, J. R., & Mitchell, S. A. (1983). *Object relations in psychoanalytic theory.* Cambridge: Harvard University Press.

Greenberg, T. M. (2009). *Psychodynamic perspectives on aging and illness.* New York: Springer.

Greenson, R. (1967). *The technique and practice of psychoanalysis.* New York: International Universities Press.

Greenson, R. (1978). *Explorations in psychoanalysis.* New York: International Universities Press.

Hartmann, H. (1939). *Ego psychology and the problem of adaptation.* New York: International Universities Press.

Hartmann, H., Kris, E., & Loewenstein, R. N. (1946). Comments on the formation of psychic structure. *Psychoanalytic Study of the Child, 2,* 11–38.

Herdt, G., & Stoller, R. J. (1990). *Intimate communications: Erotics and the study of culture.* New York/Oxford: Columbia University Press.

Horney, K. (1940). *New ways in psychoanalysis.* New York: Norton.

Horowitz, M. J. (2001). *Stress response syndromes: Personality styles and interventions.* Northvale, NJ: Jason Aronson.

Jacobs, T. J. (1991). *The use of the self. Countertransference in the analytic situation.* Madison, CT: International Universities Press.

Jones, E. (1953). *The life and work of Sigmund Freud.* New York: Basic Books.

Jung, C. (1909). *The psychology of dementia praecox.* New York: Nervous and Mental Disease Publishing Co.

Kandel, E. R. (2005). *Psychiatry, psychoanalysis, and the biology of mind.* Washington, DC: American Psychiatric Publishing, Inc.

[1] All references to Sigmund Freud are from James Strachey (Ed.). (1974). *Standard edition of the complete psychological works of Sigmund Freud.* London: Hogarth Press.

Kernberg, O. F. (1975). *Borderline conditions and pathological narcissism*. Northvale, NJ: Jason Aronson.

Kohut, H. (1971). *The analysis of the self: A systematic approach to the psychoanalytic treatment of narcissistic personality disorders*. New York: International Universities Press.

Kohut, H. (1979). The two analyses of Mr. Z. *International Journal of Psychoanalysis, 60*:3–27.

Lambert, M. J. & Bergin, A. E. (1994). The effectiveness of psychotherapy. In A. E. Bergin & S. L. Garfield (Eds.). *Handbook of psychotherapy and behavior change* (pp. 143–149). New York: Wiley.

Leary, K. (1995). "Interpreting in the dark": Race and ethnicity in psychoanalytic psychotherapy. *Psychoanalytic Psychology, 12*, 127–140.

Levenson, E. (1972). *The fallacy of understanding*. New York: Basic Books.

Luborsky, L. (1996). *The Symptom-Context Method: Symptoms as opportunities in psychotherapy*. Washington, DC: American Psychological Association.

Luborsky, L. & Crits-Christoph, P. (1998). *Understanding transference: The CCRT method* (2nd ed.). Washington, DC: American Psychological Association

Luborsky, L., Diguer, L., Luborsky, E., & Schmidt, K. (1999). "The Efficacy of Dynamic versus Other Psychotherapies." In D. Janowsky, *Psychotherapy: Indications and outcomes* (pp. 3–22). Washington, DC: American Psychiatric Press.

Luborsky, L., & Luborsky, E. (2006). *Research and psychotherapy: The vital link*. Lanham, MD: Jason Aronson.

Lyons-Ruth, K. (1991). Rapprochement or approchement: Mahler's theory reconsidered from the vantage point of recent research on early attachment relationships. *Psychoanalytic Psychology, 8*, 1–23.

Lyons-Ruth, K. (2003). The two-person construction of defenses: Disorganized attachment strategies, disorganized mental states and hostile-helpless relational processes. *Journal of Infant, Child and Adolescent Psychotherapy, 2*, 105–114.

McWilliams, N. (2004). *Psychoanalytic psychotherapy: A practitioner's guide*. New York: Guilford Press.

Mead, M. (1957). Changing patterns of parent-child relations in an urban culture. *International Journal of Psychoanalysis, 38*, 369–378.

Mitchell, S. A. (1988). *Relational concepts in psychoanalysis: An integration*. Cambridge, MA: Harvard University Press.

Orfanos, S. (2006). "On Such a Full Sea": Advances in psychoanalytic psychology. *New York State Psychologist, 8*(4):2–8.

Rendon, M. (1993). The psychoanalysis of ethnicity and the ethnicity of psychoanalysis I. *American Journal of Psychoanalysis, 53*, 109–122.

Orlinsky, D. E., Grawe, K.,& Parks, B. K. (1994). Process and outcome in psychotherapy: Nock einmal. In A. Bergin & S. Garfield, (Eds.) *Handbook of psychotherapy and behavior change*. (pp. 270–378). New York: Wiley.

PDM Task Force. (2006). *Psychodynamic diagnostic manual*. Silver Spring, MD: Alliance of Psychoanalytic Organizations.

Racker, E. (1953). A contribution to the problem of countertransference. *International Journal of Psychoanalysis, 34*, 313–324.

Rangell, L. (1963). Structural problems and intrapsychic conflict. *Psychoanalytic Study of the Child, 18*, 103–138.

Reich, W. (1949). *Character analysis*. New York: Orgone Institute Press.

Renik, O. (1995). The ideal of the anonymous analyst and the problem of self-disclosure. *Psychoanalytic Quarterly, 64*, 466–495.

Rogers, C. (1951). *Client-centered therapy*. New York: Houghton Mifflin.

Rubin, J. (1996). *Psychotherapy and Buddhism: Toward an integration*. New York: Plenum.

Safrin, J. D., & Muran, J. C. (1996). The resolution of ruptures in the therapeutic alliance. *Journal of Consulting and Clinical Psychology, 64*, 447–458.

Sarfrin, J., Muran, J., Samstag, L., & Stevens, C. (2001). Repairing alliance ruptures. *Psychotherapy: Theory, Research, Practice, Training, 38*, 406–412.

Schafer, R. (1976). *A new language of psychoanalysis*. New Haven & London: Yale University Press.

Scharff J. S., & Scharff, D. E. (1997). Object relations couple therapy. *American Journal of Psychotherapy, 51*(2), 141–173.

Schore, A. (2003). *Affect dysregulation and disorders of the self*. New York: Norton.

Schore, A. (2005). A neuropsychoanalytic viewpoint: Commentary on paper by Steven H. Knoblauch. *Psychoanalytic Dialogues, 15*(6), 829–854.

Seligman, M. (1995). The effectiveness of psychotherapy: The *Consumer Reports* study. *American Psychologist, 50*, 965–974.

Shapiro, D. (1965). *Neurotic styles*. New York: Basic Books.

Sullivan, H. S. (1953). *The interpersonal theory of psychiatry*. New York: Norton.

Sullivan, H. S. (1954). *The psychiatric interview*. New York: Norton.

Tori, C. D., & Bilmes, M. (2002). Multiculturalism and psychoanalytic psychology: The validation of defense mechanisms as a measure in an Asian population. *Psychoanalytic Psychology, 19*, 701–721.

Vaillant, G. E. (1977). *Adaptation to life*. Cambridge, MA: Harvard University Press.

Vaillant, G. E. (2002). *Aging Well*. Boston: Little, Brown.

Wachtel, E., & Wachtel, P. (1986). *Family dynamics in individual psychotherapy*. New York: Guilford Press.

Wallerstein, R. S. (1988). One psychoanalysis or many? *International Journal of Psychoanalysis, 69*, 5–21.

Westen, D. (1999). The scientific status of unconscious processes. Paper presented at the Annual Meeting of the Rapaport-Klein Study Group.

Westen, D., Novotny, C. M., & Thompson-Brenner, H. (2004). The empirical status of empirically supported psychotherapies: Assumptions, trials and reporting in clinically controlled trials. *Psychological Bulletin, 130,* 631–663.

Whiting, J. M., & Child, I. L. (1953). *Child training and personality,* New Haven: Yale University Press.

Whiting J. M., & Whiting, B. (1975). *Children of six cultures: A psycho-cultural analysis.* Cambridge: Harvard University Press.

Winnicott, D. W. (1953). Transitional objects and transitional phenomena: A study of the first not-me possession. *International Journal of Psychoanalysis, 34,* 89–97.

Winnicott, D. W. (1965). *Maturational processes and the facilitating environment.* Madison, CT: International Universities Press.

Wittkower, E. D., & Dubreuil, G. (1976). Psychoanalysis and anthropology: Some considerations. *Journal of the American Academy of Psychoanalysis, 4,* 427–432.

Zetzel, E. R. (1970). *The capacity for emotional growth: Theoretical and clinical contributions to psychoanalysis.* New York: International Universities Press.

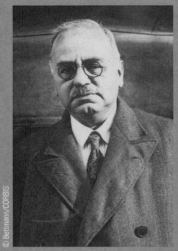

Alfred Adler, 1870–1937

3 | ADLERIAN PSYCHOTHERAPY

Harold H. Mosak and Michael Maniacci

OVERVIEW

Adlerian psychology, developed by Alfred Adler (who referred to it as Individual Psychology), views the person holistically as a creative, responsible, "becoming" individual moving toward fictional goals within his or her phenomenal field. It holds that one's life-style is sometimes self-defeating because of inferiority feelings. The individual with "psychopathology" is discouraged rather than sick, and the therapeutic task is to encourage the person to activate his or her social interest and to develop a new life-style through relationship, analysis, and action methods.

Basic Concepts

Adlerian psychology is predicated upon assumptions that differ in significant ways from the Freudian "womb" from which it emerged. Adler throughout his lifetime credited Freud with primacy in the development of a dynamic psychology. He consistently gave credit to Freud for explicating the purposefulness of symptoms and for discovering that dreams were meaningful.

The influence of early childhood experiences in personality development constitutes still another point of agreement. Freud emphasized the role of psychosexual development and the Oedipus complex, and Adler focused on the effects of children's perceptions of their family constellation and on their struggle to find a place of significance within it.

Adlerian basic assumptions can be expressed as follows:

1. All behavior occurs in a social context. Humans are born into an environment with which they must engage in reciprocal relations. The oft-quoted statement by the gestalt psychologist Kurt Lewin that "behavior is a function of person and environment" is a striking parallel to Adler's contention that people cannot be studied in isolation.

2. Individual Psychology is an interpersonal psychology. How individuals interact with the others sharing "this crust of earth" (Adler, 1931/1958, p. 6)[1] is paramount. Transcending interpersonal transactions is the development of the feeling of being a part of a larger social whole that Adler (1964b) incorporated under the heading of *Gemeinschaftsgefühl,* or social interest.

3. Adlerian psychology rejects reductionism in favor of holism. The Adlerian demotes part-functions from the central investigative focus in favor of studying the whole person and how he or she moves through life. This renders the polarities of *conscious* and *unconscious, mind* and *body, approach* and *avoidance,* and *ambivalence* and *conflict* meaningless except as subjective experiences of the whole person. That is, people behave *as if* the conscious mind moves in one direction while the unconscious mind moves in another. From the external observer's viewpoint, all part-functions are subordinate functions of the individual's goals and style of life.

4. *Conscious* and *unconscious* are both in the service of the individual, who uses them to further personal goals. Adler (1963a) treats *unconscious* as an adjective rather than as a noun. That which is unconscious is the nonunderstood. Like Otto Rank, Adler felt that humans know more than they understand. *Conflict,* defined as intrapersonal by others, is defined as a "one step forward and one step backward movement," the net effect being to maintain the individual at a point "dead center." Although people experience themselves in the throes of a conflict, unable to move, in reality they *create* these antagonistic feelings, ideas, and values because they are unwilling to move in the direction of solving their problems (Mosak & LaFevre, 1976).

5. Understanding the individual requires understanding his or her cognitive organization and life-style. The latter concept refers to the convictions individuals develop early in life to help them organize experience, to understand it, to predict it, and to control it. *Convictions* are conclusions derived from the individual's apperceptions, and they constitute a biased mode of apperception. Consequently, a *life-style* is neither right nor wrong, normal nor abnormal, but merely the "spectacles" through which people view themselves in relation to the way in which they perceive life. Subjectivity rather than so-called objective evaluation becomes the major tool for understanding the person. As Adler wrote, "We must be able to see with his eyes and listen with his ears" (1931/1958, p. 72).

6. Behavior may change throughout a person's life span in accordance with both the immediate demands of the situation and the long-range goals inherent in the life-style. The life-style remains relatively constant through life unless the convictions change through the mediation of psychotherapy. Although the definition of *psychotherapy* customarily refers to what transpires within a consulting room, a broader view of psychotherapy would include the fact that life in itself may often be psychotherapeutic.

7. According to the Adlerian conception, people are not pushed by causes; that is, they are not determined by heredity and environment. "Both are giving only the frame and the influences which are answered by the individual in regard to the styled creative power" (Ansbacher & Ansbacher, 1956). People move toward self-selected goals that they feel will give them a place in the world, will provide them with security, and will

[1] "1931/1958" indicates that the original date of publication was 1931 but that the page number refers to the reprint published in 1958.

preserve their self-esteem. Life is a dynamic striving. "The life of the human soul is not a 'being' but a 'becoming'" (Adler, 1963a, p. ix).

8. The central striving of human beings has been variously described as completion (Adler, 1931), perfection (Adler, 1964a), superiority (Adler, 1926), self-realization (Horney, 1951), self-actualization (Goldstein, 1939), competence (White, 1957), and mastery (Adler, 1926). Adler distinguishes among such strivings in terms of the direction a striving takes. If strivings are solely for the individual's greater glory, he considers them socially useless and, in extreme conditions, characteristic of mental problems. On the other hand, if the strivings are for the purpose of overcoming life's problems, the individual is engaged in striving for self-realization, in contributing to humanity, and in making the world a better place to live.

9. Moving through life, the individual is confronted with alternatives. Because Adlerians are either nondeterminists or soft determinists, the conceptualization of humans as creative, choosing, self-determined decision makers permits them to choose the goals they want to pursue. Individuals may select socially useful goals or they may devote themselves to the useless side of life. They may choose to be task oriented or they may, as does the neurotic, concern themselves with their own superiority.

10. The freedom to choose (McArthur, 1958) introduces the concepts of *value* and *meaning* into psychology. These were unpopular concepts at the time (1931) that Adler wrote *What Life Should Mean to You.* The greatest value for the Adlerian is *Gemeinschaftsgefühl,* or social interest (Ansbacher, 1968). Although Adler contends that it is an innate feature of human beings, at least as potential, acceptance of this criterion is not absolutely necessary. Mosak (1991) defines social interest as a construct rather than as an innate disposition. People possess the capacity for coexisting and interrelating with others. Indeed, the "iron logic of social living" (Adler, 1959) demands that we do so. Even in severe psychopathology, total extinction of social interest does not occur. Even people who are psychotic retain some commonality with "normal" people.

As Rabbi Akiva noted two millennia ago, "The greatest principle of living is to love one's neighbor as oneself." If we regard ourselves as fellow human beings with fellow feeling, we are socially contributive people interested in the common welfare and, by Adler's pragmatic definition of *normality,* mentally healthy (Dreikurs, 1969; Shoben, 1957).

If my feeling derives from my observation and conviction that life and people are hostile and I am inferior, I may divorce myself from the direct solution of life's problems and strive for personal superiority through overcompensation, wearing a mask, withdrawal, attempting only safe tasks where the outcome promises to be successful, and other devices for protecting my self-esteem. Adler said the neurotic in terms of movement displayed a "hesitating attitude" toward life (1964a). Also, the neurotic was described as a "yes-but" personality (Adler, 1934); at still other times, the neurotic was described as an "if only" personality (Adler, 1964a): "If only I didn't have these symptoms, I'd . . ." The latter provided the rationale for "The Question," a device Adler used for differential diagnosis as well as for understanding the individual's task avoidance.

11. Because Adlerians are concerned with process, little diagnosis is done in terms of nomenclature. Differential diagnosis between functional and organic disorder does often present a problem. Because all behavior is purposeful, a *psychogenic* symptom will have a psychological or social purpose, and an *organic* symptom will have a somatic purpose. An Adlerian would ask "The Question" (Adler, 1964a; Dreikurs, 1958, 1962), "If I had a magic wand or a magic pill that would eliminate your symptom immediately, what would be different in your life?" If the patient answers, "I'd go out more often socially" or "I'd write my book," the symptom would most likely be psychogenic. If the patient responds, "I wouldn't have this excruciating pain," the symptom would most likely be organic.

12. Life presents challenges in the form of life tasks. Adler named three of these explicitly but referred to two others without specifically naming them (Dreikurs & Mosak, 1966).

The original three tasks were those of *society, work,* and *sex.* The first has already been alluded to. Because no person can claim self-sufficiency, we are all interdependent. Not only do we need social recognition, but each of us also is dependent on the labor of other people, and they, in turn, are dependent on our contribution. Work thus becomes essential for human survival. The cooperative individual assumes this role willingly. In the sexual realm, because two different sexes exist, we must also learn how to relate to that fact. We must define our sex roles, partly on the basis of cultural definitions and stereotypes, and train ourselves to relate to the *other,* not the *opposite,* sex. Other people, of either sex, do not represent the enemy. They are our fellows, with whom we must learn to cooperate.

Fourth (Dreikurs & Mosak, 1967) and fifth tasks (Mosak & Dreikurs, 1967) have been described. Although Adler alluded to the *spiritual,* he never specifically named it (Jahn & Adler, 1964). But each of us must deal with the problem of defining the nature of the universe, the existence and nature of God, and how to relate to these concepts. Finally, we must address the task of *coping with ourselves.* William James (1890) made the distinction between the self as subject and the self as object, and it is as imperative, for the sake of mental health, that good relations exist between the "I" and the "me" as between the "I" and other people. In this task we must also deal, subjectively and reductionistically on the part of the person, with the "good me" and the "bad me."

13. Because life constantly poses challenges, living demands courage (Neuer, 1936). Courage is not an *ability* one either possesses or lacks. Nor is courage synonymous with bravery, such as falling on a grenade to save one's buddies from injury or death. *Courage* is the *willingness* to engage in risk-taking behavior either when one does not know the consequences or when the consequences might be adverse. We are all *capable* of courageous behavior, provided that we are *willing* to engage in it. Our willingness will depend on many variables, internal and external, such as our life-style convictions, our degree of social interest, the extent of risk as we appraise it, and whether we are task oriented or prestige oriented. Given that life offers few guarantees, all living requires risk taking. It would require very little courage to live if we were perfect, omniscient, or omnipotent. The question we must each answer is whether we have the courage to live despite the knowledge of our imperfections (Lazarsfeld, 1966).

14. Life has no intrinsic meaning. We give meaning to life, each of us in our own fashion. We declare it to be meaningful, meaningless, an absurdity, a prison sentence (cf., the adolescent's justification for doing as he pleases—"I didn't ask to be born"), a vale of tears, a preparation for the next world, and so on. Dreikurs (1957, 1971) maintained that the meaning of life resided in doing for others and in contributing to social life and social change. Viktor Frankl (1963) believed the meaning of life lay in love. The meaning we attribute to life will "determine" our behavior. We will behave *as if* life were really in accord with our perceptions, and therefore, certain meanings will have greater practical utility than others. Optimists will live an optimistic life, take chances, and not be discouraged by failure and adversity. They will be able to distinguish between failing and being a failure. Pessimists will refuse to be engaged with life, refuse to try, sabotage their efforts if they do make an attempt, and, through their methods of operation, endeavor to confirm their preexisting pessimistic anticipations (Krausz, 1935).

Other Systems

Students often have asked, "Do you Adlerians believe in sex, too?" The question is not always asked facetiously. Freud accorded sex the status of the master motive in behavior. Adler merely categorized sex as one of several tasks the individual is required to solve. Freud employed esoteric jargon, and Adler favored common-sense language. One story has it that a psychiatrist took Adler to task after a lecture, denigrating his approach with the criticism "You're only talking common sense," to which Adler replied, "I wish more psychiatrists did." Table 3.1 lists other differences between the theories of Freud and Adler.

TABLE 3.1   Comparison of Freud's and Adler's Concepts

Freud	Adler
1. Objective.	1. Subjective.
2. Physiological substratum for theory.	2. A social psychology.
3. Emphasized causality.	3. Emphasized teleology.
4. Reductionistic. The individual was divided into "parts" that were antagonistic toward each other: e.g., id-ego-superego, Eros vs. Thanatos, conscious vs. unconscious.	4. Holistic. The individual is indivisible. He or she is a unity, and all "parts" (memory, emotions, behavior) are in the service of the whole individual.
5. The study of the individual centers on the intrapersonal, the intrapsychic.	5. People can be understood only interpersonally and as social beings moving through and interacting with their environment.
6. The establishment of intrapsychic harmony constitutes the ideal goal of psychotherapy. "Where id was, there shall ego be."	6. The expansion of the individual, self-realization, and the enhancement of social interest represent the ideal goals for the individual.
7. People are basically "bad." Civilization attempts to domesticate them, for which they pay a heavy price. Through therapy, the instinctual demands may be sublimated but not eliminated.	7. People are neither "good" nor "bad," but as creative, choosing human beings, they may choose to be "good" or "bad" or both, depending on their life-styles and their appraisal of the immediate situation and its payoffs. Through the medium of therapy, people can choose to actualize themselves.
8. People are victims of both instinctual life and civilization.	8. People, as choosers, can shape both their internal and external environments. Although they cannot always choose what will happen to them, they can always choose the posture they will adopt toward life's stimuli.
9. Description of child development was postdictive and based not on direct observation of children but on the free associations of adults.	9. Children were studied directly in families, schools, and family education centers.
10. Emphasis on the Oedipus situation and its resolution.	10. Emphasis on the family constellation.
11. People are enemies. Others are our competitors, and we must protect ourselves from them. Theodore Reik quotes Nestroy: "If chance brings two wolves together, . . . neither feels the least uneasy because the other is a wolf; two human beings, however, can never meet in the forest, but one must think: That fellow may be a robber" (Reik, 1948, p. 477).	11. Other people are *Mitmenschen,* fellow human beings. They are our equals, our collaborators, our cooperators in life.
12. Women feel inferior because they envy men their penises. Women are inferior. Anatomy is destiny.	12. Women feel inferior because in our cultural milieu, women are undervalued. Men have privileges, rights, and preferred status, although in the current cultural ferment, their roles are being reevaluated.
13. Neurosis has a sexual etiology.	13. Neurosis is a failure of learning, a product of distorted perceptions.
14. Neurosis is the price we pay for civilization.	14. Neurosis is the price we pay for our lack of civilization.

A more extended comparison of Freud's and Adler's concepts of humankind may be found in articles by Carlson, Watts, & Maniacci (2006), H. W. von Sassen (1967), and Otto Hinrichsen (1913).

Adler and the Neo-Freudians

Adler once proclaimed that he was more concerned that his theories survive than that people remember to associate his theories with his name. His wish apparently was granted. In discussing Adler's influence on contemporary psychological theory and practice, Henri Ellenberger commented, "It would not be easy to find another author from which so much has been borrowed from all sides without acknowledgment than Adler" (1970, p. 645). However, many neo-Freudians have credited Adler with contributing to and influencing their work. In her last book, Karen Horney wrote of "neurotic ambition," "the need for perfection," and "the category of power." "All drives for glory," she wrote, "have in common the reaching out for greater knowledge, wisdom, virtue or powers than are given to human beings; they all aim at the absolute, the unlimited, the infinite" (1951, pp. 34–35). Those familiar with Adler's writings on the neurotic's perfectionistic, godlike striving will immediately be struck by the similarity in viewpoint.

Horney (1951) rejected Freud's pessimism, "his disbelief in human goodness and human growth," in favor of the Adlerian view that a person could grow and could "become a decent human being."

Others have also remarked on the resemblance between the theories of Horney and Adler; the reviewer of one Horney book wrote that Karen Horney had just written a new book by Alfred Adler (Farau, 1953).

Erich Fromm also expresses views similar to those of Adler. According to Fromm, people make choices. The attitude of the mother in child rearing is of paramount importance. Life fosters feelings of powerlessness and anxiety. Patrick Mullahy (1955) indicates that

> The only adequate solution, according to Fromm, is a relationship with man and nature, chiefly by love and productive work, which strengthens the total personality, sustains the person in his sense of uniqueness, and at the same time gives him a feeling of belonging, a sense of unity and common destiny with mankind. (pp. 251–252)

Although Harry Stack Sullivan places greater emphasis on developmental child psychology than does Adler, Sullivan's "person" moves through life in much the same manner as Adler's. Thus, Sullivan (1954) speaks of the "security operations" of the individual, a direct translation of Adler's and Lene Credner's (1930) *Sicherungen*. His "good me" and "bad me" dichotomy is, in expression if not in manner of development, essentially the same as that described by Adlerians.

So many similarities between Adler and the neo-Freudians have been noted that Gardner Murphy concluded, "If this way of reasoning is correct, neurosis should be the general characteristic of man under industrialism, a point suspected by many Freudians and, in particular, by that branch of the Freudian school (Horney and her associates) that has learned most from Adler" (1947, p. 569). A summary of such resemblances appears in Heinz and Rowena Ansbacher's *Individual Psychology of Alfred Adler* (1956), as well as in an article by Walter James (1947). Fritz Wittels (1939) has proposed that the neo-Freudians should more properly be called "neo-Adlerians," and a study by Heinz Ansbacher (1952) suggests that many traditional Freudians would concur.

Adler and Rogers

Although the therapies of Adler and Carl Rogers are diametrically opposed, their theories share many commonalities. Both are phenomenological, goal directed, and holistic.

Each views people as self-consistent, creative, and capable of change. To illustrate, Rogers (1951) postulates the following:

1. The organism reacts as an organized whole to the phenomenal field (p. 486).
2. The best vantage point for understanding behavior is from the internal frame of reference of the individual (p. 494).
3. The organism reacts to the field as it is experienced and perceived (pp. 484–485).
4. The organism has one basic tendency and striving—to actualize, maintain, and enhance the experiencing organism (p. 487).

Much of the early research on nondirective and client-centered therapy measured the discrepancy between *self-concept* and *self-ideal*. The Adlerian would describe the extent of discrepancy as a measure of inferiority feelings.

Adler and Ellis

The theories of Adler and Ellis exhibit many points of convergence. Albert Ellis (1970, 1971) finds his rational–emotive psychology to parallel that of Adler. What Adler calls basic mistakes, Albert Ellis refers to as irrational beliefs or attitudes. Both accept the notion that emotions are actually a form of thinking and that people create or control their emotions by controlling their thinking. They agree that we are not victims of our emotions but their creators. In psychotherapy, they (1) adopt similar stances with respect to unconscious motivation, (2) confront patients with their irrational ideas (basic mistakes or internalized sentences), (3) counterpropagandize the patient, (4) insist on action, and (5) constantly *encourage* patients to assume responsibility for the direction of their lives in more positive channels. The last phrase, however, reflects the major disagreement between Adler and Ellis—namely, what is "positive." Ellis puts it as follows:

> Where Adler writes, therefore, that "All my efforts are devoted towards increasing the social interest of the patient," the rational therapist would prefer to say, "Most of my efforts are devoted towards increasing the self-interest of the patient." He assumes that if the individual possesses rational self-interest he will, on both biological and logical grounds, almost invariably tend to have a high degree of social interest as well. (1957, p. 43)

Adlerian and Cognitive Therapy

Adlerian and cognitive therapy have much in common, as Beck and Weishaar (2005) acknowledge. Both are phenomenological psychologies, and both are concerned with the way individuals view the world and themselves. Both emphasize the role of cognition in emotion and behavior (Beck & Weishaar, 2005; Dreikurs, 1951; Mosak, 1985). Each posits a set of cognitive structures (for the Adlerian it is the life-style; for the cognitive therapist it is a schema). These cognitive structures *may be* (the cognitive therapist would say *are*) related to certain kinds of emotional behavior (Beck & Weishaar, 2005; Mosak, 1968). Beck and Weishaar speak of cognitive distortion and Adler of "basic mistakes." Beck and Weishaar's term is preferable, but both processes are essentially the same. The reader may wish to compare Beck's description of cognitive distortions (p. 272) and Mosak's description of basic mistakes (p. 82) in this volume.

Therapy in each system is a collaborative effort, employing what Beck and Weishaar call "collaborative empiricism, Socratic dialogue, and guided discovery" (Beck & Weishaar, 2005).

The two therapies also differ in significant ways. Cognitive therapy is not designed for personal growth, whereas Adlerians focus on personal growth even for the patient with psychopathology. Cognitive therapists narrow the types of psychopathology with which they will deal; Adlerians do not. For example, cognitive therapists do not obtain good results with people coping with psychosis (Beck & Weishaar, 2005), but Adlerians regularly treat these patients. As with Freudian analysis, a certain amount of intellectual and/or psychological sophistication on the part of the patient brings the best results from cognitive therapy. However, the Adlerian therapist has no such requirement and meets the patient's level of sophistication by speaking at the patient's level of intelligence and in the patient's idiom (Mosak & Shulman, 1963). In spite of these differences, cognitive therapy appears to be "variations on a theme by Adler," even though Beck reads better because of his use of the language of contemporary psychology rather than the archaic language of Adler and his contemporaries. Watts (2003) has provided an extensive review of Adler's influence on contemporary cognitive therapies, particularly the constructivist school. Experts from various divisions of cognitive therapy (e.g., cognitive–behavioral and constructivist) and Adlerian psychology offer their views on how the two schools of therapy have influenced and might grow from each other.

Adler and Other Systems

The many points of convergence and divergence between Adler and several of the existentialist thinkers have been noted by many writers (Birnbaum, 1961; Farau, 1964; Frankl, 1970). Phyllis Bottome had written in 1939 that "Adler was the first founder of an existence psychology" (p. 199). Given that existential psychology is not a school but a viewpoint, it is difficult to make comparisons, but interested readers may discover for themselves, in an editorial by Ansbacher (1959), the lines of continuity between Adler's ideas and existential thought.

The recognition of Adler as one of the earliest humanistic psychologists is clear. Ellis pays homage to Adler as "one of the first humanistic psychologists" (1970, p. 32). Abraham Maslow (1962, 1970) published five papers in Adlerian journals over a period of 35 years. As we have already observed, many of Adler's ideas have been incorporated by the humanistic psychologists with little awareness of Adler's contributions. "The model of man as a composite of part functions" that James Bugental (1963) questioned has been repudiated by Adlerians for more than half a century. Adlerian psychology is a value psychology (Adler wrote *What Life Should Mean to You* in 1931), as Viktor Frankl and Rollo May, among others, recognize in acknowledging their debt to Adler. Here is Frankl:

> What he [Adler] . . . achieved and accomplished was no less than a Copernican switch. . . . Beyond this, Alfred Adler may well be regarded as an existential thinker and as a forerunner of the existential-psychiatric movement. (1970, p. 38)

May expresses his debt as follows:

> I appreciate Adler more and more. . . . Adler's thoughts as I learned them in studying with him in Vienna in the summers of 1932 and 1933 led me indirectly into psychology, and were very influential in the later work in this country of Sullivan and William Alanson White, etc. (1970, p. 39)

And Abraham Maslow wrote,

> For me Alfred Adler becomes more and more correct year by year. As the facts come in, they give stronger and stronger support to his image of man. I should say that in one respect especially the times have not yet caught up with him. I refer to his holistic emphasis. (1970, p. 39)

HISTORY

Precursors

Adler's insistence that people cannot be studied in isolation but only in their social context was previously expressed by Aristotle, who referred to the human being as a *zoon politikon,* a political animal (Adler, 1959). Adler exhibits his affinity with the philosophy of stoicism, as both Ellenberger (1970) and H. N. Simpson (1966) point out. Other commentators have noted the resemblance of Adler's writings to Kant's philosophy, especially with respect to the categorical imperative, private logic, and overcoming. Adler and Nietzsche have often been compared, and much has been made of their common usage of the concept of the *will to power* (Ansbacher, 1972; Crookshank, 1933). Adler spoke of it in terms of the normal strivings for competence, however, whereas Nietzsche's references to this concept involved what Adler would call the "useless side of life." Nietzsche stressed the *Übermensch* (superman) and Adler spoke of equality. Adler further stressed *social feeling,* a concept totally alien to the Nietzschian philosophy.

Throughout history, philosophers have struggled with the mind–body problem. Psychology experienced a renaissance when psychologists and psychiatrists began to apply themselves to the study of psychosomatic syndromes. Psychosomatic and somatopsychic hypotheses were advanced to explain how emotions could influence the production of symptoms and how bodily states might create emotional or mental illness. Adler rejected such divisions. Like Kurt Lewin (1935), he rejected categorization and dichotomies. Like Jan Smuts (1961), he was a holist, and the term *Individual Psychology* was not meant to describe the psychology of the individual. It referred rather to Adler's holistic stance—that a person could be understood only as a whole, an indivisible unity. To study people atomistically was to fail to capture fully the nature of humanity. For Adler, the question was neither "How does mind affect body?" nor "How does body affect mind?" but rather "How does the individual use body and mind in the pursuit of goals?" Although Adler's *Study of Organ Inferiority and Its Psychical Compensation* (1917) might seem to contradict such statements by expressing a causalistic viewpoint, this highly original theory was formulated when Adler was a member of the Freudian circle. Later Adler added the subjective factor:

> It might be suggested, therefore, that in order to find out where a child's interest lies, we need only to ascertain which organ is defective. But things do not work out quite so simply. The child does not experience the fact of organ inferiority in the way that an external observer sees it, but as modified by his own scheme of apperception. (1969)

Perhaps the greatest influence on Adler was Hans Vaihinger's (1965) "philosophy of 'as if.'" According to Vaihinger, a fiction is "a mere piece of imagination" that deviates from reality but that is nevertheless utilitarian for the individual. Both the concept of the world and the concept of the self are subjective—fictional—and therefore in error. *Truth* is "only the most expedient error, that is, the system of ideas which enables us to act and to deal with things most rapidly, neatly, and safely, and with the minimum of irrational elements" (p. 108).

Finally, Adler's psychology has a religious tone (Adler, 1958; Jahn & Adler, 1964; Mosak, 1987c). His placement of social interest at the pinnacle of his value theory is in the tradition of those religions that stress people's responsibility for each other. Indeed, Adler maintained that "Individual Psychology makes good religion if you are unfortunate enough not to have another" (Rasey, 1956, p. 254).

Beginnings

Adler was born near Vienna on February 7, 1870, and he died while on a lecture tour in Aberdeen, Scotland, on May 27, 1937. After graduating from the University of Vienna in 1895, Adler entered private practice as an ophthalmologist in 1898. He later switched to general practice and then to neurology. During this period, Adler gave portents of his later social orientation by writing a book on the health of tailors (1898). In this respect, he may be regarded as the progenitor of industrial medicine and of community outreach.

In 1902, Adler, at Freud's invitation, joined in the latter's Wednesday evening discussion circle. Biographers agree that Adler wrote two defenses of Freud's theories, which may have gained him the invitation. Although textbooks frequently refer to Adler as a student of Freud, Adler was actually a colleague (Ansbacher, 1962; Ellenberger, 1970; Federn, 1963; Maslow, 1962). Through the next decade, Adler had one foot in and one foot out of the Freudian circle. Although his *Study of Organ Inferiority* won Freud's unqualified endorsement, Adler's introduction of the aggression instinct in 1908 met with Freud's disapproval. Not until 1923, long after Adler had discarded instinct theory, did Freud incorporate the aggressive instinct into psychoanalysis (Sicher & Mosak, 1967), at which time Adler declared, "I enriched psychoanalysis by the aggressive drive. I gladly make them a present of it!" (Bottome, 1939, p. 63).

Adler's increasing divergence from Freud's viewpoint led to discomfort and disillusion in the Vienna Psychoanalytic Society. Adler criticized Freud's sexual stance; Freud condemned Adler's ego psychology. They disagreed on (1) the unity of neuroses, (2) penis envy (sexual) versus the masculine protest (social), (3) the defensive role of the ego in neuroses, and (4) the role of the unconscious. Freud thought that Adler had not discovered anything new but had merely reinterpreted what psychoanalysis had already said. He believed that what Adler discovered was "trivial" and that it was "methodologically deplorable and condemns his whole work to sterility" (Colby, 1951). In 1911, after a series of meetings where these issues were discussed in an atmosphere of fencing, heckling, and vitriol (Brome, 1968), Adler resigned as president of the Vienna Society. Later that year, Freud forced the choice between Adler and himself. Several members of the circle expressed their sympathy for Adler by resigning and forming the Society for Free Psychoanalytic Research. The word *free* was meant to imply that this was still a psychoanalytic society, but one free of Freud.

During the next decade, with the exception of the war period, Adler and his coworkers developed the social view of the neuroses. Their focus was primarily clinical, although as early as 1908, Adler (1914) had demonstrated an interest in children, families, and education. In 1922 Adler initiated what was perhaps the first community outreach program, child-guidance centers within the community. These centers were located in public schools and were directed by psychologists who served without pay. The method, for which Adler drew much criticism, was that of public family education, a method still used in Adlerian family education centers. Twenty-eight such centers existed in Vienna until 1934, when an unfriendly government closed them. This form of center was transported to the United States by Rudolf Dreikurs and his students (Dreikurs, Corsini, Lowe, & Sonstegard, 1959). The success of these centers motivated the Vienna school authorities to invite several Adlerians to plan a school along Adlerian lines, and from this invitation emerged the school described in Oskar Spiel's *Discipline Without Punishment* (1962). The school emphasized encouragement, class discussions, democratic principles, and the responsibility of children for themselves and for each other—educational methods still in use today.

The social orientation of Adler's Individual Psychology inevitably led to interest in group methods and Adler's introduction of family therapy (1922). Dreikurs (1959) is credited with the first use of group psychotherapy in private practice.

Between World Wars I and II, Adlerian groups existed in 20 European countries and in the United States. In 1926 Adler was invited to the United States to lecture, and until 1934, when fascism took hold in Austria, he divided his time between the United States, where he was on the medical faculty of the Long Island College of Medicine, and abroad. Two of his children, Alexandra and Kurt, practiced psychiatry in New York City. With the march of Nazism, many Adlerians were forced to flee their European homelands and made the United States the center of their activities. Today, Individual Psychology societies exist in the United States, England, Canada, France, Denmark, Switzerland, Germany, Austria, the Netherlands, Greece, Italy, Israel, and Australia.

Current Status

The resurgence of the Adlerian school after the dispersion from Europe was an uphill effort. Personal hardships of refugee Adlerians were compounded by the existing psychological climate in this country. The economic depression still prevailed. The Freudian school held a near monopoly, both in the treatment area and with respect to appointments in medical schools. Some Adlerians defected; others became crypto-Adlerians. However, others persevered in retaining their identity and their optimism. Local societies were founded, and 1952 saw the formation of the American Society of Adlerian Psychology (now the North American Society of Adlerian Psychology). Several journals appeared; the major American one is the *Journal of Individual Psychology,* formerly called *Individual Psychology,* which itself was the successor of the *Individual Psychology Bulletin,* of which Dreikurs was the editor for many years. The International Association of Individual Psychology also publishes the *Individual Psychology Newsletter.*

Training institutes that offer certificates in psychotherapy, counseling, and child guidance are found in New York; Chicago; Minneapolis; Berkeley, California; San Francisco; St. Louis; Fort Wayne, Indiana; Vancouver; and Montreal. Individual courses and programs of study are offered at many universities, such as Oregon, Arizona, West Virginia, Vermont, Governors State, Southern Illinois, and Georgia State. Master's degrees based on an Adlerian curriculum are offered by Bowie State College and by the Adler School of Professional Psychology in Chicago. The latter has been accredited to offer a doctoral program in clinical psychology.

Although Adlerian psychology was once dismissed as moribund, superficial (i.e., an "ego psychology"), and suitable mainly for children, it is today considered a viable psychology.

Today's Adlerian may operate as a traditional clinician but remains innovative. For example, Joshua Bierer was a pioneer in social psychiatry (Bierer & Evans, 1969) and a leader in the day-hospital movement (1951). Therapeutic social clubs have been in operation at the Alfred Adler Mental Hygiene Clinic in New York and at Saint Joseph Hospital in Chicago. Dreikurs originated multiple psychotherapy (1950), and he, Harold Mosak, and Bernard Shulman contributed to its development (1952a, 1952b, 1982). Rudolf Dreikurs, Asya Kadis, Helene Papanek, and Bernard Shulman have made extensive contributions to group therapy. Because they prefer the goal of prevention to that of healing, Adlerians function extensively in the area of education. Manford Sonstegard, Raymond Lowe, Bronia Grunwald, Oscar Christensen, Raymond Corsini, and Loren Grey are among those responsible for applying Adlerian principles in the schools. All have been students of Dreikurs, who transported the tradition from Vienna, and who himself made a great contribution in this area. In the Adlerian social tradition, Adlerians may be involved in community outreach programs or may dedicate their efforts to the study of subjects such as drugs, aging, delinquency, religion, and poverty.

In 2008, the *Journal of Individual Psychology* (volume 64) devoted an entire issue to lesbian, gay, bisexual, and transgender individuals (Mansager, 2008). Hill, Brack, Qalinge, and Dean (2008) presented research detailing AIDS treatment in South Africa from an Adlerian perspective. Also recently published, Foley, Matheny, and Curlette (2008) have presented research detailing an Adlerian assessment of personality traits in Mainland China. In 2007, Linden presented an updated perspective of aging from an Adlerian view. Sperry and Mansager (2007) have discussed spirituality and Adlerian psychology. In yet another special issue of the *Journal of Individual Psychology,* Rasmussen (2006) has collected a series of articles updating the Adlerian view of depression. In a similar vein, Schneider, Kern and Curlette (2007) have published a special issue of the journal updating the Adlerian view of narcissism. Rotgers and Maniacci (2006) have published a volume on comparative treatments of antisocial personality disorder, with two chapters covering Adlerian perspectives.

The contemporary Adlerian finds the growth model of personality infinitely more congenial than the sickness model. The Adlerian is interested not in curing sick individuals or a sick society but in reeducating individuals and in reshaping society. Adlerians are even branching out into the Internet. Two sites of interest are www.alfredadler.org and www.adleriancounselingandtherapy.com.

Henry Stein and colleagues at the Alfred Adler Institute of San Francisco have recently completed the Alfred Adler translation project. This 12-volume set comprises newly edited and retranslated volumes of the complete clinical collected works of Alfred Adler; these translations are sorely needed to bring Adler's original writings to English-speaking audiences. The volumes are readily available via commercial bookstores, online booksellers, or through the Alfred Adler Institute of San Francisco.

PERSONALITY

Theory of Personality

Adlerian psychology is a psychology of use rather than of possession. This assumption decreases the importance of the question "How do heredity and environment shape the individual?" The functionalist, holistic Adlerian asks instead, "How does the individual use heredity and environment?" Since theirs is a psychology of use, Adlerians find it improper to employ such phrases as "He *has* social interest." People *display* social interest rather than possess it (Mosak, 1991).

For Adler, the *family constellation* constitutes the primary social environment. Every child searches for significance in this environment and competes for position within the family constellation. One sibling becomes the "best" child, another the "worst." Being favored, being one of the favored sex within the family, adopting the family values, or identifying or allying oneself with a parent or sibling may provide the grounds for the feeling of having a place. Handicaps, organ inferiorities, or being an orphan are other "position makers" for some children.

Of supreme importance is the child's position in the family constellation. Thus, it would appear that the first child usually is a conservative and the second is often a rebel. The baby is ordinarily either everyone's darling or one who stands on tiptoes to see above the preceding siblings. If these general characteristics possess any validity, at best they exist as statistical probabilities and not as defining traits. Considering the family constellation in terms of birth order or ordinal position creates the problem of characterizing, let us say, the fifth child in the family. Although the fifth child is often encountered in the therapy situation, he or she never receives any attention in the literature. Birth order, per se, also fails to take into account the gender position of the child. The children in two-sibling families in which the possible configurations are boy-boy, girl-girl, boy-girl, and girl-boy do not possess similar characteristics based on ordinal position alone (Shulman & Mosak, 1977).

The Adlerian prefers to study the family constellation in terms of the *psychological* position. A simple example illustrates this point of view. Take two siblings separated in age by 10 years. In birth order research, these would be treated as a first child and a second child. From the Adlerian point of view, the psychological position of each would *most likely* be that of an only child, with the older child *perhaps* functioning as an additional parent figure for the younger. The italicized terms *most likely* and *perhaps* are used expressly to indicate that (1) Adlerians do not recognize a causalistic, one-to-one relationship between family position and sibling traits, and (2) whatever relationship exists can be understood only in context—that is, when one knows the family climate and the total configuration of factors in the family constellation. Adler, whenever he generalized or ventured a prediction, was fond of reminding his students, "Everything could also be quite different."

The search for significance and the consequent sibling competition reflect the values of the competitive society in which we live. We are encouraged to be first, to excel, to be popular, to be athletic, to be a "real" man, to "never say die," to recall that "practice makes perfect," and to "dream the impossible dream." Consequently, each child must stake out a "territory" that includes the attributes or abilities that the child hopes will give him or her a feeling of worth. If through their evaluations of their own potency (abilities, courage, and confidence) children are convinced that they can achieve this place through useful endeavor, they will pursue "the useful side of life." Should children feel that they cannot attain the goal of having a "place" in this fashion, they will become discouraged and engage in disturbed or disturbing behavior in their efforts to find a place. For the Adlerian, the "maladjusted" child is not a "sick" child. He or she is a "discouraged" child. Dreikurs (1948, 1949) classifies the goals of the discouraged child into four groups: attention getting, power seeking, revenge taking, and declaring deficiency or defeat. Dreikurs is speaking of immediate rather than long-range goals. These are the goals of children's "misbehavior," not of all children's behavior (Mosak & Mosak, 1975b).

In the process of becoming socialized human beings, children form conclusions on the basis of their subjective experiences. Because judgment and logical processes are not highly developed in young children, many of their growing convictions contain errors or only partial "truths." Nevertheless, they accept these conclusions about themselves and others *as if* they were true. Such conclusions are subjective evaluations, biased apperceptions of themselves and of the world, rather than objective "reality." Thus, one can be truly inferior without feeling inferior. Conversely, one can feel inferior without being inferior.

The child creates a cognitive map or life-style that will assist "little me" in coping with the "big" world. The life-style includes the aspirations, the long-range goals, and a "statement" of the conditions, personal or social, that are requisite for the individual's "security." The latter are also fictions and are stated in therapy as "If only . . . , then I . . . ."

Mosak (1954) divided life-style convictions into four groups:

1. The *self-concept*—the convictions I have about who I am.
2. The *self-ideal* (Adler coined this phrase in 1912)—the convictions of what I should be or am obliged to be to have a place.
3. The *Weltbild,* or "picture of the world"—convictions about the not-self (world, people, nature, and so on) and what the world demands of me.
4. The *ethical convictions*—the personal "right–wrong" code.

When there is a discrepancy between self and ideal-self convictions ("I am short; I should be tall"), *inferiority feelings* ensue. Although an infinite variety of inferiority feelings exist, one that Adler discussed while he was still in the Freudian Society should be mentioned. This idea, the *masculine protest*, eventually led to the rift between Adler and Freud, and it assumes monumental importance in some circles today. In a culture that places a premium on masculinity, some women feel inferior because they have not been accorded the prerogatives or privileges of men ("I am woman; I should be equal to man"). But men also suffered from the masculine protest because being a man is not sufficient to provide a "place" for some men ("I am a man, but I should be a *real* man"). Because Adler believed in the equality of the sexes, he could not accept these fictions (Mosak & Schneider, 1977).

Lack of congruence between convictions in the self-concept and those in the *Weltbild* ("I am weak and helpless; life is dangerous") also results in inferiority feelings. Discrepancies between self-concept and ethical convictions ("One should always tell the truth; I lie") lead to inferiority feelings in the moral realm. Thus, the guilt feeling is merely a variant of the inferiority feeling (Mosak, 1987b).

These variations of inferiority feelings in and of themselves are not "abnormal." It would be difficult to quarrel with Adler's observations that to live is to *feel* inferior. It is only when individuals act *as if* they were inferior, develop symptoms, or behave as "sick" that we see evidence of what in the medical model would be called *pathology* and what Adlerians call *discouragement* or the *inferiority complex.* To oversimplify, the *inferiority feeling* is universal and "normal," although it may leave us uncomfortable; the *inferiority complex* reflects the discouragement of a limited segment of our society and is usually "abnormal." The former may be masked or hidden from the view of others; the latter is an open demonstration of inadequacy, or "sickness."

Using their "maps," people facilitate their movements through life. This permits them to evaluate, understand, experience, predict, and control experience. Lawrence Frank writes in this connection,

> The personality process might be regarded as a sort of rubber stamp which the individual imposes upon every situation by which he gives it the configuration that he, as an individual, requires; in so doing he necessarily ignores or subordinates many aspects of the situation that for him are irrelevant and meaningless and selectively reacts to those aspects that are personally significant. (1939, p. 392)

Although the life-style is the instrument for coping with experience, it is very largely nonconscious. The life-style comprises the cognitive organization of the individual rather than the behavioral organization. As an illustration, the conviction "I require excitement" may lead to the vocational choices of actor, racing car driver, or explorer, or to "acting out" behavior. Such a conviction may further lead to getting into jams or exciting situations, engaging in creative acts, or discovery.

Within the same life-style, one can behave usefully or uselessly. This distinction permits Adlerians (e.g., Dreikurs, 1961; Nikelly, 1971a) to distinguish between *psychotherapy* and *counseling.* The former, they maintain, has as its aim the change of life-style; the latter has as its goal the change of behavior within the existing life-style.

Because the Adlerian literature discusses the life tasks of occupation, society, and love so extensively, these tasks of life will not be elaborated on here, except for some brief comments. Lewis Way points out that "The problems they pose can never be solved once and for all, but demand from the individual a continuous and creative movement toward adaptation" (1962, pp. 179–180).

Love, as an emotion like other emotions, is cognitively based. People are not "victims" of their emotions. They create emotions to assist them in the attainment of their goals. Love is the conjunctive emotion we create when we want to move toward people.

Although the life tasks of love, occupation, and society demand solution, it is possible to avoid or postpone them if one can compensate in other areas. "Even successful persons fall into neurosis because they are not more successful" (Way, 1962, p. 206).

The *neurotic symptom* is an expression of "I *can't* because I'm sick"; the person's movement betrays the "I *won't* because my self-esteem might get hurt" (Krausz, 1959, p. 112). Although neurotics' movements are consonant with their "private logic" (Nikelly, 1971b), they still cling to "common sense." They know what they should do or feel, but they "can't." Adler referred to them as "yes-but" personalities. Eric Berne (1964) has graphically described their interpersonal maneuvers in the "Why don't you— Yes, but" game. The genesis of neurosis lies in discouragement. People avoid and postpone or take circuitous routes to solutions so they can "save face." Even when they expect or arrange to fail, they try to salvage some self-esteem. Students, fearful of failing examinations, will refrain from studying. In the event they do fail, they merely have to hold that they were lazy or neglectful but not stupid.

The psychotic's goal of superiority is often loftier than that which can be achieved by mere humans. "Individual Psychology has shown that the goal of superiority can only be fixed at such attitudes when the individual has, by losing interest in others, also lost interest in his own reason and understanding . . . common sense has become useless to him" (Adler, 1964a, pp. 128–129). Adler used "common sense" in much the same manner that Sullivan spoke of "consensual validation." In the pseudo work area, the psychotic becomes superintendent of the mental hospital. In the pseudo social area, the hypomanic patient resembles the cheerful extrovert, and the more acutely manic patient becomes a "name dropper" and "swallows up" people (Shulman, 1962). The paranoid patient pictures people as threatening and manifests a "search for glory," to use Karen Horney's (1951) phrase, by the persecutory delusion that *they* are conspiring to do something to *me*. The delusions of grandeur of psychotic depressive patients ("I'm the *worst* sinner of all time") and of the schizophrenic who claims to be Christ are some other "solutions" to the pseudo spiritual tasks. The reifying hallucinations of talking with the devil fall in this category (Adler, 1963a; Mosak & Fletcher, 1973).

The *psychologically healthy* or *normal* individual has developed social interest and is willing to commit to life and the life tasks without evasion, excuse, or "side shows" (Wolfe, 1932). This person proceeds with confidence and optimism about meeting life's challenges. There is a sense of belonging and contributing, the "courage to be imperfect," and the serene knowledge that one can be acceptable to others, although imperfect. Above all, this person rejects the faulty values that culture projects and attempts to substitute for them values more consonant with the "ironclad logic of social living." Such a person does not exist, nor will psychotherapy produce such a person. Yet this is the Adlerian ideal, and because Adler's intent was to substitute small errors for larger errors, many of these goals can be approximated in psychotherapy. Many fortunate people have the courage (Adler, 1928) and social interest to do this for themselves without therapeutic assistance.

Variety of Concepts

The simplicity of Adlerian vocabulary renders definition and interpretation generally unnecessary. Yet some differences of opinion and emphasis about Adlerian concepts remain unresolved. In terms of *life-style,* Adlerians disagree with respect to what it describes—behavioral or cognitive organization. *Social interest* (Bickhard & Ford, 1976; Crandall, 1981; Edgar, 1975; Kazan, 1978; Mosak, 1991) apparently is not a unitary concept but a cluster of feelings and behaviors (Ansbacher, 1968). Although social interest is often described as "innate," many Adlerians wonder what makes it so, given that it appears to be neither genetic nor constitutional. As one looks at the theories of Adler, Freud, and Jung, one is struck with the effort on the part of all three to "biologize" their theories. Perhaps it was the temper of the times. Perhaps it was because all three were physicians. Perhaps it resulted from the need to make their theories respectable during a period when psychoanalysis was held in low esteem. None of these theories would incur any great damage if "instincts," "social interest," and "racial unconscious" were treated as psychological constructs rather than as biological processes. Adler, having introduced the concept of *organ inferiority* with its consequent compensation, actually had proposed a biopsychological theory, but this transpired during his Freudian period. Later he substituted the *social inferiority feeling* for actual organ inferiority, and with the exception of one important article (Shulman & Klapman, 1968), Adlerians have published little on organ inferiority. Although people undoubtedly do compensate for organ inferiority, the latter is no longer the cornerstone of the Adlerian edifice.

Gardner Murphy (1947) took issue with Adler's use of compensation as the only defense mechanism. Literally, Adler's writings do read that way. On the other hand, if one reads more closely, compensation becomes an umbrella to cover all coping mechanisms. Thus Adler speaks of safeguards, excuses, projection, the depreciation tendency, creating distance, and identification. Although a Freudian might view these as defense mechanisms, the Adlerian prefers to view them as problem-solving devices the person uses to protect self-esteem, reputation, and physical self. Because Adlerians do not accept the concept of *the* unconscious, such mechanisms as repression and sublimation become irrelevant. Adlerian theory has no room for instincts, drives, libido, and other alleged movers.

Because of their mutual emphasis on behavior (movement), Adlerian psychology and behavior modification theory have been equated. This is an error. Adlerians, although interested in changing behavior, have as their major goal not behavior modification but *motivation* modification. Dreikurs writes, "We do not attempt primarily to change behavior patterns or remove symptoms. If a patient improves his behavior because he finds it profitable at the time, without changing his basic premises, then we do not consider that as a therapeutic success. We are trying to change goals, concepts, and notions" (1963, p. 79).

PSYCHOTHERAPY

Theory of Psychotherapy

All scientific schools of psychotherapy have their shares of successes and failures. A considerable number of therapies based on nonscientific foundations probably result in equivalent levels of success. In any event, regardless of its validity or endurance, any theory must be implemented within the context of the therapist–patient relationship. As Fred Fiedler (1950) has shown, therapeutic success is a function of the expertness of the therapist rather than of the therapist's orientation.

Given that the underlying psychodynamic theory is not the crucial factor in therapy, perhaps it is the special techniques that contribute to therapeutic effectiveness. This would certainly seem to have been Rogers's early position before nondirective therapy became client-centered therapy. For the early nondirective school, the creation of a warm, permissive, nonjudgmental atmosphere; reflection of feeling; and avoidance of interpretation, advice, persuasion, and suggestion were paramount in the therapeutic situation.

The Freudian assigns central importance to transference, but behavior modification therapists ignore it. To many directive therapists, content and manner of interpretation are crucial. The Adlerian emphasizes interpretation of the patient's life-style and movement.

Criteria for "getting well" correspond to the particular therapeutic emphasis. Some therapists propose depth of therapy as the decisive factor. For most Adlerians, depth of therapy does not constitute a major concern. In this connection, therapy is neither deep nor superficial except as the patient experiences it as such.

If neither theory nor the use of prescribed techniques is decisive, is it the transference relationship that makes cure possible? Or is it the egalitarian relationship? Or the warm, permissive atmosphere with the nonjudgmental therapist accepting the patient as is? Because all of these relationships are involved in various forms of both effective and ineffective therapy, we must hypothesize either that therapeutic effectiveness is a matter of matching certain therapeutic relationships to certain patients or that all therapeutic relationships possess common factors These factors—variations on the Christian virtues of faith, hope, and love—appear to be necessary, but not sufficient, conditions of effective therapy.

Faith

D. Rosenthal and Jerome D. Frank (1956) discuss the implications of faith in the therapeutic process. Franz Alexander and Thomas French state that

> As a general rule, the patient who comes for help voluntarily has this confidence, this expectation that the therapist is both able and willing to help him, before he comes to treatment; if not, if the patient is forced into treatment, the therapist must build up this feeling of rapport before any therapeutic change can be effected. (1946, p. 173)

Many therapeutic mechanisms may enhance the patient's faith. A simple explanation clarifies matters for some patients. a complex interpretation for others. The therapist's own faith in himself or herself; the therapist's appearance of wisdom, strength, and assurance; and the therapist's willingness to listen without criticism may all be used by patients to strengthen their faith.

Hope

Patients seek treatment with varying degrees of hope, running the gamut from complete hopelessness to hope for (and expectation of) everything, including a miracle. Because of the efficacy of the self-fulfilling prophecy, people *tend* to move in the direction of making their anticipations come true. Therefore, the therapist must keep the patient's hope elevated.

Because the Adlerian holds that the patient suffers from *discouragement,* a primary therapeutic technique lies in encouragement. Expression of faith in the patient, noncondemnation, and avoidance of being overly demanding may give the patient hope. The patient may also derive hope from feeling understood. Accordingly, the construction of therapy as a "we" experience where patients do not feel they stand alone, where they feel security in the strength and competency of their therapist, and where they feel some symptom alleviation may prove helpful. Patients may also gain hope from attempting some course of action they feared or did not know was available to them. Humor assists in the retention of hope (Mosak, 1987a). Lewis Way comments, "Humor such as Adler possessed in such abundance is an invaluable asset, since, if one can occasionally joke, things cannot be so bad" (1962, p. 267). Each therapist has faith in his methods for encouraging and sustaining hope. They are put to the most severe test in patients who are depressed or suicidal.

Love

In the broadest sense of love, the patient must feel that the therapist cares (Adler, 1963a, 1964a). The mere act of treating the patient may furnish such evidence by employing empathic listening, "working through" together, or having two therapists in multiple psychotherapy offering interest in the patient. Transfer of a patient to another therapist or from individual to group therapy may have a contrary effect unless it is "worked through."

However, the therapist must avoid pitfalls such as infantilizing, oversupporting, or becoming a victim of the patient when the patient accuses the therapist of not caring enough. In Adlerian group therapy, the group is conceptualized as a "reexperiencing of the family constellation" (Kadis, 1956). Thus, the therapist may be accused of playing favorites, of caring too much for one patient or too little for another.

The Adlerian theory of psychotherapy rests on the notion that psychotherapy is a cooperative educational enterprise involving one or more therapists and one or more patients. The goal of therapy is to develop the patient's social interest. To accomplish this, therapy involves changing faulty social values (Dreikurs, 1957). The subject matter of this course in reeducation is the patient—the life-style and the relationship to the life tasks. Learning the "basic mistakes" in the cognitive map, the patient has the opportunity to decide whether to continue in the old ways or to move in other directions. "The consultee must under all circumstances get the conviction in relation to treatment that he is absolutely free. He can do, or not do, as he pleases" (Ansbacher & Ansbacher, 1956, p. 341). The patient can choose between self-interest and social interest. The educational process has the following goals:

1. The fostering of social interest.
2. The decrease of inferiority feelings, the overcoming of discouragement, and the recognition and utilization of one's resources.
3. Changes in the person's life-style—that is, in her or his perceptions and goals. The therapeutic goal, as we have noted, involves transforming big errors into little ones (as with automobiles, some need a tune-up and others require a major overhaul).
4. Changing faulty motivation that underlies even acceptable behavior, or changing values.
5. Encouraging the individual to recognize equality among people (Dreikurs, 1971).
6. Helping the person to become a contributing human being.

"Students" who reach these educational objectives will feel a sense of belonging and display acceptance of themselves and others. They will feel that they can arrange, within life's limits, their own destinies. Such patients eventually come to feel encouraged, optimistic, confident, courageous, secure—and asymptomatic.

Process of Psychotherapy

The process of psychotherapy, as practiced by Adlerians, has four aims: (1) establishing and maintaining a "good" relationship; (2) uncovering the dynamics of the patient, including life-style and goals, and assessing how they affect life movement; (3) interpretation culminating in insight; and (4) reorientation.

The Relationship

A "good" therapeutic relationship is a friendly one between equals. The Adlerian therapist and the patient sit facing each other, their chairs at the same level. Many Adlerians prefer to work without a desk because distancing and separation may engender undesirable psychological sets. Having abandoned the medical model, the Adlerian looks with disfavor upon casting the doctor in the role of the actor (omnipotent, omniscient, and mysterious) and the patient in the role of the acted-upon. Therapy is structured to inform the patient that creative human beings play a role in creating their problems, that one is responsible (not in the sense of blame) for one's actions, and that one's problems are based on faulty perceptions and inadequate or faulty learning, especially of faulty values (Dreikurs, 1957). If this is so, one can assume responsibility for change. What has not been learned can be learned. What has been learned "poorly" can be replaced by better learning. Faulty perception and values can be altered and modified. From the initiation of treatment, the patient's efforts to remain passive are discouraged. The patient has an active role in the therapy. Although assuming the role of student, the patient is still an active learner responsible for contributing to his or her own education.

Therapy requires cooperation, which means alignment of goals. Noncoincidence of goals may prevent the therapy from getting off the ground, as, for example, when the patient denies the need for therapy. The initial interview(s) must not, therefore, omit the consideration of initial goals and expectations. The patient may wish to overpower the therapist or to make the therapist powerful and responsible. The therapist's goal must be to avoid these traps. The patient may want to relinquish symptoms but not underlying convictions and may be looking for a miracle. In each case, at least a temporary agreement on goals must be arrived at before the therapy can proceed. Way cautions that

> A refusal to be caught in this way [succumbing to the patient's appeals to the therapist's vanity or bids for sympathy] gives the patient little opportunity for developing serious resistances and transferences, and is indeed the doctor's only defense against a reversal of roles and against finding that he is being treated by the patient. The cure must always be a cooperation and never a fight. It is a hard test for the doctor's own balance and is likely to succeed only if he himself is free from neurosis. (1962, p. 265)

Adler (1963a) offers similar warnings against role reversal.

Because the problems of resistance and transference are defined in terms of patient–therapist goal discrepancies, throughout therapy the goals will diverge, and the common task will consist of realigning the goals so that patient and therapist move in the same direction.

The patient, in bringing a life-style to therapy, expects from the therapist the kind of response expected from all others. The patient may feel misunderstood, unfairly treated, or unloved and may anticipate that the therapist will behave accordingly. Often the patient unconsciously creates situations to invite the therapist to behave in this manner. For this reason, the therapist must be alert to what Adlerians call "scripts," and Eric Berne (1964) calls "games," and foil the patient's expectations. A patient, for example, will declare, "Have you ever seen a patient like me before?" to establish uniqueness and to challenge the therapist's competence. The therapist's response may be a straightforward, but not sarcastic, "Not since the last hour," followed by a discussion of uniqueness. Because assessment begins with the first moment of contact, the patient is generally given some interpretation, usually phrased as a guess, during the first interview. This gives the patient something to think about until the next interview. The therapist will soon find it possible to assess how the patient will respond to interpretation, to therapy, and to the therapist and will gain some glimpse of the life-style framework. The therapist does not play the patient's game, because at that game the patient is the professional, having played it successfully since childhood (although often in self-defeating fashion), whereas the therapist is a relative amateur. The therapist does not have to *win* the game but merely does not play it. Only one side wins in a tug-of-war. However, in this case, one side (the therapist) is uninterested in victories or defeats and simply doesn't pick up the end of the rope. This renders the "opponent's" game ineffective, and the two can proceed to play more productive, cooperative games (Mosak & Maniacci, 1998).

The whole relationship process increases the education of the patient. For some patients, it is their first experience of a good interpersonal relationship involving cooperation, mutual respect, and trust. Despite occasional bad feelings, the relationship can endure and survive. The patient learns that good and bad relationships do not merely happen—they are products of people's efforts—and that poor interpersonal relationships are products of misperceptions, inaccurate conclusions, and unwarranted anticipations incorporated in the life-style.

Analysis

Investigation of a patient's dynamics is divided into two parts. The therapist, first, wants to understand the patient's life-style and, second, aims to understand how the life-style affects current function with respect to the life tasks. Not all suffering stems from the patient's life-style. Many patients with adequate life-styles develop problems or symptoms in the face of intolerable or extreme situations from which they cannot extricate themselves.

Analytic investigation begins with the first moment. The way a patient enters the room, posture, and choice of seating (especially important in family therapy) all provide important clues. What the patient says and how it is said expand the therapist's understanding, especially when the therapist interprets the patient's communications in interpersonal terms, or "scripts," rather than in descriptive terms. Thus, the Adlerian translates the descriptive statement "I am confused" into the admonition "Don't pin me down." "It's a habit" conveys the declaration "And that's another thing you're not going to get me to change" (Mosak & Gushurst, 1971). The therapist assesses, follows up, and juxtaposes clues in patterns, accepting some hypotheses and rejecting others in an effort to understand the patient. As therapy progresses, the patient offers information one way or another, and the therapist pieces it together bit by bit like a jigsaw puzzle.

The Life-Style Investigation

In formal assessment procedures, the patient's family constellation is explored. The therapist obtains glimpses of what position the child found in the family and how he or she went about finding a place within the family, in school, and among peers. The second portion of the assessment consists of interpreting the patient's early recollections. An *early recollection* occurs in the period before continuous memory and may be inaccurate or a complete fiction. It represents a single event ("One day I remember . . .") rather than a group of events ("We used to . . ."). Adlerians refer to the latter as *a report* rather than a recollection. Reports are important to the therapeutic assessment process. However, they are not interpreted the same way as early recollections (Shulman & Mosak, 1988). Recollections are treated as a projective technique (Mosak, 1958). If one understands the early recollections, one understands the patient's "Story of My Life" (Adler, 1931), because people selectively recollect incidents consonant with their life-styles. The following recollection of Adler himself (1947) may serve to illustrate the consonance between his earliest recollection and his later psychological views:

> One of my earliest recollections is of sitting on a bench, bandaged up on account of rickets, with my healthy elder brother sitting opposite me. He could run, jump, and move about quite effortlessly, while for me movement of any sort was a strain and an effort. Everyone went to great pains to help me, and my mother and father did all that was in their power to do. At the time of this recollection I must have been about two years old. (p. 9)

In a single recollection, Adler refers to organ inferiority, the inferiority feeling, the emphasis on "my desire to move freely—to see all psychic manifestations in terms of movements" (p. 10), and social feeling (Mosak & Kopp, 1973).

The summary of early recollections, the story of the patient's life, permits the derivation of the patient's "basic mistakes" (Mosak & DiPietro, 2006). The life-style can be conceived as a personal mythology. The individual will behave *as if* the myths were true because, for him or her, they are true. Consequently, there are "truths" or partial "truths" in myths, and there are myths we confuse with truth. The latter are *basic mistakes*.

Basic mistakes may be classified as follows:

1. *Overgeneralizations.* "People are hostile." "Life is dangerous."

2. *False or impossible goals of security.* "One false step and you're dead." "I have to please everybody."

3. *Misperceptions of life and life's demands.* Typical convictions might be "Life never gives me any breaks" and "Life is so hard."

4. *Minimization or denial of one's worth.* "I'm stupid" and "I'm undeserving" or "I'm just a housewife."

5. *Faulty values.* "Be first even if you have to climb over others."

Finally, the therapist is interested in how the patient perceives his or her assets.

Sample Life-Style Summary

The following sample life-style summary is not intended to be a complete personality description, but it does offer patient and therapist initial hypotheses.

SUMMARY OF FAMILY CONSTELLATION

John is the younger of two children, the only boy. He grew up fatherless after age 9. His sister was so precocious that John became discouraged. Because he felt he would never become famous, he decided perhaps he could at least be notorious and brought himself to the attention of others through negative behavior. He acquired the reputation of a "holy terror." He was going to do everything his way, and nobody was going to stop him. He patterned his behavior after that of his strong, "masculine" father, from whom he learned that the toughest man wins. Because notoriety came with doing the disapproved, John early became interested in and engaged in sex. This also reinforced his feelings of masculinity. Because both parents were handicapped and yet still "made it," John apparently decided that without any physical handicaps, the sky would be the limit for him.

SUMMARY OF EARLY RECOLLECTIONS

"I run scared in life, and even when people tell me there's nothing to be scared of, I'm still scared. Women give men a hard time. They betray them, they punish them, and they interfere with what men want to do. A real man takes no crap from anybody. Somebody always interferes. I am not going to do what others want me to do. Others call that bad and want to punish me for it, but I don't see it that way. Doing what I want is merely part of being a man."

"BASIC MISTAKES"

1. John exaggerates the significance of masculinity and equates it with doing what he pleases.

2. He is not on the same wavelength as women. They see his behavior as "bad"; he sees it as only "natural" for a man.

3. He is too ready to fight, many times just to preserve his sense of masculinity.

4. He perceives women as the enemy, even though he looks to them for comfort.

5. Victory is snatched from him at the last moment.

Assets

1. He is a driver. When he puts his mind to things, he makes them work.

2. He engages in creative problem solving.

3. He knows how to get what he wants.

4. He knows how to ask a woman "nicely."

During the course of the treatment, other forms of analysis will occur. Because the therapist views the life-style as consistent, it will express itself in all of the patient's behavior—physical behavior, language and speech, fantasy productions, dreams, and interpersonal relationships, past and present. Because of this consistency, the patient may choose to express herself or himself in any or all of these media because they all express life-style. The therapist observes behavior, speech, and language closely during each interview. Sometimes the dialogue will center on the present, sometimes on the past, often on the future. Free association and chitchat, except when the latter serves a therapeutic purpose, are mostly discouraged. Although dream analysis is an integral part of psychotherapy, the patient who speaks only of dreams receives gentle dissuasion (Alexandra Adler, 1943). The analysis proceeds with an examination of the interplay between life-style and the life tasks: how the life-style affects the person's function and dysfunction vis-à-vis the life tasks.

Dreams

Adler saw the dream as a problem-solving activity with a future orientation, in contrast to Freud's view that it was an attempt to solve an old problem. The *dream* is seen by Adlerians as a rehearsal of possible future courses of action. If we want to postpone action, we forget the dream. If we want to dissuade ourselves from some action, we frighten ourselves with a nightmare.

The dream, Adler said, was the "factory of emotions." In it we create moods that move us toward or away from the next day's activities. Commonly, people say, "I don't know why but I woke up in a lousy mood today." The day before Adler died, he told friends, "I woke smiling . . . so I knew my dreams were good although I had forgotten them" (Bottome, 1939, p. 240). Just as early recollections reflect long-range goals, the dream experiments with possible answers to immediate problems. In accordance with their view of the individual's uniqueness, Adlerians reject the theory of fixed symbolism. One cannot understand a dream without knowing the dreamer, although Adler (1963b) and Erwin Wexberg (1929) do address themselves to some frequently encountered dream themes. Way admonishes,

> One is reminded again of two boys, instanced by Adler [1964a, p. 150], each of whom wished to be a horse, one because he would have to bear the responsibility for his family, the other to outstrip all the others. This should be a salutary warning against making dictionary interpretations. (1962, pp. 282–284)

The interpretation of the dream does not terminate with the analysis of the content but must include the purposive function. Dreams serve as weather vanes for treatment, bringing problems to the surface and pointing to the patient's movement. Dreikurs describes a patient who related recurrent dreams that were short and actionless, reflecting his life-style of figuring out "the best way of getting out of a problem, mostly without doing anything. . . . When his dreams started to move and become active he started to move in his life, too" (Dreikurs, 1944, p. 26).

Reorientation

Reorientation in all therapies proceeds from persuading the patient, gently or forcefully, that change is in his or her best interest. The patient's present manner of living affords "safety" but not happiness. Because neither therapy nor life offers guarantees, one must risk some "safety" for the possibility of greater happiness and self-fulfillment. This dilemma is not easily solved. Like Hamlet, the patient wonders whether it is better to "bear those ills we have than fly to others that we know not of."

Insight

Analytic psychotherapists frequently assign central importance to insight, assuming that "basic change" cannot occur in its absence. The conviction that insight must precede behavioral change often results in extended treatment, in encouraging some patients to become "sicker" to avoid or postpone change, and in increasing their self-absorption rather than their self-awareness. Meanwhile, patients relieve themselves from the responsibility of living life until they have achieved insight.

A second assumption, treasured by therapists and patients alike, distinguishes between *intellectual* and *emotional* insight (Ellis, 1963; Papanek, 1959), a dualism the holistic Adlerian experiences difficulty in accepting. This and other dualisms, such as conscious versus unconscious, undeniably exist in the patient's subjective experience. But these antagonistic forces are creations of the patient that delay action. Simultaneously, the patient can maintain a good conscience because he or she is the victim of conflicting forces or an emotional block. Solving problems is relegated to the future while the patient pursues insight. *Insight,* as the Adlerian defines it, is understanding translated into constructive action. It reflects the patient's understanding of the purposive nature of behavior and mistaken apperceptions, as well as an understanding of the role both play in life movement. So-called intellectual insight merely reflects the patient's desire to play the game of therapy rather than the game of life.

Interpretation

The Adlerian therapist facilitates insight mainly by interpreting ordinary communications, dreams, fantasies, behavior, symptoms, the patient–therapist transactions, and the patient's interpersonal transactions. The emphasis in interpretation is on purpose rather than cause, on movement rather than description, on use rather than possession. Through interpretation, the therapist holds up a mirror for the patient.

The therapist relates past to present only to indicate the continuity of the maladaptive life-style, not to demonstrate a causal connection. The therapist may also use humor (Mosak, 1987a) or illustrate with fables (Pancner, 1978), anecdotes, and biography. Irony may prove effective, but it must be handled with care. The therapist may "spit in the patient's soup," a crude expression for exposing the patient's intentions in such a way as to make them unpalatable. The therapist may offer the interpretation directly or in the form of "Could it be that . . .?" or may invite the patient to make interpretations. Although timing, exaggeration, understatement, and accuracy are technical concerns of any therapist, they are not emphasized by the Adlerian therapist, who does not view the patient as fragile.

Other Verbal Techniques

Advice is often frowned upon by therapists. Hans Strupp relates, "It has been said that Freud, following his own recommendations, never gave advice to an analysand on the couch but did not stint with the commodity from the couch to the door" (1972, p. 40).

Wexberg (1929/1970) frowned on giving advice to a patient, but the Adlerian therapist freely gives advice, as did Freud, taking care, however, not to encourage dependency. In practice, the therapist may merely outline the alternatives and let the patient make the decision. This invitation develops faith in self rather than faith in the therapist. On the other hand, the therapist may offer direct advice, taking care to encourage the patient's self-directiveness and willingness to stand alone.

Given that Adlerians consider the patient discouraged rather than sick, it is no surprise that they make extensive use of encouragement. Enhancing the patient's faith in self, "accentuating the positive and eliminating the negative," and keeping up the patient's hope all contribute to counteracting discouragement. The patient who "walks and falls" learns it is not fatal and can get up and walk again. Therapy also counteracts the patient's social values, thus altering his or her view of life and helping give meaning to it. Moralizing is avoided, although therapists must not deceive themselves into believing their system has no value orientation. The dialogue concerns "useful" and "useless" behavior rather than "good" and "bad" behavior.

The therapist avoids rational argument and trying to "out-logic" the patient. These tactics are easily defeated by the patient who operates according to the rules of *psycho-logic* (private logic) rather than formal logic. Catharsis, abreaction, and confession may afford the patient relief by freeing him or her from carrying the burden of "unfinished business," but as has been noted (Alexander & French, 1946), these may also be a test of whether the patient can place trust in the therapist.

Action Techniques

Adlerians regularly use role playing, talking to an empty chair (Shoobs, 1964), the Midas technique (Shulman, 1962), the behind-the-back technique (Corsini, 1953), and other action procedures to assist the patient in reorientation. The extent of use is a function of the therapist's preference, training, and readiness to experiment with the novel.

Mechanisms of Psychotherapy

The Therapist as Model

The therapist represents values the patient may attempt to imitate. Adlerian therapists represent themselves as being "for real," fallible, able to laugh at themselves, caring— models for social interest. If the therapist can possess these characteristics, perhaps the patient can, too, and many patients emulate their therapists, whom they use as referents for normality (Mosak, 1967).

Change

There comes a time in psychotherapy when analysis must be abandoned and the patient must be encouraged to move forward. Insight has to give way to decisive action.

Some of the techniques Adlerians use to elicit change are described below and by Mosak and Maniacci (1998). They are not panaceas, nor are they used indiscriminately. The creative therapist will improvise techniques to meet the needs of the therapeutic moment and will remember, above all, that people are more important than techniques and strategies. The therapist who loses sight of these cautions is a technician who does all the "right" things but is never engaged in a human encounter with another human being.

Acting "As If"

A common patient refrain in treatment is "If only I could . . ." (Adler, 1963a). Adlerian therapists often request that for the next week the patient act "as if." The patient may protest that it would only be an act and therefore phony. We explain that all acting is not phony pretense, that one can try on a role as one might try on a suit. It does not change the person wearing the suit, but sometimes with a handsome suit of clothes, one may feel differently and perhaps behave differently, thus becoming a different person.

Task Setting

Adler (1964a) gave us the prototype for task setting in his treatment of depressives:

> To return to the indirect method of treatment: I recommend it especially in melancholia. After establishing a sympathetic relation I give suggestions for a change of conduct in two stages. In the first stage my suggestion is "Only do what is agreeable to you." The patient usually answers, "Nothing is agreeable." "Then at least," I respond, "do not exert yourself to do what is disagreeable." The patient, who has usually been exhorted to do various uncongenial things to remedy this condition, finds a rather flattering novelty in my advice, and may improve in behavior. Later I insinuate the second rule of conduct, saying that "it is much more difficult and I do not know if you can follow it." After saying this I am silent, and look doubtfully at the patient. In this way I excite his curiosity and ensure his attention, and then proceed, "If you could follow this second rule you would be cured in fourteen days. It is helpful to consider from time to time how you can give another person pleasure. It would very soon enable you to sleep and would chase away all your sad thoughts. You would feel yourself to be useful and worthwhile."
>
> I receive various replies to my suggestion, but every patient thinks it is too difficult to act upon. If the answer is, "How can I give pleasure to others when I have none myself?" I relieve the prospect by saying, "Then you will need four weeks." The more transparent response, "Who gives *me* pleasure?" I counter with what is probably the strongest move in the game, by saying, "Perhaps you had better train yourself a little thus: Do not actually DO anything to please anyone else, but just think out how you COULD do it." (pp. 25–26)

The tasks are relatively simple and are set at a level at which patients can sabotage the task, but they cannot fail and then scold the therapist.

> The patient must understand that not the physician but life itself is inexorable. He must understand that ultimately [he will have] to transfer to practical life that which has been theoretically recognized. . . . But from the physician he hears no word of reproach or of impatience, at most an occasional kindly, harmless, ironical remark. (p. 101)

A 50-year-old man who professed "genuine" intention to get married but simultaneously avoided women was instructed to seek one meaningful contact with a woman (how to do so was up to him) every day. After raising many objections, he complained, "But it's so hard! I'll get so tired out I won't be able to function." The therapist good-humoredly relented and informed him, "Since God rested on the seventh day, I can't ask you to do more than God. So you need carry out the task only six days a week."

One form of task setting that Adler introduced is called *antisuggestion* by Wexberg (1929) and *paradoxical intention* by Frankl (1963). This method, used nonclinically by Knight Dunlap (1933), was labeled *negative practice.* The symptomatic patient unwittingly reinforces symptoms by fighting them, by saying, "Why did this have to happen to *me?*" The insomniac keeps one eye open to observe whether the other is falling asleep. To halt this fight, the patient is instructed to intend and even increase that which he or she is fighting against.

Creating Images

Adler was fond of describing patients with a simple phrase—for example, "the beggar as king." Other Adlerians give patients similar shorthand images that confirm the adage that "one picture is worth a thousand words." Remembering this image, the patient can remember goals and, in later stages, can learn to use the image to laugh at self. One over-ambitious patient, labeled "Superman," one day began to unbutton his shirt. When the therapist made inquiry, the patient laughingly replied, "So you can see my blue shirt with the big 'S' on it." Another patient, fearing sexual impotence, concurred with the therapist's observation that he had never seen an impotent dog. The patient advanced as explanation: "The dog just does what he's supposed to do without worrying about whether he'll be able to perform." The therapist suggested that at his next attempt at sexual intercourse, before he made any advances, he should smile and say inwardly, "Bow wow." The following week, the patient informed the members of his group, "I bow wowed."

Catching Oneself

When patients understand personal goals and want to change, they are instructed to catch themselves "with their hand in the cookie jar." Patients may catch themselves in the midst of their old behavior but still feel incapable of doing anything about it at the moment. With additional practice, they learn to anticipate situations in time to avoid them.

The Push-Button Technique

This method, effective with people who feel they are victims of their disjunctive emotions, involves requesting patients to close their eyes, to re-create a pleasant incident from past experience, and to note the feeling that accompanies this image. Then they are asked to re-create an unpleasant incident of hurt, humiliation, failure, or anger and to note the accompanying feeling. Following this, the patient re-creates the first scene again. The lesson Adlerians try to teach clients is that they can create whatever feeling they wish merely by deciding what they will think about. One is the creator, not the victim, of emotions. To be depressed, for example, requires *choosing* to be depressed. We try to impress patients with their power for self-determination. This method, devised for clinical use by Mosak (1985), has been the subject of experimental investigation by Brewer (1976), who found it an effective technique in treating state depression.

The "Aha" Experience

The patient who gains awareness in treatment and increases participation in life recurrently has "aha" or "eureka" experiences. With this greater understanding, the patient generates self-confidence and optimism, resulting in increased encouragement and willingness to confront life's problems with commitment, compassion, and empathy.

Post-therapy

After therapy is over, the patient can implement newly acquired learning. Operationally, the goal of therapy may be defined as making the therapist superfluous. If therapist and patient have both done their jobs well, the goal will have been achieved.

APPLICATIONS

Who Can We Help?

Although Adler, like the other *Nervenärzte* ("nerve doctors") of his era, conducted one-to-one psychotherapy, his own social orientation moved him out of the consulting room and into the community. Although he never relinquished his clinical interests, he concurrently was an educator and a social reformer. Joost Meerloo, a Freudian, eulogizes Adler with his confession:

> As a matter of fact, the whole body of psychoanalysis and psychiatry is imbued with Adler's ideas, although few want to acknowledge this fact. We are all plagiarists, though we hate to confess it. . . . The whole body of social psychiatry would have been impossible without Adler's pioneering zest. (1970, p. 40)

Clinical

All the early pioneers in psychotherapy treated neurotics. Psychotics were considered not amenable to psychotherapy because they could not enter into a transference relationship. Adlerians, unencumbered by the concept of transference, treated psychotics regularly.

Henri Ellenberger (1970, p. 618) suggests that "among the great pioneers of dynamic psychiatry, Janet and Adler are the only ones who had personal clinical experience with criminals, and Adler was the only one who wrote something on the subject from his direct experience." An Adlerian, Ernst Papanek (1971), of whom Claude Brown (1965) wrote so glowingly in *Manchild in the Promised Land,* was director of Wiltwyck School (a reform school). Mosak set up a group therapy program at Cook County Jail in Chicago employing paraprofessionals as therapists (O'Reilly, Cizon, Flanagan, & Pflanczer, 1965). The growth model implicit in Adlerian theory has prompted Adlerians to see human problems in terms of people's realizing themselves and becoming fellow human beings. Much "treatment" then is of "normal" people with "normal" problems. A therapy that does not provide the client with a philosophy of life, whatever else it may accomplish in the way of symptom eradication or alleviation, behavior modification, or insight, is an incomplete therapy. Hence the Adlerian is concerned with the client's problems of living and existence. Deficiency, suffering, and illness do not constitute the price of admission to Adlerian therapy. One may enter therapy to learn about oneself, to grow, and to actualize oneself.

Social

Adler's interests were rather catholic. In the area of education, he believed in prevention rather than cure and founded family education centers. Dreikurs and his students (Dreikurs et al., 1959) have founded family education centers throughout the world. Offshoots of these centers include hundreds of parent study groups (Soltz, 1967). In addition, professional therapists have used a variety of methods for teaching child-rearing practices (Allred, 1976; Beecher & Beecher, 1966; Corsini & Painter, 1975; Dreikurs, 1948; Dreikurs & Soltz, 1964; Painter & Corsini, 1989).

Adler himself wrote on social issues and problems such as crime, war, religion, group psychology, Bolshevism, leadership, and nationalism. Among contemporary Adlerians (Angers, 1960; Clark, 1965, 1967a, 1967b; Elam, 1969a, 1969b; Gottesfeld, 1966; Hemming, 1956; La Porte, 1966; Lombardi, 1969; Nikelly, 1971c), the "newer" social problems of protest, race, drugs, and social conditions, as well as the "newer" views of religion (Mosak, 1987b), have been added to the Adlerians' previous interests.

Treatment

One can hardly identify a mode of treatment in which some Adlerian is not engaged. From a historical standpoint, the initial Adlerian modality was one-to-one psychotherapy. Many Adlerians still regard individual psychotherapy as the treatment of choice. Adlerians have demonstrated willingness to undertake treatment with any who sought their services (Watts & Carlson, 1999).

Dreikurs, Mosak, and Shulman (1952a, 1952b, 1982) introduced *multiple psychotherapy,* a format in which several therapists treat a single patient. It offers constant consultation between therapists, prevents the emotional attachment of a patient to a single therapist, and obviates or dissolves impasses. Countertransference reactions are minimized. Flexibility in the number of therapist roles and models is increased. Patients are more impressed or reassured when two therapists independently agree. The patient also may benefit from the experience of observing disagreement between therapists and may learn that people can disagree without loss of face.

Multiple therapy creates an atmosphere that facilitates learning. Therapeutic impasses and problems of dependency are resolved more easily. These include the responsibility for self, therapist–transference reactions, and termination. In the event that therapist and patient do not hit it off, the patient does not become a therapeutic casualty and is merely transferred to the second therapist.

In the mid-1920s, Dreikurs (1959) initiated group therapy in private practice. This application was a natural evolution from the Adlerian axiom that people's problems are always social problems. Group therapy finds considerable adherents among Adlerians. Some Adlerian therapists regard group therapy as the method of choice either on practical grounds (e.g., fees, large numbers of patients to be treated, etc.) or because they believe that human problems are most effectively handled in the group social situation. Others use group therapy as a preface to individual therapy or to wean patients from intensive individual psychotherapy. A number of therapists combine individual and group psychotherapy in the conviction that this combination maximizes therapeutic effect (Papanek, 1954, 1956). Still other therapists visualize the group as assisting in the solution of certain selected problems or with certain types of populations. Co-therapist groups are very common among Adlerians.

An offshoot of group treatment is the therapeutic social club in a mental hospital, as initiated by the British Adlerian, Joshua Bierer. Although these clubs possess superficial similarities to Abraham Low's recovery groups (Low, 1952) and to halfway houses in that all attempt to facilitate the patient's reentrance into society, the therapeutic social club emphasizes the "social" rather than the "therapeutic" aspects of life, taking the "healthy" rather than the "sick" model.

Psychodrama has been used by Adlerians, sometimes as separate therapy, sometimes in conjunction with another therapeutic modality (Starr, 1977).

Marriage counseling has figured prominently in Adlerian activities. Adlerians defied the trend of the times and preferred to treat the couple as a unit rather than as separate individuals. To "treat" merely one mate may be compared to having only half the dialogue of a play. Seeing the couple together suggests that they have a joint relationship problem rather than individual problems and invites joint effort in the solution of these problems. The counselor can observe and describe their interaction (Mozdzierz & Lottman, 1973; Pew & Pew, 1972). Married couples group therapy (Deutsch, 1967) and married couples study groups are two more settings for conducting marriage counseling. Phillips and Corsini (1982) and Dinkmeyer and Carlson (1989) have written self-help books designed to be used by married people who are experiencing trouble in their marriage.

In the early 1920s, Adler persuaded the Viennese school administration to establish child-guidance centers. The social group was the primary vehicle for treatment (Adler,

1963a; Alexandra Adler, 1951; Seidler & Zilahi, 1949). Dreikurs wrote several popular books and many articles (Dreikurs, 1948; Dreikurs & Grey, 1968; Dreikurs & Soltz, 1964) to disseminate this information to parents and teachers, and today thousands of parents are enrolled in study groups where they obtain supplementary information on child rearing.

Adler's preventive methods in schools were adopted by educators and school counselors who used them in individual classes and schools and, in one case, in an entire school system (Mosak, 1971). The methods were originally applied in the Individual Psychological Experimental School in Vienna (Birnbaum, 1935; Spiel, 1962) and have been elaborated on in this country (Corsini, 1977, 1979; Dinkmeyer & Dreikurs, 1963; Dreikurs, 1968, 1972; Dreikurs, Grunwald, & Pepper, 1982; Grunwald, 1954).

With respect to broader social problems, Dreikurs devoted the last part of his life to the problem of interindividual and intergroup conflict resolution. Much of this work was performed in Israel and has not been reported. Kenneth Clark, a former president of the American Psychological Association, has devoted much of his career to studying and providing recommendations for solutions for problems of African-Americans, as have Harry Elam (1969a, 1969b) and Jacqueline Brown (1976).

The Setting

Adlerians function in every imaginable setting: the private-practice office, hospitals, day hospitals, jails, schools, and community programs. Offices do not need any special furnishings but reflect either the therapist's aesthetic preferences or the condition of the institution's budget. No special equipment is used, except perhaps for special projects. Although voice recordings are a matter of individual choice, they are sometimes maintained as the patient's file.

In the initial interviews, the therapist generally obtains the following kinds of information (in addition to demographic information):

1. Was the patient self-referred?

2. Is the patient negative about treatment? If the patient is reluctant, "conversion" is necessary if therapy is to proceed.

3. What does the patient come for? Is it treatment to alleviate suffering? If so, suffering from what? Some new patients are "supermarket shoppers" who announce the number of therapists who have helped them already. Their secret goal is to be perfect. Unless such a patient's fictional goal is disclosed, today's therapist may be the latest of many therapists about whom the patient will be telling the next one.

4. What are the patient's expectations about treatment?

5. What are the patient's expectations about outcome? Perfection? Failure? A solution for a specific problem without any major personality alterations? Immediate cure?

6. What are the patient's goals in psychotherapy? We must distinguish between stated goals—to get well, to learn about self, to be a better spouse and parent, to gain a new philosophy of life—and nonverbalized goals—to remain sick, to punish others, to defeat the therapist and sabotage therapy, to maintain good intentions without changing.

The patient may also resist in order to depreciate or defeat the therapist because the patient lacks the courage to live on the useful side of life and fears that the therapist might nudge him or her in that direction. The intensification of such escape methods may become most pronounced during the termination phase of treatment, when the patient realizes he or she must soon face the realistic tasks of life without the therapist's support.

Tests

Routine physical examinations are not required by Adlerians, in view of the therapy's educational orientation. Nevertheless, many patients do have physiological problems, and Adlerians are trained to be sensitive to the presence of these problems. The therapist who suspects such problems will make referrals for physical examination.

Adlerians are divided on the issue of psychological testing. Most Adlerians avoid nosological diagnosis, except for nontherapeutic purposes such as filling out insurance forms. Labels are static descriptions that ignore the *movement* of the individual. They describe what the individual *has,* but not how he or she moves through life.

Regine Seidler placed more faith in projective testing than in so-called objective tests, maintaining that the latter are actually subjective tests because "the *subjective attitude* of each and every individual toward any given test necessarily renders the test nonobjective" (1967, p. 4). Objective tests were more useful to her as measures of test-taking attitude than as measures of what the test was purportedly measuring.

Early recollections serve as a test for Adlerians, assisting them in the life-style assessment, and Mosak & DiPietro (2006) have published a manual for interpreting them. Younger Adlerians employ many conventional tests and some unconventional ones for diagnostic purposes as well as in the treatment of the patient.

The BASIS-A Inventory (Wheeler, Kern, & Curlette, 1993), more formally known as the Basic Adlerian Scales for Interpersonal Success, is a 65-item test grounded in Adlerian principles. It measures individuals along five dimensions: Belonging-Social Interest, Going Along, Taking Charge, Wanting Recognition, and Being Cautious. In addition, there are five supporting scales that help round out the personality picture: Harshness, Entitlement, Liked by All, Striving for Perfection, and Softness. This instrument has been used in dozens of research studies (Kern, Gormley, & Curlette, 2008), and has become widely used to supplement the life-style assessment procedure commonly used by more traditionally trained clinicians.

The Therapist

The Adlerian therapist ideally is an authentically sharing, caring person. Helene and Ernst Papanek write,

> The therapist participates actively. Without playing any sharply defined "role," he shows warmth toward and a genuine interest in the patient and encourages especially his desire for change and betterment. The relationship itself has a purpose: to help the patient help himself. (1961, p. 117)

Adlerian therapists remain free to have feelings and opinions and to express them. Such expression in a spontaneous way permits patients to view therapists as human beings. If therapists err, they err—but then the patient may learn the courage to be imperfect from this experience (Lazarsfeld, 1966). The experience may also facilitate therapy.

Therapists must not inject evaluation of their own worth into the therapy; rather, they must do their therapeutic job without concern for prestige, not reveling in successes or becoming discouraged by failures. Otherwise, they may bounce like a rubber ball from therapy hour to therapy hour or perhaps even within the same hour. The therapist's worth depends not on external factors but on what lies within the self. The therapist is task oriented rather than self oriented.

Therapists reveal themselves as persons. The concept of the *anonymous therapist* is foreign to Adlerian psychology. Such a role would increase social distance between therapist and patient, interfering with the establishment of an egalitarian, human relationship. The "anonymous therapist" role was created to facilitate the establishment of a transference relationship, and because the Adlerian rejects the transference concept as Freud formulated it, maintaining such a posture would be irrelevant, if not harmful, to the relationship. Dreikurs (1961) deplored the prevalent attitude among therapists of not coming too close to patients because it might affect the therapeutic relationship adversely. Shulman (Wexberg, 1929/1970, p. 88) defines the role of the therapist as that of "a helping friend." Self-revelation can occur only when therapists feel secure, at home with others, unafraid to be human and fallible, and thus unafraid of their patients' evaluations, criticism, or hostility (compare Rogers's "congruence").

Is the Adlerian therapist judgmental? In a sense, all therapists are judgmental in that therapy rests upon some value orientation: a belief that certain behavior is better than other behavior, that certain goals are better than other goals, that one organization of personality is superior to another form of organization. However, given that two cardinal principles of the Adlerian intervention are caring and encouragement, a critical or judgmental stance is best avoided.

Patient Problems

If the therapist does not like the patient, it raises problems for a therapist of any persuasion (Fromm-Reichman, 1949). Some therapists merely do not accept such patients. Still others feel they ought not to have (or ought to overcome) such negative feelings and therefore accept the patient for treatment, which often leads to both participants "suffering." It appears difficult to have "unconditional positive regard" for a patient you dislike. Adlerians meet this situation in the same manner other therapists do.

Seduction problems are treated as any other patient problem. The secure therapist will not become frightened, panic, or succumb. If the patient's activities nevertheless prevent the therapy from continuing, the patient may be referred to another therapist. Flattery problems are in some ways similar and have been discussed elsewhere (Berne, 1964; Mosak & Gushurst, 1971).

Suicide threats are always taken seriously (Ansbacher, 1961, 1969). Alfred Adler warned, however, that our goal is "to knock the weapon out of his hand" so the patient cannot make us vulnerable and intimidate us at will with his threats. As an example, he recounts that "A patient once asked me, smiling, 'Has anyone ever taken his life while being treated by you?' I answered him, 'Not yet, but I am prepared for this to happen at any time'" (Ansbacher & Ansbacher, 1956, pp. 338–339). Kurt Adler postulates "an underlying rage against people" in suicide threats and believes that this goal of vengefulness must be uncovered. He "knocks the weapon out of the patient's hand" as follows:

> Patients have tested me with the question of how would I feel if I were to read of their suicide in the newspaper. I answer that it is possible that some reporter hungry for news would pick up such an item from a police blotter. But, the next day, the paper will already be old, and only a dog perhaps may honor their suicide notice by lifting a leg over it in some corner. (1961, p. 66)

Alexandra Adler (1943), Lazarsfeld (1952), Pelzman (1952), Boldt (1994), and Zborowski (1997) discuss problems beyond the scope of this chapter.

Evidence

Until very recently, little research had emerged from the Adlerian group. Like most European clinicians, European Adlerians were suspicious of research based on statistical methods. A complicating factor was the *idiographic* (case method) approach on which Adlerians relied. Even now, statisticians have not developed appropriate sophisticated methods for idiographic studies. The research methods lent themselves well to studies of causal factors, but the Adlerian rejected causalism, feeling that causes can only be imputed (and therefore disputed) in retrospective fashion but that they contributed little to the understanding of humans.

The most often-cited studies involving Adlerian psychology were conducted by non-Adlerians. Fred Fiedler (1950) compared therapeutic relationships in psychoanalytic, nondirective, and Adlerian therapy. He found that there was greater similarity between therapeutic relationships developed by experts of the three schools than between expert and less expert therapists within the same school. Crandall (1981) presented the first large-scale investigation of an Adlerian construct. Using his Social Interest Scale, Crandall found positive correlations between social interest and optimism about human nature, altruism, trustworthiness, being liked, and several measures of adjustment and well-being. Because of the number of ways in which social interest has been defined (Bickhard & Ford, 1976; Crandall, 1981; Edgar, 1975; Kazan, 1978; Mosak, 1991), his study represents a valuable contribution to the understanding of this concept.

A joint research study conducted by the (Rogerian) Counseling Center of the University of Chicago and the Alfred Adler Institute of Chicago examined the effects of time limits in psychotherapy (Shlien, Mosak, & Dreikurs, 1962). Patients of both groups of therapists were given 20 interviews, and the groups were compared with each other and with two control groups. The investigators reported changes in self-ideal correlations. These correlations improved significantly and, according to this measure, suggest that time-limited therapy "may be said to be not only *effective* but also twice as *efficient* as time-unlimited therapy" (p. 33).

Follow-up of these patients in both experimental groups indicated that the gains were retained one year later.

Much of the research in family constellation has been done by non-Adlerians. Charles Miley (1969) and Lucille Forer (1977) have compiled bibliographies of this literature. The results reported are contradictory, probably because non-Adlerians treat birth order as a matter of ordinal position and Adlerians consider birth order in terms of psychological position (Mosak, 1972). Walter Toman (1970) recognized this distinction in his many studies of the family constellation.

Ansbacher (1946) and Mosak (1958) have also distinguished between Freudian and Adlerian approaches to the interpretation of early recollections. Robin Gushurst (1971) provides a manual for interpreting and scoring one class of recollections. His reliability studies demonstrate that judges can interpret early-recollection data with high interjudge reliability. He also conducted three validity studies to investigate the hypothesis that life goals may be identified from early-recollection data and found that he could do this with two of his three experimental groups. Whereas Fiedler compared therapists of different orientations, Heine (1953) compared patients' reports of their experiences in Adlerian, Freudian, and Rogerian therapy. Taylor (1975) has written an excellent review of some early-recollection validity studies.

Adlerian psychology would undoubtedly benefit from more research. With the shift in locus from Europe to the United States, with the accelerated growth of the Adlerian school in recent years, with the introduction of more American-trained Adlerians into academic settings, and with the development of new research strategies suitable for idiographic data, there is increasing integration of Adlerians into research activities. A summary of these activities appears in articles by Watkins (1982, 1983) and Watkins and Guarnaccia (1999).

Westen, Novotny, and Thompson-Brenner (2004) have recently argued that the emphasis on empirically supported treatments is misplaced, for many reasons. Among other things, proponents of ESTs advocate something they call empirically informed treatments. The change is more than terminological. Rather than advocating empirically supported treatments per se, they advocate investigating techniques that could be used by clinicians across treatments, regardless of orientation. If this were to be done, books such as Mosak and Maniacci's (1998) would be useful in supplying a range of techniques (i.e., tactics) that could be investigated across a range of situations. As Westen, Novotny, and Thompson-Brenner discuss, if techniques were empirically supported, treatments then would be empirically informed, even if the theories themselves were not. Additionally, they advocate tailoring treatment much more specifically to the personality pattern of clients, and not simply to symptoms and behaviors, a point long emphasized by the Adlerian concept of life-style.

Kern, Gormley, and Curlette (2008) have presented an invaluable summary of findings that used an Adlerian-based instrument, the BASIS-A, in more than 40 research studies across a wide range of issues (from the years 2000 through 2006). As the personality inventory continues to gain wider use, more research is expected, reversing a once unfortunate but common trend in Adlerian psychology that overlooked the importance of research. Similarly, Eckstein and Kern (2002) have summarized research in Adlerian psychology, with a special emphasis upon birth order research, citing more than 250 different studies.

Psychotherapy in a Multicultural World

Psychotherapy is an interpersonal transaction. For Adlerians especially, it entails the meeting of two worlds, the therapist's and the client's. This meeting requires both respect and tact.

In a multicultural world, psychotherapy can be perceived as intrusive. One of the reasons for such a perception is the therapist's insensitivity to the world view of the client. However, Adlerians have an answer to this dilemma: the life style assessment. Through the process of asking about the early family situation, including the family dynamics, values, interactions, and the social, academic, and religious factors of development, Adlerians quickly become sensitized to the particulars of an individual's development. In fact, the life style assessment process is typically a quick course in multiculturalism during which the client teaches the therapist about his or her culture. In the course of numerous life style assessments the authors have conducted with clients from several countries (including, but not limited to, China, Ghana, Ireland, Iraq, Iran, Israel, South Africa, Thailand, Japan, Italy, Columbia, England, France, Turkey and Germany), the client has served as instructor to us, the therapists, in what were key factors in his or her development. The life style assessment served as a bridge between cultures.

CASE EXAMPLE

Background

The patient was a 53-year-old, Vienna-born man who had been in treatment almost continuously with Freudian psychoanalysts, both in the United States and abroad, since he was 17. With the advent of tranquilizers, he had transferred his allegiances to psychiatrists who treated him with a combination of drugs and psychotherapy and finally with drugs alone. When he entered Adlerian treatment, he was being maintained by his previous therapist on an opium derivative and Thorazine. He failed to tell his previous therapist of his decision to see us and also failed to inform us that he was still obtaining medication from his previous therapist.

The treatment process was atypical in the sense that the patient's "illness" prevented our following our customary procedure. Having over the years become therapy-wise, he invested his creativity in efforts to run the therapy. Cooperative effort was virtually impossible. In conventional terms, the co-therapists, Drs. A and B, had their hands full dealing with the patient's resistances and "transference."

Problem

When the patient entered treatment, he had taken to bed and spent almost all his time there because he felt too weak to get up. His wife had to be constantly at his side or he would panic. Once she was encouraged by a friend to attend the opera alone. The patient wished her a good time and then told her, "When you return, I shall be dead." His secretary was forced into conducting his successful business. Everyone was forced into "the emperor's service." The price he paid for this service was intense suffering in the form of depression, obsessive-compulsive behavior, phobic behavior (especially agoraphobia), divorce from the social world, somatic symptoms, and invalidism.

Treatment

The patient was seen in multiple psychotherapy by Drs. A and B, but both therapists were not present at each interview. We dispensed with the life-style assessment because the patient had other immediate goals. It seemed to us from the patient's behavior that he probably had been raised as a pampered child and that he was using "illness" to tyrannize the world and to gain exemption from the life tasks. If these guesses were correct, we anticipated he would attempt to remain "sick," would resist giving up drugs, and would demand special attention from his therapists. As part of the treatment strategy, the therapists decided to wean him from medication, to give him no special attention, and not to be manipulated by him. Given that he had undergone analysis over a period of more than three decades, the therapists thought he could probably produce a better analysis of his problems than they could. For this reason, interpretation was kept at a minimum. The treatment plan envisaged a tactical and strategic, rather than interpretive, approach.

Some excerpts from the therapists' notes on the early part of treatment follow.

March 8

Dr. B wanted to collect life-style information but the patient immediately complained that he wanted to terminate. He said his previous therapist, Dr. C, had treated him differently. Therapist B was too impersonal. "You won't even give me your home phone number. You aren't impressed by my illness. Your treatment is well meaning but it won't help. Nothing helps. I'm going to go back to Dr. C and ask him to put me in the hospital. He gave me advice and you are so cruel by not telling me what to do."

March 19

Relatively calm. Compares B with Dr. C. Later compares B with A. Favors B over Dr. C because he respects former's strength. Favors B over A because he can succeed in ruffling latter but not former. Talk centers about his use of weakness to overpower others.

March 22

Telephones to say he must be hospitalized. Wife left him [untrue] and secretary left him [it turns out she went to lunch]. Would B come to his office to see him? B asks him to keep appointment in B's office. Patient races about office upset. "I'm sweating water and blood." When B remains calm, patient takes out bottle of Thorazine and threatens to take all. Next he climbs up on radiator, opens window (17th floor), jumps back, and says, "No, it's too high." "You don't help me. Why can't I have an injection?" Then he informs B that B is a soothing influence. "I wish I could spend the whole day with you." B speaks softly to patient and patient speaks quietly. Patient asks for advice about what to do this weekend. B gives antisuggestion and tells him to try to worry as much as he can. He is surprised and dismisses it as "bad advice."

March 29

B was sick on March 26, so patient saw A. "It was useless." No longer worried about state hospital. Thinks he will now wind up as bum because he got drunk last week. His secretary gave him notice but he hopes to keep her "by taking abuse. No one treats a boss like she treats me." Got out of bed and worked last week. Went out selling but "everyone rejected me." When B indicates that he seems to be better, he insists he's deteriorating. When B inquires how, he replies paradoxically, "I beat out my competitors this week."

April 2

Has habit of sticking finger down throat to induce vomiting. Threatens to do so when enters office today. B tells patient about the logical consequences of his act—he will have to mop up. Patient withdraws finger. "If you would leave me alone, I'd fall asleep so fast." B leaves him alone. Patient angrily declaims, "Why do you let me sleep?"

April 9

Too weak even to telephone therapist. If wife goes on vacation, he will kill himself. How can he survive with no one to tell him to eat, to go to bed, to get up? "All I do is vomit and sleep." B suggests that he tyrannizes his wife as he did his mother and sister. He opens window and inquires, "Shall I jump?" B recognizes this as an attempt to intimidate rather than a serious threat and responds, "Suit yourself." Patient closes window and accuses, "You don't care either." Asks whether he can see A next time and before receiving answer, says, "I don't want him anyway." Follows this with "I want to go to the state hospital. Can you get me a private room?" At end of interview falls to knees and sobs, "Help me! Help me to be a human being."

April 12

Enters, falls to knees, encircles therapist's knees, whimpers, "Help me!" So depressed. If only he could end it all. B gives him Adler's suggestion to do one thing each day that would give someone pleasure. Patient admits behaving better. Stopped annoying secretary and let her go home early because of bad weather. Agitation stops.

April 15

Didn't do anything this weekend to give pleasure. However, he did play cards with wife. Took her for drive. Sex with wife for "first time in a long time." B gives encouragement and then repeats "pleasure" suggestion. He can't do it. Calm whole hour. Says his wife has told him to discontinue treatment. Upon inquiry, he says she didn't say exactly that but had said, "I leave it up to you."

April 19

Wants B to accompany him back to his office because he forgot something. Wants shorter hour this week and longer one next week. "Dr. C let me do that." When B declines, he complains, "Doctor, I don't know what to do with you anymore."

April 23

Wouldn't consider suicide. "Perhaps I have a masochistic desire to live." B suggests he must be angry with life. He responds that he wants to be an infant and have all his needs gratified. The world should be a big breast and he should be able to drink without having to suck [probably an interpretation he had received in psychoanalysis]. Yesterday he had fantasy of destroying the whole city.

This weekend he helped his wife work in the garden. He asks for suggestions for weekend. B and patient play "yes-but." B does so deliberately to point out game (cf. Berne's "Why don't you . . .? Yes but" [1964]) to patient. Patient then volunteers possibility of clay modeling. B indicates this may be good choice in that patient can mold, manipulate, and "be violent."

April 29

Had birthday last week and resolved to turn over new leaf for new year but didn't. Cries, "Help me, help me." Depreciates B. "How much would you charge me to come to my summer home? I'm so sick, I vomited blood." When B tells him if he's that sick, hospitalization might be advisable, he smiles and says, "For money, you'd come out." B and patient speak of attitude toward B and attitude toward his father. Patient depreciates both, possibly because he could not dominate either.

May 1

Didn't think he could make it today because he was afraid to walk on street. Didn't sleep all night. So excited, so upset [he seems calm]. Perhaps he should be put in hospital, but then what will happen to his business?

"We could sit here forever and all you would tell me is to get clay. Why don't you give me medicine or advice?" B points out that the patient is much stronger than any medication, as evidenced by number of therapists and treatments he has defeated.

He says he is out of step with world. B repeats an earlier interpretation by A that the patient wants the world to conform to him and follows with statement about his desire to be omnipotent, a desire that makes him feel weak and simultaneously compensates for his feelings of weakness. He confirms with "All Chicago should stand still so I could have a holiday. The police should stop at gunpoint anyone who wants to go to work. But I don't want to. I don't want to do anything anymore. I want a paycheck but I don't want to work." B remarks on shift from "I can't" to "I don't want to." Patient admits and says, "I don't want to get well. Should I make another appointment?" B refers decision back to him. He makes appointment.

May 6

"I'm at the end, dying with fear [enumerates symptoms]. Since five this morning I'm murdering ———— and ————. Such nice people and I'm murdering them and I'm electrocuted. And my secretary and wife can't stand it anymore. Take me to a state hospital. I don't want to go. Take me. I'm getting crazy and you don't help me. Help me, *Lieber Doktor!* I went to the ladies' room twice today to get my secretary and the girls complained to the building office. I'm not above the rules. I knew I violated them. My zipper was down again [he frequently "forgets"] and I just pulled it up before you came in today." B agrees that state hospital might be appropriate if he is becoming "crazier." "Then my wife will divorce me. It's terrible. They have bars there. I won't go. I'm not that bad yet. Why, last week I went out and made a big sale!" B suggests he "practice" his fears and obsessions.

May 8

Seen by A and B, who did summary of his family constellation. It was done very tentatively because of the meager information elicited.

May 13

Complains about symptoms. He had taken his wife to the movies but "was too upset to watch it." He had helped with the raking. Returns to symptoms and begging for Thorazine. "How will I live without Thorazine?" B suggests they ought to talk about how to live. He yells, "With your quiet voice, you'll drive me crazy." B asks, "Would you like me to yell at you like your father did?" "I won't talk to you anymore." "*Lieber Gott,* liberate me from the evil within me." Prays to everyone for help. B counters with "Have you ever solicited your own help?" Patient replies, "I have no strength, I could *cry.* I could shout. I don't have strength. Let me vomit."

May 15

Demands Thorazine or he will have heart attack. B requests a future autobiography. Responds "I don't anticipate anything" and returns to Thorazine question. B points out his real achievement in staying off Thorazine. Patient mentions price in suffering. B points out that this makes it an even greater achievement. Patient accepts idea reluctantly. B points out that they are at cross-purposes because patient wants to continue suffering but have pills; B's goal is to have him stop his suffering. "I want pills." B offers clay. "Shit on your clay."

May 20

Must have Thorazine. Has murderous and self-castrating fantasies. Tells A that A does not know anything about medicine. Dr. C did. Why don't we let him go back to Dr. C? A leaves room with patient following. After three to four minutes patient returns and complains, "You call this treatment?" Dr. A points out demand of patient to have own way. He is a little boy who wants to be big but doesn't think he can make it. He is a pampered tyrant. A also refers to patient's favorite childhood game of lying in bed with sister and playing "Emperor and Empress."

Patient points out innate badness in himself. A points out he creates it. Patient talks of hostility and murder. A interprets look on his face as taking pride in his bad behavior. Patient picks up letter opener, trembles, then grasps hand with other hand but continues to tremble. A tells him that this is a spurious fight between good and evil, that he can decide how he will behave.

He kneaded clay a little while this weekend.

May 22

Last weekend he mowed lawn, tried to read but "I'm nervous. I'm talking to you like a human being but I'm not really a human being." Raw throat. Fears might have throat cancer. Stopped sticking finger down throat to vomit as consequence. Discussion of previously expressed ideas of "like a human being." Fantasy of riding a boat through a storm. Fantasy of A being acclaimed by crowd and patient in fantasy asking B, "Are you used to A getting all the attention?" Complains about wife and secretary, neither of whom will any longer permit tyrannization.

June 3

Relates fantasy of being magician and performing unbelievable feats at the White House. He asked the President whether he was happily married and then produced the President's ring. Nice weekend. Made love to wife at his initiative. Grudgingly admits enjoying it.

June 10

"Ignored my wife this week." Yet he took initiative and they had sex again. Both enjoyed it but he was afraid because he read in a magazine that sex is a drain on the heart. At work secretary is angry. After she checks things, he rechecks. Pledged to God today he wouldn't do it anymore. He'll only check one time more. Outlines several plans for improving business "but I don't have the strength." Wants to cut down to one interview per week because he doesn't get well and can't afford to pay. B suggests that perhaps he is improving if he wants to reduce the number of sessions. Patient rejects and agrees to two sessions weekly.

June 24

Talks about fears. B tells him he will go on vacation next week. He accepts it calmly although he had previously claimed to be unendurably upset. Patient tells B that he has given up vomiting and masturbation, saying, "You have enormous influence on me." B encourages by saying patient made the decision by himself.

Sept. 4

[Patient was not seen during August because he went on a "wonderful" vacation.] Stopped all medication except for occasional use of a mild tranquilizer his family physician prescribed. Able to read and concentrate again. Has surrendered his obsessive ruminations. He and his secretary get along without fighting although she doesn't like him. He is punctual at the office. He and wife get along well. He is more considerate of her. Both are sexually satisfied.

B and patient plan for treatment. Patient expresses reluctance, feeling that he has gone as far as he can. After all, one psychoanalyst said that he was hopeless and had recommended a lobotomy, so this was marked improvement. B agreed, telling patient that if he had considered the patient hopeless, he would not have undertaken treatment, nor would he now be recommending continuation. "What kind of treatment?" B tells him that no external agent (e.g., medicine, lobotomy) will do it, that his salvation will come from within, that he can choose to live life destructively (and self-destructively) or constructively. He proposes to come weekly for four weeks and then biweekly. B does not accept the offer.

Sept. 17

Since yesterday his symptoms have returned. Heart palpitations.

Sept. 25

Took wife to dinner last night. Very pleasant. Business is slow and his obligations are heavy but he is working. He has to exert effort not to backslide. B schedules double interview. Patient doesn't want to see A. It will upset him. He doesn't see any sense in seeing B either but since B insists. . . . Heart palpitations disappeared after last interview. Expresses realistic concerns today and has dropped usual frantic manner. Wants biweekly interviews. B wants weekly. Patient accepts without protest.

As therapy continued, the patient's discussion of symptoms was superseded by discussion of realistic concerns. Resistance waned. When he entered treatment, he perceived himself as a good person who behaved badly because he was "sick." During therapy, he saw through his pretenses and settled for being "a bad guy." However, once he understood his tyranny and was able to accept it, he had the opportunity to ask himself how he preferred to live his life—usefully or uselessly. Because the therapists used the monolithic approach (Alexander & French, 1946; Mosak & Shulman, 1963), after resolving the issue of his tyranny, therapy moved on to his other "basic mistakes," one at a time. The frequency of interviews was decreased, and termination was by mutual agreement.

Follow-Up

The patient improved, remaining off medication. When he devoted himself to his business, it prospered to the point where he could retire early. He moved to a university town, where he studied archaeology, the activity he liked best in life. His relationship with his wife improved, and they traveled abroad. Because of the geographical distance between them, the therapists and the patient had no further contact.

SUMMARY

Adlerian theory may be described as follows:

1. Its approach is social, teleological, phenomenological, holistic, idiographic, and humanistic.

2. Its underlying assumptions are that (a) the individual is unique, (b) the individual is self-consistent, (c) the individual is responsible, (d) the person is creative, an actor, a chooser, and (e) people in a soft-deterministic way can direct their own behavior and control their destinies.

3. Its personality theory takes as its central construct the life-style, a system of subjective convictions held by the individual that contains his or her self-view and world view. From these convictions, other convictions, methods of operation, and goals are derived. The person behaves as if these convictions were true and uses his life-style as a cognitive map with which he explores, comprehends, prejudges, predicts, and controls the environment (the life tasks). Because the person cannot be understood in a vacuum but only in his or her social context, the interaction between the individual and the individual's life tasks is indispensable for the purpose of fully comprehending that individual.

4. "Psychopathology," "mental illness," and similar nomenclature are reifications and perpetuate the *nominal fallacy,* "the tendency to confuse naming with explaining" (Beach, 1955). The "psychopathological" individual is a discouraged person. Such people either have never developed or have lost their courage with respect to meeting the life tasks. With their pessimistic anticipations, they create "arrangements"—evasions, excuses, sideshows, symptoms—to protect their self-esteem, or they may "cop out" completely.

5. Because people's difficulties emanate from faulty perceptions, learnings, values, and goals that have resulted in discouragement, therapy consists of an educative or re-educative endeavor in which two equals cooperatively tackle the educational task. Many of the traditional analytic methods have been retained, although they are understood, and sometimes used, differently by the Adlerian. The focus of therapy is encouragement of the individual. The individual learns to have faith in self, to trust, and to love. The ultimate, *ideal* goal of psychotherapy is to release people's social interest so they may become fellow human beings, cooperators, and contributors to the creation of a better society. Such patients can be said to have actualized themselves. Because therapy is learning, everyone can change. On the entrance door of the Guidance Clinic for Juvenile Delinquency in Vienna was the inscription "It is never too late" (Kramer, 1947).

Adlerian psychology has become a viable, flourishing system. Neglected for several decades, it has in recent years acquired respectability. Training institutes, professional societies, family education centers, and study groups continue to proliferate. With Adlerians being trained in universities rather than solely in institutes, they are writing more and doing research. Non-Adlerians are also engaged in Adlerian research. The previously rare Adlerian dissertation has become more commonplace. Currently, Adlerians are moving into society to renew their attention to the social issues Adler raised 70 years ago—poverty, war, conflict resolution, aggression, religion, substance abuse, and social cooperation. As Way puts it, "We shall need not only, as Adler says, more cooperative individuals, but a society better fitted to fulfill the needs of human beings" (1962, p. 360).

Complementing the Adlerians' endeavors are individuals and groups who have borrowed heavily from Adler, often without acknowledgment or awareness. Keith Sward, reviewing Alexander and French's *Psychoanalytic Therapy* (1946), writes,

> The Chicago group would seem to be Adlerian through and through. . . . The Chicago Institute for Psychoanalysis is not alone in this seeming rediscovery of Rank and Adler. Psychiatry and psychology as a whole seem to be drifting in the same direction. . . . Adler has come to life in other vigorous circles, notably in the publications of the "Horney" school. (1947, p. 601)

We get glimpses of Adler in the Freudian ego-psychologists, neo-Freudians, existential systems, humanistic psychologies, cognitive and constructivist psychologies, person-centered theory, rational emotive therapy, integrity therapy, transactional analysis, and reality therapy. This does not mean that Adlerian psychology will eventually disappear through absorption into other schools of psychology, for, as the motto of the Rockford, Illinois, Teacher Development Center claims, "Education is like a flame. . . . You can give it away without diminishing the one from whom it came." As Joseph Wilder writes in his introduction to *Essays in Individual Psychology* (Adler & Deutsch, 1959), "Most observations and ideas of Alfred Adler have subtly and quietly permeated modern psychological thinking to such a degree that the proper question is not whether one is Adlerian but how much of an Adlerian one is" (p. xv).

ANNOTATED BIBLIOGRAPHY

Ansbacher, H. L., & Ansbacher, R. (Eds.). (1964). *Individual psychology of Alfred Adler* (2nd ed.). New York: Harper Torchbooks.
An almost encyclopedic collection of Adler's writings, this volume displays both the great variety of topics that commanded his attention and the evolution of his thinking. Because of the nature of the construction of this book, it is imperative that the reader read the preface.

Carlson, J., Watts, R. E., & Maniacci, M. (2006). *Adlerian therapy: Theory and practice.* Washington, DC: American Psychological Association.
This is the newest book on Adlerian psychotherapy. Topics such as the therapeutic relationship; individual, couple, group, and family counseling and therapy; assessment and psychological testing; and personality development are covered in detail. Many updated references are included, as well as lists of Adlerian intervention videos that are available.

Manaster, G. J., & Corsini, R. J. (1982). *Individual psychology.* Itasca, IL: F. E. Peacock.
This is the first textbook of Adlerian psychology written in English by two students of Rudolf Dreikurs. Corsini was the former editor of the *Journal of Individual Psychology,*

and Manaster succeeded him. Written in a much simpler style than the Ansbacher and Ansbacher text (1956), this book covers more or less the same materials. Two features make it unique: It contains the most nearly complete Adlerian psychotherapy case summary published to date, and there is a section abstracting the more important research studies published in the field of Adlerian psychology.

Mosak, H. H., & Maniacci, M. (1999). *A primer of Adlerian psychology.* Philadelphia: Brunner/Mazel.
A more recent textbook than Manaster and Corsini (1982), the *Primer* discusses the basic assumptions of Adlerian psychology, life-style, the life tasks as well as their applications in psychotherapy, child guidance, parent education, schools, marriage counseling, and social advocacy.

Mosak, H. H., & Maniacci, M. (1998). *Tactics in counseling and psychotherapy.* Itasca, IL: F. E. Peacock.
The authors present a variety of tactics that may serve as interventions for both Adlerians and non-Adlerians. These tactics aim to answer such questions as "What do I do when my patient . . .?" Various differential diagnosis, encouragement, confrontation, and countertactics are among the methods described and illustrated.

CASE READINGS

Adler, A. (1929). The case of Miss R: The interpretation of a life study. New York: Greenberg.

Adler does an interlinear interpretation of the case study of a patient who in his time would have been labeled "psychasthenic." The patient is also agoraphobic. Since Adler did not treat this patient, the course of therapy is unknown. However, we can observe how Adler constructs a life-style, as well as his understanding of the patient's approach to the life tasks.

Adler, A. (1964). *The case of Mrs. A.: The diagnosis of a life style.* In H. L. Ansbacher & R. R. Ansbacher (Eds.), *Superiority and social interest* (pp. 159–190). Evanston, IL: Northwestern University Press (1969). [Also Chicago: Alfred Adler Institute.] (Original work published in 1931.) [Reprinted in D. Wedding & R. J. Corsini (Eds.) (1979). *Great cases in psychotherapy.* Itasca, IL: F. E. Peacock.]

This publication is similar to the one discussed above and interprets the case study of an obsessive–compulsive woman who fears that she will kill her children.

Ansbacher, H. L. (1966). Lee Harvey Oswald: An Adlerian interpretation. *Psychoanalytic Review, 53,* 379–390.

The psychodynamics of John F. Kennedy's assassin are presented from the Adlerian point of view.

Dreikurs, R. (1959). A record of family counseling sessions. In R. Dreikurs, R. Lowe, M. Sonstegard, & R. J. Corsini (Eds.), *Adlerian family counseling* (pp. 109–152). Eugene, OR: University of Oregon Press.

Two sessions of family counseling conducted by Rudolf Dreikurs and Stefanie Necheles are presented.

The identified patient, a 9-year-old boy, is described by his parents as an angry child.

Frank, I. (1981). My flight toward a new life. *Journal of Individual Psychology, 37*(1), 15–30.

A young anorexic woman describes the course of her eating problem as well as the various treatments, Adlerian and non-Adlerian, that she underwent until the problem was resolved.

Manaster, G. J., & Corsini, R. J. (1982). *Individual psychology.* Itasca, IL: F. E. Peacock.

Chapter 17 offers verbatim excerpts of a course of therapy for a man who in dualistic fashion perceives himself as conflicted, ambivalent, and self-contradictory.

Mosak, H. H. (1972). Life-style assessment: A demonstration based on family constellation. *Individual Psychology, 28,* 232–247.

A verbatim description of a life-style assessment done in public demonstration is presented. The subject is a teenage girl who feels that she is the sole "non-very" person in a "very" family.

Mosak, H. H., & Maniacci, M. (2011). The case of Roger. In D. Wedding & R. J. Corsini (Eds.), *Case studies in psychotherapy.* Belmont, CA: Brooks/Cole.

This case history, which was specifically written to complement this chapter, illustrates many of the methods, techniques, and principles of Adlerian psychotherapy. Careful reading of the case should help the student more fully appreciate how an Adlerian actually proceeds in therapy.

REFERENCES

Adler, Alexandra. (1943). Problems in psychotherapy. *American Journal of Individual Psychology, 3,* 1–5.

Adler, Alexandra. (1951). Alfred Adler's viewpoint in child guidance. In E. Harms (Ed.), *Handbook of child guidance.* New York: Child Care Publications.

Adler, Alfred. (1898). *Gesundheitsbuch für das Schneidergewerbe.* Berlin: C. Heymanns.

Adler, A. (1914). *Das Zärtlichkeitsbedürfnis des Kindes.* In A. Adler & C. Furtmüller (Eds.), *Heilen und Bilden.* München: Reinhardt.

Adler, A. (1917). *Study of organ inferiority and its psychical compensation.* New York: Nervous and Mental Disease Publishing Co.

Adler, A. (1922). *Erziehungsberatungsstellen.* In A. Adler & C. Furtmüller (Eds.), *Heilen und Bilden.* München: Reinhardt.

Adler, A. (1926/1972). *The neurotic constitution.* Freeport, NY: Books for Libraries Press.

Adler, A. (1928). On teaching courage. *Survey Graphic, 61,* 241–242.

Adler, A. (1931/1958). *What life should mean to you.* New York: Capricorn Books.

Adler, A. (1934). Lecture to the Medical Society of Individual Psychology, London. *Individual Psychology Pamphlets, 13,* 11–24.

Adler, A. (1947). How I chose my career. *Individual Psychology Bulletin, 6,* 9–11.

Adler, A. (1959). *Understanding human nature.* New York: Premier Books.

Adler, A. (1963a). Contributions to the theory of hallucinations. In A. Adler, *The practice and theory of individual psychology* (pp. 51–58). Paterson, NJ: Littlefield, Adams.

Adler, A. (1963b). Dreams and dream interpretations. In A. Adler, *The practice and theory of individual psychology* (pp. 214–226). Paterson, NJ: Littlefield, Adams.

Adler, A. (1964a). *Problems of neurosis.* New York: Harper & Row.

Adler, A. (1964b). *Social interest: A challenge to mankind.* New York: Capricorn Books.

Adler, A. (1969). *The science of living.* New York: Doubleday Anchor Books.

Adler, K. A. (1961). Depression in the light of individual psychology. *Journal of Individual Psychology, 17,* 56–67.

Adler, K. A., & Deutsch, D. (Eds.) (1959). *Essays in individual psychology.* New York: Grove Press.

Alexander, F., & French, T. M. (1946). *Psychoanalytic therapy.* New York: Ronald Press.

Allred, G. H. (1976). *How to strengthen your marriage and family.* Provo, UT: Brigham Young University Press.

Angers, W. P. (1960). Clarifications toward the rapprochement between religion and psychology. *Journal of Individual Psychology, 16,* 73–76.

Ansbacher, H. L. (1946). Adler's place today in the psychology of memory. *Journal of Personality, 15,* 197–207.

Ansbacher, H. L. (1952). "Neo-Freudian" or "Neo-Adlerian"? *American Journal of Individual Psychology, 10,* 87–88. [Also in *American Psychologist* (1953), *8,* 165–166.]

Ansbacher, H. L. (1959). The significance of the socioeconomic status of the patients of Freud and of Adler. *American Journal of Psychotherapy, 13,* 376–382.

Ansbacher, H. L. (1961). Suicide: Adlerian point of view. In N. L. Farberow & E. S. Schneidman (Eds.), *The cry for help.* New York: McGraw-Hill.

Ansbacher, H. L. (1962). Was Adler a disciple of Freud? A reply. *Journal of Individual Psychology, 18,* 126–135.

Ansbacher, H. L. (1968). The concept of social interest. *Journal of Individual Psychology, 24,* 131–141.

Ansbacher, H. L. (1969). Suicide as communication: Adler's concept and current applications. *Journal of Individual Psychology, 25,* 174–180.

Ansbacher, H. L. (1972). Adler's "striving for power," in relation to Nietzsche. *Journal of Individual Psychology, 28,* 12–24.

Ansbacher, H. L., & Ansbacher, R. (Eds.). (1956). *The individual psychology of Alfred Adler.* New York: Basic Books.

Beach, F. A. (1955). The descent of instinct. *Psychological Review, 62,* 401–410.

Beck, A. T., & Weishaar, M. E. (2005). Cognitive therapy. In R. J. Corsini & D. Wedding (Eds.), *Current psychotherapies* (pp. 238–268). Belmont, CA: Wadsworth.

Beecher, W., & Beecher, M. (1966). *Parents on the run.* New York: Agora Press.

Berne, E. (1964). *Games people play.* New York: Grove Press.

Bickhard, M. H., & Ford, B. L. (1976). Adler's concept of social interest. *Journal of Individual Psychology, 32,* 27–49.

Bierer, J. (1951). *The day hospital, an experiment in social psychiatry and synthoanalytic psychotherapy.* London: H. K. Lewis.

Bierer, J., & Evans, R. I. (1969). *Innovations in social psychiatry.* London: Avenue Publishing.

Birnbaum, F. (1935). The Individual Psychological Experimental School in Vienna. *International Journal of Individual Psychology, 1,* 118–124.

Birnbaum, F. (1961). Frankl's existential psychology from the viewpoint of Individual Psychology. *Journal of Individual Psychology, 17,* 162–166.

Boldt, R. (1994). *Lifestyle types and therapeutic resistance: An Adlerian model for prediction and intervention of characterological resistance in therapy.* Unpublished Psy.D. dissertation. Chicago: Adler School of Professional Psychology, Chicago, Illinois.

Bottome, P. (1939). *Alfred Adler: A biography.* New York: Putnam.

Brewer, D. H. (1976). *The induction and alteration of state depression: A comparative study.* Unpublished doctoral dissertation. University of Houston.

Brome, V. (1968). *Freud and his early circle.* New York: William Morrow.

Brown, C. (1965). *Manchild in the promised land.* New York: Signet Books.

Brown, J. F. (1976). Parallels between Adlerian psychology and the Afro-American value system. *Individual Psychologist, 13,* 29–33.

Bugental, J. F. T. (1963). Humanistic psychology: A new breakthrough. *American Psychologist, 18,* 563–567.

Carlson, J., Watts, R. E., & Maniacci, M. (2006). *Adlerian therapy: Theory and practice.* Washington, DC: American Psychological Association.

Clark, K. B. (1965). Problems of power and social change: Toward a relevant social psychology. *Journal of Social Issues, 21,* 4–20.

Clark, K. B. (1967a). *Dark ghetto.* New York: Harper Torchbooks.

Clark, K. B. (1967b). Implications of Adlerian theory for understanding of civil rights problems and action. *Journal of Individual Psychology, 23,* 181–190.

Colby, K. M. (1951). On the disagreement between Freud and Adler. *American Imago, 8,* 229–238.

Corsini, R. J. (1953). The behind-the-back technique in group psychotherapy. *Group Psychotherapy, 6,* 102–109.

Corsini, R. J. (1977). Individual education. *Journal of Individual Psychology, 33,* 295–349.

Corsini, R. J. (1979). Individual education. In E. Ignas & R. J. Corsini (Eds.), *Alternative educational systems* (pp. 200–256). Itasca, IL: F. E. Peacock.

Corsini, R. J., & Painter, G. (1975). *The practical parent.* New York: Harper & Row.

Crandall, J. E. (1981). *Theory and measurement of social interest.* New York: Columbia University Press.

Credner, L. (1930). Sicherungen. *Internationale Zeitschrift für Individual Psychologie, 8,* 87–92. [Translated as Safeguards (1936). *International Journal of Individual Psychology, 2,* 95–102.]

Crookshank, F. G. (1933). Individual Psychology and Nietzsche. *Individual Psychology Medical Pamphlets, 10,* 7–76.

Deutsch, D. (1967). Group therapy with married couples. *Individual Psychologist, 4,* 56–62.

Dinkmeyer, D. C., & Carlson, J. (1989). *Taking the time for love.* Englewood Cliffs, NJ: Prentice-Hall.

Dinkmeyer, D., & Dreikurs, R. (1963). *Encouraging children to learn: The encouragement process.* Englewood Cliffs, NJ: Prentice-Hall.

Dreikurs, R. (1944). The meaning of dreams. *Chicago Medical School Quarterly, 5*(3), 4–7.

Dreikurs, R. (1948). *The challenge of parenthood.* New York: Duell, Sloan & Pearce.

Dreikurs, R. (1949). The four goals of children's misbehavior. *Nervous Child, 6,* 3–11.

Dreikurs, R. (1950). Techniques and dynamics of multiple psychotherapy. *Psychiatric Quarterly, 24,* 788–799.

Dreikurs, R. (1951). The function of emotions. *Christian Register, 130*(3), 11–14, 24.

Dreikurs, R. (1957). Psychotherapy as correction of faulty social values. *Journal of Individual Psychology, 13,* 150–158.

Dreikurs, R. (1958). A reliable differential diagnosis of psychological or somatic disturbances. *International Record of Medicine, 171,* 238–242.

Dreikurs, R. (1959). Early experiments with group psychotherapy. *American Journal of Psychotherapy, 13,* 882–891.

Dreikurs, R. (1961). The Adlerian approach to therapy. In M. I. Stein (Ed.), *Contemporary psychotherapies* (pp. 80–94). Glencoe, IL: The Free Press.

Dreikurs, R. (1962). Can you be sure the disease is functional? *Consultant* (Smith, Kline & French Laboratories).

Dreikurs, R. (1963). Psychodynamic diagnosis in psychiatry. *American Journal of Psychiatry, 119,* 1045–1048.

Dreikurs, R. (1968). *Psychology in the classroom.* New York: Harper & Row.

Dreikurs, R. (1969). Social interest: The basis of normalcy. *The Counseling Psychologist, 1,* 45–48.

Dreikurs, R. (1971). *Social equality: The challenge of today.* Chicago: Henry Regnery.

Dreikurs, R. (1972). Technology of conflict resolution. *Journal of Individual Psychology, 28,* 203–206.

Dreikurs, R., Corsini, R. J., Lowe, R., & Sonstegard, M. (1959). *Adlerian family counseling.* Eugene, OR: University of Oregon Press.

Dreikurs, R., & Grey, L. (1968). *Logical consequences.* New York: Meredith.

Dreikurs, R., Grunwald, B., & Pepper, F. C. (1982). *Maintaining sanity in the classroom* (2nd ed.). New York: Harper & Row.

Dreikurs, R., & Mosak, H. H. (1966). The tasks of life. I. Adler's three tasks. *Individual Psychologist, 4,* 18–22.

Dreikurs, R., & Mosak, H. H. (1967). The tasks of life. II. The fourth life task. *Individual Psychologist, 4,* 51–55.

Dreikurs, R., Shulman, B. H., & Mosak, H. H. (1952a). Patient-therapist relationship in multiple psychotherapy. I. Its advantages to the therapist. *Psychiatric Quarterly, 26,* 219–227.

Dreikurs, R., Mosak, H. H., & Shulman, B. H. (1952b). Patient-therapist relationship in multiple psychotherapy. II. Its advantages for the patient. *Psychiatric Quarterly, 26,* 590–596.

Dreikurs, R., Shulman, B. H., & Mosak, H. H. (1982). *Multiple psychotherapy.* Chicago: Alfred Adler Institute.

Dreikurs, R., & Soltz, V. (1964). *Children: The challenge.* New York: Duell, Sloan & Pearce.

Dunlap, K. (1933). *Habits: Their making and unmaking.* New York: Liveright.

Eckstein, D., & Kern, R. (2002). *Psychological fingerprints: Lifestyle assessment and interventions* (5th ed.). Dubuque: Kendall/Hunt.

Edgar, T. (1975). Social interest—another view. *Individual Psychologist, 12,* 16–24.

Elam, H. (1969a). Cooperation between African and Afro-American, cultural highlights. *Journal of the National Medical Association, 61,* 30–35.

Elam, H. (1969b). Malignant cultural deprivation, its evolution. *Pediatrics, 44,* 319–326.

Ellenberger, H. F. (1970). *The discovery of the unconscious.* New York: Basic Books.

Ellis, A. (1957). Rational psychotherapy and Individual Psychology. *Journal of Individual Psychology, 13,* 38–44.

Ellis, A. (1963). Toward a more precise definition of "emotional" and "intellectual" insight. *Psychological Reports, 13,* 125–126.

Ellis, A. (1970). Humanism, values, rationality. *Journal of Individual Psychology, 26,* 37–38.

Ellis, A. (1971). Reason and emotion in the Individual Psychology of Adler. *Journal of Individual Psychology, 27,* 50–64.

Farau, A. (1953). The influence of Alfred Adler on current psychology. *American Journal of Individual Psychology, 10,* 59–76.

Farau, A. (1964). Individual psychology and existentialism. *Individual Psychologist, 2,* 1–8.

Federn, E. (1963). Was Adler a disciple of Freud? A Freudian view. *Journal of Individual Psychology, 19,* 80–81.

Fiedler, F. E. (1950). A comparison of therapeutic relationships in psychoanalytic, non-directive and Adlerian therapy. *Journal of Consulting Psychology, 14,* 436–445.

Foley, Y.C., Matheny, K.B., & Curlette, W. (2008). A cross-generational study of Adlerian personality traits and life satisfaction in Mainland China. *Journal of Individual Psychology, 64,* 324–338.

Forer, L. K. (1977). Bibliography of birth order literature of the 1970s. *Journal of Individual Psychology, 33,* 122–141.

Frank, L. K. (1939). Projective methods for the study of personality. *Journal of Personality, 8,* 389–413.

Frankl, V. E. (1963). *Man's search for meaning.* New York: Washington Square Press.

Frankl, V. E. (1970). Forerunner of existential psychiatry. *Journal of Individual Psychology, 26,* 38.

Fromm-Reichman, F. (1949). Notes on personal and professional requirements of a psychotherapist. *Psychiatry, 12,* 361–378.

Goldstein, K. (1939). *The organism.* New York: American Book Co.

Gottesfeld, H. (1966). Changes in feelings of powerlessness in a community action program. *Psychological Reports, 19,* 978.

Grunwald, B. (1954). The application of Adlerian principles in a classroom. *American Journal of Individual Psychology, 11,* 131–141.

Gushurst, R. S. (1971). *The reliability and concurrent validity of an idiographic approach to the interpretation of early recollections.* Unpublished doctoral dissertation. University of Chicago.

Heine, R. W. (1953). A comparison of patients' reports on psychotherapeutic experience with psychoanalytic, non-directive, and Adlerian therapists. *American Journal of Psychotherapy, 7,* 16–23.

Hemming, J. (1956). *Mankind against the killers.* London: Longmans, Green.

Hill, M. B., Brack, G., Qalinge, L., & Dean, J. (2008). Adlerian similarities to a Sangoma Treating AIDS in South Africa. *Journal of Individual Psychology, 64,* 310–323.

Hinrichsen, O. (1913). Unser Verstehen der seelischen Zusammenhänge in der Neurose and Freud's and Adler's Theorien. *Zentralblätter für Psychoanalyse, 3,* 369–393.

Horney, K. (1951). *Neurosis and human growth.* London: Routledge & Kegan Paul.

Jahn, E., & Adler, A. (1964). Religion and Individual Psychology. In H. L. Ansbacher & R. Ansbacher (Eds.), *Superiority and social interest.* Evanston, IL: Northwestern University Press. [Reprinted in *Individual Psychology,* 1987, *43*(4), 522–526.]

James, W. (1890). *Principles of psychology.* New York: Holt.

James, W. T. (1947). Karen Horney and Erich Fromm in relation to Alfred Adler. *Individual Psychology Bulletin, 6,* 105–116.

Kadis, A. L. (1956). Re-experiencing the family constellation in group psychotherapy. *American Journal of Individual Psychology, 12,* 63–68.

Kazan, S. (1978). Gemeinschaftsgefühl means caring. *Journal of Individual Psychology, 34,* 3–10.

Kern, R., Gormley, L., & Curlette, W.L. (2008). BASIS-A Inventory empirical studies: Research findings from 2000 to 2006. *Journal of Individual Psychology, 64,* 280–309.

Kramer, H. D. (1947). Preventive psychiatry. *Individual Psychology Bulletin, 7,* 12–18.

Krausz, E. O. (1935). The pessimistic attitude. *International Journal of Individual Psychology, 1,* 86–99.

Krausz, E. O. (1959). The commonest neurosis. In K. A. Adler & D. Deutsch (Eds.), *Essays in individual psychology* (pp. 108–118). New York: Grove Press.

La Porte, G. H. (1966). Social interest in action: A report on one attempt to implement Adler's concept. *Individual Psychologist, 4,* 22–26.

Lazarsfeld, S. (1952). Pitfalls in psychotherapy. *American Journal of Individual Psychology, 10,* 20–26.

Lazarsfeld, S. (1966). The courage for imperfection. *Journal of Individual Psychology, 22,* 163–165.

Lewin, K. (1935). *A dynamic theory of personality.* New York: McGraw-Hill.

Linden, G. W. (2007). Special essay: An Adlerian view of aging. *Journal of Individual Psychology, 63,* 387–398.

Lombardi, D. M. (1969). The special language of the addict. *Pastoral Psychology, 20,* 51–52.

Low, A. A. (1952). *Mental health through will training.* Boston: Christopher.

Mansager, E. (Ed.). (2008). Affirming lesbian, gay, bisexual, and transgender individuals [Special issue]. *Journal of Individual Psychology, 64*(2).

Maslow, A. H. (1962). Was Adler a disciple of Freud? A note. *Journal of Individual Psychology, 18,* 125.

Maslow, A. H. (1970). Holistic emphasis. *Journal of Individual Psychology, 26,* 39.

May, R. (1970). Myth and guiding fiction. *Journal of Individual Psychology, 26,* 39.

McArthur, H. (1958). The necessity of choice. *Journal of Individual Psychology, 14,* 153–157.

Meerloo, J. A. M. (1970). Pervasiveness of terms and concepts. *Journal of Individual Psychology, 26,* 40.

Miley, C. H. (1969). Birth-order research, 1963–1967: Bibliography and index. *Journal of Individual Psychology, 25,* 64–70.

Mosak, H. H. (1954). The psychological attitude in rehabilitation. *American Archives of Rehabilitation Therapy, 2,* 9–10.

Mosak, H. H. (1958). Early recollections as a projective technique. *Journal of Projective Techniques, 22,* 302–311. [Also in G. Lindzey & C. S. Hall (Eds.). (1965). *Theories of personality: Primary sources and research.* New York: Wiley.]

Mosak, H. H. (1967). Subjective criteria of normality. *Psychotherapy, 4,* 159–161.

Mosak, H. H. (1968). The interrelatedness of the neuroses through central themes. *Journal of Individual Psychology, 24,* 67–70.

Mosak, H. H. (1971). Strategies for behavior change in schools: Consultation strategies. *Counseling Psychologist, 3,* 58–62.

Mosak, H. H. (1972). Life style assessment: A demonstration based on family constellation. *Journal of Individual Psychology, 28,* 232–247.

Mosak, H. H. (1985). Interrupting a depression: The pushbutton technique. *Individual Psychology, 41*(2), 210–214.

Mosak, H. H. (1987a). *Ha ha and aha: The role of humor in psychotherapy.* Muncie, IN: Accelerated Development.

Mosak, H. H. (1987b). Guilt, guilt feelings, regret and repentance. *Individual Psychology, 43*(3), 288–295.

Mosak, H. H. (1987c). Religious allusions in psychotherapy. *Individual Psychology, 43*(4), 496–501.

Mosak, H. H. (1991). "I don't have social interest": Social interest as construct. *Individual Psychology, 47,* 309–320.

Mosak, H. H., & DiPietro, R. (2006). *Early recollections: Interpretative methods and applications.* New York: Routledge.

Mosak, H. H., & Dreikurs, R. (1967). The life tasks. III. The fifth life task. *Individual Psychologist, 5,* 16–22.

Mosak, H. H., & Fletcher, S. J. (1973). Purposes of delusions and hallucinations. *Journal of Individual Psychology, 29,* 176–181.

Mosak, H. H., & Gushurst, R. S. (1971). What patients say and what they mean. *American Journal of Psychotherapy, 3,* 428–436.

Mosak, H. H., & Kopp, R. (1973). The early recollections of Adler, Freud, and Jung. *Journal of Individual Psychology, 29,* 157–166.

Mosak, H. H., & LaFevre, C. (1976). The resolution of "intrapersonal conflict." *Journal of Individual Psychology, 32,* 19–26.

Mosak, H. H., & Maniacci, M. P. (1998). *Tactics in counseling and psychotherapy.* Itasca, IL: F. E. Peacock.

Mosak, H. H., & Mosak, B. (1975b). Dreikurs' four goals: The clarification of some misconceptions. *Individual Psychologist, 12*(2), 14–16.

Mosak, H. H., & Schneider, S. (1977). Masculine protest, penis envy, women's liberation and sexual equality. *Journal of Individual Psychology, 33,* 193–201.

Mosak, H. H., & Shulman, B. H. (1963). *Individual psychotherapy: A syllabus.* Chicago: Alfred Adler Institute.

Mozdzierz, G. J., & Lottman, T. J. (1973). Games married couples play: Adlerian view. *Journal of Individual Psychology, 29,* 182–194.

Mullahy, P. (1955). *Oedipus: Myth and complex.* New York: Evergreen.

Murphy, G. (1947). *Personality: A biosocial approach to origins and structure.* New York: Harper.

Neuer, A. (1936). Courage and discouragement. *International Journal of Individual Psychology, 2,* 30–50.

Nikelly, A. G. (1971a). Basic processes in psychotherapy. In A. G. Nikelly (Ed.), *Techniques for behavior change* (pp. 27–32). Springfield, IL: Charles C Thomas.

Nikelly, A. G. (1971b). Developing social feeling in psychotherapy. In A. G. Nikelly (Ed.), *Techniques for behavior change* (pp. 91–95). Springfield, IL: Charles C Thomas.

Nikelly A. G. (1971c). The protesting student. In A. G. Nikelly (Ed.), *Techniques for behavior change* (pp. 159–164). Springfield, IL: Charles C Thomas.

O'Reilly, C., Cizon, E., Flanagan, J., & Pflanczer, S. (1965). *Men in jail.* Chicago: Loyola University.

Painter, G., & Corsini, R. J. (1989). *Effective discipline in the home and the school.* Muncie, IN: Accelerated Development.

Pancner, K. R. (1978). The use of parables and fables in Adlerian psychotherapy. *Individual Psychologist, 15,* 19–29.

Papanek, E. (1971). Delinquency. In A. G. Nikelly (Ed.), *Techniques for behavior change* (pp. 177–183). Springfield, IL: Charles C Thomas.

Papanek, H. (1954). Combined group and individual therapy in private practice. *American Journal of Psychotherapy, 8,* 679–686.

Papanek, H. (1956). Combined group and individual therapy in the light of Adlerian psychology. *International Journal of Group Psychotherapy, 6,* 135–146.

Papanek, H. (1959). Emotion and intellect in psychotherapy. *American Journal of Psychotherapy, 13,* 150–173.

Papanek, H., & Papanek, E. (1961). Individual Psychology today. *American Journal of Psychotherapy, 15,* 4–26.

Pelzman, O. (1952). Some problems in the use of psychotherapy. *Psychiatric Quarterly Supplement, 26,* 53–58.

Pew, M. L., & Pew, W. (1972). Adlerian marriage counseling. *Journal of Individual Psychology, 28,* 192–202.

Phillips, C. E., & Corsini, R. J. (1982). *Give in or give up.* Chicago: Nelson–Hall.

Rasey, M. I. (1956). Toward the end. In C. E. Moustakas (Ed.), *The self: Explorations in personal growth* (pp. 247–260). New York: Harper.

Rasmussen, P. R. (Ed.). (2006). Anxiety and depression [Special issue]. *Journal of Individual Psychology, 62* (4).

Reik, T. (1948). *Listening with the third ear.* New York: Farrar, Straus & Cudahy.

Rogers, C. R. (1951). *Client-centered therapy.* Boston: Houghton Mifflin.

Rosenthal, D., & Frank, J. D. (1956). Psychotherapy and the placebo effect. *Psychological Bulletin, 53,* 294–302.

Rotgers, F., & Maniacci, M. (Eds.). (2006). *Antisocial personality disorder: A practitioner's guide to comparative treatments.* New York Springer.

Schneider, M. F., Kern, R.M., & Curlette, W. L. (Eds.). (2007). Narcissism, imagery, early recollections, and social interest [Special issue]. *Journal of Individual Psychology, 63*(2).

Seidler, R. (1967). The individual psychologist looks at testing. *Individual Psychologist, 5,* 3–6.

Seidler, R., & Zilahi, L. (1949). The Vienna child guidance clinics. In A. Adler & Associates, *Guiding the child* (pp. 9–27). London: Allen & Unwin.

Shlien, J. M., Mosak, H. H., & Dreikurs, R. (1962). Effect of time limits: A comparison of two psychotherapies. *Journal of Counseling Psychology, 9,* 31–34.

Shoben, E. J., Jr. (1957). Toward a concept of normal personality. *American Psychologist, 12,* 183–189.

Shoobs, N. E. (1964). Role-playing in the individual psychotherapy interview. *Journal of Individual Psychology, 20,* 84–89.

Shulman, B. H. (1962). The meaning of people to the schizophrenic and the manic-depressive. *Journal of Individual Psychology, 18,* 151–156.

Shulman, B. H., & Klapman, H. (1968). Organ inferiority and psychiatric disorders in childhood. In E. Harms (Ed.), *Pathogenesis of nervous and mental diseases* (pp. 49–62). New York: Libra.

Shulman, B. H., & Mosak, H. H. (1977). Birth order and ordinal position. *Journal of Individual Psychology, 33,* 114–121.

Shulman, B. H., & Mosak, H. H. (1988). *Manual for lifestyle assessment.* Muncie, IN: Accelerated Development.

Sicher, L., & Mosak, H. H. (1967). Aggression as a secondary phenomenon *Journal of Individual Psychology, 23,* 232–235.

Simpson, H. N. (1966). *Stoic apologetics.* Oak Park, IL: Author.

Smuts, J. C. (1961). *Holism and evolution.* New York: Viking Press.

Soltz, V. (1967). *Study group leader's manual.* Chicago: Alfred Adler Institute.

Sperry, L., & Mansager, E. (2007). The relationship between psychology and spirituality: An initial taxonomy for spiritually oriented counseling and psychotherapy. *Journal of Individual Psychology, 63,* 359–370.

Spiel, O. (1962). *Discipline without punishment.* London: Faber & Faber.

Starr, A. (1977). *Psychodrama.* Chicago: Nelson-Hall.

Strupp, H. H. (1972). Freudian analysis today. *Psychology Today, 6,* 33–40.

Sullivan, H. S. (1954). *The psychiatric interview.* New York: Norton.

Sward, K. (1947). Review. [Review of K. Horney, *Our inner conflicts.*] *Science,* December 1, 600–601.

Taylor, J. A. (1975). Early recollections as a projective technique: A review of some recent validation studies. *Journal of Individual Psychology, 31,* 213–218.

Toman, W. (1970). Never mind your horoscope, birth order rules all. *Psychology Today, 4,* 45–48, 68–69.

Vaihinger, H. (1965). *The philosophy of "as if."* London: Routledge & Kegan Paul.

Von Sassen, H. W. (1967). Adler's and Freud's concepts of man: A phenomenological comparison. *Journal of Individual Psychology, 23,* 3–10.

Watkins, C. E., Jr. (1982). A decade of research in support of Adlerian psychological theory. *Individual Psychology, 38*(1), 90–99.

Watkins, C. E., Jr. (1983). Some characteristics of research on Adlerian theory, 1970–1981. *Individual Psychology, 39*(1), 99–110.

Watkins, C. E., & Guarnaccia, C. A. (1999). The scientific study of Adlerian psychology. In R. E. Watts & J. Carlson (Eds.), *Interventions and strategies in counseling and psychotherapy* (pp. 207–230). Philadelphia: Accelerated Development.

Watts, R. E. (Ed.). (2003). *Adlerian, cognitive and constructivist therapies: An integrative dialogue.* New York: Springer.

Watts, R. E., & Carlson, J. (Eds.). (1999). *Interventions and strategies in counseling and psychotherapy.* Philadelphia: Accelerated Development.

Way, L. (1962). *Adler's place in psychology.* New York: Collier Books.

Westen, D., Novotny, C. M., & Thompson-Brenner, H. (2004). The empirical status of empirically supported psychotherapies: Assumptions, findings, and reporting in controlled clinical trials. *Psychological Bulletin, 130,* 631–663.

Wexberg, E. (1929). *Individual Psychology.* London: Allen & Unwin.

Wexberg, E. (1929/1970). *Individual psychological treatment.* Chicago: Alfred Adler Institute. (Original published in 1929.)

Wheeler, M. S., Kern, R. M., & Curlette, W.L. (1993). *BASIS-A Inventory.* Highlands, NC: TRT.

White, R. W. (1957). Adler and the future of ego psychology. *Journal of Individual Psychology, 13,* 112–124.

Wittels, F. (1939). The neo-Adlerians. *American Journal of Sociology, 45,* 433–445.

Wolfe, W. B. (1932). *How to be happy though human.* London: Routledge & Kegan Paul.

Zborowski, R. (1997). *The phenomenon of transference: An Adlerian perspective.* Unpublished Psy.D. dissertation, Adler School of Professional Psychology, Chicago, Illinois.

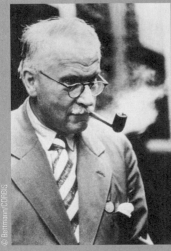

Carl Jung, 1875–1961

4 | ANALYTICAL PSYCHOTHERAPY

Claire Douglas

OVERVIEW

Analytical psychology, the psychodynamic system and personality theory created by Carl Gustav Jung, builds on Freud's and Adler's perspectives, offering an expanded view of humanity's personal and collective realities. Analytical psychotherapy offers a map of the human psyche that encompasses conscious and unconscious elements, including both a transpersonal (archetypal) and a personal layer in the unconscious. The goals of psychotherapy are reintegration, self-knowledge, and individuation, with a heartfelt awareness of the human condition, individual responsibility, and a connection to the transcendent replacing a wounded, one-sided, rationalistic, and limited sense of self. Therapy taps into the healing and self-regulating potential of the psyche by means of a profound encounter between the interacting personalities of patient and therapist.

Basic Concepts

The cornerstone of Jung's psychological system is his concept of the psyche, the inner realm of personality that balances the outer reality of material objects. Jung defined *psyche* as a combination of spirit, soul, and idea; he viewed psychic reality as the sum of the conscious and unconscious processes. According to Jung, this inner world influences biochemical processes in the body, affects the instincts, and determines one's perception of outer reality. Jung proposed that physical matter can be known only through a person's psychic images of outside reality; thus, what people perceive is in large part determined by who they are.

113

The reality of the psyche was Jung's working hypothesis, confirmed through material he gathered from fantasy, myth, image, and the behavior of individual people. Jung mapped the psyche in terms of a whole made up of balancing and compensatory opposites. Key aspects of his map of the psyche are a personal and collective unconscious as well as a personal and collective consciousness.

Jung's description of the personal unconscious is similar to Freud's, but more extensive. In Jungian theory, an individual's personal unconscious contains not only material unacceptable to one's ego and superego and therefore repressed, but also material unimportant to the psyche, temporarily or permanently dropped from consciousness. It also contains undeveloped parts of one's personality not yet ready for or admitted to consciousness, as well as elements rising from the collective unconscious.

Collective unconscious is Jung's term for the vast, hidden psychic resource shared by all human beings. Jung discovered the collective unconscious through his patients' disclosures, his own self-analysis, and cross-cultural studies. He found the same basic motifs expressed in fantasies, dreams, symbols, or myths. Images that emerge out of the collective unconscious are shared by all people but modified by their personal experiences. Jung called these motifs archetypal images and depicted the collective unconscious as organized in underlying patterns.

An *archetype* is an organizing principle, a system of readiness, and a dynamic nucleus of energy. As an organizing principle, an archetype is analogous to the circuitry pattern in the brain that orders and structures reality; as a system of readiness, it parallels animals' instincts; as a dynamic nucleus of energy, it propels a person's actions and reactions in a patterned way. Jung believed that humans have an inherited predisposition to form their personalities and to view reality according to universal inner patterns.

Archetypes can be seen as pathways along whose course energy flows from the collective unconscious into consciousness and action. Jung wrote that there were as many archetypal images in the collective unconscious as there were typical situations in life, and that they have appeared in individual experience from time immemorial and will reappear in the future whenever analogous situations arise. Some archetypal patterns that became a major focus of Jung's work and a fertile source for popular psychology are the Heroic Quest; the Night Sea Journey; the Inner Child (often seen as the childlike part of one's own personality) and Divine Child; the Maiden, Mother, and Goddess; the Wise Old Man; and the Wild Man.

Whereas the collective unconscious reveals itself to a person by means of such archetypal images, the personal unconscious makes itself known through *complexes*. Archetypal images flow from the collective unconscious into the personal unconscious by means of a *complex* (a sensitive, energy-filled cluster of emotions, such as an attitude toward one's father or anyone resembling him). Jung's idea of the complex came from his research on the Word Association Test. Jung would read a list of words aloud, asking subjects to respond with the first word that came to their minds; he then repeated the list, with the subjects attempting to recall their initial responses. Jung noticed pauses, failures to respond or remember, and bodily reactions, and he believed that such variations revealed sensitive, hidden areas. Jung named these reactions complexes— emotionally charged associations of ideas and feelings that act as magnets to draw a net of imagery, memories, and ideas into their orbit.

Jung believed the complex to be so important that when he broke with Freud and looked for a name for his form of psychoanalysis, his first choice was Complex Psychology. Freud and Adler adopted Jung's terminology of the complex, but Jung's formulation was far richer than those of his colleagues. Jung believed that even though a complex may have restricting, upsetting, or other disturbing consequences in some instances, it can also be positive, serving to bring matters of importance to consciousness. Complexes demand personal confrontation and response that can promote a person's development and growth. One can relate to a complex positively by meeting its demand, but this takes hard psychological work. Many people try to manage a complex by projecting its contents: A man with a negative mother complex, for instance, may see all women in an exaggeratedly negative light. (*Projection* means attributing to another person something that really belongs to one's own personality.) Another way a person may try to avoid a complex is by repression. Thus, a woman with a negative mother complex may cut herself off from all that she considers feminine so as not to resemble her mother in any way. Another woman with a mother complex might perceive herself as an all-good, "earth mother" type of woman. In more extreme cases, a complex may overpower an individual so that the person loses touch with reality, becoming psychotic; a psychotic woman who has a mother complex may believe she is Mother Nature and the mother of everything and everybody on earth.

Rather than seeing the unconscious as something that needs to be cleaned out and made conscious, Jung felt that individuals grow toward wholeness when both conscious and unconscious parts of the mind work in harmony. Because of this natural movement toward balance and self-healing, Jung concluded that neurosis contained the seeds of its own cure and had the energy to bring about growth and healing. The Jungian analyst serves as a catalyst to promote balance growth, and integration.

Other Systems

Jung's theories have influenced contemporary religious, cultural, and sociological thought, as well as art, literature, and drama. Nevertheless, psychology in general, and modern psychotherapeutic systems in particular, frequently overlook or ignore Jung's influence. There are many reasons for this, including the difficulty of Jung's writing style and the bitter parochialism of some early psychoanalysts. The situation is compounded by the tendency of psychologists to believe what they have *heard* about Jung rather than reading what he wrote. Today's psychologists receive a rigorously scientific education that often leads them to fear "soft" science and to avoid a system that they have been told is mystical. In reality, the pragmatism of Jung's practical and inclusive approach to psychotherapy has contributed much to the general field of psychology. To ignore one of the three great early psychodynamic theoreticians of the twentieth century is to travel with an incomplete map of the human psyche.

Jung started to develop his own form of psychoanalysis and to treat patients before he met Freud. However, his debt to Freud is great. Perhaps most important to Jung were Freud's exploration of the unconscious through free association, his focus on the significance of dreams, and his stress on the role of early childhood experiences in the formation of personality (Davis, 2008; Ellenberger, 1981). Jung constructed a map of these areas that became broader and more inclusive than Freud's.

Jung focused on the complex as the royal road to the unconscious, whereas Freud emphasized the importance of dreams. Yet dreams play a more significant role in Jung's system than in Freud's, since Jung saw dreams as more meaningful than simple wish-fulfillments, requiring a more thorough and well-rounded technique of dream analysis. For Jung, Freud's Oedipus complex was only one of many possible complexes and not necessarily the most important one. Sexuality and aggression, rather than being the sole channels for the expression of libido, were only two of its many possible routes. Neurosis had many causes, including, but not limited to, sexual problems. Perhaps the most salient difference between Freud and Jung resulted from Jung's belief that the quest for meaning was as strong a need as the sex drive.

Jung believed that certain people would profit most from a Freudian analysis, others from an Adlerian analysis, and still others from a Jungian analysis. He viewed Adler's theory of dreams as similar to his own. Both theories held that dreams could reveal what an individual wanted not to recognize in himself or herself (what Jung called the *shadow* aspects of the personality). Both Jung and Adler believed that dreams reveal the underlying pattern of the way an individual relates to the world. Adler and Jung also stressed the importance of first memories, and of fulfilling life tasks and one's duties to society. Jung taught that unless these tasks were fulfilled, neurosis would result. They both met the individual patient on a more equal footing than Freud. Freud had his patients lie on a couch and free associate, but Jung and Adler sat face-to-face with their patients. Finally, both Adler and Jung believed that psychotherapy should look to the future as well as to the past. Jung's ideas of life goals and forward-looking (teleological) energy are similar to Adler's views.

Life-span psychologists owe much to Jung. Erik Erikson's life stages, Lawrence Kohlberg's stages of moral development, and Carol Gilligan's reevaluation and redefinition of Kohlberg's work to reflect women's development—all express Jung's ideas of individuation over the life span. Jung's theories inspired Henry A. Murray's Needs-Press Theory of Personology, and Jung's encouragement of fantasies inspired the Thematic Apperception Test (Christiana Morgan, its first author, and Murray were analyzed by Jung). Gestalt therapy can be seen as an extension of Jung's method of dream interpretation. Jungians such as E. C. Whitmont and Sylvia Perera (1992) use a combination of gestalt enactment and active imagination (a conscious exploration of one's fantasies) as core analytic tools. J. L. Moreno's psychodrama reflects Jung's encouragement of patients' enacting their dreams and fantasies; Moreno's ideas of role and of surplus reality mirror Jung's belief in a pluralistic psyche composed of many archetypal images and possible roles.

Harry Stack Sullivan's *good me* and *bad me* reflect Jung's concepts of positive and negative *shadow* (the rejected or unrecognized parts of one's personality). Alexander Lowen's bioenergetic theory follows Jung's theory of typology, and Jung's four functions of *thinking, feeling, sensation,* and *intuition* loosely parallel Lowen's hierarchy of personality functions. Holistic therapies of all varieties, from the Adlerian to the most modern, share with Jung the idea of a person made up of many parts in service to the whole, with the individual having a normal urge toward growth and healing. Self-actualizing theories, such as those derived from Abraham Maslow's work, stress the forward-looking and optimistic parts of Jung's psychology, and the person-centered psychology of Carl Rogers echoes Jung's human interest and personal devotion to his patients. Jung (1935a) insisted on the human quality in analysis, emphasizing the integrity of the patient who "inasmuch as he is an individual . . . can only become what he is and always was . . . the best thing the doctor can do is lay aside his whole apparatus of methods and theory" (p. 10) in order to be with the patient as a fellow human being.

Theories that have emerged from neo-Freudian ego psychology, such as Melanie Klein's and Erich Fromm's theories, share so much with Jungian thought that they cross-fertilize each other and are producing a vigorous hybrid. Jungians have pointed out the similarity of their constructs to Jung's original formulations in realms such as the description of infancy and its tasks, the internalization of parts of others' personalities, projections, and the death instinct (e.g., Maduro & Wheelwright, 1977; Solomon, 2009). Barbara Stephens (1999) sees the following Jungian themes fertilizing post-Freudian thought: the centrality of self and subjective experience; countertransference as helpful analytic data; the role of symbol and symbol formation; the importance of primitive (and infantile) affective states; and Freudian feminists' focus on desire as a significant conduit of integration and healing.

Jung's emphasis on the value of being as well as doing, and his deep trust in religious or mystical feelings, are similar to many Asian psychotherapies (Young-Eisendrath, 2008; Higuchi, 2009). Jung's method for incubating fantasies in active imagination is a directed meditation. Jung lectured widely on Asian systems of thought, comparing them to his own theories; perhaps his most cogent lecture was on yoga in relation to the analysis of one of his patients (Douglas, 1997b).

HISTORY

Precursors

Carl Gustav Jung (1875–1961), the eldest son of a clergyman, grew up in the German-speaking part of Switzerland during the final quarter of the nineteenth century. His mother came from a family of theologians; his father's father, a physician, had also been a renowned poet, philosopher, and classical scholar. Jung received a thorough education embedded not only in the Protestant theological tradition but also in classical Greek and Latin literature. He was influenced especially by the pre-Socratic philosopher Heraclitus, by the mystic Jacob Boehme, by romantic philosophy and psychiatry, and by Asian philosophy. During an era that marked the rise of scientific positivism, Jung's teachers emphasized a rational, optimistic, and progressive view of human nature. Nevertheless, Jung was drawn instead to romanticism, which valued the irrational, the occult, the mysterious, and the unconscious. Romanticism had a more pessimistic view of human nature than positivism did. According to romantic philosophy, humans were divided and polarized; they yearned for a unity and wholeness that had been lost. This yearning manifested itself through the desire to plumb the depths of the natural world as well as the individual soul (Douglas, 2008).

Romantic philosophy underlay nineteenth-century anthropology, linguistics, and archaeology, as well as research on sexuality and the inner worlds of the mentally ill—all topics that interested Jung. Romanticism also manifested itself in the exploration of parapsychological phenomena and the occult.

Tracing the specific sources of Jung's ideas would require many chapters (see especially Bair, 2003, Bishop, 2009, and Shamdasani, 2003). Perhaps the best brief coverage is by Henri Ellenberger (1981), who stresses Jung's debt to romantic philosophy and psychiatry. The theories of Goethe, Kant, Schiller, and Nietzsche were influential in forming Jung's style of thinking in terms of opposites.

Jung's fellow townsman, Johann Bachofen, was interested in the religious and philosophical importance of myths and the meaning of symbols. Nietzsche had borrowed Bachofen's concept of a Dionysian–Apollonian duality, which Jung adopted in turn. (Dionysius stood for the sensual side of life, and Apollo represented the rational.) Nietzsche shared with Jung a sense of the tragic ambiguity of life and the presence of good and evil in every human interaction. Nietzsche's ideas about the origin of civilization, humanity's moral conscience, and the importance of dreams, together with his concern about evil, influenced Jung. Nietzsche's description of the Shadow, the Persona, the Superman, and the Wise Old Man were taken up by Jung as specific archetypal images.

Carl Gustav Carus and Arthur Schopenhauer also influenced Jung. Carus had written about the creative and healing functions of the unconscious 50 years before Freud or Jung. Carus outlined a tripartite model of the unconscious that prefigured Jung's concepts of the archetypal, collective, and personal unconscious. Schopenhauer possessed a view of life that attracted Jung. Both wrote about the irrational in human psychology, as well as the role played by human will, repression, and the power of the instincts. Schopenhauer and Nietzsche inspired Jung's theory of archetypes; also influential was Schopenhauer's emphasis on imagination, the role of the unconscious, the reality of evil, and the importance of dreams. Both Schopenhauer and Jung were interested in moral issues and in Eastern philosophy, and both believed in the possibility of personal wholeness.

Ellenberger (1981) traces Jung's psychotherapeutic emphasis on transference and countertransference (*transference* refers to feelings the patient projects onto the analyst and *countertransference* to the ways in which the analyst is influenced by patients' projections) to a chain of thought that originated in the exorcism of devils, wound through Anton Mesmer's theory of animal magnetism, and led to the early-nineteenth-century use of hypnosis by Pierre Janet to cure mental illness. Janet also influenced Jung through his classifications of mental diseases and his interest in multiple personality and fixed ideas. For Janet, as for Jung, the dedication of the doctor and the personal harmony between doctor and patient were major elements in cures.

Beginnings

Jung wrote, "Our way of looking at things is conditioned by what we are" (1929/1933/1961, p. 335). He believed all psychological theories were subjective, reflecting the personal history of their founders. Jung's parents had been raised in prosperous city families and were well educated; their discontent with their life in the poor rural parish of Kesswil, where Jung's father served as a country pastor, affected Jung's childhood. Jung described his youth as lonely. Until he went to high school, his companions were mostly uneducated farm children. His early experience with peasants brought out a practical and earthy side of Jung that balanced his tendency toward introspection (Jung, 1965).

Jung was close to his mother. He experienced her as having two sides. One side was intuitive, with an interest in parapsychology that he feared; the other side was warm and maternal, which comforted him. In his mind, Jung split her into a daytime/nighttime, good/bad person. Jung's later efforts to integrate these contrasting aspects of his mother found form in his emphasis on the importance of the Hero's quest to free himself from the Terrible Mother, as well as his depiction of powerful feminine archetypal images. Jung's unsatisfactory relationship with his father may have led to his later problems with men, especially male mentors and other authority figures.

Throughout his life, Jung was interested in and attracted to women. He married a woman with an earthy side similar to his mother's, but he remained captivated by intuitive women whom he described as his lost feminine half. In his autobiography, Jung remembered a nursemaid who took care of him when his mother was hospitalized for several months. This nurse became the prototype for a series of women who were to fascinate and inspire him. The parapsychological experiments of Jung's cousin, Helene Preiswerk, became the subject of his medical school dissertation. Her influence was seminal to the development of Jung's theories.

Much of Jung's reading during his university and medical school years concerned multiple personality, trance states, hysteria, and hypnosis. He brought this interest to his coursework and to his lectures to fellow students, as well as to his dissertation. His fascination with these subjects, and his reading of Richard von Krafft-Ebing's study of sexual psychopathology propelled Jung into psychiatry (Jung, 1965). Soon after Jung finished his dissertation, he started work under Eugen Bleuler at the Burgholzli Psychiatric Hospital, then a famous center for research on mental illness. Jung lived at the Burgholzli Hospital from 1902 to 1909 and became intimately involved with the daily lives of mentally disturbed patients. Their inner worlds intrigued him, and his exploration of the symbolic universe of one of his schizophrenic patients, Babette, was a major source of Jung's study on schizophrenia, *The Psychology of Dementia Praecox* (1907/1960). At the Burgholzli, Jung developed and administered a number of psychological tests. His Word Association Test studies (1904–1907) gained him renown. These studies were the first demonstration of the reality of the unconscious. This work led Jung to begin a correspondence with Sigmund Freud.

Freud appreciated Jung's contributions to psychoanalytic theory and accepted Jung as his heir apparent. He appointed Jung president of the International Psychoanalytic Association and editor of the *Jahrbuch,* the first psychoanalytic journal. The two men traveled together to the United States in 1909 to lecture on their respective views of psychoanalysis at Clark University. Jung considered himself Freud's collaborator, not his disciple. Divergent perceptions, as well as their conflicting personalities, caused them to sever their alliance. Jung brought about his inevitable break with Freud through writing *The Psychology of the Unconscious* (1911, revised in 1956 as *Symbols of Transformation*).

In this book, Jung set forth his own form of psychoanalysis, in which myth, cultural history, and personal psychology were interwoven; he also redefined *libido* more comprehensively than had Freud. During this period, Jung married and then left the Burgholzli for private practice. He began to train his followers in his own method, and his wife, Emma Jung, became one of the first analytical psychotherapists.

After his break with Freud, Jung suffered a period of extreme introversion that Ellenberger (1981) called a creative illness. At this time, a third in the series of women who inspired him, his former patient and a future analyst, Toni Wolff, served as Jung's guide for his descent into the unconscious. Jung acknowledged his debt to her, as well as to the women who were the subjects of his first three books, and to his female patients when he wrote, "What this psychology owes to the direct influence of women . . . is a theme that would fill a large volume. I am speaking here not only of analytical psychology but of the beginnings of psychopathology in general" (Jung, 1927/1970, p. 124). He added that "I have had mainly women patients, who often entered into the work with extraordinary conscientiousness, understanding and intelligence. It was essentially because of them that I was able to strike out on new paths in therapy" (Jung, 1965, p. 145).

Jung's emergence from his period of creative introversion was signaled by the 1921 publication of his *Psychological Types.* Its inspiration came from Jung's reflection on the destructive antagonism among Freud, Adler, and himself. Jung made his private peace with them by creating a system of typology that allowed for and explained the different ways each experienced and reacted to the world.

Current Status

Interest in Jungian psychology is growing as the incompleteness of positivistic science becomes more apparent and the world becomes increasingly complex. In spite of the dismissal of analytical psychology by some pragmatic psychologists, the fact that analytical psychology answers a strong need for many people can be seen in the growing number of Jungian professional training institutes and analysts. As of 2009, the International Association for Analytical Psychology had 2929 certified analyst members in 45 countries, 51 professional societies (19 in the United States), and 19 developing groups. There are Jungian study groups and analytical psychology clubs that thrive both in cities that have professional societies and in many places not large enough to have institutes, and there are increasing numbers of people who call themselves Jungian-oriented therapists but have not gone through an institute's rigorous training. Professional journals are associated with specific institutes; among the more important ones are the British *Journal of Analytical Psychology;* San Francisco's *Jung Journal: Culture and Psyche;* the Los Angeles Institute's *Psychological Perspectives;* the New York Institute's *Journal of Jungian Theory and Practice;* Chicago's series of *Chiron* monographs on clinical practice; and the post-Jungian journal of archetypal studies, *Spring.* Important non-English journals include the *Cahiers de Psychologie Jungienne* from Paris, the *Zeitschrift für Analytische Psychologie* from Berlin, and Rome's *La Rivista di Psicologia Analitica.*

Training varies from institute to institute and country to country. Although Jung accepted lay analysts, the trend toward increasing professionalism grows. In the United States, institutes most often accept physicians, clinical psychologists, and social workers for training. Jung was the first psychoanalyst to insist that an analyst be personally analyzed. The cornerstone of Jungian training remains a thorough analysis over many years, often with two different analysts. Six or more years of case supervision comes next in importance (Crowther, 2009; Mathers, 2009; Sherwood, 2009). Coursework in the

United States commonly takes 4 years and involves seminars that provide a thorough grounding in clinical theory and practice (from both a Jungian and a neo-Freudian perspective), dream analysis, and archetypal psychology. Extensive personal reviews, oral and written examinations, and a clinical dissertation are generally required for professional certification as a Jungian analyst. The average length of training is 6 to 8 years though some newer groups are shortening training in Jungian psychotherapy to about 4 years.

There is an exciting ferment within Jungian studies at this time. Interest in child analysis, group work, body work, and art therapy is increasing, as is a concomitant interest in a hybrid of Jungian psychology and post-Freudian's object relations theory that focuses on the analysis of early childhood development and early childhood wounds (Cambray & Carter, 2004). *Object relations* is an unfortunate term for the way people relate to other people. This hybrid is becoming increasingly popular, especially in the United States and the United Kingdom. Others are revising or discarding the more time- or culture-bound aspects of Jung's theory. Two examples are a Jungian psychology of women that fits the reality of contemporary women and a reformulation of Jung's anima-animus concept. *Anima* is a feminine archetypal image most often represented through the feminine part of a man; *animus* is a masculine archetypal image most often represented through the masculine part of a woman. Jungians are currently reassessing what were once held to be traditionally "masculine" and "feminine" characteristics and are reappraising Jungian typological theory. There is also an extension of archetypal theory to images relevant to contemporary life, both in scholarly works and in popular works that reach a wide and receptive audience. There has been a gradual easing of the bad feelings and jealousy that divided the various schools of depth psychology since Freud, Adler, and Jung parted ways. Thus, for example, the National Accreditation Association for Psychoanalysis includes depth psychologists and institutes from many different, and formerly opposing, schools, and the British *Journal of Analytical Psychology* gives a yearly conference that is sponsored by the American Psychoanalytical Foundation and Jungian Institutes in Chicago and New York.

PERSONALITY

Theory of Personality

Jung's theory of personality rests on the concept of a dynamic unity of all parts of a person. The psyche is made up of conscious and unconscious components with connections to the *collective unconscious* (underlying patterns of images, thoughts, behaviors, and experiences). According to Jungian theory, our conscious understanding of who we are comes from two sources: the first derives from encounters with social reality, such as the things people tell us about ourselves, the second from what we deduce from our observations of others. If others seem to agree with our self-assessment, we tend to think we are normal; if they disagree, we tend to see ourselves, or to be seen by others, as abnormal.

In addition, each individual has a personal unconscious. This is an area of personality that cannot be understood directly and can be approached only indirectly through dreams and through analysis. The personal unconscious is affected by what Jung called the collective unconscious, an inherited human factor that expresses itself in the personal unconscious through archetypal images and complexes.

Thus, in effect, there are two aspects to the human psyche. One is an accessible side referred to as consciousness, comprising one's senses, intellect, emotions, and desires, and the other is an inaccessible side—the personal unconscious—containing elements of personal experience we have forgotten or denied, as well as elements of the collective unconscious that can be discerned through archetypal images and complexes.

Jung defined the Self as archetypal energy that orders and integrates the personality, an encompassing wholeness out of which personality evolves. The Self is the goal of personal development. The infant starts in a state of initial wholeness, as a unitary Self that soon fragments into subsystems. Through this fragmentation, mind and consciousness develop; over the course of a lifetime, the healthy personality then reintegrates at a higher level of development.

The most important fragment of the Self, the ego, first appears as the young child gains some sense of identity as an independent being. The ego in early life is like an island of consciousness set in an ocean of personal and unconscious material. The island grows in size and definition as it gathers and digests the deposits from the sea around it. This ego becomes the "I"—an entity comprising everything a person believes himself or herself to be, including thoughts, feelings, wants, and bodily sensations. The ego, as the center of consciousness, mediates between the unconscious realm and the outer world. Part of human psychological development consists of creating a strong and resilient ego that can filter stimuli from each of these domains without identifying with or being overcome by either side.

The *personal shadow* balances the ego in the personal unconscious. The shadow contains everything that could or should be part of the ego but that the ego denies or refuses to develop. The personal shadow can contain both positive and negative aspects. Shadow elements often appear in dreams in attacking or frightening forms of the same gender as the dreamer; they also erupt into consciousness through projection onto hated or envied individuals or groups. The personal shadow tends to be the vehicle through which archetypal images of evil emerge out of the collective unconscious, such as when, for instance, a mob gets carried away in mindless acts of violence. Confronting shadow material, making it and one's response to it conscious, can reclaim important parts of the personality to consciousness; these are essential tasks for the mature personality.

Jung believed in the reality of evil and viewed it as an increasing problem in the world. Jung felt that humans could confront evil by becoming conscious of it and aware of archetypal, inherited images of absolute evil. He thought that responsibly facing human evil meant becoming conscious of what is in one's own shadow, confronting archetypal images of evil instead of being overwhelmed by them, and taking personal responsibility for one's own evil propensities and actions rather than projecting shadow material and complexes onto other people, groups, or nations.

The *persona* is the public "face" of an individual in society. Jung named the persona for the Greek theatrical mask that hid the actor's face and indicated the part he chose to play. The persona shields the ego and reveals appropriate aspects of it, smoothing the individual's interactions with society. The development of an adequate persona allows for the privacy of thoughts, feelings, ideas and perceptions, as well as for modulation in the way they are revealed. Just as people can identify with their egos, they can identify with their persona, believing they really *are* the role they have chosen to play.

Jung believed that the task of the first part of life was strengthening the ego, taking one's place in the world in relationships with others, and fulfilling one's duty to society. The task of the second half of life was to reclaim undeveloped parts of oneself, fulfilling these aspects of personality more completely. He called this process *individuation* and believed this life task drew many of his older patients into analysis. By individuation, Jung did not mean perfection; the idea refers to completion and wholeness, including acceptance of the more negative parts of one's personality and adoption of an ethical, though individual, response to them. Fordham (1996) and many other contemporary Jungians believe that individuation does not have to wait until middle age. Jung's emphasis on individuation as the task of the second half of life further differentiated his personality theory from Freud's because it allowed for growth and transformation throughout the life cycle. The mid-life crisis, looked at in this way, becomes a challenging opportunity for further development.

Part of the process of individuation concerns not only assimilation of personal shadow material but also awareness and integration of the contrasexual elements in the psyche—what Jung called the *anima* (an archetypal image of the feminine) and *animus* (an archetypal image of the masculine), which serve as bridges to the unconscious. The form and character of the archetypal images of anima and animus are highly individual, based on a person's experience of the opposite sex, cultural assumptions, and the archetype of the feminine or masculine. Since so much about gender and gender roles is in flux today, current images no longer match those of Jung's time and are changing as culture and experience change (Douglas, 2006). Contemporary reevaluation of this concept holds much promise for a reappraisal of homosexuality as a natural occurrence.

Typology is one of the most important and best-known contributions Jung made to personality theory. In *Psychological Types* (1921/1971), Jung describes varying ways in which individuals habitually respond to the world. Two basic responses are *introversion* and *extraversion.* Jung saw introversion as natural and basic. Energy for the introvert flows predominantly inward, with reality being the introvert's reaction to an event, object, or person. Introverts need solitude to develop and maintain their rich inner worlds; they value friendship, having few but deep relationships with others. The extravert's reality, on the other hand, consists of objective facts or incidents. The extravert connects with reality mainly through external objects. Whereas the introvert adapts outer reality to inner psychology, the extravert adapts himself or herself to the environment and to people. Extraverts usually communicate well, make friends easily, and have a great deal of libido for interactions with other people. Jung described nations as well as people as being either predominantly introverted or extraverted. For instance, he saw Switzerland as basically introverted and the United States not only as primarily extraverted but also as tending to look on introversion as unhealthy.

In his theory of typology, Jung went on to divide personality into functional types, based on people's tendency to perceive reality primarily through one of four mental functions: *thinking, feeling, sensation,* and *intuition.* Each of these four functions can be experienced in an extraverted or an introverted way. According to Jung,

> For complete orientation all four functions should contribute equally: thinking should facilitate cognition and judgment, feeling should tell us how and to what extent a thing is important or unimportant for us, sensation should convey concrete reality to us through seeing, hearing, tasting, sensing, etc., and intuition should enable us to divine the hidden possibilities in the background, since these too belong to the complete picture of a given situation. (1921/1971, p. 518)

According to Jung, a thinker finds rules, assigns names, makes classifications, and develops theories; a feeling person puts a value on reality, often by liking or disliking something; a sensing type uses the five senses to grasp inner or outer reality; and an intuitive person has hunches that seem to penetrate into past and future reality, as well as an ability to pick up accurate information from the unconscious of another person.

Most people seem to be born with one of these four primary functions dominant. The dominant function is used more than the others and is developed more fully. Often a secondary function will develop as the person matures, while a third but weaker function—such as feeling for the thinker, or sensation for the intuitive person—remains shadowy and undeveloped. Jung stressed the importance of the least-developed function. Largely unconscious, it is often seen first in shadow and animus/anima subpersonalities. This undeveloped function causes trouble when it breaks into consciousness, but it can also bring creativity and freshness, appearing when the mature personality feels lifeless and spent.

People tend to develop one primary attitude and function and then rely on these, sometimes inappropriately. For instance, a predominantly thinking type tends always to consider the facts of the case when it may be better simply to understand that something is right or wrong, good or bad, worthy of acceptance or rejection.

Everyone has access to all four functions as well as to introversion and extraversion. Part of personality development, according to Jungians, consists of first refining one's predominant type and then cultivating one's less-evolved functions. In life-span development, the secondary function matures after the first and is followed by the third; the blooming of the least-developed function comes last and can be a source of great creativity in the latter part of life. It is important to stress that typological theory is a blueprint or map far clearer than the terrain of the personality itself, which is full of individual differences.

Variety of Concepts

Opposites

Jung (1976) wrote, "Opposites are the ineradicable and indispensable preconditions for all psychic life" (p. 169). In line with the dualistic theories of his day, Jung saw the world in terms of paired opposites such as good and evil, light and dark, positive and negative. He designed his personality theory with *consciousness* opposing the *unconscious, masculine* opposing *feminine,* the *good aspects* of an archetypal image opposing the *bad* (e.g., the *Nourishing* opposing the *Devouring* Mother), *ego* opposing *shadow,* and so on. These opposites engage in active struggle, and personality development takes place through the tension this conflict produces in the psyche. For instance, a woman's conscious sexuality may war with her animus figure, who may appear in her dreams as a negative and judgmental male cleric. Caught in the conflict, she may go from one pole to the other and may develop neurotic symptoms from the split. Through bringing the fight between her eroticism and her spirituality into awareness, attentively following it, and allowing both sides their voice in fantasies and therapy, the woman may increase her consciousness and thus integrate the opposing sides of her sexuality and her religious feelings at a higher level of awareness.

Enantiodromia

This word refers to Heraclitus' law that everything sooner or later turns into its opposite. To illustrate enantiodromia, Jung liked to tell the story of the man who laughed on the way up a precipitous mountain path and cried on the easy way down. While climbing, he anticipated the effortless descent, but while ambling down, he remembered the difficult ascent he had made. Jung believed enantiodromia governed the cycles of human history as well as personal development. He thought that one could escape such cycles only through consciousness. Jung's belief in Heraclitus' law underlies his theory of compensation.

Compensation

Jung not only divided the world into paired opposites but also formed a theory built on the idea that just as the opposites lay in dynamic balance, so everything in the personality balanced or supplemented its opposite in a self-regulatory way. Jung referred to this tendency as compensation. Thus, the personal unconscious balances an individual's consciousness, giving rise in dreams, fantasies, or somatic symptoms to its opposite; the more rigidly one holds the conscious position, the more strongly will its opposite appear in images or symbols and break through into consciousness. Thus, someone who consciously identifies with a harshly judgmental spirituality may have a prostitute figure active in his or her unconscious who, if further repressed, may induce a scandalous alliance in the outer world.

The Transcendent Function

Jung called reconciling symbols, or images that form bridges between opposites, compensatory or transcendent functions. These symbols synthesize two opposing attitudes or conditions in the psyche by means of third forces different from both but uniting the two. Jung used the word *transcendent* because the image or symbol went beyond, as well as mediated between, the two opposites, allowing a new attitude or relationship between them. Bringing the opposites of one's conscious ego and the personal unconscious together generates a conflict in the personality that is highly charged and full of energy. The specific image that appears at the height of a seemingly unsolvable conflict between two opposites seems both unexpected and inevitable, holding an energy-filled charge capable of uniting and reconciling the opposing sides. The woman whose animus male cleric warred with her womanly sexuality had a fantasy in which she was crowned with grape leaves and led a snake to the foot of an altar; the snake slithered up the cross and wrapped itself about it (Douglas, 2006). The crown of grape leaves was an emblem of sensuality, while the snake on the cross (connected with feminine energy in many myths, the most familiar being Eve and the Garden of Eden) reconciled the woman's opposing sides in a surprising new form of union.

Mandala

Jung defined the mandala as a symbol of wholeness and of the center of the personality. The word *mandala* comes from the Sanskrit word for a geometric figure in which a circle and square lie within each other, and each is further subdivided. The mandala usually had religious significance. A mandala often appears in dreams, both as a symbol of wholeness and as a compensatory image during times of stress. An example of a mandala is shown in Figure 4.1.

Preoedipal Development

In contrast to Freud's stress on the oedipal phase of personality development, Jung focused on *preoedipal experience.* He was one of the first psychoanalysts to stress the importance of early mother-child interactions. The initial relationship between mother and child affects personality development at its most basic and profound level. Jung paid far more attention to this stage and its problems than to the father-son complications of the Oedipus complex. He placed the archetypal image of the Good Mother/Bad Mother at the center of an infant's experience.

Development of Consciousness

Jungian theory holds that the infant follows the pattern of the development of consciousness in general, first experiencing total merger with the mother in a state of primordial fusion, then partially splitting off from her through perceiving her as sometimes all good and sometimes all bad. The child follows humanity's general historical development, emerging into self-awareness in a patriarchal stage where the father and male values are paramount. This stage affects girls as well as boys and is considered a stumbling block to women's development. When the ego is firmly in place, however, a person can integrate

FIGURE 4.1   __Mandala__

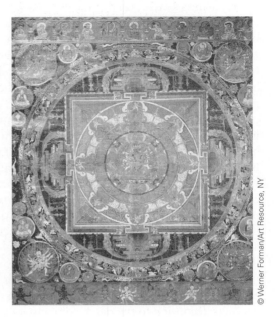

© Werner Forman/Art Resource, NY

the mother world and father world, uniting both energies to become a more complete personality (Jung, 1934a/1970; Ulanov, 2007; Whitmont, 1997).

Psychopathology

Psychopathology derives in large part from problems and conflicts that arise in early mother-child relationships but is made worse by other stresses. The psyche directs attention to such disharmony and calls out for a response. Since the psyche is a self-regulating system, pathological symptoms derive from the frustrated urge toward wholeness and often contain within themselves the clue to their own healing (Hollis, 2008). Thus, for instance, extreme switches between love and hate for the same person often typify an individual with borderline personality disorder and call attention to faulty infantile development.

Defense Mechanisms

Defense mechanisms are seen as attempts of the psyche to survive the onslaught of complexes. They can represent normal as well as destructive modes of protection. Jung felt that any rigidly held defense caused an imbalance and would become increasingly pathological if its calls for attention were ignored. *Regression,* for example, is a defense that becomes pathological only when a person remains stuck in it. Jung felt that regression was often a natural and necessary period of consolidation and regeneration that could herald an individual's subsequent personal growth.

PSYCHOTHERAPY

Theory of Psychotherapy

To Sigmund Freud's predominantly analytic, reductive system, Carl Jung added a synthesis that included the psyche's purposiveness. According to Jung, the personality not only has the capacity to heal itself but also becomes enlarged through experience.

Jung (1934b/1966) built his system of psychotherapy on four tenets: (1) the psyche is a self-regulating system, (2) the unconscious has a creative and compensatory component, (3) the doctor-patient relationship plays a major role in facilitating self-awareness and healing, and (4) personality growth takes place at many stages over the life span.

Jung found that neurosis tends to appear when a person slights or shrinks back from some important worldly or developmental task. A neurosis is a symptom of disturbance in the personality's equilibrium; thus, the whole personality has to be considered, not only the symptom of distress. Rather than concentrating on isolated symptoms, the psychotherapist looks for an underlying complex. The symptom and the complex are important clues that both hide and reveal "the patient's secret, the rock against which he is shattered" (Jung, 1965, p. 117). Jung stated that when therapists discover their patients' secrets, they have the key to treatment.

Overt symptoms, dreams, and fantasies can reveal to the analyst a complex hidden from the patient's consciousness. Analytical psychotherapists deal with secrets, complexes, and neuroses by tracking their roots to past events and traumas, by seeing how they interfere with present functioning especially in the relationship between doctor and patient, and by recognizing the archetypal patterns that emerge into consciousness through the action of complexes.

Analytical psychotherapy also deals with "the mental and moral conflicts of normal people" (Jung, 1948/1980, p. 606). Jung differentiated normal from pathological conflicts according to the degree of consciousness a person has of the conflict and the amount of power exerted by the underlying complex. The level of dissociation between conscious and unconscious content reflects the intensity of the disturbance and the amount of pathology. Jung lectured frequently on his psychotherapeutic theory, yet he also declared that the practice of psychotherapy "does not involve intellectual factors only, but also feeling values and above all the important question of human relationship" (Jung, 1948/1980, p. 609). The dialogue and partnership between patient and analyst probably play the most essential roles in therapy. Jung himself was a notably effective therapist who followed the tenets of his theory, adapting it to the needs of each of his cases. This interaction between theory and the personal equation gives creative energy to analytical psychology as a whole and particularly to its practice of psychotherapy.

Analytical psychotherapy is, in essence, a dialogue between two people undertaken to facilitate growth, healing, and a new synthesis of the patient's personality at a higher level of functioning. By means of the analytic relationship, one works through personal problems and gains greater understanding of one's inner and outer worlds. Because of the importance of this relationship, the therapist's character, training, development, and individuation are crucial to the healing process. Jung insisted not only on the training analysis of the analyst but also on constant self-examination by the analyst. Next, and equal in importance, he valued the therapist's respect for patients, care for their values, and "supreme tact and . . . artistic sensitiveness" toward psychic material (Jung, 1934b/1966, p. 169). Jung wrote of the therapist's need to consider the patient from many angles, including a sociocultural one: "Psychic modes of behavior are, indeed, of an eminently historical nature. The psychotherapist has to acquaint himself not only with the personal biography of his patient, but also with the mental and spiritual assumptions prevalent in his milieu, both present and past, where traditional and cultural influences play a part and often a decisive one" (Jung, 1957, pp. vii–viii).

Through his emphasis on the mutual influence of the two people in therapy, Jung was one of the first psychoanalysts to focus on both transference and countertransference phenomena. Rather than viewing therapy as something done by one person to another, Jung acknowledged that the therapist needs to be affected before transformation can occur in the patient. Jung emphasized the influence of the patient's unconscious on the analyst as well as the need for the analyst to be open to this power. The therapist's own analysis and continued self-examination are essential if the therapist is going to maintain a beneficial role.

The psychotherapeutic process can (and often should) stop when specific goals are reached or specific problems are overcome. Nevertheless, analytical psychotherapy in its most complete form has the goal of self-actualization—helping patients discover and live up to their full potential. Thus, Jungian psychotherapy goes beyond the resolution of complexes, the strengthening of the conscious mind, and ego development, to include a larger comprehension of the psyche. Through this process, patients achieve greater personal self-knowledge and the capacity for improved relationships with themselves, with others, and with the world at large.

Michael Fordham (1996) and his followers have enriched Jung's basic theory of psychotherapy by carefully observing young children's behavior and by analyzing children and childhood, focusing on the primary infantile wounds behind complexes. A growing number of Jungians stress the analysis of early childhood experiences, including the analysis of fantasy material. They also stress the value of verbal interpretation and explanations of present behavior. This approach has resulted in a synthesis of Jungian psychotherapy with neo-Freudian, often Kleinian, psychoanalysis.

Another major movement in Jungian psychotherapy questions the value of verbal interpretation as the primary mode of analysis. Instead, the patient's affect, feelings, and body awareness are emphasized, and therapists are more likely to use the traditionally feminine realm of subjective and shared experience (Douglas, 2006; Ulanov, 2007). Wilmer (1986) finds emotion to be the core subject matter in a therapeutic setting where patient and therapist meet as equals. Sullivan (1989), Siegelman (1990, 2002, 2003), and Chodorow (1997, 2006) focus on the importance of subjective feelings. They emphasize the analyst's empathy, free-floating or hovering attention, and shared metaphoric images. They also provide a theoretical base for what has been a neglected but important aspect of analytical psychotherapy.

John Beebe (1992) stresses "active passivity," in which the analyst opens himself or herself to the wide range of stimuli emitted by the patient. Beebe points out that infringements on a person's privacy inevitably occur in psychotherapy, since its subject matter concerns sensitive secrets about which one is often ashamed. These secrets, when sensitively examined, may lead to the recall and healing of early infringements of bodily or psychological space. Because of sensitive subject matter, therapists need to adhere to an ethical code that honors and respects the integrity of their patients' boundaries (also see Zoja, 2007). Beebe suggests that ethical principles in psychotherapy derive from the necessity of protecting patients' self-esteem while also protecting the integrity of the therapeutic setting and the beliefs that are essential for progress in analytical psychotherapy.

These views remain faithful to Jung's ideas of the primacy of patients and also preserve Jung's belief that the principal aim of psychotherapy is ultimately neither curing nor alleviating patients' unhappiness but increasing patients' self-respect and self-knowledge. A sense of peace and a greater capacity for both suffering and joy can accompany this expanded sense of self, and patients become more likely to take personal responsibility for their behavior.

Process of Psychotherapy

Psychotherapy takes place among fallible equals; however, Andrew Samuels's (2001) term *asymmetrical mutuality* may be preferred to *equals* inasmuch as it acknowledges the differing roles and responsibilities of patients and analysts. Jung (1933/1966) delineated four stages in the process of psychotherapy: *confession, elucidation, education,* and *transformation.*

Confession

The first stage, confession, is a cathartic recounting of personal history. During this stage, the patient shares conscious and unconscious secrets with the therapist, who serves as a nonjudgmental, empathic listener. Jung found that confession brought the basic material of psychotherapy to the surface. Confession makes people feel less like outcasts, restoring them to their place in the human community. The analyst facilitates this process through an accepting attitude that drains the poison of guilt at the same time that it releases emotions long held hostage. The process of confession does, however, tend to bind the patient to the therapist through transference.

Elucidation

During elucidation, the therapist draws attention to the transference relationship as well as to dreams and fantasies in order to connect the transference to its infantile origins. The goal of this stage is insight on both affective and intellectual levels. Jung describes the successful outcome of this procedure as leading to a person's "normal adaptation and forbearance with his own shortcomings: these will be his guiding moral principles, together with freedom from sentimentality and illusion" (Jung, 1933/1966, p. 65).

Education

The third stage, education, moves the patient into the realm of the individual as an adapted social being. Whereas confession and elucidation primarily involve exploring the personal unconscious, education is concerned with persona and ego tasks. At this stage the therapist encourages the patient to develop an active and health-promoting role in everyday life. Insight, previously mostly intellectual, is now translated into responsible action.

Transformation

Many people stop therapy at the completion of the first three stages, but Jung noted that some clients seemed impelled to go further, especially people in the second half of life. The transference does not go away for these patients, even though its infantile origins have been thoroughly explored. These people feel a desire for greater knowledge and insight leading them toward the final stage—*transformation*. Jung described this as a period of self-actualization; the person in this stage values unconscious as well as conscious experience. The archetypal image of the Self appears in the transference as well as in dream and fantasy; this archetypal image of wholeness inspires the patient to become a uniquely individual self, encompassing all that he or she can be, yet without losing a sense of responsible integrity.

In this most Jungian of stages, the transference-countertransference becomes even more profound, and what happens to the patient "must now happen to the doctor, so that his personality shall not react unfavorably on the patient. The doctor can no longer evade his own difficulty by treating the difficulties of others" (Jung, 1933/1966, p. 74). The analyst often has to face a challenge in his or her own life before something changes in the patient. Jung gave an example that occurred when he was becoming quite famous and was treating a woman patient who worshiped him. Nothing changed until he realized that he had become too removed from his patients and was starting to feel superior to this one especially; he then dreamed he was kneeling before her as though she were a female divinity. With this, he was brought back to reality, and the analysis started to progress again.

Jung spent the latter part of his career explaining this stage through a series of analogies to alchemy. He found that the symbols and processes of medieval alchemy were comparable to those of the psychotherapeutic process in that alchemists most often worked in pairs and left records showing that they were examining their own psyches while trying to transform some base material, through a series of stages, into gold. Jung's inclusion of self-realization as part of the process broadened the scope of psychology immeasurably, bringing analytical psychotherapy into the area of human potential, consciousness study, and field theory.

Jung became increasingly interested in the transformative stage and gathered much of the material in his case studies from it. He found that the transference and dream symbols went from the personal to the archetypal during this stage. Jung illustrated the process with the case study of a patient who projected a personal father image onto Jung in the first three stages of her therapy. When she got to the transformative stage, however, her dreams of him as her good father changed. Now she dreamed of a giant father figure towering over a field of ripe wheat; as she nestled in the palm of this giant's hand, he rocked her in rhythm with the blowing wind. Jung interpreted this as an archetypal image of the Great Father in the form of a vegetation god and declared that it, along with the ripeness of the wheat, signaled that the patient was entering the final stage of analysis (Jung, 1935b/1966).

Jung noted that each stage of the analytical process seems to be accompanied by a sense of finality, as if it were a goal in itself. Although each stage can be a temporary goal or the endpoint of a partial analysis, all four belong in a complete analysis. The stages overlap and can be concurrent, with no stage excluding the others, because neither their order nor their duration is fixed.

Mechanisms of Psychotherapy

Analysis of the Transference

Jungian psychotherapists agree with all practitioners of depth psychology that transference plays a crucial role throughout therapy; however, the idea takes on a different resonance and complexity in Jungian theory. In his Tavistock Lectures (Jung, 1935c/ 1980), Jung described four stages of analysis of the transference itself. In the first stage, transference projections onto the therapist mirror the personal history of the patient. Patients, in working through each of their earlier relationships, relate to the analyst as though he or she were the problematic person. This is an invaluable aid to therapy, because it allows for regression and brings the past into the consulting room. The three goals at this stage are to have one's patients realize that the projections belong to themselves and not to others, withdraw the projections from the analyst, and integrate them as conscious parts of the patient's own personalities. Jung, writing about this first stage, said, "to establish a really mature attitude, [the patient] has to see the *subjective value* of all these images which seem to create trouble for him. He has to assimilate them into his own psychology; he has to find out in what way they are part of himself" (Jung, 1933/1966, p. 160).

Jung expanded the scope of transference by considering its sociocultural and archetypal components. These impersonal aspects are also projected onto the therapist. During the second stage of the analysis of the transference, patients learn to discriminate between the personal and the impersonal contents they project onto the therapist; they determine what belongs to their own psyches and what belongs to the collective realms of culture and archetype. The impersonal cannot be assimilated, but the act of projecting it can be stopped. In the case of the woman who dreamed of the Giant Vegetation God, Jung helped her see that this image was a transpersonal one reflecting a need for her personal connection to her image. When she had seen the differences among what belonged to her, what to Jung, and what to the impersonal archetypal image of the Great Father, she could establish a more healing relationship with the image's power.

In the third stage of analyzing the transference, the personal reality of the analyst becomes differentiated from the image assigned him or her by the patient. At this stage, the patient can begin to relate to the therapist as a normal human being, and the personality of the therapist plays a pivotal role. In the final stage, as the transference is resolved and greater self-knowledge and self-realization take place, a truer evaluation of the therapist emerges, along with a more straightforward and empathic connection between patient and therapist.

Active Imagination

To help his patients get in touch with unconscious material, Jung taught a form of meditative imagery based on his own self-analysis. This came to be known as active imagination.

The process calls for clearing the mind and concentrating intensely, so that inner images can be activated. The patient watches these, always returning his or her mind to them until movement is observed, upon which the patient enters into the scene, becoming part of the picture or action. Patients are instructed to pay relaxed meditative attention to what is going on. After the images stop, patients are to write, draw, paint, or even dance the story (Chodorow, 2006; Douglas, 2008; Salman, 2009). The starting point for the exercise of active imagination can be a mood, a complex, an obsessive thought or feeling, or an image from a dream (Chodorow, 1997, 2006). Active imagination allows unconscious images to reveal themselves with little conscious intervention, yet it is more focused than dreams because of the presence of a witnessing consciousness.

Therapists today emphasize that a patient must have a strong ego if unconscious images are to be dealt with in this way. Unless and until a stronger ego is present, the personal daily reality of the patient is the main focus of therapy; archetypal images or fantasies, if they appear, need to be grounded in a more objective, down-to-earth, and personal way than through active imagination.

Dream Analysis

Not all people remember their dreams, nor do all people who enter Jungian therapy discuss their dreams. The perspective offered by a dream does, however, often compensate for the one-sidedness of the waking ego. Dreams, according to Jung, don't necessarily conceal, as in the traditional Freudian view, nor do they always denote unfulfilled wishes, nor can they be interpreted according to a standard symbology. They are accurate renderings of something to which one may need to pay attention and take as seriously as a conscious event. Dreams may represent wishes and fears; they often express impulses the dreamer either represses or finds impossible to voice; they can also point to solutions to both exterior and interior problems. They are of great value in exposing a patient's hidden inner life, and through their evolving symbolic imagery, they reveal changes occurring in the patient's psyche. For example, at the start of therapy, a woman may dream of hostile men breaking into her house. As she deals with past traumas and begins to explore and integrate her own masculine energy, these malevolent male figures slowly change. In the latter part of a long dream series, the figures often turn into friends, helpers, and guides. Their positive and helpful behavior markedly contrasts with their earlier threatening demeanor. By watching the archetypal images of the unconscious through dreams, the personality is able to regulate itself.

An analytical psychotherapist looks for the role a dream may play in relation to the patient's conscious attitude. The therapist often explores the dream first on the objective level, considering in what ways it accurately portrays an actual person or situation.

A dream is then probed for what it reveals about the patient's own behavior and character (Mattoon, 2006). Jung gave the example of a young man who dreamed of a headstrong father smashing a car. Jung first investigated the objective reality but found little that resonated with his patient. On the subjective level, however, the dream compensated for the boy's tendency to overidealize his father and any other man in a position of authority as well as to ignore the heedless part of himself (Jung, 1934c/1966). In treating this patient, a Jungian therapist would ascertain whether something akin to the image might be shadowing the therapy—for instance, whether either the therapist or the patient was recklessly endangering the analysis by their attitudes or actions. In dream analysis, the unconscious and the dream are relied on far more than the therapist's interpretation (Bosnak, 1996). Jung believed that if the interpretation was not accurate, another dream would inevitably correct the faulty understanding.

Types of Dreams

The initial dream, recurrent dreams, dreams containing shadow material, and dreams about the therapist or therapy are especially useful to the therapist. The initial dream at or near the start of therapy may indicate the path that a particular therapy may take and the type of transference that may occur. For instance, a short and unsuccessful therapy was predicted by an initial dream in which a female patient dreamed her therapist neither looked at nor listened to her but admired a beautiful jade figurine instead. The patient switched to a different analyst and then dreamed she was a baby panther being roughly groomed by the mother panther. This initial dream boded well for the course of the new therapy. Although the patient experienced some pain from what she felt was the therapist's fierce mothering, over the course of the therapy the patient regained a connection to her instinctual nature and discovered her own feminine power.

Recurrent dreams, especially those from early childhood, suggest problematic complexes and/or a repressed traumatic event. In trauma, the dream remains a photographic replay. Over the course of the therapy, the dreams change from flashback accuracy to less realistic and more neutral imagery and finally include scenarios in which the patient exerts some control (Kalsched, 2009; Wilmer, 1986). Dreams that contain rage, violence, or immoral conduct provide a clearer illustration of the patient's shadow than the therapist might perceive (Kalsched, 1996). This is because the material comes from the patient, with the unconscious part of the personality commenting on another part. Dreams about the therapist, the setting, or the therapy itself bring to light transference feelings of which the patient is either unaware or fearful. They provide symbols and language for both the patient and the analyst (Douglas, 2006; Whitmont & Perera, 1992).

Dreams can block therapy as well as advance it. This happens when patients bring in a flood of dream material and use it to fill up the therapy hour; when they prefer to remain in their dream worlds rather than to confront life; or when they distance themselves from the dream by refusing to engage their emotions or feelings (Whitmont & Perera, 1992; Mattoon, 2006). The therapist can observe this behavior for a while and then, at an appropriate moment, bring the situation to the patient's attention and explore the reasons for these defensive maneuvers.

APPLICATIONS

Who Can We Help?

There is wide latitude in the types of patients Jungians see and the forms of therapy they employ. Jungian therapists treat people of all ages and cultures, at all levels of functioning. Analytical therapy is suitable for people facing the common problems of life and accompanying symptoms of stress, anxiety, depression, and low self-esteem. It is also useful in dealing with people who have severe personality disorders or psychoses. What problems an analytical psychotherapist chooses to treat depends on that analyst's personality, ability, and training. Specific types of therapists seem to attract specific patients, yet each patient creates a different situation. The therapist's technique must be flexible enough to adapt to the particular patient and situation, and firm enough that the therapist works within his or her limits of expertise.

Some of the most interesting applications of analytical psychotherapy involve people with severe personality disorders; hospital and follow-up care of psychotics; and treatment of post-traumatic stress, disturbed children, the aging, the sick, and those gravely ill, dying, or preparing for death. Some Jungian therapists specialize in short-term psychodynamic psychotherapy, treating substance abusers, battered women, or the sexually abused. Some analysts integrate feminism with Jungian theory, often attracting patients who are reevaluating traditional gender roles or dealing with sexual trauma. Innovative work is also being done with people who have creative, religious, relationship, or sexual problems.

People who have undergone other depth analyses are increasingly undergoing a Jungian analysis because they feel their earlier analysis did not touch a dimension of their psyche. So, too, some Jungians, especially those who were more archetypally analyzed, seek some form of object relations therapy to fill gaps in their own self-knowledge.

Patients who adapt well to talking cures are those who are capable of introspection and have the ability to regress and yet maintain a working alliance with the therapist. Analytical psychotherapists working with people who have less intact egos, such as borderline personalities, adapt their technique to focus on supportive ego building. Other patients may need to remain in any one of the first three stages of therapy—confession, elucidation, and education—so that they can learn to live more easily in the human community, have better relationships with others, and establish and maintain themselves through meaningful work.

Analytical psychotherapy is singularly beneficial for people undergoing a midlife crisis and concerned with the problems of the second half of life, in old age or illness, or confronting death (Godsil, 2000). Dieckmann (1991) mentions three types of people who are drawn toward the process of individuation at midlife: those who find deep meaning within themselves and want to explore their inner worlds further; those who realize they have failed to reach the goals of their youth or who find these goals insufficient or no longer compelling; and those who have reached their goals and are confronting problems that accompanied worldly success. Because the scope of Jung's theory is so wide and concerns final causes as well as the status quo, many who look for more profound meaning in their lives and who are concerned with people's impact on each other and on the world's survival are also drawn to analytical psychotherapy.

Treatment

Jung was open to a wide variety of modalities, settings, and styles in his treatment of patients. Today, analytical psychotherapy most often takes place at a regular time and place, for a set fee. The encounter is often face to face, with therapist and patient both seated, though many analysts use a couch from time to time or as a matter of course.

Jungian analysts also work with body movement, dramatization, art, sandtrays, or an eclectic mixture of these methods. Just as the primary mode of therapy varies among analysts, so too does the timing. Most often, sessions in the United States are for 45 to 50 minutes once or twice per week, although three times is not uncommon; the more Kleinian-oriented therapists prefer four to five times a week. The timing varies and often includes more frequent and shorter visits for hospitalized clients, disturbed children, and the ill or severely impaired.

The impact of managed care on the modality and length of treatment has led to some experimentation with brief therapy. It has also resulted in many more analysts practicing entirely outside the managed-care system. The effect of these changes on the types of patient seen has yet to be studied.

Group Therapy

As an adjunct to and amplification of individual therapy, individuals sometimes meet in groups of approximately 6 to 10 people. Members are usually patients of the analyst who runs the group, although some analysts will accept referrals. The meetings customarily take place once a week and run for about 90 minutes. The group is usually carefully selected to create a balance of gender, typology, age, and type of problem. Some therapists run single-issue or single-gender groups, though an eclectic mixture of patients is more common. Undergoing group therapy has been suggested or required of an analyst in training. Patients need adequate ego strength because the situation is apt to be confrontive as well as supportive. Group therapy has been found to be particularly suitable for introverts drawn to Jungian psychotherapy. It is also recommended for patients who tend to intellectualize or aestheticize their analysis or otherwise defend themselves from their feelings and for those who have been unable to translate what they have learned in private therapy into real life.

Group work focuses on therapeutic issues through discussions, dream analysis, active imagination, psychodrama, gestalt, and bioenergetic modalities. The group is most effective, however, when complexes become active and particular issues come to life through the various clashes, alliances, and confrontations between and among members of the group. Participating in group therapy allows individuals to experience themselves interacting with others, experiencing their shared humanity as they reality-test, reveal themselves, and give clarifying feedback. Within the group, patients must agree to confidentiality. Whether patients socialize between meetings is up to the group and the particular therapist.

During the course of the meetings, the individual tends to project his or her own shadow (that part of the personality that people cannot acknowledge in themselves) onto the group, while the group inevitably picks up on parts of the personality that the individual conceals. Resistances are often more visible in a group than in private therapy and can be dealt with more easily. The group reconstellates the family, so issues of family dynamics arise, including a re-creation of sibling rivalries or problems of an individual's position within the family. Each member of the group, therefore, is able to work on family issues in a way not possible in individual therapy. Transference issues with the analyst can be transferred to the group and worked on in this arena as well. An analyst's shadow can also be seen more clearly in the group. Patients who have felt the analyst to be too powerful in individual therapy may be able to express feelings toward the therapist in group work. Patients who have gone through group therapy remark on the difficulty of the process, as well as on the depth of feeling engendered through the group's acceptance of their most vulnerable or wounded sides. They report a greater feeling of resiliency, more ease in social settings, and more acceptance of themselves after group work.

Family and Marital Therapy

Jungian analysts often use some mode of analytical family therapy or refer their patients to such therapy. Analysts will see the couple or family sometimes as a unit and sometimes separately or will do conjoint family work. The use of Jungian terminology, especially the concepts of typology, *anima* and *animus, shadow,* and *projection,* forms a language through which the family or couple can discern and reflect on their own dynamics.

Therapists often administer a typology test to the couple or family members. Through its interpretations, family members realize that one source of their differences may be a typology problem. Dissimilarities can be accepted and worked with more easily when interpreted as a typological clash, and knowledge of each family member's particular mixture of attitude and function types—introversion and extraversion, thinking, feeling, sensation, and intuition—can lead to improved family communication. Individual family members often have different typological ways of perceiving reality, and people often choose partners with a typology opposite to their own.

Analysts working with families and couples emphasize family dynamics caused by members' shadow and animus/anima projections onto other family members. Fights arise when a family member projects these, believing the other person is behaving in ways that really belong to the accuser's own shadow or anima/animus. Thus, a predominantly thinking-type man might fall prey to inferior feelings and fight his wife through moodiness while accusing her of his own sulkiness, and she, if she is predominantly a feeling type, might defend herself with theoretical arguments and blame her husband for her own judgmental stance. An argument of this sort is doomed to failure. Scapegoating of a specific individual frequently takes place when the scapegoated person is typologically different from the rest of the family or when the scapegoated person reminds a spouse or parent of a disliked parent or sibling.

Body/Movement Therapy

Jung encouraged patients to engage in active imagination through body movement or dance (Monte, 2009). Jung found that by using his own body to mirror the gestures of his psychotic and withdrawn patients at the Burgholzli, he could better understand feelings they were trying to communicate. He found that the body stores, holds, experiences, and communicates psychological and emotional experience as much as, if not more than, words. Joan Chodorow (1997, 2006) has described movement as a type of active imagination that, in therapy, accompanies and is followed by discussion. She found that the transference, as well as trauma, early or crisis experiences, grief, dreams, fantasies, feelings, and moods, can be embodied and expressed in movement. As the patient moves, the therapist observes or serves as a mirror moving along with the patient.

Art Therapy

Jung often suggested that a patient draw or paint an image from a dream or from active imagination. During his own self-analysis, Jung painted his dream and fantasy images; he perceived therapeutic value in doing this, in playing with stones like a child, and (later) in sculpting in stone and carving at his retreat in Bollingen. Jung encouraged his patients to do the same in their own analysis through painting, sculpting, and other form-giving methods that provided a feeling and image through which the contents of the unconscious could find expression. He felt this was especially valuable for people who were out of touch with their feelings or who tried to deal with their experience solely through logic.

Analytical psychotherapy encourages art in therapy as a conscious way to express elements of the unconscious. Art therapy is especially useful in working through and integrating traumatic material when isolated images and feeling states tend to explode into consciousness. The expression of these images or feeling states through art releases their archetypal power and "domesticates" them in a way that gives the survivor a sense of control.

Art therapy is also useful in overcoming mental blocks or side-stepping an overly one-sided consciousness. The point of the therapy is not to produce a finished or aesthetically pleasing object but to allow an active dialogue with the unconscious.

Sandtray Therapy

This method was inspired by Jung's construction of stone "villages" during his self-analysis and then was further developed by Dora Kalff, who combined Jung's ideas with Margaret Lowenfeld's World Technique. In Kalff's adaptation, a rectangular box measuring approximately $30 \times 20 \times 3$ inches is filled with sand and becomes a miniature world that a child or adult can shape and form, meanwhile arranging any of the hundreds of figurines the analyst provides. In therapy, the sandtray becomes a world through which complexes, pain, trauma, moods, emotions, and feelings are given expression. Use of the sandtray, like other forms of active imagination, provides a bridge to the unconscious; during the process, the child or adult can also recover undeveloped elements of his or her character (Bradway, Chambers, & Chiaia, 2005). Sand-play studies document the efficacy of the procedure (Bradway & McCoard, 1997). Over the course of therapy, the trays show a progressive change from a primitive and disorganized state, through images representative of vegetation, animals the shadow and the human, toward more order, peacefulness, and integration. Symbols appearing toward the end of therapy often have a mandala form and tend to evoke a holy feeling.

Sandtray therapy with children is useful as a structured and healing form of free play that promotes the child's ego development and unblocks hidden feelings. In adults, it returns the patient to a world of childhood play where lost parts of the personality can again come alive and contribute to self-healing.

Child Analysis

Children pick up and reflect what is going on in their surroundings. This happens to such a degree that Jung once analyzed a parent through the dreams and nightmares of his son. Training in child analysis is required at a growing number of Jungian Institutes and is based on core work by the Jungian analysts Frances Wickes, Erich Neumann, Dora Kalff, and Edith Sullwold. Treatment is based on the theory that children have within themselves what they need for a natural process of growth and self-healing to occur. The process works by providing a safe environment in which the therapist serves as witness, participant, and ally, who not only treats the child but also intervenes appropriately so that the child's family and life situation can be improved. During therapy, the child slowly learns to integrate and humanize potentially overwhelming archetypal images. Children's therapy is similar to adults' analytical psychotherapy, but it uses a wider variety of tactile and nonverbal modalities. A child finds expression for dreams, fantasies, and fears through sandtray therapy, arts and crafts, clay modeling, musical instruments, and body movement, as well as through stories and myths. The therapist provides boundaries and a safe space so that the child can work out problems, strengthen ego and resilience, and become more self-accepting, independent, and better functioning.

Post-Traumatic Stress

In 1934, in a letter to a Dr. Birnie, Jung wrote of the profound biological (as well as psychological) changes that can follow the experience of an overwhelming trauma. He went on to write about repetitive dreams and the way the unconscious keeps bringing the trauma up as if to search for its healing through repetition. Modern research on post-traumatic stress disorder (PTSD) supports Jung's observations and documents similar physical and psychological changes in survivors of wars, abuse, torture, and other overwhelming situations. Werner Engel (1986) has described his work with Nazi concentration camp survivors and their long-lasting feelings of guilt. He states that the power of Jungian psychotherapy lies in the curative value of patient and therapist listening together to a patient's horrors, combined with a belief in self-healing and the application of archetypal theory.

Henry Wilmer (1986) studied 103 patients suffering from PTSD subsequent to their Vietnam service, focusing on their repetitive nightmares. He believed that such photographic repetition must have a psychological and/or biological purpose. He shared the pain of one PTSD patient as expressed through his dreams and experience. Accompanying the patient in a receptive, noninterpretive way, Wilmer watched as the patient's nightmares finally began to change. The patient started to wake up, not caught in the frozen repetition of a flashback, but in tears. Healing took place when the patient mourned what had happened, found meaning in his experience, and finally saw his role in the dream shift into one in which he could actively change the outcome.

Donald Kalsched (1996, 2009) found that severe trauma during childhood can produce an internalization of the traumatizer that remains active in the now-adult psyche. He observes that the patients' self-attacking internal figures initially serve to defend the psyche but gradually change, over the course of therapy, until these isolating defenses are no longer needed.

Increasing numbers of individual Jungian analysts are helping traumatized populations around the world (Murray Stein, personal communication). For instance: Heyong Shen, a Chinese analyst, took his students and volunteer analysts from other countries to help set up sandtray centers in schools and orphanages after the 2008 earthquake in China. Eva Pattis and others have done the same in townships of Africa and Ethiopia, while some Zurich analysts are delivering Jungian oriented therapy services to refugees and traumatized people in Afghanistan and the Balkans. This indicates a new and growing urge to widen the response of Jungians to our increasingly troubled world.

The Treatment of Psychosis

Jung as a psychiatrist treated a full range of severe mental problems. He discerned a pattern and internal logic in the psychotic utterances and fantasies of patients he treated and concluded that the personality of the patient in a psychosis is dominated by a complex split from reality and/or is overwhelmed by (and identifies with) archetypal images that belong to the collective unconscious. Jung believed that the psychotic's upheaval led to distinct psychosomatic changes as well as to chemical changes in the brain. He also speculated that some bodily toxin might produce the psychosis. Today, analytical treatment of psychosis includes listening for the meaning or metaphor behind the symptom so that psychotics' mental worlds and imagery can be used in their healing. Group work, a safe living environment, and art therapy are valuable adjuncts to psychotherapy, as is medication. All help build an environment in which patients can emerge from their chaotic and mythic worlds and prepare for a more regular life. A minority of analytical therapists believe that medication blunts the regression of a psychotic person and prevents the individual from working through the psychosis. Some therapists have run types of home-based therapy, where patients and therapists interact in a homelike setting throughout the day. They report the successful treatment of a schizophrenic episode without the use of drugs and with no relapse; however, no long-range study of this form of therapy has been done.

Evidence

Evaluation of the Therapist

Training and supervisory assessment: A Jungian analyst undergoes a rigorous training program during which he or she is assessed and evaluated in classes, in case seminars, in individual supervision, and through appearances before various committees that closely monitor the quality of candidates' patient care as well as their self-knowledge.

A combination of clinical and theoretical exams and a written case study and/or thesis round out training based on the depth of the candidate's own analysis. Participation in peer supervision, in monthly meetings of individual analytic societies, regional yearly meetings, and international meetings is combined with reading or writing articles in various Jungian clinical journals. Each society of Jungian analysts has education and ethics committees that monitor and review the quality of care that therapists deliver.

Evaluation of Therapy

The most convincing and conclusive studies evaluating particular forms of psychodynamic psychotherapy conclude that therapy is more beneficial than no therapy, but that the type of therapy is less important than the quality of the person who delivers it and the match, and/or empathic bond, between patient and therapist. Thus, followers of a specific modality can make only modest claims for their theory's value, even though therapists' and patients' belief in that theory enhances positive outcomes.

The evaluation of the success of analytical psychotherapy comes from clinical observation, mainly through single case studies. In them, as well as in patients' reports, the patient's quality of life usually improves slowly over the course of the therapy. Dreams can be evaluated in terms of the evolution of the types of images and in terms of changes in their affective content over the course of the analysis. For example, nightmares usually cease, and their terrifying images or threatening figures slowly change into more benign or friendly ones. A specific dream may indicate that the time for the termination of therapy has arrived; this could be as graphic as a dream in which the patient bids good-bye to the therapist before a positive move or journey, or as subtle as one in which the patient not only acquires a piece of beautiful fabric she once dreamed her therapist owned but is now weaving her own material as well.

Subjective assessment is also meaningful: The improving patient reports symptom relief, looks more alive, has more energy, and often can release and experience blocked or untapped channels of creativity. Relationships with other people improve markedly. The process of growth becomes independent of the therapist when patients start to do their own work between sessions, master new and enriching habits of introspection and self-examination, pay attention to their dreams and fantasies, and deal with themselves and others with integrity. An analytical psychotherapist would agree with Freud that learning to love and to work is the key to measuring the outcome of a successful analysis. Jungians would also want to see their patients develop a more intimate knowledge of, a relationship with, and responsibility for all aspects of their psyche. This development often leads patients to grapple with philosophical and religious questions about the meaning of existence, including their personal responsibility to the world in which they find themselves and which they will pass on to others.

Evaluation of Theory

Both qualitative and quantitative studies have examined Jung's theories (Kast, 2009), most especially of typology. These types, or personality dimensions, consist of the two basic attitudes of introversion and extraversion and the four functions of thinking, feeling, intuition, and sensation. We all have these qualities to different degrees, but we often prefer one mode to the others. The *Myers-Briggs* and the *Grey-Wheelwright* typology tests ascertain a person's predominant attitude and function, as well as the relative amounts of each attitude and function in an individual's personality (Beebe, 2006). Both tests are questionnaires that follow Jung's original formulations, determining a person's degree of introversion and extraversion, as well as his or her relative preference for the thinking, feeling, sensing, and intuitive modes of experiencing reality. The tests give a more rounded view of character than simply looking at a single function or attitude. The Myers-Briggs adds questions to determine whether one perceives things first (as Jung wrote of sensates and intuitives) or judges them first (as both feelers and thinkers do). It yields 16 different personality types. Many analysts find these typology tests especially beneficial when working with couples. By indicating differences in the ways in which people of differing types tend to interpret their environment, they provide an objective explanation for many problems in communication. The theory is now undergoing major assessment and review (Beebe, 2006).

Jung used statistics in his Word Association Tests to display evidence of his theory of complexes. Some analysts make use of these association tests to uncover material in patients who have difficulties with self-exploration. Projective tests such as the Rorschach test and the Thematic Apperception Test (TAT), which are based on Jung's theories of complex and projection, are also used. Contemporary studies of the validity of projective tests have been less persuasive, but the tests themselves still prove clinically useful. *The Journal of Analytical Psychology* has a research section, as well as a directory of research in analytical psychology, and sponsors a yearly conference.

A major contribution to the science of Analytical Psychology has come about through recent discoveries in neuroscience. Infant research and infant observation have mapped the development of self-awareness and the crucial importance of relational dynamics, whereas trauma and its healing are being measured in analysis of brain MRIs (Wilkinson, 2006;). Daniel Shore (2006), in his foreword to Wilkinson's book, states that these more accurate models of development have generated "a deeper understanding of change processes within the unconscious mind that potentially occur over all later stages of the lifespan, including models of change within the psychotherapeutic context" (p. vii).

Hester Solomon (2000) goes so far as to conclude that these discoveries are synthesizing "archetypal theory, the ethological basis of attachment theory, psychoanalytic object relations theory, and Jungian development theory, all of which can be hard-grounded in the skin-to-skin, brain-to-brain neurobiological interconnectedness between the infant and its primary caregiver" (p. 136). Therapy is being measured for the best ways to accomplish repair (Wilkinson, 2003; 2006).

Psychotherapy in a Multicultural World

Multiculturalism can be seen through the growing number of South American, Asian, and Eastern European Institutes and Jungian societies; the small but growing number of Asian, African-American, Hispanic, gay, lesbian, and feminist analysts in the United States; and a newly active attention in training and in journals to multicultural, gender, and aging issues. Samuels, for example, in *Politics on the Couch* (2001) calls for psychotherapists to develop a sense of sociocultural reality and responsibility with clients and in the community at large, while Singer and Kimbles (2004), in *The Cultural Complex,* examine the source and nature of group conflict from a Jungian perspective. An important new book, *Jungian Psychoanalysis* (Stein, in press), has chapters on cultural complexes in the process of analysis or psychotherapy, on the influence of gender and sexuality on therapy, on the influence of culture (in this case Japanese culture), and a study of therapy with a person with a congenital physical disability.

Along with this important and growing emphasis, there is also a backlash among more conservative Jungians who argue that Jung's original words—even when considered socioculturally suspect by today's standards—should not be reinterpreted or "watered down" by contemporary standards or cross-fertilization but, rather, should be accepted and taught as he first presented them. Some Jungian institutes are experiencing a paradigm shift, accompanied by fruitful ferment and discussion (see Casement, 2009, Douglas, 2008, and Withers, 2003 for a discussion of these issues); other institutes have split into two or more groups because of this disagreement.

CASE EXAMPLE

Rochelle, a divorced white woman in her mid-thirties, taught at a community college. Her self-consciousness and anxiety brought her into analysis, as did the nightmares that had plagued her since childhood. She was drawn to Jungian psychotherapy because of a lifelong interest in dreams and a love of myths and fairy tales. She had been in therapy before (it had started off well but ended in disappointment), and she wondered if working with a female analyst this time would make a difference.

During the initial stages of therapy, Rochelle settled into twice-weekly sessions. The following facts emerged during the first months of treatment, often in association with dream material. She remembered little about her childhood except having had an active fantasy and dream life and having been happiest alone, outdoors, or daydreaming. Her family life had been chaotic. For several years while she was in grade school, partly because of her father's illness, Rochelle was sent by her mother to live with a series of relatives. Later she was dispatched to a girls' boarding school, where she did well. She was a good student who was active in student government. Rochelle had earned her own living since she was 18, putting herself through college with a scholarship and a series of part-time jobs.

She reported being close to neither parent but having more negative feelings toward her mother, blaming her for neglect. Rochelle had a form of negative mother complex expressed in her determination to do everything in a way opposite to the way her mother did things. Rochelle kept clear of her mother psychically through the development of her thinking function, especially in academic work, in which she excelled. She typified Jung's further description of this type of unmothered daughter as being awkward, lacking body awareness, and suffering from a variety of uterine problems; in Rochelle's case, a hysterectomy had been suggested.

Even though Rochelle most often appeared to be dryly rationalistic, there was also a charged emotional component in her personality that revealed itself in the outbursts of tears that accompanied early therapy sessions. Her therapist gave Rochelle typology tests. Rochelle was found to be markedly introverted, with thinking as her primary function followed by intuition; sensation and feeling were conspicuously low. Rochelle gained comfort from reading about these types and learning that she behaved fairly typically for a person with an undeveloped and primitive feeling function.

In the initial stages of therapy, Rochelle exhibited a strong idealizing transference and worked hard during the hour, although it felt to her therapist as if she were encased in ice. (The therapist was primarily an introverted sensation type and so tended to experience things first as inner images or sensations rather than as ideas or emotions.) However, Rochelle took great pleasure in having someone listen to the story of her life and take her dreams seriously. Her therapist kept interpretations to a minimum and directed attention as much as possible to Rochelle's daily life. Rochelle could not accept anything that seemed like criticism from her analyst but flourished under the analyst's empathic reflection of her feelings; gradually she started to look more relaxed and attractive as she felt herself valued and nurtured.

Rochelle had one or two women friends but had trouble relating to men. She tended to fall in love rapidly, idealizing the man and often negating her own interests to meet his and to help him with his career. Overidealization and a romantic belief in living happily ever after, however, soon turned into hypercriticism and rejection, withdrawal, and flight. Some of these dynamics in her personal life started to appear in the consulting room. Compliance and admiration marked Rochelle's conscious relationship to her therapist, but she seemed to be always on guard. The therapist's countertransference was a strong bodily feeling of distance, at times as if her patient were miles away across the room or vanishing. There was something almost desperate behind the exaggeratedly "Jungian" quality and quantity of the material Rochelle brought to her therapy hour.

It was as if Rochelle were trying very hard to produce what she thought her therapist would want, without noticing her therapist's efforts to focus on Rochelle's anxiety symptoms and her outer life. The therapist used the dream material sparingly, primarily as a doorway into the reality of Rochelle's experience. Rochelle concealed from herself her contempt for her analyst's continued emphasis on the here and now and her focus on Rochelle's physical and psychological condition. When this was brought to Rochelle's attention, she responded with a fierce burst of anger that brought the pain of her negative mother complex to the surface. There ensued a number of months of transference in which Rochelle attacked the analyst as the negative mother while the analyst subjectively felt the misery Rochelle had experienced under her mother's care.

Despite the negative transference, however, Rochelle kept turning up for sessions. In response to the therapist's support of Rochelle's sensation function and her need for autonomy, she sought out a second opinion concerning her hysterectomy and found that it was not indicated. Rochelle also started to pay attention to her body. About nine months after her decision not to undergo the operation, she enrolled in a dance class upon learning from an acquaintance that her analyst liked to dance.

The analyst did not interpret her behavior but held it in the back of her mind. She continued to pay a hovering, almost free-floating attention to Rochelle's behavior and words, as well as to the images and sensations they brought up in her own mind. She noticed that the feeling quality in the room was growing warmer but still contained chilling voids that seemed to parallel Rochelle's own recollection of her past. The therapist felt a sense of foreboding building up with each visit, as though Rochelle were accompanied by some chaotic and unspecific feeling of violence.

Rochelle attended a weekend dance/movement seminar at the local Jungian Institute; at the following session, as she started to describe a nightmare, her nose started to bleed. A look of horror came over Rochelle's face as she experienced the first of a series of flashbacks accompanied by recurrent nightmares. They concerned the sexual attacks she had endured as a child after she had been sent to live with a relative who was an elder in their church. He had coerced her into secrecy under the threat of God's wrath, and he had explained the blood on the child's bedclothes to the housekeeper as the result of a nosebleed.

Initially in therapy, Rochelle had professed herself untouched by this molestation, but now its full emotional impact flooded her. The slow recall of discrete images and memories marked a critical point in therapy. Rochelle fell into a depression and entered a needy and fearful regression during which her sessions were increased to four times a week. At this time, Rochelle made considerable use of the clay, art materials, and sandtray that her analyst kept in her office. Most of the emotional history of her trauma came first through her hands; only later could it be put into words. It took many more months before the splits in Rochelle's feeling recall were slowly filled in and the story of her early life emerged in a more or less linear way. Rochelle now looked to her therapist as a positive mother figure and felt entirely safe only in the therapy room and its boundaries, although she lashed out at her therapist for causing her to feel the reality of her memories and for taking away the lovely dreams into which she had escaped.

In her regression, Rochelle found weekends and holidays intolerable but got through them by borrowing a small figure from the sandtray. Her analyst felt great tenderness for her patient as she witnessed Rochelle's experience and shared her pain. She allied herself with her patient's efforts to recall secrets that had long been repressed. She let them unfold in their own order and time, without questioning or probing. Sometimes the therapist felt drained by the quantity of pain that was now flooding the room and struggled with herself to neither block it nor silence Rochelle. For both analyst and patient, these were difficult times in the analysis, as both experienced the surfacing of the agony that Rochelle had not been able to permit herself to feel before. The therapist found herself increasingly inclined to comfort Rochelle and was tempted to break her own boundary rules by extending the hour or letting Rochelle stay on for a cup of tea. She considered how much of her response was countertransference and how much represented something she needed to process further in herself. The analyst knew how crucial it was for her to symbolically hold the transference in this charged arena and not act it out; she also knew that part of the force field generated by Rochelle's initial trauma came from the dangerous pull toward repetition that Rochelle and many trauma survivors experience. In order to check that she completely understood her own countertransference issues, the analyst went into supervision with a senior analyst. Through weeks of self-confrontive work, the analyst gained a deeper understanding of the powerfully destructive pull to reenactment that makes trauma survivors all too often fall victim to reinjury. Both Rochelle and her therapist succeeded in maintaining their boundaries without cutting off the current between them. [See Douglas (1997a, 2006), Kalsched (1996, 2009), and Rutter (1997) for a further discussion of this important subject from a Jungian standpoint.]

Shortly after her therapist had completed her own self-examination, Rochelle emerged from her depression and started intensive work on the transference on a different level. This was accompanied by Rochelle's reading about goddesses and images of powerful female archetypes. At this point, work on the archetypal image of incest started to accompany the personal work. Rochelle came into the session one day with an Irish myth that she said both terrified and fascinated her. For a time, its analogies with her own trauma became the focus of much of Rochelle's interest, as she and the therapist began to use the myth as a common metaphor. This caused renewed work on Rochelle's childhood abuse at a deeper but also more universal level.

The myth was about a girl named Saeve, whose relative, a Druid named Dark, pursued her. Unable to escape his advances, she turned herself into a deer and vanished into the woods. Three years later a hero, Fionn, found her and led her to his castle, where she turned back into a beautiful young woman. They lived completely enraptured with each other until Fionn had to leave for battle. Soon after Fionn's departure, Saeve thought she saw him returning; she raced out of the castle to meet him but realized too late that it was the Druid disguised as Fionn. He tapped her with his hazel rod and turned her back into a deer, and they vanished.

Rochelle used this fairy tale to picture her own neurotic patterns of behavior. Through the story, she could start to view them objectively, without shame. The myth gave form and an image to the damage she had experienced from too potent and too early experience of an invasive other. Rochelle gained a feeling for her own horrors through her feelings for Saeve; she also began to understand her defense of splitting off from reality (becoming a deer) when scared and vanishing into daydreams. The story also helped Rochelle comprehend why she seemed incapable of maintaining a relationship, turning every lover from a Fionn into a Druid. Eventually she even recognized that she had internalized the church elder into an inner negative animus who kept judgmentally assaulting her.

As Rochelle's therapy progressed, she stopped turning against the childlike parts of herself that needed to idealize someone as all-good, and she started to forgive herself for what had happened to her. She also started to understand the protective value of splitting off from an intolerable reality and assuming a deerlike disguise. As she did this, that particular defense started to drop away. Rochelle also grew to understand her desire for a savior: What she had experienced was so vile (the touch of the Druid) that what she longed for became impossibly pure (Fionn). She also better understood her self-consciousness and fear of people, as well as her feelings of loneliness; she felt she had lived much of her life alone as a deer in the woods hiding in disguise, flight, and illusion instead of being able to maintain relationships.

Her therapist's accompanying Rochelle on this voyage of discovery allowed her the time to look at the world in terms of the separation and division of opposites: the blackest of villains versus the noblest of heroes. Rochelle realized that she was repeatedly searching for Fionn, the hero, protector, and savior, whom she inevitably scanned for the slightest defect. And just as inevitably, when he showed a failing or two, she looked upon him as an all-evil Druid. She then escaped in deer disguise and in a split-off little-girl vulnerability, yet behind her meltingly doelike softness lay a self-destructive, self-hating, abusive, rapist animus tearing at her sad child's soul. On the other side, her inner hero tended to become icily rational or heady; he drove Rochelle into unmercifully heroic activity and disdained the dark, sensual, unmaidenly feminine inside her. The Druid animus brutalized her inner child-maiden and the deer, while the virtuous animus punished her for the very brutalization she experienced.

At this point Rochelle became kinder to herself. She stopped ricocheting from one opposite to the other and stopped mistaking the dark for the light or turning someone she had thought good into bad as soon as he made a mistake. Her impaired relations with others slowly started to heal as she allowed her therapist to be neither all-light nor all-dark but intermingled. Through confronting and fighting with her analyst, Rochelle started to regain some of her own darkly potent female energy. Now she also started to be able to claim her own needs in a relationship, rather than disguising herself as an all-giving woman.

Assimilation of her shadow, not identification with it, grounded Rochelle. Her nightmares lessened in intensity after a watchful and self-contained black cat, whom Rochelle associated with her therapist, started to appear in her dreams sitting on a round rug and silently witnessing the dream's turmoil. Rochelle felt that the female cat figure symbolized something old and complex, as if it held attributes of both a Wise Woman and a Terrible Mother in its centered witnessing. From this center and with the continued empathic witnessing support of her therapist, Rochelle's inner and outer lives gradually changed as she mulled over her life history and her powerfully archetypal myth and dream material. It was not enough for her to experience something of this intensity in the consulting room; she needed to see what the images meant in her own life. As Rochelle slowly reclaimed and integrated the cat, the animus figures, and finally the good-enough mother analyst in herself, the black cat figure in her dreams assumed a human form. Rochelle decided to leave an analysis that had taken three and a half years; there followed a newly creative turn in her work, and she also risked loving a quiet and fallible man. Over the next few years, Rochelle returned to her therapy for brief periods in times of crisis or as her complexes reappeared, but she generally could rely on her inner therapist for recentering herself.

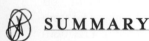

SUMMARY

Jung pioneered an approach to the psyche that attracts a growing number of people through its breadth of vision and its deep respect for the individual. Rather than pathologizing, Jung looked for the meaning behind symptoms, believing that symptoms held the key to their own cure. Jung discovered methods and techniques for tapping into the self-healing potential in human beings and taught a process that engages therapist and patient alike in a profound and growth-promoting experience. Jung's purpose was to assist psychological development and healing by involving all aspects of the personality.

Analytical personality theory provides a map of the psyche that values the unconscious as much as consciousness, seeing each as complementing the other. In the personal realm, the personal conscious (the ego or I) and persona (the social mask) are matched with the personal unconscious. The personal unconscious contains things repressed, forgotten, or at the verge of consciousness, as well as the personal shadow (what the ego does not accept in itself) and the animus and anima (ego-alien contrasexual elements). The impersonal or collective unconscious can never be known, but it can be pictured as a vast deposit that flows into the personal unconscious and consciousness by means of archetypal images: propensities, motifs, and forms common to all humanity. The interface between the collective and personal unconscious may represent the most archaic and least-mapped layer of the psyche. Complexes grow in this interface. Complexes are energy-filled constellations of psychic elements that have an archetypal core and erupt into consciousness, often in an autonomous way. They are both personal and impersonal. The personal unconscious is created by the individual and ultimately is his or her personal responsibility. Since the collective unconscious is innate and impersonal, it would be an error for the individual to claim its powers or in any way identify with its contents. The unconscious itself is completely neutral and becomes dangerous only to the degree that the ego has a wrong relationship to it or represses it. The impersonal realm is home also to the collective consciousness, the giant matrix of the outer world in which an individual lives his or her life.

The archetype of the Self encompasses the personal unconscious and conscious and a bit of the other realms as they impinge on or seep into the personal. A newborn infant is immersed in the self; it soon splits (or deintegrates) into fragments of ego, consciousness, and unconscious. The task of psychotherapy is to consolidate the ego and let the psyche heal and responsibly enlarge itself so that all the parts of the self can develop, reintegrate, and maintain a more balanced and less egocentric relationship with each other. In analytical psychotherapy, it is not enough to understand these concepts and their activity; they must be felt experientially by the individual in relation to the past and as they come into play in the therapy room through transference and countertransference. The new understanding then needs to be lived so that the individual can participate in life with integrity. To this end, experiential methods of analytical psychotherapy are especially valuable, as is the therapist's inclusion of the feminine dimension of receptive empathy, groundedness, nurturing, and ability to hold the personality as it develops. This generative approach allows growth and healing to take place alongside what can be gained from insight and interpretation.

Analytical psychotherapy stresses the patient-therapist encounter as one that involves empathy, trust, openness, and risk. Through the interaction of the two personalities and the quality of this relationship, the self-regulating and healing potential of the personality can come into play, repairing old wounds while allowing the individual to grow in self-knowledge. This is why analytical psychotherapy stresses the quality, training, analysis, and continuing self-analysis of therapists.

Depth psychotherapy, as it is understood today, is less than a century old. Jung often wrote of psychology being in its infancy, and he believed no one map of its realm could be complete. Depth-oriented psychotherapeutic systems of all types contain more similarities than differences. The systems reflect the language and style of their creator and attract those of like mind. It is as if all the founders of the varied schools have drawn slightly different maps of the same terrain—the human psyche. Although the particular style of these maps varies, those that are still useful have more and more in common as original rivalries are forgotten and each is freer to borrow what it needs from the others. At the same time, a specifically Jungian map may be best for one person, whereas someone else may need an Adlerian, a Rogerian, a neo-Freudian, or some other map.

Jungian psychology is especially inclusive, because its four stages of therapy cover essential elements of the others' theories while adding a particular emphasis on wholeness, completion, and individuation. Analytical psychotherapy allows room for the depths of the collective unconscious and the width of humanity's collective history, art, and culture, while grounding itself solidly in the particular individual at a particular time and place. It is a rich and diverse system that rests on a theory whose practice undergoes constant transformation as the experience and needs of the individual and society both change.

ANNOTATED BIBLIOGRAPHY

Primary Sources

Jung, C. G. (1954–1991). *The collected works of C. G. Jung.* (22 volumes). Princeton, NJ: Princeton University Press.

See especially the following:

Jung, C. G. (1957). *The practice of psychotherapy. Collected works,* Vol. 16.
This collection of Jung's essays and lectures includes both basic and in-depth discussions of Jung's methods and techniques of psychotherapy. Part One concerns general problems in psychotherapy and clearly differentiates Jung's theory and practice from those of Freud and Adler. Part Two examines specific topics such as abreaction, Jungian dream analysis, and transference. Most of the book is highly suitable for general study; however, the article on the transference is steeped in Jung's alchemical studies and is somewhat arcane.

Jung, C. G. (1935/1956). *Two essays on analytical psychology. Collected works,* Vol. 17.
A clear, succinct portrayal of the basic concepts of analytical psychology, this book also gives a good account of the early history of depth psychology. Part One sets out Jung's ideas on the psychology of the unconscious, clearly differentiating the personal from the impersonal unconscious. Part Two deals with the ego and its relationship to the personal and collective unconscious and to the task of integration and individuation.

Secondary Sources

Dougherty, N.J. and West, J. J. (2007). *The matrix and meaning of character: An archetypal and developmental approach.* New York: Routledge.
Surveys all the DSM-IV personality disorders and discusses nine character structures from a Jungian perspective.

Douglas, C. (2006). *The old woman's daughter.* College Station, Texas A&M University Press.
Reflecting Jungian theory in its development and in practice, this book presents and reclaims the importance of a feminine as well as a masculine way of doing therapy and being in the world. Chapter Three traces the development of a Jungian body-aware, nurturing, and receptively attuned way of doing therapy that values nonverbal and early-attachment states. Chapter Four includes a long case study of the analysis of a middle-aged man integrating his masculine and feminine sides.

Kalsched, D. (1998). Archetypal affect, anxiety and defense in patients who have suffered early trauma. In A. Casement (Ed.), *Post-Jungians today: Key papers in contemporary analytical psychology* (pp. 83–102). New York: Routledge.
Kalsched discusses the ways in which the psyche internalizes trauma and demonstrates the self's role in defending the psyche. He describes the way a self-care system often keeps the trauma victim at the mercy of sadistic, self-attacking internal figures and dreams. Kalsched considers dreams and dream images about these terrifying "dark forces," as well as a dream that demonstrated a core positive side to a patient's psyche and an opening toward healing. After a historical overview of depth psychologists' work on primitive anxiety and defense, he ends with a discussion of the transformation possible in therapy.

Papadopolous, R. K. (2006). *The handbook of Jungian psychology: Theory, practice, applications.* New York: Routledge.
This clear and concise delineation of the basic tenets of analytical psychology and its current developments is authored by many (often British) authorities. Part One sets out Jung's basic theory in seven chapters covering Jung's epistemology, the unconscious, archetypes, shadow, anima/animus, psychological types, and the self. Part Two concerns therapy, Part Three applications to other fields. Each chapter discusses Jung's position, his major innovations, and the relevance of his theories; developments since Jung's time; and the current status of analytical psychology and trends for future development.

Rosen, D. (2002). *Transforming depression: Healing the soul through creativity.* York Beach, ME: Nicholas-Hays.
A practical book on treating depression and suicide that offers a creative way for therapists to help their clients turn away from self-destruction and hopelessness and toward a more meaningful life. The book is a good overview of crisis points and suicidality—as well as of current diagnosis and treatment—from biological, sociological, psychological, and spiritual perspectives. Part Three of the book is particularly useful to the clinician; it follows in detail the treatment of four patients and illustrates Rosen's theory put into practice.

Sedgwick, D. (2001). *Introduction to Jungian psychotherapy: The therapeutic relationship.* Philadelphia: Taylor and Francis.
This is a detailed account of analytical psychotherapy that focuses on the unique relationship between patient and therapist. Sedgwick's well-argued thesis is that this relationship constitutes the main healing factor in psychotherapy. He demonstrates this belief using both traditional Jungian theory and such post-Freudians as Bion, Klein, Kohut, and Winnicott. A clear, concise, and grounded basic teaching text on clinical issues, it is especially thorough on transference and countertransference in therapy and on ways to set up and maintain the practical components of a good therapeutic relationship. Clinical examples are particularly well chosen.

Singer, T., and Kimbles, S. (Eds.). (2004). *The cultural complex: Contemporary Jungian perspectives on psyche and society.* New York: Brunner-Routledge.
This is a key book written by academics and analysts from many countries and cultures. It examines the psychological nature of conflict from a Jungian perspective and presents a clear picture of its source in both personal and cultural complexes. It looks at cultural complexes historically as played out in Jung, Freud, and their followers' quarrel. It examines racism with an excellent case history. Its strongest chapters focus on the way collective and personal trauma fuel cultural complexes.

Withers, R. (2003). *Controversies in analytical psychology.* New York: Brunner-Routledge.

Eleven mostly clinical differences of approach in current analytical practice are discussed by 24 Jungian analysts or psychotherapists. Some of the issues debated are the prospects for a Jung/Klein synthesis; the status of developmental theory; working with the transference; the role of interpretation; frequency of sessions and keeping the analytic frame; integrating the body/mind split; and political, religious, and gender issues, as well as a rare discussion of the heterosexual framing of most theory and how this might affect homosexual analysts and patients.

Young-Eisendrath, P., and Dawson, T. (Eds.). (2008). *The Cambridge companion to Jung.* 2nd ed. Cambridge, Eng. and New York: Cambridge University Press.

A critical introduction to Jung's theory and work and their importance to current psychotherapy, this book is divided into three parts. Part One discusses Jung's ideas and their context. Part Two examines Jungian psychology in practice, with chapters on archetypal, developmental, and classical approaches to psychotherapy and a case study discussed from these three vantage points. Part Three addresses analytical psychology in contemporary society, literature, gender studies, politics, and religion.

CASE READINGS

Abramovich, H. (2002). Temenos regained: Reflections on the absence of the analyst. *Journal of Analytical Psychology, 47*(4), 583–598.

Two cases are used to illustrate boundary and containment issues. The first and lengthier discussion is of a woman who needed to preserve the analytic container while her therapist was away for several months. The case is explored in much detail, and a novel and healing way to provide a holding space is found. Abramovich's discussion of maternal reverie and maternal holding in therapy is of special interest. In the second case, the patient has a chance extra-analytic encounter with his therapist, who exits quickly. The patient perceives Abramovich's sacrifice of his self-interest as an effort to preserve the patient's space; he contrasts it with the way someone in his household took advantage of him over many years. For the first time, the patient could experience a safe place both within and outside of the therapy.

Beebe, J., McNeely, D., and Gordon, G. (2008). The case of Joan: Classical archetypal, and developmental approaches. In Young-Eisendrath and Dawson (Eds.), *Cambridge companion to Jung* (pp. 185–219). Cambridge, UK: Cambridge University Press.

Three analysts focus on the study of a 40-year-old woman suffering from an eating disorder, each with an emphasis on a different style of Jungian therapy.

Douglas, C. (2006). The case of Bruce. In C. Douglas, *The old woman's daughter.* College Station, Texas A&M University Press.

This case study demonstrates the way a Jungian therapist uses dream and analytical work to help a client overcome a midlife crisis through the reintegration of cut-off aspects of himself, especially his feminine side. The case highlights issues of transference and countertransference. [Reprinted in D. Wedding and R. J. Corsini (Eds.). (2011). *Case studies in psychotherapy.* Belmont, CA: Brooks/Cole.]

Jung, C. G. (1968). An analysis of a patient's dream. *Analytical psychology: Its theory and practice.* New York: Pantheon.

This analysis of a patient's dream is taken from one of Jung's speeches. It demonstrates the ways in which dreams can be used to support clinical inferences.

Kalsched, D. (1996). The inner world of trauma in a diabolical form, and further clinical illustrations of the self care system. In *The inner world of trauma: Archetypal defenses of the personal spirit,* Chapters One and Two (pp. 11–67). London and New York: Routledge.

Important case reading on trauma and post-traumatic stress, the two chapters present a series of nine cases, discussed and interpreted, in which early childhood trauma has produced similar defenses, repetition compulsions, and self-care systems that further isolate and attack each of the patients. Healing is shown as occurring in a similar manner across all cases.

Kimbles, S. L. (2004). A cultural complex operating in the overlap of clinical and cultural space. In T. Singer, and S. Kimbles, (Eds.), *The Cultural Complex: Contemporary Jungian perspectives on psyche and society* (pp. 199–211). New York: Brunner-Routledge.

The relationship between personal complexes and a cultural complex is explored in the analysis of a patient and analyst of different races and genders. The material is clearly portrayed through the dreams and fantasies of the patient and through the dynamics of transference/countertransference as experienced by the analyst.

REFERENCES

Bair, D. (2003) *Jung: A biography.* Boston: Little Brown.

Beebe, J. (1992). *Integrity in depth.* College Station, TX: Texas A&M University Press.

Beebe, (2006). Psychological types. In R. Papadopolous (Ed.), *The handbook of Jungian psychology* (pp. 130–152). New York: Routledge.

Bishop, P. (2009). *Analytics psychology and german classical aesthetics: Goethe, Schiller, and Jung.* Vol. 2, The constellation of the self. London: Routledge.

Bosnak, R. (1996). *Tracks in the wildernesss of dreaming: Explorung interior landscape through practical dreaming.* New York: Delta.

Bradway, K., & McCoard, B. (1997). *Sandplay—Silent workshop of the psyche.* New York: Routledge.

Bradway, K., Chambers, L., & Chiaia, M. E. (2005). *Sandplay in three voices: Images, relationship, the numinous.* London: Routledge.

Cambray, J., and Carter, L. (Eds.). (2004). *Analytical psychology: Contemporary perspectives in Jungian analysis.* New York: Brunner-Routledge.

Casement, A. (in press). Training programs. In M. Stein (Ed.), *Jungian psychoanalysis.* Chicago: Open Court.

Chodorow, J. (2006). Active Imagination. In R. Papadopolous (Ed.), *The handbook of Jungian psychology* (pp. 215–243). New York: Routledge.

Chodorow, J. (Ed.). (1997). *Jung on active imagination.* Princeton: Princeton University Press.

Crowther, C. (in press). Supervision. In M. Stein (Ed.), *Jungian psychoanalysis.* Chicago: Open Court.

Davis, D. (2008). Freud, Jung, and psychoanalysis. In P. Young-Eisendrath and T. Dawson (Eds.), *The Cambridge companion to Jung,* 2nd ed. (pp. 39–55). Cambridge, UK: Cambridge University Press.

Dieckmann, H. (1991). *Methods in analytical psychology.* Wilmette, IL: Chiron.

Dougherty, M. (in press). Interpretation of pictures. In M. Stein (Ed.), *Jungian psychoanalysis.* Chicago: Open Court.

Douglas, C. (1997a). After such violence: A reconceptualization of Jung's incest theory. In M. A. Mattoon, (Ed.), *Zurich 95: Open questions in analytical psychology.* Einsiedeln, Switzerland: Daimon Verlag.

Douglas, C. (1997b). Introduction. In C. G. Jung, *The visions seminar* (pp. ix–xxxiii). Princeton: Princeton University Press.

Douglas, C. (2006). *The old woman's daughter: Reimaging the mother archetype.* College Station: Texas A&M University Press.

Douglas, C. (2008). The historical context of analytical psychology. In P. Young-Eisendrath and T. Dawson (Eds.), *The Cambridge companion to Jung,* 2nd ed. (pp. 17–36). Cambridge, UK: Cambridge University Press.

Ellenberger, H. (1981). *The discovery of the unconscious.* New York: Basic Books.

Engel, W. H. (1986). Postscript. *Quadrant, 19*(1), 62.

Fordham, M. (1996). *Analyst-patient interaction: Collected papers on technique.* New York: Routledge.

Godsil, G. (2000). Winter's ragged hand: Creativity in the face of death. In E. Christopher & H. Solomon (Eds.), *Jungian thought in the modern world* (pp. 244–263). London: Free Association Books.

Higuchi, K. (in press). Jungian psychoanalysis in the context of Japanese culture. In M. Stein (Ed.), *Jungian psychoanalysis.* Chicago: Open Court.

Hollis, J. (2008). *Why good people do bad things: Understanding our darker selves.* New York, NY: Penguin.

Jung, C. G. (1904–1907/1973). Studies in word association. In *Experimental researches. Collected works,* Vol. 2 (pp. 3–482). Princeton: Princeton University Press.

Jung, C. G. (1907/1960). Psychology of dementia praecox. In *The psychogenesis of mental disease. Collected works,* Vol. 3 (pp. 1–151). Princeton: Princeton University Press.

Jung, C. G. (1911/1956). *The psychology of the unconscious.* Revised as *Symbols of transformation. Collected works,* Vol. 5. Princeton: Princeton University Press.

Jung, C. G. (1921/1971). *Psychological types. Collected works,* Vol. 6. Princeton: Princeton University Press.

Jung, C. G. (1927/1970). Woman in Europe. In *Civilization in transition. Collected works,* Vol. 10 (pp. 113–133). Princeton: Princeton University Press.

Jung, C. G. (1929/1933/1961). Freud and Jung: Contrasts. In *Freud and psychoanalysis. Collected works,* Vol. 4 (pp. 333–340). Princeton: Princeton University Press.

Jung, C. G. (1933/1966). Problems of modern psychotherapy. In *The practice of psychotherapy. Collected works,* Vol. 16. (pp. 53–75). Princeton: Princeton University Press.

Jung, C. G. (1934a/1970). *The development of personality. Collected works,* Vol. 17. Princeton: Princeton University Press.

Jung, C. G. (1934b/1966). The state of psychotherapy today. In *The practice of psychotherapy. Collected works,* Vol. 16 (pp. 157–173). Princeton: Princeton University Press.

Jung, C. G. (1934c/1966). The practical use of dream analysis. In *The practice of psychotherapy. Collected works,* Vol. 16 (pp. 139–161). Princeton: Princeton University Press.

Jung, C. G. (1935a/1966). Principles of practical psychotherapy. In *The practice of psychotherapy. Collected works,* Vol. 16 (pp. 3–20). Princeton: Princeton University Press.

Jung, C. G. (1935b/1966). The relations between the ego and the unconscious. In *Two essays on analytical psychology. Collected works,* Vol. 7 (pp. 132–134). Princeton: Princeton University Press.

Jung, C. G. (1935c/1980). The Tavistock lectures. In *Symbolic life: Miscellaneous writings. Collected works,* Vol. 18 (pp. 1–182). Princeton: Princeton University Press.

Jung, C. G. (1948/1980). Techniques of attitude change conducive to world peace. In *The symbolic life. Collected works,* Vol. 18 (pp. 606–613). Princeton: Princeton University Press.

Jung, C. G. (1957). *The practice of psychotherapy. Collected works,* Vol. 16. Princeton: Princeton University Press.

Jung, C. G. (1965). *Memories, dreams, reflections.* New York: Vintage.

Jung, C. G. (1976). *Mysterium Coniunctionis. Collected works,* Vol. 14. Princeton: Princeton University Press.

Kalsched, D. (1996). *The inner world of trauma: Archetypal defenses of the personal spirit.* New York: Routledge.

Kalsched, D. (in press). Working with trauma in analysis. In M. Stein (Ed.), *Jungian psychoanalysis.* Chicago: Open Court.

Kast, V. (in press). Research. In M. Stein (Ed.), *Jungian psychoanalysis.* Chicago: Open Court.

Maduro, R., & Wheelwright, J. B. (1977). Analytical psychology. In R. Corsini (Ed.), *Current personality theories* (pp. 83–124). Itasca, IL: F. E. Peacock.

Mathers, D. (Ed.) (2009). *Vision and supervision: Jungian and post-Jungian perspectives.* London: Routledge.

Mattoon, M. A. (2006). Dreams. In R. Papadopolous (Ed.), *The handbook of Jungian psychology* (pp. 244–260). New York: Routledge.

Monte, C. (in press). The body and movement in analysis. In M. Stein (Ed.), *Jungian psychoanalysis.* Chicago: Open Court.

Papadopolous, R. (Ed.). (2006). *The handbook of Jungian psychology.* New York: Routledge.

Rutter, P. (1997). *Sex in the forbidden zone: When men in power—therapists, doctors, clergy, teachers, and others—betray women's trust.* New York: Ballantine Books.

Salman, S. (in press). Active imagination. In M. Stein (Ed.), *Jungian psychoanalysis.* Chicago: Open Court.

Samuels, A. (2001). *Politics on the couch: Citizenship and the internal life.* New York: Karnac Books.

Shamdasani, S. (2003) *Jung and the making of modern psychology.* Cambridge: Cambridge University Press.

Sherwood, D. (in press). Training analysis. In M. Stein (Ed.), *Jungian psychoanalysis.* Chicago: Open Court.

Shore, D. (2006). Foreword. In M. Wilkinson, *Coming into mind: The mind-brain relationship: A Jungian clinical perspective* (pp. vii–xii). New York: Routledge.

Siegelman, E. Y. (1990). *Metaphor and meaning in psychotherapy.* New York: Guilford Press.

Siegelman, E. Y. (2002). The analyst's love: An exploration. *Journal of Jungian theory and practice, 3*(I), 19–33.

Siegelman, E. Y. (2003). "Amo, Amas, Amat." *San Francisco Jung Institute Library Journal, 22*(I), 19–28.

Singer, T., and Kimbles, S. (Eds.). (2004). *The cultural complex: Contemporary Jungian perspectives on psyche and society.* New York: Brunner-Routledge.

Solomon, H. (2000). Recent development in the neurosciences. In E. Christopher and H. Solomon (Eds.), *Jungian thought in the modern world* (pp. 126–136). London: Free Association Books.

Solomon, H. (in press). Ethics in analysis. In M. Stein (Ed.), *Jungian psychoanalysis.* Chicago: Open Court.

Stein, M. (Ed.). (in press). *Jungian psychoanalysis.* Chicago: Open Court.

Stephens, B. D. (1999). The return of the prodigal: The emergence of Jungian themes in post-Freudian thought. *Journal of Analytical Psychology, 44*(2), 197–220.

Sullivan, B. S. (1989). *Psychotherapy grounded in the feminine principle.* Wilmette, IL: Chiron.

Ulanov, A. (2007). *The unshuttered heart: Opening to aliveness and deadness in the self.* Nashville, TN: Abingdom Press.

Whitmont, E. C. (1997). *Return of the goddess.* New York: Continuum.

Whitmont, E. C., & Perera, S. (1992). *Dreams, a portal to the source.* New York: Routledge.

Wilkinson, M. (2003). Undoing trauma: Contemporary neuroscience—a clinical perspective, *Journal of Analytical Psychology, 48*(2), 235–253.

Wilkinson, M. (2006). *Coming into mind: The mind-brain relationship: A Jungian clinical perspective.* New York: Routledge.

Wilmer, H. A. (1986). The healing nightmare: A study of the war dreams of Vietnam combat veterans. *Quadrant, 19*(1), 47–61.

Withers, R. (2003). *Controversies in analytical psychology.* New York: Brunner-Routledge.

Young-Eisendrath, P. (2008). Jung and Buddhism: Refining the dialogue. In P. Young-Eisendrath and T. Dawson (Eds.), *The Cambridge companion to Jung,* 2nd ed. (pp. 235–51). Cambridge, UK: Cambridge University Press.

Zoja, L. (2007). *Ethics in analysis: Philosophical perspectives and their application in therapy.* College Station: Texas A&M University Press.

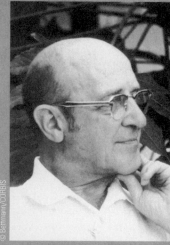

Carl R. Rogers, 1902–1987

5 | CLIENT–CENTERED THERAPY

Nathaniel J. Raskin, Carl R. Rogers, and Marjorie C. Witty

OVERVIEW

In 1940, at a conference for educators and psychologists at the University of Minnesota, Carl Ransom Rogers presented his revolutionary theory of therapy. Since that time, his theory has variously been called nondirective therapy, client-centered therapy, and the person-centered approach. Rogers's hypothesis states that a congruent therapist who expresses attitudes of unconditional positive regard and empathic understanding within a genuine relationship will catalyze psychotherapeutic personality change in a vulnerable, incongruent client. This hypothesis has been confirmed over decades in work with individuals of all ages, and with couples, families, and groups. The democratic, nonauthoritarian values inherent in this theory result in an approach to therapy that honors the persons' right to self-determination and psychological freedom.

Basic Concepts

The Person

The foundation of the approach is grounded in the perspective of human persons as active, self-regulating organisms. "[T]he image of the human being as a *person*" differentiates client-centered theory from approaches which reduce the person to diagnostic categories (Schmid, 2003, p. 108).

Based on the work of Kurt Goldstein (1934/1959) and his own observations of clients, Rogers postulated that all living organisms are dynamic processes motivated by an inherent tendency to maintain and enhance themselves. This *actualizing tendency* functions continually and holistically throughout all subsystems of the organism. Rogers (1980) speculated that the actualizing tendency is part of a more general *formative tendency,* observable in the movement toward greater order, complexity, and interrelatedness that occurs in stars, crystals, and microorganisms as well as in human beings. Persons are constantly evolving toward greater complexity, fulfilling those potentials that preserve and enhance themselves.

The Therapist

The client-centered therapist trusts the person's inner resources for growth and self-realization, in spite of his or her impairments or environmental limitations. The therapist's belief in the client's inherent growth tendency and right to self-determination is expressed, in practice, through commitment to "the nondirective attitude" (Raskin, 1947, 1948; Rogers, 1951). If the aims of psychotherapy are to free the person for growth and development, one cannot employ disempowering means in the service of emancipatory ends.

To be a client-centered therapist is to risk meeting the client as a person, to be of service in an authentic, collaborative relationship. It is the difference between *using* techniques to achieve certain ends and *being* oneself in relation to another person.

To undertake to develop as a client-centered therapist, one must be willing to take on the discipline of learning to be an open, authentic, empathic person who implements these attitudes in the relationship. Rogers described this empathic orientation as a "way of being" (Rogers, 1980). In client-centered therapy, unconditional positive regard and empathic understanding are neither techniques nor aspects of a professional role. To be effective, they must be real. The discipline consists of inhibiting the desire to show power, to use the client in any way, or to view the client in terms of reductionist categories that diminish the person's status as a human (Grant, 1995).

The Relationship

Psychotherapy outcome research supports Rogers's hypothesis that the therapeutic *relationship* accounts for a significant percentage of the variance in positive outcome in all theoretical orientations of psychotherapy (Asay & Lambert, 1999, p. 31).

In practice, the therapist's implementations of the therapeutic attitudes creates a climate of freedom and safety. Within this climate, the client is the active narrator of meanings, goals, intentions. The client propels the process of self-definition and differentiation. Bohart elucidates the client's active, self-healing activities which, in interaction with the therapist-provided conditions, promote positive change. In this interactive, synergistic model, the client actively co-constructs the therapy (Bohart, 2004, p. 108).

Because both the therapist and the client are unique persons, the relationship that develops between them cannot be prescribed by a treatment manual. It is a unique, unpredictable encounter premised on the response of the therapist to a person who seeks help. Client-centered therapists tend to be spontaneously responsive and accommodating to the requests of clients whenever possible. This willingness to accommodate requests—by answering questions, by changing a time or making a phone call on behalf of a client—originates in the therapist's basic trust in and respect for the client.

On a practical level, practitioners of client-centered therapy trust that individuals and groups are fully capable of articulating and pursuing their own goals. This has special meaning in relation to children, students, and workers, who are often viewed as requiring constant guidance and supervision. The client-centered approach endorses the person's right to choose or reject therapy, to choose a therapist whom he or she thinks may be helpful (sometimes a person of the same age, race, gender, or sexual orientation), to choose the frequency of sessions and the length of the therapeutic relationship, to speak or to be silent, to decide what needs to be explored, and to be the architect of the therapy process itself. Clients can talk about whatever they wish, whatever is present for them at the current moment. Similarly, when the therapeutic conditions are present in a group and when the group is trusted to find its own way of being, group members tend to develop processes that are right for them and to resolve conflicts within time constraints in the situation.

The Core Conditions

Congruence

Congruence, unconditional positive regard, and *empathic understanding of the client's internal frame of reference* are the three therapist-provided conditions in client-centered therapy. There is a vast literature investigating the efficacy of what have grown to be called "the core conditions" (Patterson, 1984). Although they are distinguishable, these three attitudes function holistically as a gestalt in the experience of the therapist (Rogers, 1957).

Congruence represents the therapist's ongoing process of assimilating, integrating, and symbolizing the flow of experiences in awareness. Rogers states, "To me being congruent means that I am aware of and willing to represent the feelings I have at the moment. It is being real and authentic in the moment" (Baldwin, 1987, p. 51).

A psychotherapist who is aware of the inner flow of experiencing and who is acceptant toward these inner experiences can be described as integrated and whole. Thus, even when the therapist experiences a lack of empathic understanding or even dislike for the client, if these experiences are allowed into awareness without denial or distortion, the therapist meets Rogers's condition of congruence (Brodley, 2001, p. 57). The therapist's congruence usually manifests itself in the outward appearance of transparency or genuineness and in the behavioral quality of relaxed openness. As therapist congruence persists over time, the client learns that the therapist's apparent openness is genuine and that the therapist is not covertly "up to" anything regarding the client.

Unconditional Positive Regard

The therapist enters into a relationship with the client hoping to experience *unconditional positive regard* for the client. This construct refers to a warm appreciation or prizing of the other person. The therapist accepts the client's thoughts, feelings, wishes, intentions, theories, and attributions about causality as unique, human, and appropriate to the present experience. The client may be reserved or talkative, may address any issue, and may come to whatever insights and resolutions are personally meaningful. Ideally, the therapist's regard for the client will not be affected by these particular choices, characteristics, or outcomes. Complete, unswerving unconditionality is an ideal, but in seeking to realize this ideal attitude, therapists find that their acceptance, respect, and appreciation for clients deepens with the growth of understanding.

The therapist's ability to experience unconditional positive regard toward a particular client, which is reliably present over time, is a developmental process involving a commitment to eschew judgmental reactions and to learn to inhibit critical responses that often emerge in common life situations. The novice therapist makes a commitment to expand his or her capacity for acceptance, to challenge his or her automatic judgments and biases, and to approach each client as a unique person doing the best he or she can under circumstances as they perceive them and that are affecting them even though they may not be aware of them.

Basic concepts on the client side of the process include *self-concept, locus of evaluation,* and *experiencing.* In focusing on what is important to the person seeking help, client-centered therapists soon discovered that the person's perceptions and feelings about self were of central concern (Raimy, 1948; Rogers, 1951, 1959b). A major component of one's self-concept is self-regard, often lacking in clients who seek therapeutic help. Some of the earliest psychotherapy research projects showed that when clients were rated as successful in therapy, their attitudes toward self became significantly more positive (Sheerer, 1949). More recent research underscores this important aspect of positive therapy outcome.

Ryan and Deci's self-determination theory (SDT) has stimulated numerous studies demonstrating that psychological well-being is associated with the satisfaction of basic needs for autonomy, competence, and relatedness, conceptions that are integrally related to Rogers's notion of the *fully functioning person* (Deci & Ryan, 1985, 1991). The client-centered therapist's experiencing of the core conditions expressed as a gestalt and informed by the nondirective attitude creates an optimal environment for the expression of these basic needs that enhance self-determination for both therapist and client (Ryan & Deci, 2000).

> Comparisons between people whose motivation is *authentic* (literally, self-authored or endorsed) and those who are merely *externally controlled* for an action typically reveal that the former, relative to the latter, have more interest, excitement, and confidence which in turn is manifest both as enhanced performance, persistence, and creativity (Deci & Ryan, 1991; Sheldon, Ryan, Rawsthorne, & Ilardi, 1997) and as heightened vitality (Nix, Ryan, Manly, and Deci, 1999), self-esteem (Deci & Ryan, 1995), and general well-being (Ryan, Deci, & Grolnick, 1995). This is so even when people have the same level of perceived competence or self-efficacy for the activity. (Ryan & Deci, 2000, p. 69)

Rogers's group also found that clients tended to progress along a related dimension termed *locus of evaluation.* As they gained self-esteem, they tended to shift the basis for their standards and values from other people to themselves. People commonly began therapy overly concerned with what others thought of them; that is, their locus of evaluation was external. With success in therapy, their attitudes toward others, as toward themselves, became more positive, and they were less dependent on others for their values and standards (Raskin, 1952).

A third central concept in client-centered therapy is *experiencing,* a dimension along which many but not all clients improved (Rogers, Gendlin, Kiesler, & Truax, 1967), shifting from a rigid mode of experiencing self and world to one of greater openness and flexibility.

The therapeutic attitudes and the three client constructs described in this section have been carefully defined, measured, and studied in scores of research projects relating therapist practice to the outcome of psychotherapy. There is considerable evidence that when clients perceive unconditional positive regard and empathic understanding in a relationship with a congruent therapist, their self-concepts become more positive and realistic, they become more self-expressive and self-directed, they become more open and free in their experiencing, their behavior is rated as more mature, and they cope more effectively with stress (Rogers, 1986a).

Other Systems

Client-centered therapy evolved predominantly out of Rogers's own experience as a practitioner. There are both important differences and conceptual similarities between the person-centered approach and other personality theories.

Self-actualization, a concept central to person-centered theory, was advanced most forcefully by Kurt Goldstein. His holistic theory of personality emphasizes that individuals must be understood as totalities that strive to actualize themselves (Goldstein, 1934/1959). Goldstein's work and ideas prefigured those of Abraham Maslow, a founder of humanistic psychology, who opposed Freudian and stimulus/response interpretations of human nature, asserting instead that persons seek out meaning, valuing, transcendence, and beauty.

Heinz Ansbacher, a leading proponent of Adlerian theory, joined Maslow (1968) and Floyd Matson (1969) in recognizing a host of theories and therapists "united by six basic premises of humanistic psychology":

1. People's creative power is a crucial force, in addition to heredity and environment.
2. An anthropomorphic model of humankind is superior to a mechanomorphic model.
3. Purpose, rather than cause, is the decisive dynamic.
4. The holistic approach is more adequate than an elementaristic one.
5. It is necessary to take humans' subjectivity, their opinions and viewpoints, and their conscious and unconscious fully into account.
6. Psychotherapy is essentially based on a good human relationship (Ansbacher, 1977, p. 51).

Among those subscribing to such beliefs were Alfred Adler, William Stern, and Gordon Allport; the gestalt psychologists Max Wertheimer, Wolfgang Kohler, and Kurt Koffka; the neo-Freudians Franz Alexander, Erich Fromm, Karen Horney, and Harry Stack Sullivan; post-Freudians such as Judd Marmor and Thomas Szasz; phenomenological and existential psychologists such as Rollo May; the cognitive theorist George A. Kelly, and of course Carl Rogers (Ansbacher, 1977).

Meador and Rogers (1984) distinguished client-centered therapy from psychoanalysis and from behavior modification in these terms:

> In psychoanalysis the analyst aims to interpret connections between the past and the present for the patient. In client-centered therapy, the therapist facilitates the client's discoveries of the meanings of his or her own current inner experiencing. The psychoanalyst takes the role of a teacher in interpreting insights to the patient and encouraging the development of a transference relationship, a relationship based on the neurosis of the patient. The person-centered therapist presents him- or herself as honestly and transparently as possible and attempts to establish a relationship in which he or she is authentically caring and listening.
>
> In client-centered therapy, transference relationships may begin, but they do not become full-blown. Rogers has postulated that transference relationships develop in an evaluative atmosphere in which the client feels the therapist knows more about the client than the client knows about him- or herself, and therefore the client becomes dependent, repeating the parent–child dynamic of the past.

Person-centered therapists tend to avoid evaluation. They do not interpret for clients, do not question in a probing manner, and do not reassure or criticize clients. Person-centered therapists have not found the transference relationship, [which is] central to psychoanalysis, a necessary part of a client's growth or change.

In behavior therapy, *behavior change* comes about through external control of associations to stimuli and the consequences of various responses. In practice, if not in theory, behavior therapy *does* pay attention to the therapy relationship; however, its major emphasis is on specific changes in behaviors. In contrast, person-centered therapists believe behavior change evolves from within the individual. Behavior therapy's goal is symptom removal. It is not particularly concerned with the relationship of inner experiencing to the symptom under consideration, or with the relationship between the therapist and the client, or with the climate of their relationship. It seeks to eliminate the symptom as efficiently as possible using the principles of learning theory. Obviously, this point of view is quite contrary to person-centered therapy, which maintains that fully functioning people rely on inner experiencing to direct their behavior. (Meador & Rogers, 1984, p. 146)

Raskin (1974), in a study comparing Rogers's therapy with those of leaders of five other orientations, found that client-centered therapy was distinctive in providing empathy and unconditional positive regard. Psychoanalytically oriented and eclectic psychotherapists agreed with client-centered theory on the desirability of empathy, warmth, and unconditional positive regard, but examples of rational emotive, psychoanalytically oriented, and Jungian interviews were ranked low on these qualities.

This study provided a direct comparison of audiotaped samples of therapy done by Rogers and Albert Ellis, the founder of rational emotive behavior therapy (REBT). Among 12 therapist variables rated by 83 therapist-judges, the only one on which Rogers and Ellis were alike was Self-Confident. The therapy sample by Rogers received high ratings on the following dimensions: Empathy, Unconditional Positive Regard, Congruence, and Ability to Inspire Confidence. The interview by Ellis was rated high on the Cognitive and Therapist-Directed dimensions. Rogers was rated low on Therapist-Directed, and Ellis received a low rating on Unconditional Positive Regard.

This research lends support to the following differences between client-centered therapy and rational emotive behavior therapy.

1. Unlike REBT, the person-centered approach greatly values the therapeutic relationship.

2. Rational emotive therapists provide much direction, whereas the person-centered approach encourages the client to determine direction.

3. Rational emotive therapists work hard to point out deficiencies in their clients' thought processes; person-centered therapists accept and respect their clients' ways of thinking and perceiving.

4. Client-centered therapy characteristically leads to actions chosen by the client; rational emotive methods include "homework" assignments by the therapist.

5. The person-centered therapist relates to the client on a feeling level and in a respectful and accepting way; the rational emotive therapist is inclined to interrupt this affective process to point out the irrational harm that the client may be doing to self and to interpersonal relationships.

Although Rogers and Ellis have very different philosophies and methods of trying to help people, they share some very important beliefs and values:

1. A great optimism that people can change, even when they are deeply disturbed

2. A perception that individuals are often unnecessarily self-critical and that negative self-attitudes can become positive

3. A willingness to put forth great effort to try to help people, both through individual therapy and through professional therapy and nontechnical writing

4. A willingness to demonstrate their methods publicly

5. A respect for science and research

Similar differences and commonalities are found when Rogers is compared to other cognitive therapists, such as Aaron Beck.

HISTORY

Precursors

One of the most powerful influences on Carl Rogers was learning that traditional child-guidance methods in which he had been trained did not work very well. At Columbia University's Teachers College, he had been taught testing, measurement, diagnostic interviewing, and interpretive treatment. This was followed by an internship at the psychoanalytically oriented Institute for Child Guidance, where he learned to take exhaustive case histories and do projective personality testing. It is important to note that Rogers originally went to a Rochester child-guidance agency believing in this diagnostic, prescriptive, professionally impersonal approach, and only after actual experience did he conclude that it was not effective. As an alternative, he tried listening and following the client's lead rather than assuming the role of the expert. This worked better, and he discovered some theoretical and applied support for this alternative approach in the work of Otto Rank and his followers at the University of Pennsylvania School of Social Work and the Philadelphia Child Guidance Clinic.

One particularly important event was a three-day seminar in Rochester with Rank (Rogers & Haigh, 1983). Another was his association with a Rankian-trained social worker, Elizabeth Davis, from whom "I first got the notion of responding almost entirely to the feelings being expressed. What later came to be called the reflection of feeling sprang from my contact with her" (Rogers & Haigh, 1983, p. 7).

Rogers's therapy practice and, later, his theory grew out of his own experience. At the same time, a number of links to Otto Rank are apparent in Rogers's early work.

The following elements of Rankian theory bear a close relationship to principles of nondirective therapy.

1. The individual seeking help is not simply a battleground of impersonal forces such as the id and superego, but has personal creative powers.

2. The aim of therapy is acceptance by the individual of self as unique and self-reliant.

3. In order to achieve this goal, the client rather than the therapist must become the central figure in the therapeutic process.

4. The therapist can be neither an instrument of love, which would make the client more dependent, nor an instrument of education, which attempts to alter the individual.

5. The goals of therapy are achieved by the client not through an explanation of the past, which the client would resist if interpreted, and which, even if accepted, would lessen responsibility for present adjustment, but rather through experiencing the present in the therapeutic situation (Raskin, 1948, pp. 95–96).

Rank explicitly, eloquently, and repeatedly rejected therapy by technique and interpretation:

Every single case, yes every individual hour of the same case, is different, because it is derived momentarily from the play of forces given in the situation and immediately applied. My technique consists essentially in having no technique, but in utilizing as much as possible experience and understanding that are constantly converted into skill but never crystallized into technical rules which would be applicable ideologically. There is a technique only in an ideological therapy where technique is identical with theory and the chief task of the analyst is interpretation (ideological), not the bringing to pass and granting of experience. (1945, p. 105)

Rank is obscure about his actual practice of psychotherapy, particularly the amount and nature of his activity during the treatment hour. Unsystematic references in *Will Therapy, Truth and Reality* (1945) reveal that, despite his criticism of educational and interpretive techniques and his expressed value of the patient being his or her own therapist, he assumed a position of undisputed power in the relationship.

Beginnings

Carl Ransom Rogers was born in Oak Park, Illinois, on January 8, 1902. Rogers's parents believed in hard work, responsibility, and religious fundamentalism and frowned on activities such as drinking, dancing, and card playing. The family was characterized by closeness and devotion but did not openly display affection. While in high school, Carl worked on the family farm, and he became interested in experimentation and the scientific aspect of agriculture. He entered the University of Wisconsin, following his parents and older siblings, as an agriculture major. Rogers also carried on his family's religious tradition. He was active in the campus YMCA and was chosen to be one of 10 American youth delegates to the World Student Christian Federation's Conference in Peking, China, in 1922. At that time he switched his major from agriculture to history, which he thought would better prepare him for a career as a minister. After graduating from Wisconsin in 1924 and marrying Helen Elliott, a childhood friend, he entered the Union Theological Seminary. Two years later, and in part as a result of taking several psychology courses, Rogers moved "across Broadway" to Teachers College, Columbia University, where he was exposed to what he later described as "a contradictory mixture of Freudian, scientific, and progressive education thinking" (Rogers & Sanford, 1985, p. 1374).

After Teachers College, Rogers worked for 12 years at a child-guidance center in Rochester, New York, where he soon became an administrator as well as a practicing psychologist. He began writing articles and became active at a national level. His book *The Clinical Treatment of the Problem Child* was published in 1939, and he was offered a professorship in psychology at Ohio State University. Once at Ohio State, Rogers began to teach newer ways of helping problem children and their parents.

In 1940, Rogers was teaching an enlightened distillation of the child-guidance practices described in *The Clinical Treatment of the Problem Child*. From his point of view, this approach represented a consensual direction in which the field was moving and was evolutionary rather than revolutionary. The clinical process began with an assessment, including testing children and interviewing parents; assessment results provided the basis for a treatment plan. In treatment, nondirective principles were followed.

Rogers's views gradually became more radical. His presentation at the University of Minnesota on December 11, 1940, entitled "Some Newer Concepts in Psychotherapy," is the single event most often identified with the birth of client-centered therapy. Rogers decided to expand this talk into a book titled *Counseling and Psychotherapy* (1942). The book, which included an electronically recorded eight-interview case, described the generalized process in which a client begins with a conflict situation and a predominance of negative attitudes and moves toward insight, independence, and positive attitudes. Rogers hypothesized that the counselor promoted such a process by avoiding advice and interpretation and by consistently recognizing and accepting the client's feelings. Research corroborating this new approach to counseling and psychotherapy was offered, including the first (Porter, 1943) of what soon became a series of pioneering doctoral dissertations on the process and outcomes of psychotherapy. In a very short time, an entirely new approach to psychotherapy was born, as was the field of psychotherapy research. This approach and its accompanying research led to the eventual acceptance of psychotherapy as a primary professional function of clinical psychologists.

After serving as director of counseling services for the United Service Organizations during World War II, Rogers was appointed professor of psychology at the University of Chicago and became head of the university's counseling center. The 12 years during which Rogers remained at Chicago were a period of tremendous growth in client-centered theory, philosophy, practice, research, applications, and implications.

In 1957, Rogers published a classic paper entitled "The necessary and sufficient conditions of therapeutic personality change." Congruence, unconditional positive regard, and empathic understanding of the client's internal frame of reference were cited as three essential therapist-offered conditions of therapeutic personality change. This theoretical statement applied to all types of therapy, not just the client-centered approach. It was followed by his "magnum opus," the most comprehensive and rigorous formulation of his theory of therapy, personality, and interpersonal relationships (Rogers, 1959b).

Rogers's philosophy of the "exquisitely rational" nature of the behavior and growth of human beings was further articulated and related to the thinking of Søren Kierkegaard, Abraham Maslow, Rollo May, Martin Buber, and others in the humanistic movement whose theories were catalyzing a "third force" in psychology, challenging the dominance of behaviorism and psychoanalysis.

As the practice of client-centered therapy deepened and broadened, the therapist was also more fully appreciated as a person in the therapeutic relationship. Psychotherapy research, which had begun so auspiciously at Ohio State, continued with investigations by Godfrey T. Barrett-Lennard (1962), John Butler and Gerard Haigh (1954), Desmond Cartwright (1957), Eugene Gendlin (1961), Nathaniel Raskin (1952), Julius Seeman (1959), John Shlien (1964), and Stanley Standal (1954), among others.

At Ohio State, there was a sense that client-centered principles had implications beyond the counseling office. At Chicago, this was made most explicit by the empowerment of students and the counseling center staff. About half of Rogers's *Client-Centered Therapy* (1951) was devoted to applications of client-centered therapy, with additional chapters on play therapy, group therapy, and leadership and administration.

In 1957, Rogers accepted a professorship in psychology and psychiatry at the University of Wisconsin. With the collaboration of associates and graduate students, a massive research project was mounted, based on the hypothesis that hospitalized schizophrenics would respond to a client-centered approach (Rogers et al., 1967). Two relatively clear conclusions emerged from a complex maze of results: (1) the most successful patients were those who had experienced the highest degree of accurate empathy, and (2) it was the client's, rather than the therapist's, judgment of the therapy relationship that correlated more highly with success or failure.

Rogers left the University of Wisconsin and full-time academia and began living in La Jolla, California, in 1964. He was a resident fellow for four years at the Western Behavioral Sciences Institute and then, starting in 1968, at the Center for Studies of the Person. In more than two decades in California, Rogers wrote books on a person-centered approach to teaching and educational administration, on encounter groups, on marriage and other forms of partnership, and on the "quiet revolution" that he believed would emerge with a new type of "self-empowered person." Rogers believed this revolution had the potential to change "the very nature of psychotherapy, marriage, education, administration, and politics" (Rogers, 1977). These books were based on observations and interpretations of hundreds of individual and group experiences.

A special interest of Rogers and his associates was the application of a person-centered approach to international conflict resolution. This resulted in trips to South Africa, Eastern Europe, and the Soviet Union, as well as in meetings with Irish Catholics and Protestants and with representatives of nations involved in Central American conflicts (Rogers & Ryback, 1984). In addition to Rogers's books, a number of valuable films and videotapes have provided data for research on the basic person-centered hypothesis that individuals and groups who have experienced empathy, congruence, and unconditional positive regard will go through a constructive process of self-directed change.

Current Status

Since 1982, there have been biennial international forums on the person-centered approach, meeting in Mexico, England, the United States, Brazil, the Netherlands, Greece, and South Africa. Alternating with these meetings have been international conferences on client-centered and experiential psychotherapy in Belgium, Scotland, Austria, Portugal, and the United States.

In September 1986, five months prior to his death, Rogers attended the inaugural meeting of the Association for the Development of the Person-Centered Approach (ADPCA) held at International House on the campus of the University of Chicago. At this meeting, which was to be the last Carl Rogers attended, the idea for a workshop on the person-centered approach was developed. The workshop, organized by Jerold Bozarth, Professor Emeritus at University of Georgia, and several graduate students, began a week after Carl Rogers's death on February 4, 1987. It was held in Warm Springs, Georgia, February 11–15, 1987, at the Rehabilitation Institute, where Franklin Roosevelt was treated after being struck by polio. Forty participants, including Barbara Brodley, Chuck Devonshire, Nat Raskin, David Spahn, and Fred Zimring, among others, came from Georgia, Florida, Illinois, Kansas, and Nevada. The group expressed its appreciation to Jerold Bozarth for allowing it to find its own direction and develop its own process. Workshops have been held annually at Warm Springs since 1987, and this nondirective climate has been maintained over the years. In addition to the Warm Springs Workshop, the ADPCA meets annually and can be accessed online at www. adpca.org. The association is composed of persons in many different occupations; educators, nurses, psychologists, artists, and business consultants are all part of this growing community of persons interested in the potential of the approach.

The *Person-Centered Review,* "an international journal of research, theory, and application," was initiated by David Cain in 1986. The journal has an editorial board made up of scholars and practitioners from around the world. In 1992, the *Review* was succeeded by the *Person-Centered Journal,* co-edited by Jerold Bozarth and Fred Zimring.

Raskin (1996) formulated significant steps in the evolution of the movement from individual therapy in 1940 to the concept of community in the 1990s.

In 2000, the World Association for Person-Centered and Experiential Psychotherapy and Counseling (WAPCEPC) was founded at the International Forum for the Person-Centered Approach in Portugal. This association consists of psychotherapists, researchers, and theorists from many countries and actively seeks to reassert the revolutionary nature of a person-centered approach. Association activities, conference schedules, and membership information may be found online at www.pce-world.org.

This organization has launched the peer-reviewed journal *Person-Centered and Experiential Psychotherapy* (PCEP), which publishes empirical, qualitative, and theoretical articles of broad interest to humanistic practitioners and researchers. Full-text articles are available online for the PCEP back to 2001. For a more thorough review of the current status of the person-centered approach, see Howard Kirschenbaum's and April Jourdan's (2005) article "The Current Status of Carl Rogers and the Person-Centered Approach."

PERSONALITY

Theory of Personality

Rogers moved from a lack of interest in psychological theory to the development of a rigorous 19-proposition "theory of therapy, personality, and interpersonal relationships" (Rogers, 1959b). On one level, this signified a change in Rogers's respect for theory. On another, this comprehensive formulation can be understood as a logical evolution. His belief in the importance of the child's conscious attitudes toward self and self-ideal was central to the test of personality adjustment he devised for children (Rogers, 1931). The portrayal of the client's growing through a process of reduced defensiveness and of self-directed expansion of self-awareness was described in a paper on the processes of therapy (Rogers, 1940). Rogers wrote here of a gradual recognition of a real self with its childish, aggressive, and ambivalent aspects, as well as more mature components. As data on personality changes in psychotherapy started to accumulate rapidly, with the objective analyses of verbatim interviews, Rogers found support for his belief that the facts are always friendly, despite some results that did not support his hypotheses.

Rogers expanded his observations into a theory of personality and behavior that he described in *Client-Centered Therapy* (1951). This theory is based on 19 basic propositions:

1. Every individual exists in a continually changing world of experience of which he or she is the center.

2. The organism reacts to the field as it is perceived. This perceptual field is, for the individual, "reality."

3. The organism reacts as an organized whole to this phenomenal field.

4. The organism has one basic tendency and striving—to actualize, maintain, and enhance the experiencing organism.

5. Behavior is basically the goal-directed attempt of the organism to satisfy its needs as experienced, in the field as perceived.

6. Emotion accompanies and in general facilitates such goal-directed behavior, the kind of emotion being related to the seeking versus the consummatory aspects of the behavior, and the intensity of the emotion being related to the perceived significance of the behavior for the maintenance and enhancement of the organism.

7. The best vantage point for understanding behavior is from the internal frame of reference of the individual.

8. A portion of the total perceptual field gradually becomes differentiated as the self.

9. As a result of interaction with the environment, and particularly as a result of evaluational interaction with others, the structure of self is formed—an organized, fluid, but consistent conceptual pattern of perceptions of characteristics and relationships of the "I" or the "me," together with values attached to these concepts.

10. The values attached to experiences, and the values that are a part of the self-structure, in some instances are values experienced directly by the organism, and in some instances are values introjected or taken over from others, but perceived in distorted fashion, as though they had been experienced directly.

11. As experiences occur in the life of the individual, they are (a) symbolized, perceived, and organized into some relationship to the self, or (b) ignored because there is no perceived relationship to the self-structure, or (c) denied symbolization or given a distorted symbolization because the experience is inconsistent with the structure of the self.

12. Most of the ways of behaving that are adopted by the organism are those that are consistent with the concept of self.

13. Behavior may, in some instances, be brought about by organismic experiences and needs that have not been symbolized. Such behavior may be inconsistent with the structure of the self, but in such instances the behavior is not "owned" by the individual.

14. Psychological maladjustment exists when the organism denies to awareness significant sensory and visceral experiences, which consequently are not symbolized and organized into the gestalt of the self-structure. When this situation exists, there is a basis for potential psychological tension.

15. Psychological adjustment exists when the concept of the self is such that all the sensory and visceral experiences of the organism are, or may be, assimilated on a symbolic level into a consistent relationship with the concept of self.

16. Any experience that is inconsistent with the organization or structure of self may be perceived as a threat, and the more of these perceptions there are, the more rigidly the self-structure is organized to maintain itself.

17. Under certain conditions, involving primarily complete absence of any threat to the self-structure, experiences that are inconsistent with it may be perceived and examined, and the structure of self revised to assimilate and include such experiences.

18. When the individual perceives all his sensory and visceral experiences and accepts them into one consistent and integrated system, then he is necessarily more understanding of others and more accepting of others as separate individuals.

19. As the individual perceives and accepts into his self-structure more of his organismic experiences, he finds that he is replacing his present value system—based so largely on introjections that have been distortedly symbolized—with a continuing organismic valuing process. (pp. 481–533)

Rogers comments that

> This theory is basically phenomenological in character, and relies heavily upon the concept of the self as an explanatory construct. It pictures the end-point of personality development as being a basic congruence between the phenomenal field of experience and the conceptual structure of the self—a situation which, if achieved, would represent freedom from internal strain and anxiety, and freedom from potential strain; which would represent the maximum in realistically oriented adaptation; which would mean the establishment of an individualized value system having considerable identity with the value system of any other equally well-adjusted member of the human race. (1951, p. 532)

Further investigations of these propositions were conducted at the University of Chicago Counseling and Psychotherapy Research Center in the early 1950s in carefully designed and controlled studies. Stephenson's (1953) Q-sort technique was used to measure changes in self-concept and self-ideal during and following therapy and in a no-therapy control period. Many results confirmed Rogers's hypotheses; for example, a significant increase in congruence between self and ideal occurred during therapy, and changes in the perceived self resulted in better psychological adjustment (Rogers & Dymond, 1954).

Rogers's personality theory has been described as growth-oriented rather than developmental. Although this description is accurate, it does not acknowledge Rogers's sensitivity to the attitudes with which children are confronted, beginning in infancy:

> While I have been fascinated by the horizontal spread of the person-centered approach into so many areas of our life, others have been more interested in the vertical direction and are discovering the profound value of treating the infant, during the whole birth process, as a person who should be understood, whose communications should be treated with respect, who should be dealt with empathically. This is the new and stimulating contribution of Frederick Leboyer, a French obstetrician who . . . has assisted in the delivery of at least a thousand infants in what can only be called a person-centered way. (Rogers, 1977, p. 31)

Rogers goes on to describe the infant's extreme sensitivity to light and sound, the rawness of the skin, the fragility of the head, the struggle to breathe, and the like, along with the specific ways in which Leboyer has taught parents and professionals to provide a beginning life experience that is caring, loving, and respectful.

This sensitivity to children was further expressed in Rogers's explanation of his fourth proposition (The organism has one basic tendency and striving—to actualize, maintain, and enhance the experiencing organism):

> The whole process (of self-enhancement and growth) may be symbolized and illustrated by the child's learning to walk. The first steps involve struggle, and usually pain. Often it is true that the immediate reward involved in taking a few steps is in no way commensurate with the pain of falls and bumps. The child may, because of the pain, revert to crawling for a time. Yet the forward direction of growth is more powerful than the satisfactions of remaining infantile. Children will actualize themselves, in spite of the painful experiences of so doing. In the same way, they will become independent, responsible, self-governing, and socialized, in spite of the pain which is often involved in these steps. Even where they do not, because of a variety of circumstances, exhibit the growth, the tendency is still present. Given the opportunity for clear-cut choice between forward-moving and regressive behavior, the tendency will operate. (Rogers, 1951, pp. 490–491)

One of Rogers's hypotheses about personality (Proposition 8) was that a part of the developing infant's private world becomes recognized as "me," "I," or "myself." Rogers described infants, in the course of interacting with the environment, as building up concepts about themselves, about the environment, and about themselves in relation to the environment.

Rogers's next suppositions are crucial to his theory of how development may proceed either soundly or in the direction of maladjustment. He assumes that very young infants are involved in "direct organismic valuing," with very little or no uncertainty. They have experiences such as "I am cold, and I don't like it," or "I like being cuddled," which may occur even though they lack descriptive words or symbols for these organismic experiences. The principle in this natural process is that the infant positively values those experiences that are perceived as self-enhancing and places a negative value on those that threaten or do not maintain or enhance the self.

This situation changes once children begin to be evaluated by others (Holdstock & Rogers, 1983). The love they are given and the symbolization of themselves as lovable children become dependent on behavior. To hit or to hate a baby sibling may result in the child's being told that he or she is bad and unlovable. The child, to preserve a positive self-concept, may distort experience.

> It is in this way . . . that parental attitudes are not only introjected, but . . . are experienced . . . in distorted fashion, *as if* based on the evidence of one's own sensory and visceral equipment. Thus, through distorted symbolization, expression of anger comes to be "experienced" as bad, even though the more accurate symbolization would be that the expression of anger is often experienced as satisfying or enhancing. . . . The "self" which is formed on this basis of distorting the sensory and visceral evidence to fit the already present structure acquires an organization and integration which the individual endeavors to preserve. (Rogers, 1951, pp. 500–501)

This type of interaction may sow the seeds of confusion about self, self-doubt, and disapproval of self, as well as reliance on the evaluation of others. Rogers indicated that these consequences may be avoided if the parent can accept the child's negative feelings and the child as a whole, while refusing to permit certain behaviors such as hitting the baby.

Variety of Concepts

Various terms and concepts appear in the presentation of Rogers's theory of personality and behavior that often have a unique and distinctive meaning in this orientation.

Experience

In Rogers's theory, the term *experience* refers to the private world of the individual. At any moment, some experience is conscious; for example, we feel the pressure of the keys against our fingers as we type. Some experiences may be difficult to bring into awareness, such as the idea "I am an aggressive person." People's actual awareness of their total experiential field may be limited, but each individual is the only one who can know it completely.

Reality

For psychological purposes, reality is basically the private world of individual perceptions, although for social purposes, reality consists of those perceptions that have a high degree of consensus among local communities of individuals. Two people will agree on the reality that a particular person is a politician. One sees her as a good woman who wants to help people and, on the basis of this reality, votes for her. The other person's reality is that the politician appropriates money to win favor, so this person votes against her. In therapy, changes in feelings and perceptions will result in changes in reality as perceived. This is particularly fundamental as the client is more and more able to accept "the self that I am now."

The Organism's Reacting as an Organized Whole

A person may be hungry but, because of a report to complete, skips lunch. In psychotherapy, clients often become clearer about what is important to them, resulting in behavioral changes directed toward the clarified goals. A politician may choose not to run for office because he decides that his family life is more important. A client with a disabling condition is more open to the changed circumstances of her life with the illness and is better able to care for herself in terms of rest and self-care.

The Organism's Actualizing Tendency

This is a central tenet in the writings of Kurt Goldstein, Hobart Mowrer, Harry Stack Sullivan, Karen Horney, and Andras Angyal, to name just a few. The child's painful struggle to learn to walk is an example. It is Rogers's belief and the belief of most other personality theorists that in the absence of external force, individuals prefer to be healthy rather than sick, to be free to choose rather than having choices made for them, and in general to further the optimal development of the total organism. Deci and Ryan's (1985, 1991) formulation of self-determination theory (SDT) has stimulated a number of recent empirical studies investigating situations that support or constrain intrinsic motivation, which is a natural feature of human living. Ryan and Deci describe this human capacity:

> Perhaps no single phenomenon reflects the positive potential of human nature as much as intrinsic motivation, the inherent tendency to seek out novelty and challenges, to extend and exercise one's capacities, to explore, and to learn. . . . [T]he evidence is now clear that the maintenance and enhancement of this inherent propensity requires supportive conditions, as it can be fairly readily disrupted by various non-supportive conditions. . . . [T]he study of conditions which facilitate versus undermine intrinsic motivation is an important first step in understanding sources of both alienation and liberation of the positive aspects of human nature. (Ryan & Deci, 2000, p. 70)

In Rogers's theory, the actualizing tendency functions as an axiom and is not subject to falsification. In the therapy situation, it is a functional construct for the therapist, who can conceive of the client as attempting to realize self and organism, especially when the client's behavior and ways of thinking appear self-destructive or irrational. In these situations, the client-centered therapist's trust in the client's self-righting, self-regulatory capacities may be sorely tested, but holding to the hypothesis of the actualizing tendency supports the therapist's efforts to understand and to maintain unconditionality toward the client. (Brodley, 1999c)

The Internal Frame of Reference

This is the perceptual field of the individual. It is the way the world appears to us from our own unique vantage point, given the whole continuum of learnings and experiences we have accumulated along with the meanings attached to experience and feelings. From the client-centered point of view, apprehending this internal frame provides the fullest understanding of why people behave as they do. It is to be distinguished from external judgments of behavior, attitudes, and personality.

The Self, Concept of Self, and Self-Structure

> These terms refer to the organized, consistent, conceptual gestalt composed of perceptions of the characteristics of the "I" or "me" and the perceptions of the relationships of the "I" or "me" to others and to various aspects of life, together with the values attached to these perceptions. It is a gestalt available to awareness although not necessarily in awareness. It is a fluid and changing process, but at any given moment it . . . is at least partially definable in operational terms. (Meador & Rogers, 1984, p. 158)

Symbolization

This is the process by which the individual becomes aware or conscious of an experience. There is a tendency to deny symbolization to experiences at variance with the concept of self; for example, people who think of themselves as truthful will tend to resist the symbolization of an act of lying. Ambiguous experiences tend to be symbolized in ways that are consistent with self-concept. A speaker lacking in self-confidence may symbolize a silent audience as unimpressed, whereas one who is confident may symbolize such a group as attentive and interested.

Psychological Adjustment or Maladjustment

Congruence, or its absence, between an individual's sensory and visceral experiences and his or her concept of self defines whether a person is psychologically adjusted or maladjusted. A self-concept that includes elements of weakness and imperfection facilitates the symbolization of failure experiences. The need to deny or distort such experiences does not exist and therefore fosters a condition of psychological adjustment. If a person who has always seen herself as honest tells a white lie to her daughter, she may experience discomfort and vulnerability. For that moment there is incongruence between her self-concept and her behavior. Integration of the alien behavior—"I guess sometimes I take the easy way out and tell a lie"—may restore the person to congruence and free the person to consider whether she wants to change her behavior or her self-concept. A state of psychological adjustment means that the organism is open to his or her organismic experiencing as trustworthy and admissible to awareness.

Organismic Valuing Process

This is an ongoing process in which individuals freely rely on the evidence of their own senses for making value judgments. This is in contrast to a fixed system of introjected values characterized by "oughts" and "shoulds" and by what is supposed to be right or wrong. The organismic valuing process is consistent with the person-centered hypothesis of confidence in the individual and, even though established by each individual, makes for a highly responsible socialized system of values and behavior. The responsibility derives from people making choices on the basis of their direct, organismic processing of situations, in contrast to acting out of fear of what others may think of them or what others have taught them is "the way" to think and act.

The Fully Functioning Person

Rogers defined those who can readily assimilate organismic experiencing and who are capable of symbolizing these ongoing experiences in awareness as "fully functioning" persons, able to experience all of their feelings, afraid of none of them, allowing awareness to flow freely in and through their experiences. Seeman (1984) has been involved in a long-term research program to clarify and describe the qualities of such optimally functioning individuals. These empirical studies highlight the possession of a positive self-concept, greater physiological responsiveness, and an efficient use of the environment.

PSYCHOTHERAPY

Theory of Psychotherapy

Rogers's theory of therapeutic personality change posits that if the therapist experiences unconditional positive regard and empathic understanding of the client's communications from the viewpoint of the internal frame of reference of the client, and succeeds in communicating these attitudes in the relationship with the client, then the client will respond with constructive changes in personality organization (Rogers, 1957, 1959b). Watson points out that

> If the client perceives the therapist as ungenuine, then the client will not perceive the therapist as communicating the other two conditions. It follows from this hypothesis that the client's perception of the therapist's congruence is one of the necessary and sufficient conditions for effective therapy. (Watson, 1984, p. 19)

When the core conditions are realized to some degree by the therapist (of any theoretical orientation), studies demonstrate that these qualities may be perceived by the client within the first several interviews. Changes in self-acceptance, immediacy of experiencing, directness of relating, and movement toward an internal locus of evaluation may occur in short-term intensive workshops or even in single interviews.

After a four-day workshop of psychologists, educators, and other professionals conducted by Rogers and R. C. Sanford in Moscow, participants reported their reactions. The following is a typical response:

> This is just two days after the experience and I am still a participant. I am a psychologist, not a psychotherapist. I have known Rogers's theory but this was a process in which we were personally involved. I didn't realize how it applied. I want to give several impressions. First was the effectiveness of this approach. It was a kind of process in which we all learned. Second, this process was moving, without a motor. Nobody had to lead it or guide it. It was a self-evolving process. It was like the Chekhov story where they were expectantly awaiting the piano player and the piano started playing itself. Third, I was impressed by the manner of Carl and Ruth [Sanford]. At first I felt they were passive. Then I realized it was the silence of understanding. Fourth, I want to mention the penetration of this process into my inner world. At first I was an observer, but then the approach disappeared altogether. I was not simply surrounded by this process, I was absorbed into it! It was a revelation to me. We started moving. I wasn't simply seeing people I had known for years, but their feelings. My fifth realization was my inability to control the flow of feelings, the flow of the process. My feelings tried to put on the clothes of my words. Sometimes people exploded; some even cried. It was a reconstruction of the system of perception. Finally, I want to remark on the high skill of Carl and Ruth, of their silences, their voices, their glances. It was always some response and they were responded to. It was a great phenomenon, a great experience. (Rogers, 1987, pp. 298–299)

This kind of experience speaks against the perception of the person-centered approach as safe, harmless, innocuous, and superficial. It is intended to be safe, but clearly it can also be powerful.

Empathic Understanding of the Client's Internal Frame of Reference

Empathic understanding in client-centered therapy is an active, immediate, continuous process with both cognitive and affective aspects. Raskin, in an oft-quoted paper written in 1947, describes this process.

> At this level, counselor participation becomes an active experiencing with the client of the feelings to which he gives expression, the counselor makes a maximum effort to get under the skin of the person with whom he is communicating, he tries to get within and to live the attitudes expressed instead of observing them, to catch every nuance of their changing nature; in a word, to absorb himself completely in

the attitudes of the other. And in struggling to do this, there is simply no room for any other type of counselor activity or attitude; if he is attempting to live the attitudes of the other, he cannot be diagnosing them, he cannot be thinking of making the process go faster. Because he is another, and not the client, the understanding is not spontaneous but must be acquired, and this through the most intense, continuous and active attention to the feelings of the other, to the exclusion of any other type of attention. (Raskin, 1947/2005, pp. 6–7)

The accuracy of the therapist's empathic understanding has often been emphasized, but more important is the therapist's interest in appreciating the world of the client and offering such understanding with the willingness to be corrected. This creates a process in which the therapist gets closer and closer to the client's meanings and feelings, developing an ever-deepening relationship based on respect for and understanding of the other person. Brodley (1994) has documented the high proportion (often as high as 80 to 90%) of "empathic understanding responses" in Rogers's therapy transcripts. Brodley's research has shown that Rogers's therapy was highly consistent throughout his career and did not waver from his trust in the client and his commitment to the principle of nondirectivity.

Unconditional Positive Regard

Other terms for this condition are warmth, acceptance, nonpossessive caring, and prizing.

> When the therapist is experiencing a positive, nonjudgmental, acceptant attitude toward whatever the client *is* at that moment, therapeutic movement or change is more likely. It involves the therapist's willingness for the client to *be* whatever immediate feeling is going on—confusion, resentment, fear, anger, courage, love, or pride. . . . When the therapist prizes the client in a total rather than a conditional way, forward movement is likely. (Rogers, 1986a, p. 198)

Congruence

Rogers regarded congruence as

> the most basic of the attitudinal conditions that foster therapeutic growth. [It] does not mean that the therapist burdens the client with all of his or her problems or feelings. It does not mean that the therapist blurts out impulsively any attitudes that come to mind. It does mean, however, that the therapist does not deny to himself or herself the feelings being experienced and that the therapist is willing to express and to be open about any persistent feelings that exist in the relationship. It means avoiding the temptation to hide behind a mask of professionalism. (Rogers & Sanford, 1985, p. 1379)

Relationship Therapeutic Conditions

There are three other conditions in addition to the "therapist-offered" conditions of empathy, congruence, and unconditional positive regard (Rogers, 1957).

1. The client and therapist must be in psychological contact.
2. The client must be experiencing some anxiety, vulnerability, or incongruence.
3. The client must perceive the conditions offered by the therapist.

Rogers described the first two as preconditions for therapy. The third, the reception by the client of the conditions offered by the therapist, is sometimes overlooked but is essential. Research relating therapeutic outcome to empathy, congruence, and unconditional positive regard based on external judgments of these variables is supportive of the person-centered hypothesis. If the ratings are done by clients themselves, the relationship to outcome is stronger. Orlinsky and Howard (1978) reviewed 15 studies relating client perception of empathy to outcome and found that 12 supported the critical importance of perceived empathy. More recently, Orlinsky, Grawe, and Parks (1994), updating the original study by Orlinsky and Howard, summarized findings from 76 studies investigating the relationship between positive regard and therapist affirmation and outcome. Out of 154 findings from these studies, 56% showed the predicted positive relationship, and when patients' ratings were used, the figure rose to 65%. As Watson (1984) points out, the theory requires the client's perception of the attitudes, so in any outcome research, the client is the most legitimate judge of the therapist's attitudes (1984, p. 21).

Process of Psychotherapy

The practice of client-centered therapy is a distinctive practice by virtue of a thoroughgoing respect for the client as the architect of the therapy (Witty, 2004). This commitment differentiates client-centered therapy from psychoanalytic models and cognitive behavioral approaches that have *a priori* goals for the client. It distinguishes the approach from other humanistic therapies that involve directing the client to focus on particular experiences such as emotion-focused, focusing-oriented, and experiential orientations within the humanistic framework.

In the client-centered approach, therapy begins immediately, with the therapist trying to understand the client's world in whatever way the client wishes to share it. The first interview is not used to take a history, to arrive at a diagnosis, to determine whether the client is treatable, or to establish the length of treatment.

The therapist respects clients, allowing them to proceed in whatever way is comfortable for them, listening without prejudice and without a private agenda. The therapist is open to either positive or negative feelings, to either speech or silence. The first hour may be the first of hundreds or it may be the only one; this is for the client to determine. If the client has questions, the therapist tries to recognize and respond to whatever feelings are implicit in the questions. "How am I going to get out of this mess?" may be the expression of the feeling "My situation seems hopeless." The therapist will convey recognition and acceptance of this statement. If this question is actually a plea for suggestions, the therapist first clarifies the question. If the therapist has an answer, he or she will give it. Often, we may not really know an answer, in which case the therapist explains why. Either one simply doesn't know or doesn't yet have sufficient understanding to formulate an answer. There is a willingness to stay with the client in moments of confusion and despair. Reassurance and advice-giving are most often not helpful and may communicate a subtle lack of confidence in the client's own approach to his or her life difficulties. Brodley and other client-centered practitioners (1999a) agree that the attitude that leads the therapist to reassure and support the client is often a reflection of the therapist's own anxiety. There are no rules, however; in some cases, spontaneous reassurances may be given. It depends on the relationship and on the freedom and confidence of the therapist.

Principled nondirectiveness in practice requires that the therapist respond to the client's direct questions simply out of respect (Grant, 1990). In the case example later in this chapter, there are examples of the therapist responding directly to the client's questions. Learning to answer questions in ways that are consistent with nondirectiveness is an aspect of client-centered therapy as a discipline, since in everyday life, we are often eager to assert our own frame of reference and readily jump in with answers. Brodley explains:

> The nondirective attitude in client-centered work implies that questions and requests should be respected as part of the client's rights in the relationship. These rights are the client's right to self-determination of his or her therapeutic content and process, and the client's right to direct the manner of the therapist's participation within the limits of the therapist's philosophy, ethics, and capabilities. The result of the therapist's respect towards these client rights is a collaborative relationship (see Natiello, 1994).
>
> This conception of the client's rights in the relationship is radically different from that of other clinical approaches. In other approaches, to a greater or lesser extent depending upon the theory, the therapist paternalistically decides whether or not it will be good for the client to have his or her questions answered or requests honored. The client-centered approach eschews decision making for the client. (Brodley, 1997, p. 24)

Regard is also demonstrated through discussion of options such as group therapy and family therapy, in contrast to therapists of other orientations who "put" the client in a group or make therapy conditional on involvement of the whole family. In this approach, the client is a vital partner in determining the nature of the therapy, the frequency, the length of time he or she wishes to invest in the work. On all issues pertaining to the client, the client is regarded as the best expert.

In a paper given at the first meeting of the American Academy of Psychotherapists in 1956, Rogers (1959a) presented "a client-centered view" of "the essence of psychotherapy." He conceptualized a "molecule" of personality change, hypothesizing that "therapy is made up of a series of such molecules, sometimes strung rather closely together, sometimes occurring at long intervals, always with periods of preparatory experiences in between" (p. 52). Rogers attributed four qualities to such a "moment of movement":

(1) It is something which occurs in this existential moment. It is not a *thinking* about something, it is an *experience* of something at this instant, in the relationship.

(2) It is an experiencing that is without barriers, or inhibitions, or holding back.

(3) The past "experience" has never been completely experienced.

(4) This experience has the quality of being acceptable and capable of being integrated with the self-concept.

Mechanisms of Psychotherapy

Broadly speaking, there are two theoretical perspectives that try to account for change in the person's concept of self that ultimately results in more effective functioning. The traditional paradigm, which is common to most psychotherapies, including client-centered therapy, asserts that change is the product of "unearthing" hidden or denied feelings or experiences that distort the concept of self, resulting in symptoms of vulnerability and anxiety.

In the course of development, most children learn that their worth is conditional on good behavior, moral or religious standards, academic or athletic performance, or undecipherable factors they can only guess at. In the most severe cases, the child's subjective reality is so consistently denied as having any importance to others that the child doubts the validity of his or her own perceptions and experiences. Rogers describes this process as "acquiring conditions of worth" and the resulting self as "incongruent." For persons whose own attempts at self-definition and self-regulation have met with harsh conditions of worth, the act of voicing a preference or a feeling or an opinion is the first step in establishing selfhood and personal identity. From the perspective of the traditional theory, such a person has suppressed his or her own feelings and reactions habitually for long periods of time. The popularized image is one of a "murky swamp" of unexplored "forgotten" experiences.

There arises, however, the issue of how "feelings" that heretofore have been "hidden" or "not in awareness" exist as "entities." The traditional model has pictured these problematic feelings paradoxically as both existent (coming from the past) and yet nonexistent until symbolized in awareness (felt for the first time when expressed). This paradox requires resolution because logic demands it and because of the issue of where to direct our empathic understanding when we are listening to clients' narratives.

Fred Zimring, a colleague of Rogers, clarifies the problem: "If the therapist attends to material not in the client's awareness, the therapist is not in the client's internal frame of reference and so would not be fulfilling an important 'necessary' condition" (Zimring, 1995, p. 36). Additionally, how can we know what is not in the client's awareness until the client tells us? Zimring presents a new paradigm that unifies Rogers's theory of the necessary and sufficient conditions with the therapeutic practice of empathic understanding, which avoids the problematic notion of hidden or unknown feelings (1995). A much abbreviated version of his work is summarized here.

Zimring asserts that human beings become persons only through interaction with other persons and that this process takes place within a particular culture. If you were born into a Western culture, the notion of the "buried conflict" is part of your cultural legacy. There is some pathological entity "inside" that needs to be brought into the light of awareness. Whether it is the wounded "inner child" or "repressed memories" or one's "abandonment issues," the underlying assumption holds that until one is able to make the unconscious conscious, psychological maladjustment will persist.

By contrast, Zimring posits that each of us does, in fact, live within a phenomenological context akin to Rogers's notion of the inner frame of reference, but that that context is always "under construction." The self in this sense is a *perspective* that crystallizes and dissolves constantly in each moment of each new situation. It is a dynamic property arising from interactions between the person and the situation, rather than a static, private entity. Zimring explains:

> As mentioned above, the old paradigm assumes that our experience is determined by inner meanings and reactions. Thus, if we feel bad, it is assumed that we are not aware of some internal meaning which is affecting our experience. In the new paradigm our experience is seen as having a different source: experience is seen as coming from the context in which we are at the moment. We feel differently when in one context rather than in the other. (1995, p. 41)

Zimring explains that in the Western context, we tend to think in terms of an "inside" and an "outside." But actually we construct both the subjective, reflexive internal world and the objective, everyday world; that is, we interact with our own unique internal representations of both of these contexts. Persons differ in their awareness and access to the inner subjective context. This is understandable, given Rogers's explication of the ways in which the person's absorption of harsh conditions of worth tend to degrade or erase the significance of subjective experience. Zimring (1995) gives an example of a client he was working with who had little access to the subjective context at all:

> Most of the time these people see themselves as part of the objective world. When forced to describe something that may have subjective dimensions, they will emphasize the objective aspect of the thing described. A man described

how he cried on the anniversary of his daughter's death. When asked how he felt when he was crying, he responded, "I hoped I could stop." In the client-centered situation, this person may be seen as the "difficult" client (the difficulty is not in the client but rather in the therapist's unrealistic expectation that the client "should" be talking about a subjective world). In other therapy contexts, this client is seen as defensive. The present analysis gives rise to a different description. Here, this client is seen as not having *developed* a reflexive, subjective world. (1995, p. 42)

Because, within the subjective context, "it is the quality of the reaction to which we are attending, its fresh presentness, personal relevance and aliveness" (Zimring, p. 41), we are, in that moment, free from the defining criteria of the objective context that is governed by logic, causation, success, or failure. Experience of the subjective context gives access to the inner locus of evaluation and the freedom from moralistic or pathologizing judgments (in the specific way Zimring is defining it). We can enter the objective context in our own inner representations, for instance, by picturing being blamed for losing a championship game by missing the last free throw and how we might deal with such a humiliating disappointment. But it is only when "I" attend to my feeling of disappointment with myself instead of reacting to the "me" that I can be said to have access to the subjective context and to allow the feeling to change.

Thus, Zimring is describing two different types of internal contexts: the objective context that is stressed in our culture as significant and meaningful, and the subjective context having little real-world value. Thinking of oneself as an object, as "me," is to inhabit an objective transactional state, whereas while thinking as a subject, as "I," is to inhabit a subjective transactional state. Client-centered therapists, by attending to and carefully attempting to understand the person's narrative (even though the narrative may be a story of what happened to the "me" at the basketball game), tacitly validate the subjective context, eventually strengthening the person's subjective context itself and access to it.

The theory presented here assumes the self to be existing in the discourse that occurs in reaction to the phenomenological and social context, assumes a self that exists in perspective and in action, rather than a self that exists as an entity that determines action. This view of self implies a new view of the processes of change of self. This view is that the self changes from a change in perspective and discourse not from a discovery of the hidden, true self. . . . [T]he self changes, as feelings do, when we develop a new context. (1995, p. 47)

For some clients, establishing contact with their own subjective inner context within the facilitative interpersonal context of client-centered therapy may prove a difficult transition that may take time. Eventually, their access to that context and their ability to express it may increase. The self (the "I") that was available to the person only within therapy begins to appear in other contexts. An Asian American woman client of the third author recently said, "I was actually facing up to my father's anger. He was yelling at me that I was 'unfriendly,' meaning I wasn't doing what he wanted me to do. I could hardly recognize myself!"

It now is clearer why the client's perception of the therapist-provided conditions is so critical in achieving progress in therapy. Validation of the client's internal frame of reference (or, in Zimring's terms, the subjective context) is a serendipitous by-product of the process of interaction between the client who is communicating and the therapist's empathic responses. As the client perceives himself or herself as being received as unique and particular, as not being "made into an instance of anything else, be it a social category, a psychological theory, a moral principle, or whatever" (Kitwood, 1990, p. 6), the person's experience of being a self is strengthened and changed. Zimring explains that empathic understanding allows the client to "change from being in the Me to being in the I state which also grows the I":

> [W]e are responding to the unique aspects of the person, to those aspects in which we are most individual. In responding to these, in checking with the person to see if our responses are valid, in our assumption that these unique aspects of the person are important truths, we are demonstrating our belief in the validity of the person's intentions and inner world. Once this happens, once people begin to believe in the validity of their intentions and inner world, of their internal frame of reference, they begin to respond from an internal rather than from an external frame of reference. When we see ourselves as I or agent rather than Me or object, our experience changes. (Zimring, 2000, p. 112)

Client-centered therapy, in common with other therapeutic approaches, aims to enhance the life functioning and self-experience of clients. Unlike other therapies, however, client-centered therapy does not use techniques, treatment planning, or goal setting to achieve these ends. Brodley states:

> It may seem strange, but the therapeutic benefits of client-centered work are serendipitous in the sense that they are not the result of the therapist's concrete intentions when he or she is present with or expressively communicating with the client. The absence of intentional goals pursued for clients seems to me to be essential for some of the therapeutic benefits of the approach. Specifically, the nondirectivity inherent in the therapist's expressive attitude helps protect the client's autonomy and self-determination. It has the effect of promoting the client's experience as the architect of the therapy. . . . Client-centeredness, in its nondirectivity and expressiveness—being profoundly nondiagnostic and concretely not a means to any ends—has an exceptional power to help without harming. (Brodley, 2000, pp. 137–138)

APPLICATIONS

Who Can We Help?

Since client-centered therapy is not *problem*-centered but *person*-centered, clients are not viewed as instances of diagnostic categories who come into therapy with "presenting problems" (Mearns, 2003). When the therapist meets the other person as a human being worthy of respect, it is the emergent collaborative relationship that heals, not applying the correct "intervention" to the "disorder" (Natiello, 2001). Of course, clients come to therapy for a reason, and often the reason involves "problems" of some kind. But the point is that problems are not assumed and are not viewed as instances of *a priori* categories. Mearns clarifies this stance:

> Each person has a unique "problem" and must be treated as unique. The definition of the problem is something the client does, gradually symbolizing different facets under the gentle facilitation of the therapist; the client's work in "defining the problem" *is* the therapy. This is the same reasoning behind Carl Rogers's statement that the therapy is the diagnosis. "In a very meaningful and accurate sense, therapy is diagnosis, and this diagnosis a process which goes on in the experience of the client, rather than in the intellect of the clinician." (Mearns, 2003, p. 90; Rogers, 1951, p. 223)

This philosophy of the person leads us in the direction of appreciating each person as a dynamic whole. Human lives are processes evolving toward complexity, differentiation, and more effective self/world creation. In contrast, the medical model sees persons in terms of "parts"—as problematic "conflicts," "self-defeating" behaviors, or "irrational cognitions." Proponents of client-centered therapy see problems, disorders, and diagnoses as constructs that are generated by processes of social and political influence in the domains of psychiatry, pharmaceuticals, and third-party payers as much as by *bona fide* science.

Another common misconception of client-centered therapy concerns the applicability of the approach. Critics from outside the humanistic therapies dismiss this approach as (1) biased toward white, Western, middle-class, verbal clients, and thus ineffective for clients of less privileged social class, clients of color, or those who live in collectivist cultures; (2) superficial, limited, and ineffective, particularly with "severe disorders" such as Axis II personality disorders; and (3) utilizing only the technique of "reflection" and thus failing to offer clients "treatments" of proven effectiveness. Students of this approach who wish to investigate both the critiques and the refutations are referred to several recent works: Bozarth's *Person-Centered Therapy: A Revolutionary Paradigm* (1998), Brian Levitt's *Embracing Non-directivity* (2005), and Moodley, Lago, and Talahite's *Carl Rogers Counsels a Black Client* (2004). In their analysis of Rogers's work with a black client, Mier and Witty defend the adequacy of the theory insofar as constructs such as experiencing and the client's internal frame of reference are held to apply universally. Tension or limitations in cross-cultural therapy dyads arise from the personal limitations and biases of the therapist (Mier & Witty, 2004, p. 104).

In therapy, some clients may define self fundamentally by their group identity—e.g., family or kinship relations, religion, or tribal customs. Many persons, at some points in their lives, may define themselves in terms of other types of group affiliation (e.g., "I am a transsexual," "I am a trauma survivor," "I'm a stay-at-home Mom"). These definitions of self tend to emerge in the therapy relationship and are accepted and understood as central to the client's personal identity. However, it is an error to suppose that client-centered therapists aim to *promote* autonomy, independence, or other Western social values such as individualism and self-reliance. Respect for and appreciation of clients precludes therapists' formulating goals. Consultation offers the opportunity for therapists to examine biases of all types and to progress toward greater openness and acceptance of clients' culture, religious values, and traditions.

Feminist scholars of therapy both within the humanistic tradition and from the psychodynamic traditions have criticized client-centered therapy as focusing only on the individual without educating the client to the political context of her problems. Although it is true that client-centered therapists do not have psychoeducational goals for clients, these writers fail to recognize the ways in which social and political perspectives emerge in client-centered relationships. The recent work of Wolter-Gustafson (2004) and Proctor and Napier (2004) shows the convergence between the client-centered approach and the more recent "relational" and feminist therapies.

In an interview with Baldwin shortly before his death in 1987, Rogers made the following statement that illustrates the consistency with which he endorsed the nondirective attitude: "[T]he goal has to be within myself, with the way I am. . . . [Therapy is effective] when the therapist's goals are limited to the process of therapy and not the outcome" (quoted in Baldwin, 1987, p. 47).

Occasionally, clients who are veterans of the mental health system may have incorporated clinical diagnoses into their self-concepts and may refer to themselves in those terms. For example, "I guess I suffer from major depression. My psychiatrist says I'm like a plane flying with only one engine." Even though client-centered therapists do not view clients through a diagnostic lens, this self-description is to be understood and accepted, like any other aspect of the client's self-definition. It should be noted that this kind of self-categorization can be an instance of an external locus of evaluation in which a naïve and uncritical client has taken a stock label and applied it to himself or herself, or, conversely, it may represent a long, thoughtful assessment of one's experience and history, thus being a more truly independent self-assessment. If the client describes herself as "crazy" or "psychotic," the client-centered therapist would not say, "Oh, don't be so hard on yourself. You're not crazy." We put our confidence in the process of the therapy over time to yield more self-accepting and accurate self-appraisals on the part of the client, rather than telling the client how to think because his or her thinking is clearly wrong.

Although client-centered therapy is nondiagnostic in stance, client-centered therapists work with individuals diagnosed by others as psychotic, developmentally disabled, panic disordered, bulimic, and the like, as well as with people simply seeking a personal growth experience. This assumption that the therapy is generally applicable to anyone, regardless of diagnostic label, rests on the belief that the person is always more—that it is the person's expression of self and his or her relation between self and disorder, self and environment, that we seek to understand. Rogers states unequivocally that the diagnostic process is unnecessary and "for the most part, a colossal waste of time" (Kirschenbaum & Henderson 1989, pp. 231–232). Rogers elaborates on the issue:

> Probably no idea is so prevalent in clinical work today as that one works with neu-rotics in one way, with psychotics in another; that certain therapeutic conditions must be provided for compulsives, others for homosexuals, etc. . . . I advance the concept that the essential conditions of psychotherapy exist in a single configuration, even though the client or patient may use them very differently . . . [and that] it is [not] necessary for psychotherapy that the therapist have an accurate psychological diagnosis of the client. . . . [T]he more I have observed therapists . . . the more I am forced to the conclusion that such diagnostic knowledge is not essential to psychotherapy. (Kirschenbaum & Henderson, 1989, pp. 230–232)

When therapists do not try to dissuade clients from asking direct questions by suggesting that clients should work on finding their own answers, clients may occasionally request help from the therapist. Although there is some disagreement within the person-centered therapeutic community about answering questions, many client-centered therapists believe that following the client's self-direction logically requires responding to the client's direct questions. Depending on the question, such therapists might offer their thinking, which could include diagnostic observations, in the interest of providing the client with access to alternatives, including pharmacotherapy, behavioral interventions and the like. But, crucially, these offerings emerge from the client's initiative, and therapists have no stake in gaining "compliance" from the client with their offerings.

Client-centered therapists have worked successfully with a myriad of clients with problems in living, including those of psychogenic, biogenic, and sociogenic origins. The common thread is the need to understand the client's relationship to the problem, illness, or self-destructive behavior; to collaborate with the client in self-healing and growth; and to trust that the client has the resources to meet the challenges he or she faces. No school of psychotherapy can claim to cure schizophrenia or alcoholism or to extract someone from an abusive relationship. But within a partnership of respect and acceptance, the client's inner relation to the behavior or negative experience changes in the direction of greater self-acceptance and greater self-understanding, which often leads to more self-preserving behavior.

In spite of the stereotype of client-centered therapy as applicable only to "not-too-severe" clients, a number of client-centered scholars and practitioners have written about the success of this approach with clients whose lives have been severely afflicted with "mental illness." For example, Garry Prouty's work with clients who are described as "psychotic" is described in his book *Theoretical Evolutions in Person-Centered/ Experiential Therapy* (1994). Lisbeth Sommerbeck, a Danish clinician, in her book *The Client-Centered Therapist in Psychiatric Contexts: A Therapist's Guide to the Psychiatric Landscape and its Inhabitants,* presents the issues she deals with as a client-centered therapist in a psychiatric setting in which her colleagues treat "patients" from the traditional medical model (Sommerbeck, 2003).

In contrast to long-term therapy, the current trend with persons diagnosed with schizophrenia has focused on social skills training, occupational therapy, and medication. It is rare for such a person to experience the potency of a client-centered relationship in which she or he is not being prodded to "comply" with a medication regimen, to exhibit "appropriate" behavior and social skills, and to follow directives that are supposedly in the person's interest as defined by an expert. In the client-centered relationship, the person can express her or his own perceptions that the medication isn't helping, without the immediate response "But you know that if you stop the medication, you will end up back in the hospital." This respect of the person's inner experience and perceptions empowers the person as someone with authority about self and experience. This is not to deny the positive aspects of skills training, psychotropic medications, and psychiatry. If medications and programs really do help, clients can be trusted to *elect* to utilize them; if they are *forced* to do so by their families and therapists and by institutions of the state, they are being treated paternalistically, as less than fully capable of deciding their own course in life.

A case that stuck in Rogers's memory over the years was that of "James," part of the Wisconsin study of chronically mentally ill patients (Rogers et al., 1967). In the course of a detailed description of two interviews with this patient, a "moment of change" is described in which the patient's hard shell is broken by his perception of the therapist's warmth and caring, and he pours out his hurt and sorrow in anguished sobs. This breakthrough followed an intense effort by Rogers, in two interviews a week for the better part of a year, to reach this 28-year-old man, whose sessions were filled with prolonged silences of up to 20 minutes. Rogers stated, "We were relating as two . . . genuine persons. In the moments of real encounter the differences in education, in status, in degree of psychological disturbance, had no importance—we were two persons in a relationship" (Rogers et al., 1967, p. 411). Eight years later, this client telephoned Rogers and reported continued success on his job and general stability in his living situation, and he expressed appreciation for the therapeutic relationship with Rogers (Meador & Rogers, 1984).

This account emphasizes the person-centered rather than problem-centered nature of this approach. Rogers often stated his belief that what was most personal was the most universal. The client-centered approach respects the various ways in which people deal with fear of being unlovable, fear of taking risks, fear of change and loss and the myriad nature of problems in living. Understanding the range of differences among us, Rogers saw that people are deeply similar in our wish to be respected and loved, our hope for belonging, for being understood, and our search for coherence, value, and meaning in our lives.

Client-centered therapists are open to a whole range of adjunctive sources of help and provide information to clients about those resources if asked. These would include self-help groups, other types of therapy, exercise programs, medication, and the like, limited only by what the therapist knows about and believes to be effective and ethical. The attitude toward these psychoeducational procedures and treatments is not one of *urging* the client to seek out resources of any kind but, rather, to suggest them in a spirit of "you can try it and see what you think." The client is always the ultimate arbiter of what is and what is not helpful and of which professionals and institutions are life-enhancing and which are disempowering.

Since the therapist is open to client initiatives, clients may at times wish to bring in a partner, spouse, child, or other person with whom they are having a conflict. Client-centered therapists are flexible and are often open to these alternative ways of working collaboratively with clients. The ethical commitment, however, is to the client, and it may be appropriate to refer others for couple or family therapy within the client-centered framework. A number of authors (including Nathaniel Raskin, Ferdinand van der Veen, Kathryn Moon and Susan Pildes, John McPherrin, Ned Gaylin, and Noriko Motomasa) have written about working with couples and families in the person-centered/client-centered approach.

This lack of concern with a person's "category" can be seen in person-centered cross-cultural and international conflict resolution. Empathy is provided in equal measure for Catholics and Protestants in Northern Ireland (Rogers & Ryback, 1984) and for black South Africans and whites in South Africa (Rogers, 1986b). Conflict resolution is fostered when the facilitator appreciates the attitudes and feelings of opposing parties, and then the stereotyping of one side by the other is broken down by the protagonists' achievement of empathy. Marshall Rosenberg, a student of Rogers at the University of Wisconsin, has developed an important approach to conflict that he calls "non-violent communication" (Rosenberg, 1999). This approach to communication implements the client-centered conditions in ways that do not dehumanize the other person or group.

Treatment

The person-centered approach has been described particularly in the context of individual psychotherapy with adults, its original domain. The broadening of the "client-centered" designation to "the person-centered approach" stemmed from the generalizability of client-centered principles to child, couple, and family work, the basic encounter group, organizational leadership, parenting, education, medicine, nursing, and forensic settings. The approach is applicable in any situation where the welfare and psychological growth of persons is a central aim. People who have institutional responsibility learn—often by trial and error—to implement the core conditions guided by the principle of nondirectiveness. For example, a graduate student in clinical psychology described going to the cell of an inmate he was seeing in therapy. He addressed the man as "Mr." and invited him to join him for the hour, giving him the power to refuse to talk if he didn't want to or feel up to it. This courteous treatment was such a contrast to the ways the man was treated by the prison guards that he wrote the student a long letter after the conclusion of the therapy, expressing his gratitude for being treated like a human being. Thus, even when clients are involuntarily mandated to "treatment," it is possible to function consistently from the core conditions.

Play Therapy

Rogers deeply admired Jessie Taft's play therapy with children at the Philadelphia Child Guidance Clinic, and he was specifically impressed by her ability to accept the negative feelings verbalized or acted out by the child, which eventually led to positive attitudes in the child. One of Rogers's graduate student associates, Virginia Axline, formulated play therapy as a comprehensive system of treatment for children. Axline shared Rogers's deep conviction about self-direction and self-actualization and, in addition, was passionate about helping fearful, inhibited, sometimes abused children develop the courage to express long-buried emotions and to experience the exhilaration of being themselves.

She used play when children could not overcome the obstacles to self-realization by words alone.

Axline made major contributions to research on play therapy, group therapy with children, schoolroom applications, and parent–teacher as well as teacher–administrator relationships. She also demonstrated the value of play therapy for poor readers, for clarifying the diagnosis of mental retardation in children, and for dealing with race conflicts in young children (Axline, 1947; Rogers, 1951).

Ellinwood and Raskin (1993) offer a comprehensive chapter on client-centered play therapy that starts with the principles formulated by Axline and shows how they have evolved into practice with parents and children. Empathy with children and adults, respect for their capacity for self-directed change, and the congruence of the therapist are emphasized and illustrated. More recently, Kathryn Moon has clarified the nondirective attitude in client-centered work with children (Moon, 2002).

Client-Centered Group Process

Beginning as a one-to-one method of counseling in the 1940s, client-centered principles were being employed in group therapy, classroom teaching, workshops, organizational development, and concepts of leadership less than 10 years later. Teaching, intensive groups, and peace and conflict resolution exemplify the spread of the principles that originated in counseling and psychotherapy.

Classroom Teaching

In Columbus, while Rogers was beginning to espouse the nondirective approach, he accepted the role of the expert who structured classes and graded students. At Chicago, he began to practice a new philosophy, which he later articulated in *Freedom to Learn:*

> I ceased to be a teacher. It wasn't easy. It happened rather gradually, but as I began to trust students, I found they did incredible things in their communication with each other, in their learning of content material in the course, in blossoming out as growing human beings. Most of all they gave me courage to be myself more freely, and this led to profound interaction. They told me their feelings, they raised questions I had never thought about. I began to sparkle with emerging ideas that were new and exciting to me, but also, I found, to them. I believe I passed some sort of crucial divide when I was able to begin a course with a statement something like this: "This course has the title 'Personality Theory' (or whatever). But what we do with this course is up to us. We can build it around the goals we want to achieve, within that very general area. We can conduct it the way we want to. We can decide mutually how we wish to handle these bugaboos of exams and grades. I have many resources on tap, and I can help you find others. I believe I am one of the resources, and I am available to you to the extent that you wish. But this is our class. So what do we want to make of it?" This kind of statement said in effect, "We are *free* to learn what we wish, *as* we wish." It made the whole climate of the classroom completely different. Though at the time I had never thought of phrasing it this way, I changed at that point from being *a teacher* and *evaluator,* to being *a facilitator of learning*—a very different occupation. (1983, p. 26)

The change was not easy for Rogers. Nor was it easy for students who were used to being led and who thus experienced the self-evaluation method of grading as strange and unwelcome.

The Intensive Group

The early 1960s witnessed another important development, the intensive group. Rogers's move to California in 1964 spurred his interest in intensive groups, and in 1970 he published a 15-step formulation of the development of the basic encounter group. Rogers visualized the core of the process, the "basic encounter," as occurring when an individual in the group responds with undivided empathy to another in the group who is sharing and also not holding back. Rogers conceptualized the leader's or facilitator's role in the group as exemplifying the same basic qualities as the individual therapist; in addition, he thought it important to accept and respect the group as a whole, as well as the individual members. An outstanding example of the basic encounter group can be seen in the film *Journey into Self,* which shows very clearly the genuineness, spontaneity, caring, and empathic behavior of co-facilitators Rogers and Richard Farson (McGaw, Farson, & Rogers, 1968).

Peace and Conflict Resolution

Searching for peaceful ways to resolve conflict between larger groups became the cutting edge of the person-centered movement in the 1980s. The scope of the person-centered movement's interest in this arena extends from interpersonal conflicts to conflicts between nations. In some instances, opposing groups have met in an intensive format with person-centered leadership. This has occurred with parties from Northern Ireland, South Africa, and Central America. A meeting in Austria on the "Central American Challenge" included a significant number of diplomats and other government officials (Rogers, 1986d). A major goal accomplished at this meeting was to provide a model of person-centered experiences for diplomats in the hope that they would be strengthened in future international meetings by an increased capacity to be empathic. Rogers (1987) and his associates also conducted workshops on the person-centered approach in Eastern Europe and the Soviet Union.

Rogers offered a person-centered interpretation of the Camp David Accords and a proposal for avoiding nuclear disaster (Rogers & Ryback, 1984). One notion is central to all these attempts at peaceful conflict resolution: When a group in conflict can receive and operate under conditions of empathy, genuineness, and caring, negative stereotypes of the opposition weaken and are replaced by personal, human feelings of relatedness (Raskin & Zucconi, 1984).

Evidence

Although clients almost never ask us to produce empirical evidence to support our claim that client-centered therapy will succeed in helping them, the question is entirely legitimate and one we should be capable of answering. To be a therapist is to represent oneself as a professional who is successful at helping. If one fails to help, there is an ethical responsibility to give the client an accounting for the failure (Brodley, 1974).

While the medical model of "treatment" is antithetical to client-centered philosophy and practice, objective, empirical research is not. Humanistic scholars see the links between theoretical models of therapy, research methods, and the practice of therapy as complex, plural, and not inevitable because they necessarily issue from differing philosophies of science and epistemologies. The fundamental question is posed: What is the relationship between scientific research findings and practice? What *should* the relationship be?

Support for Empiricism

Carl Rogers was a committed researcher and student of the therapy process, and he received the Distinguished Scientific Contribution Award from the American

Psychological Association in 1957. He said that it was the award he valued over all others. Client-centered scholars and researchers continue to be interested in finding answers to the questions of the efficacy and effectiveness of the client-centered approach. However, large-scale quantitatively focused studies have been lacking in recent decades, even though theoretical, philosophical, ethical, and naturalistic qualitative studies have burgeoned in the *Person-Centered Review* and *The Person-Centered Journal,* the *Person-Centered and Experiential Psychotherapy Journal,* and *Journal of Humanistic Psychology,* among many others, including non-English journals. Research in process-experiential therapy is an exception, as is the research being conducted in Germany (Eckert, Hoger & Schwab, 2003). Client-centered therapy also has strong support, albeit indirect support, from "common-factors" research efforts.

Common Factors

Saul Rosenzweig (1936) first hypothesized that outcome in psychotherapy might be due to factors that all therapies have in common (such as the personal characteristics of the therapist, the resources of the client, and the potency of the therapeutic relationship), rather than to techniques specific to theoretical orientations. This hypothesis was termed the *Dodo Bird conjecture.*

The character of the Dodo Bird appears in *Alice in Wonderland.* The animals decided to have a race to dry off after they were soaked by Alice's tears. Because they ran in all directions, the race had to be suspended. The animals appealed to the Dodo Bird for a decision. The Dodo Bird ruled as follows: "Everybody has won and all must have prizes!" The conclusion that all major psychotherapies, in fact, yield comparable effect sizes (measures of effectiveness) is often referred to as the *Dodo Bird effect.*

Decades of meta-analyses strongly support the Dodo Bird effect, refuting the idea that specific schools of therapy and their specific techniques are more important than the common factors (Elliott, 1996, 2002; Lambert, 2004; Luborsky, Singer, & Luborsky, 1975; Smith & Glass, 1977; Wampold, 2006). Interestingly, even therapies that are based on radically different philosophies and values show similar effect sizes in terms of successful outcome in studies utilizing widely varying outcome measures.

The elements that constitute outcome can be categorized as either therapeutic or extratherapeutic. In the first category we find effects that issue from the therapist, the therapeutic relationship, and the specific techniques associated with the particular therapeutic orientation. In the case of client-centered therapy, the therapist's experienced attitudes and communication of the attitudes, and the client's perception of these attitudes, are hypothesized to be the necessary and sufficient conditions that are causal factors leading to positive outcome. Therapeutic effects also include the impact of specific techniques that are sometimes utilized by nondirective client-centered therapists if clients suggest their use and if the therapist is competent in the particular technique. Lambert's 1992 study estimated that the variance in outcome attributed to therapeutic factors is approximately 30%; that attributed to techniques was about 15%. Placebo or expectancy effects represent 15% of the variance in outcome. (Client variables account for the remaining 40%.) This describes a situation in which the client has reason to expect that the therapy is going to make a positive difference in his or her life situation and experience simply by virtue of undertaking the therapy process with some degree of commitment.

Extratherapeutic factors include the environment of the client, the various vulnerabilities and problems he or she is dealing with, the presence or absence of adequate social support, and any particular events (such as losses or other changes) that influence the course of therapy. This category also includes client factors described by Bohart, such as the person's own creative resources and ability to direct his or her decisions, resilience or hardiness, and life experience in solving problems in living and the client's own active utilization of the therapy experience (Bohart, 2006, pp. 223–234). This factor is estimated at 40% of the overall variance. Clearly, the client and the numerous variables that make up the internal and external realities of the client's situation contribute greatly to the therapy outcome equation (Bohart, 2004).[2]

If a client is not in therapy voluntarily, is hostile toward the process and the therapist, and is noncommittal about attending sessions, the likelihood of positive outcome diminishes. By contrast, a client who enters the relationship feeling a strong need to obtain help, who is open and willing to give therapy a try, who is consistent in following through in attending sessions, and who is capable of relating to the therapist is much more likely to benefit from the experience. This tradition of what is called common-factors research has yielded strong, very consistent findings supportive of the therapy relationship as a principal source of therapeutic change. Such research has also found that techniques, though not negligible, contribute much less to the actual outcome. Many clinicians, however, have resisted the common-factors position, insisting that their techniques are the difference which makes the difference.

Bozarth (2002), along with many others who support a contextual or common-factors position, opposes the idea that specific techniques (most often cognitive behavioral or other behavioral approaches) are crucial to therapeutic success. Further, he argues that this idea, which he calls the "specificity myth"—i.e., the belief that specific disorders require specific "treatments"—is a fiction. Bruce Wampold's (2001) book *The Great Psychotherapy Debate,* in which he reviews and reanalyzes many meta-analytic studies, supports Bozarth's assessment. Wampold concludes that the famous Dodo Bird verdict has been robustly and repeatedly confirmed. Wampold reiterates his findings in a more recent review (2006).

Despite the work of Wampold and others, resistance to the Dodo Bird verdict continues. New schools of thought and accompanying techniques produce income and status in the field of psychology, leading to a proliferation of "treatments" for an ongoing proliferation of "disorders" on which various practitioners announce themselves as experts. But in the big picture of psychotherapy outcome, the evidence strongly supports a contextual model of therapy in which, as Wampold points out, the specific ingredients are important only as aspects of the entire healing context (2001, p. 217).

Evidence for the Core Conditions

The client-centered approach can confidently claim evidentiary support for the core conditions and for the impact on outcome when the client's perception of the conditions is utilized as an outcome measure (this was part of Rogers's original hypothesis that the client must perceive the therapist-experienced conditions in order to derive benefit).

Truax and Mitchell's (1971) analysis of 14 studies with 992 total participants studied the association between the core conditions and outcome. Sixty-six significant findings correlated positively with outcome, and there was one significant negative correlation (Kirschenbaum & Jourdan, 2005, p. 41).

C. H. Patterson's "Empathy, Warmth and Genuineness: A Review of Reviews" (1984) critiques conclusions from many studies of the core conditions conducted in the 1970s and 1980s. Patterson concludes that in many studies in which client-centered therapy was either the experimental or the control condition, the therapists were not experienced

---

[2] Bohart argues that theories of therapy, including client-centered therapy, posit the therapist as the "engine of change," failing to credit the client's considerable capacities as a self-healer.

client-centered therapists. Researchers either knowingly or unknowingly equated client-centered therapy with active listening or simple repeating back what the client says, and, consequently, did not meet the requirements of the theory of the conditions necessary for change in psychotherapy. In spite of this, many studies produced positive results supporting the approach. Patterson speculates that the measures of outcome would probably have been substantially more significant had the therapists involved been committed to working from Rogers's premise and had developed their ability to realize the attitudinal conditions (Patterson, 1984). His review also notes the bias against client-centered therapy in many reviews, in spite of the actual positive evidence under review.

Orlinsky and Howard (1986) reviewed numerous studies focusing on relationship variables and clients' perception of the relationship. They found that generally between 50 and 80% of the substantial number of findings in this area were significantly positive, indicating that these dimensions were very consistently related to patient outcome. This was especially true when process measures were based on patients' observations of the therapeutic relationship. (Orlinsky & Howard, 1986, p. 365)

Orlinsky, Grawe, and Parks (1994), updating the original study by Orlinsky and Howard, summarized findings from 76 studies investigating the relationship between positive regard and therapist affirmation and outcome. Out of 154 findings from these studies, 56% showed the predicted positive relationship; when patients' ratings were used, the figure rose to 65%.

Bohart, Elliott, Greenberg, and Watson (2002) conducted a large meta-analytic study of empathy and outcome, surveying studies from 1961 through 2000. These studies involved 3,026 clients and yielded 190 associations between empathy and outcome. A medium effect size of .32 was found, which indicates a meaningful correlation. With regard to these last two studies, we must remember that studies of only one of the core conditions do not test Rogers's client-centered model of therapy; rather, all six of the necessary and sufficient conditions must be accounted for in the research design (Watson, 1984). Even so, positive correlations between outcome and empathy and between outcome and positive regard are partially supportive of the model.

A recent study by process-experiential researchers illustrates some of the difficulties in assessing client-centered therapy. Greenberg and Watson's (1998) study of experiential therapy for depression compares process-experiential interventions (in the context of the core conditions) to the client-centered relationship conditions. Basically, the study showed the equivalence of the relationship conditions with process-experiential interventions for depression. Although process-directivity received some support in long-term follow-up, the treatments did not differ at termination or at 6-month follow-up (Greenberg & Watson, 1998). Once again, however, because the "client-centered" experimental condition in this study was operationalized with a manual, the comparison condition does not represent client-centered therapy. Bohart comments about this particular study:

> It is true, in a sense, that client-centered therapy has been manualized (Greenberg and Watson, 1998). I have personally seen these manuals. They are very well done, but what they create is an excellent *analogue* of client-centered therapy mapped into a different intellectual universe. They do not fully represent client-centered therapy as I understand it. Again, the very concept of following a manual is antithetical to the basic nature of client-centered therapy. To manualize an approach like client-centered therapy reminds me a little bit of Cinderella's sister who tries to fit into the glass slipper by cutting off part of her foot. One can do it, and one can even make it fit, but would it not be better to find a scientific glass slipper that truly fits the phenomenon being studied instead of mangling it to fit it into one that doesn't? (Bohart, 2002, p. 266)

In pointing out the problems with studying client-centered therapy not as a treatment package but as a unique relationship, we are not denying the importance of finding adequate ways to conduct research on this approach (see Mearns & McLeod, 1984). Newer models are emerging from the humanistic research community that hold promise for more adequate assessments of this model, such as Elliott's single-case hermeneutic design, Bohart's adjudicational model, Rennie's studies of client experience while in the therapy hour, and many qualitative studies that have emerged in the past two decades.

Most recently, Elliott and Freire (2008; Elliott, 2002) conducted an expanded meta-analysis of humanistic therapies (including client-centered, process-experiential, focusing-oriented, and emotion-focused therapies) that assessed nearly 180 outcome studies. Their analyses examined 203 client samples from 191 studies, 14,000 people overall. Their findings follow.

1. Person-centered/experiential therapies are associated with large pre–post change. Average effect size was 1.01 standard deviations (considered a very large effect).

2. Posttherapy gains in person-centered therapies are stable; they are maintained over early (less than 12 months) and late (12 months) follow-ups.

3. In randomized clinical trials with untreated control clients, clients who participate in person-centered/experiential therapies generally show substantially more change than comparable untreated clients (controlled effect size of .78 standard deviations).

4. In randomized clinical trials with comparative treatment control clients, clients in humanistic therapies generally show amounts of change equivalent to clients in nonhumanistic therapies, including CBT. (Elliott, 2002, pp. 71–72; Elliott & Freire, 2008).

Elliott and Freire conclude that their meta-analytic studies show strong support for person-centered/experiential therapy, even when compared to cognitive behavioral approaches. In some studies where CBT appears to have an edge over person-centered therapy, this advantage disappeared when they controlled for researcher allegiance (experimenter bias).

Evidence for the Self–Determining Client

The work of Ryan and Deci and colleagues supports the view of the person as intrinsically motivated toward autonomy, competence, and relatedness—that is, the active client as described by Bohart and Tallman (1999). The literature focusing on subjective well-being (SWB), hardiness and resilience, and self-determination and psychological well-being (PWB) supports the image of the active, generative, meaning-making person whom Rogers observed in his own therapy, which led him to postulate the actualizing tendency as the sole motive in human life.

Empirically Supported Treatments

In 1995, a Society of Clinical Psychology (Division 12) Task Force on Promotion and Dissemination of Psychological Procedures of the American Psychological Association (now known as the APA Division 12 Science and Practice Committee) was charged with identifying those "treatments" that warranted the description "empirically validated." This initiative followed on similar efforts in medicine to identify "best practices." The reasoning behind the effort to identify best practices for particular disorders such as bulimia, obsessive-compulsive disorder, depression, and generalized anxiety disorder, among others, seems straightforward. Are certain types of therapy more effective than others in helping people suffering with these problems? When this question and its implications are explored in depth, however, many difficulties arise, and addressing them has led to greater clarity about the epistemological assumptions informing research studies.

The empirically supported treatments (EST) movement urges use of the "gold standard" research design utilized by pharmaceutical companies when testing the efficacy of new medications. This design calls for random sampling of subjects and random assignment to experimental and control groups using double-blind procedures so that neither the clinician nor the patient knows which group receives the active medication. Since double-blind procedures are not possible in testing therapeutic efficacy (because the therapist is aware of which is the "active" treatment), there is the immediate confound of researcher allegiance unless therapists committed to one orientation are compared to therapists equally committed to another.

Additional difficulties arise in deciding what the control will consist of and how it will be administered. Wampold (2001) argues that any control group must be a *bona fide* psychological treatment, not just a wait-list or group case management condition. Attrition from randomization is a common problem in randomized clinical trials (RCTs). Elliott (1998) has raised the issue of underpowered studies in which the numbers of subjects are too low to outweigh allegiance effects and other threats to validity.

As Wampold (2006) cautions, the fact that a "treatment" has not met the criteria to be labeled an empirically supported treatment does not mean that many therapeutic approaches are not just as effective as those treatments that have been studied using the Task Force's criteria. Wampold (2001) argues as follows:

> Simply stated, the conceptual basis of the EST movement is embedded in the medical model of psychotherapy and thus favors treatments more closely aligned with the medical model, such as behavioral and cognitive treatments. . . . As a result of this medical model bias, humanistic and dynamic treatments are at a distinct disadvantage, regardless of their effectiveness. . . . In the larger context . . . giving primacy to an EST ignores the scientific finding that all treatments studied appear to be uniformly beneficial as long as they are intended to be therapeutic. . . . Although apparently harmless, the EST movement has immense detrimental effects on the science and practice of psychotherapy, as it legitimates the medical model of psychotherapy when in fact treatments are equally effective. (pp. 215–216)

From the point of view of client-centered therapy research, the problem with many studies that focus on only one of the core conditions is that the client-centered model Rogers proposed is not being tested. Rogers proposed that the therapist-provided conditions/attitudes function holistically as a single gestalt, with the client perceiving the levels of the presence of the conditions in a succession of percepts and related inferences about the therapist's relation to her or him. Many studies of empathy, particularly those from other orientations, are, we believe, studying a somewhat different condition. A congruent, nondirective client-centered therapist who has no goals for the client, who is experiencing some level of positive regard, and who aims to empathically understand the communications of the client from within the frame of reference of the client is a different phenomenon from the therapist who deliberately sets out to establish a "therapeutic alliance" *in order to* establish bonds, tasks, and goals. Indeed, Rogerian therapy is a wholly different phenomenon from studies where "nondirective therapy" is used as a control in which the therapist uses empathic responses. These studies show nothing valid (pro or con) about true client-centered therapy. In spite of these methodological flaws and definitional differences, studies from a psychodynamic perspective also support the association between positive regard and outcome (Farber & Lane, 2002, p. 191).

Strong support exists for empathic understanding and positive regard, whereas the results of studies of congruence are more ambiguous. Part of the problem in studying congruence results from confusion about definitions. Many researchers, including person-centered investigators, seem to define congruence behaviorally as achieving transparency through self-disclosure. In fact, although Rogers advocated for client-centered therapists' freedom to be real and personal in the relationship, he didn't advocate saying whatever comes into one's mind. Only when the therapist has a "persistent feeling" should he or she consider raising the issue with the client. The necessity of maintaining the other core conditions influences how and when the therapist brings in his or her own frame of reference.

In research, congruence should be defined as an inner state of integration that naturally fluctuates throughout a session, in concert with the experienced attitudes of unconditional positive regard and empathy. The therapeutic attitudes combine into a gestalt as the therapist attends to the narrative of the client. Therapist congruence must be assessed primarily by the therapist; the client may evaluate whether he or she perceived the therapist as sincere, genuine, and transparent, but those evaluations are inferences based on the therapist's verbal and nonverbal behavior, not on congruence itself. Watson (1984) has argued that Rogers's 1957 hypothesis (which he intended to apply to all therapies) has not really been tested adequately. With some few exceptions, this is still the case more than two decades since Watson's meticulous examination of the data available on client-centered therapy in 1984.

Alternatives to the strategies of studying persons as objects, as the final repository of the action of independent variables, are humanistic research paradigms in which clients are co-investigators of the therapy process. Guidelines detailing these approaches can be found in a document produced by a Task Force for the Development of Practice Recommendations for the Provision of Humanistic Psychosocial Services from the APA Division of Humanistic Psychology (2005; www.apa.org/divisions/div32/draft.html).

For a more comprehensive survey (from the humanistic side) of the issues involved in the EST controversy, see Bohart (2002); Elliott, Greenberg, and Lietaer (2004); Kirschenbaum and Jourdan (2005); Norcross, Beutler, and Levant (2006); Wampold (2006; 2001); and Westen, Novotny, and Thompson-Brenner (2004), among others. A recent book edited by Norcross, Beutler, and Levant, *Evidence-based Practices in Mental Health: Debate and Dialogue on the Fundamental Questions* (2006), is a wide-ranging collection of articles debating the EST movement and challenging the RCT research model, as well as arguing for its continuing significance.

Psychotherapy in a Multicultural World

If the reader has followed Rogers's arguments against the "specificity hypothesis," it will come as no surprise to find that client-centered therapists have reacted with skepticism to arguments supporting the necessity of culture-specific approaches to each racial, cultural or ethnic group, gender identity, sexual orientation, or social class identity. Attempts to sensitize student therapists to cultural differences have often led to simplistic stereotypes about differing groups. We argue that within-group differences may exceed between-group differences, that groups' self-definitions are constantly under construction, and that similarly, group members are usually members of multiple groups leading to ever-increasing permutations of identity (Patterson, 1996).

A client-centered approach does not assume "difference" except as the client asserts how he or she experiences self as different. At the same time, those of us working from this approach understand that each person is completely unique in terms of what his or her history, ethnicity, religion or lack of it, and racial identity(ies) mean. The task, as always, is empathic understanding of the client's communicated meanings about self and about the world he or she perceives and constructs.

Does this mean that client-centered therapy has a "one size fits all" approach? The answer is complex. We answer "yes" to the extent that *uniqueness of the person is a universal.* We answer "no" in order to counteract the prevalent color-blind assertion that "We're all human beings!" This seemingly benign assertion has masked many covert biases that therapists whose master statuses are dominant and "unmarked" have carried into therapy. The multicultural therapy movement has served to sensitize and challenge this kind of status quo thinking and practice. Client-centered therapists are just as prone to bias as therapists of differing theoretical orientations. We suspect that there is a qualitative difference in the empathic understanding process of the therapist who has been challenged on his or her biases and the therapist who is still denying them. Research has yet to be done regarding this contention, but it seems to us very likely that the quality and depth of empathy are affected by the therapist's own growth of understanding about his or her location in the various social hierarchies of dominance.

Our basic practice remains true to the core conditions no matter who our client may be. We also assert that our ability to form an initial therapeutic relationship depends upon our own openness to and appreciation of and respect for all kinds of difference.

CASE EXAMPLE

It has always been characteristic of the person-centered approach to illustrate its principles with verbatim accounts. This has the advantage of depicting the interaction between therapist and client exactly and gives readers the opportunity to agree or to differ with the interpretation of the data. The following interview took place in Szeged, Hungary, at a Cross-Cultural Workshop, in July of 1986. John Shlien, former colleague and student of Rogers, had convened a group to learn about client-centered therapy, and Dr. Barbara Temaner Brodley, who had practiced client-centered therapy for more than 30 years at that time, volunteered to do a demonstration interview. A young European woman who had recently earned a master's degree in the United States volunteered to be the client. There were several English-speaking participants in the observing group and 8 or 10 Hungarians. The Hungarian participants clustered together in a corner so as not to disturb the interview while they were receiving a simultaneous translation. The interview was scheduled for 20 minutes, more or less, depending on the client's wishes.

The Demonstration Interview[3]

Barbara: Before we start I'd like to relax a little bit. Is that all right with you? (Spoken to the Client) I would like to say to the group that I'm going to attempt to empathically understand my client, to do pure empathic following. As I have the need, I will express my empathic understanding of what she says, and expresses, to me about her concerns and herself. (Turns to Client) I want you to know that I am also willing to answer any questions that you might ask. (C: O.K.) If it happens that you have a question.

[3] Reproduced with permission from Fairhurst, I. (Ed). (1999). *Women writing in the person-centered approach,* Ross-on-Wye, UK: PCCS Books.

C1:   You are my first woman therapist. Do you know that?

T1:   I didn't know.

C2:   And that's important for me because . . . uh . . . it sort of relates to what I'm going to talk about. Which has been going on in my mind since I decided to spend
the summer in Europe. (T: Uhm-hm) Um . . . I spent the last two years in the
United States studying, and (pause) when I left ******* in 1984, I was not the
same person I am right now.

T2:   Something has happened to you.

C3:   A lot of things have happened to me! (laughs). And, I'm coming back to Europe
this summer primarily to see my parents again. When I had left ******* two
years ago, I had left in a state of panic. Promising almost never to go back. Promising never to see them again. And . . .

T3:   Escaping and going *to* something.

C4:   Yeah, yeah, yeah. Getting away from . . . and I had never expected that I would
reach this point, that I would be able to go back and see them again.

T4:   Uhm-hm. You were so sure, then.

C5:   I was *angry*. (T: Uhm-hmm) I was *so angry*. And it's good for me that I'm taking
all this time before I go back to *******. I mean this workshop now, and then
I'm going to travel. And then I'm going to go to ******* at a certain point in
August. (T: Uhm-hmm) But sometimes, I just, I'm struck by the fact that, *gosh,*
I'm going to see them again, and how would that be? How will that be?

T5:   You're making it gradual and yet at a certain point you will be there, (C: Uh-huh)
and what will that be? (C: Uh-huh) Is? . . . you have, uh, an . . . anticipation or
fear (C: Yeah) or (C: Yeah) something like that.

C6:   Yeah, and I guess . . . I was thinking about my mother the other day, and . . .
I realized, in the States, I realized that she and I had a very competitive
relationship. And . . . it was interesting, but three days ago in Budapest I saw a
lady in the street who reminded me of my mother. But my mother—not at the
age which she has right now—but my mother 20 years from now. And, I don't
know why. I was so struck by that because I saw my mother being old and, and,
weak. So she was not this powerful, domineering person that she used to be in
******* who I was so much afraid of.

T6:   Uhm-hm. But old and weakened and diminished . . .

C7:   Diminished. That's the word. (T: Uhm-hm.) That's the word. (Begins to cry).

T7:   It moved you to think of that, that she would (C: Yeah.) be so weak and
diminished.

C8:   And I think there was something in that lady's eyes that reminded me of my
mother which (voice breaks; crying) I was not aware of when I was in *******.
And it was fear. (T: Uh-huh) I saw fear in the woman's eyes. (T: Fear) Yeah. And,
I was not aware of that.

T8:   You mean, when you saw this woman who resembled your mother but 20 years
from now, you saw in this woman's eyes something you had not realized was, in
fact, in the eyes of your mother. (C: Yeah) And that was the quality of fear. And
that had some great impact on you.

C9:   Yeah. Because I felt that this woman needed me. (Crying) (Pause) It feels good
that I am crying now. (T: Uhm-hm) I'm feeling very well that I am crying . . .
(T: Uhm-hm)

T9:   (Pause) It was a sense of your mother in the future, and that your mother *will*
need you.

C10:   You got it! The future stuff. It's not the present stuff. (Pause) It feels right here.
(She places her hand over her abdomen.)

T10:   The feeling is that your mother will have—has—fear and will have great need for you, (C: Yeah.) later on.

C11:   Yeah. (Pause) And as I am going back to *******, I don't know if I'm ready to, if I'm ready to take care of her. I don't know if I'm ready to see that need expressed by her. (Continuing to cry)

T11:   Uhm-hm, uhm-hm, uhm-hm. (Pause) You're afraid that when you get there, that will be more present in her. Or you will see it more than you did before, now that you've seen this woman. And that that will be a kind of demand on you, and you're afraid you're not ready to meet that.

C12:   That's it, yeah, and it's gotten too much for me. Or, right now in Hungary, I perceive it as being too much. (Crying continues)

T12:   Uhm-hm. At least, you're saying you're not sure how you will feel there, but it feels now like if that comes forth, if you see that, you, you, won't be able to . . . (C: Take it.) respond—be able to take it.

C13:   Yeah, yeah. It was interesting. I kept looking at her, you know. And it's like I was staring at her and she was staring at me. She was Hungarian. She didn't know why I was looking at her and I didn't know why I was looking at her either. But it's like I wanted to take all of her in, and make her mine, and prepare myself. And suddenly I realized that all this anger I had was gone. There was nothing left. It was gone. (Crying)

T13:   Uhm-hm. You mean, as you and this older woman looked at each other, and you had the meaning that it had for you about your mother, you wanted to—at that moment—you wanted to take her in and to give to her. To somehow have her feel that you were receiving her.

C14:   Yeah. (Expressed with a note of reservation)

T14:   The important thing is that . . . out of that you realized that you weren't afraid of your mother anymore, you weren't afraid of her dominance or . . .

C15:   Yeah. Yeah.

T15:   And that's a kind of incredible—(C: Discovery)—discovery and an incredible phenomenon that that (C: Yeah) fear and oppression could drop away so suddenly.

C16:   And I guess, another feeling that I had also was, I felt sorry for her.

T16:   Your mother.

C17:   Yeah. (Pause) And I don't like feeling sorry for her at all. (Crying) I used to a lot. For a long time when I loved somebody I used to feel sorry for them at the same time. I couldn't split those two things. (Pause) I don't know what I'm trying to say right now . . . I don't know if I'm trying to say that I felt that I was loving her or that I was feeling sorry for her or both.

T17:   There's a quality—pity . . . or feeling sorry for her that was strong but which you did not like. And then you don't know whether there was a quality of love that was part of that pity?

C18:   Yeah.

T18:   So both the feelings are mixed and confusing (C: Yeah) and then the reactions of—of having the sympathy and then having the (C: Uh-huh) pulling back (C: Uh-huh) from it.

C19:   And I don't know if the woman did really resemble my mother or if it was my wish to make her resemble my mother. Maybe I'm ready (pause) ready to get there. I'm ready to see my mother as a person, and not—I can't put a word because I don't know how I was perceiving my life so far. But I had never perceived her as a woman in the street, just a woman, just another woman in the street, (her voice quakes with feeling) vulnerable and anxious and needy, and scared (softly).

T19: And you don't know whether you had changed and therefore saw—experienced this woman from the change, of being open to seeing all of that in your mother. (C: That's right) Or whether she really—when you looked at her—looked very much like your mother and how *she* would look. Is that right? (C: Yeah) You don't know which?

C20: Yeah.

T20: I guess then, that the really important thing is that you saw her, your mother, in your mind through this woman in a completely new way, as a person, as vulnerable, as afraid, as in need.

C21: Uhm-hm, uhm-hm. And that made me feel more human . . .

T21: Made *you* feel more human. (C: Uh-huh) To see *her* as more human (C: Also) made you feel more human in yourself.

C22: Yeah.

T22: Uhm-hm, because the force of how she *had* been to you—the tyrant or something . . .

C23: She had a lot of qualities. Some of them I don't remember anymore.

T23: But not a whole person to you, not a vulnerable person.

C24: Uhm-hm. (Pause) I said at the beginning that you were my first woman therapist. (T: Uhm-hm) I was avoiding women therapists like hell. (T: Uhm-hm) All the therapists I had were men so far and now I know why. I can't put why to words but I know why.

T24: That some of your feelings about *her* made you avoid a woman therapist and choose men?

C25: Yeah. (Pause) And lots of other things. But at this point, um, I, I'm perceiving everybody as another person, and that makes me feel more of a person as well.

T25: Uhm-hm. You're perceiving everybody (C: Everybody) as more rounded . . . um . . . (C: Yeah) including the therapist.

C26: Therapists were big—were a big thing for me for a long time. Very big authority figures and stuff like that. (T: Uhm-hm) So I guess I was afraid that a woman therapist—a woman therapist was very threatening to me. (T: Uhm-hm) Four years ago, three years ago. But at this point I feel everybody's a person.

T26: Everybody's a person. So that among the many transformations that have occurred since you left home (C: Yeah) for the United States. That's a big one. (C: That was . . .) That people have become persons to you instead of figures of various sorts.

C27: Absolutely true. I *mean* that's absolutely *right*. And it happened after I left *****.

T27: Uhm-hm.

C28: And I feel . . . (Looking toward group).

T28: And you feel it's about time?

C29: (Client nods.) Thank you.

T29: You're welcome. Thank *you*. (Client leans towards therapist and they embrace with affection and smiles.)

C30: Thank you very much. (They continue to embrace.)

Brodley comments about the interview:

> When I evaluate client-centered therapy interviews, I make a basic distinction between errors of understanding and errors of attitude. Errors of attitude occur when the therapist's intentions are other than maintaining congruence, unconditional positive regard and empathic understanding or other than a nondirective attitude. For example, when the therapist is distracted and failing to try to empathically understand the client. Or when the therapist is emotionally disturbed and unsettled.

Or when the therapist has lost unconditional acceptance and reveals this in the tone or content of his communications. Errors of understanding occur when the therapist is attempting to acceptantly and empathically understand, but misses or misinterprets what the client is getting at and trying to express. In this brief interview my volunteer client was in her mid-twenties and I was in my late fifties when the interview took place. It is impossible to know how much influence on the content of the interview resulted from my age being close to the client's mother's age. I do know that we had a good chemistry, were attracted to each other. The client and I had briefly encountered each other the evening before the interview and after the interview, she told me she had experienced a positive reaction to me (as I had toward her) and that she volunteered because I was to be the therapist. In the session I was emotionally open to her and felt strong feelings as she unfolded her narrative. One of our Hungarian observers told me after the interview, "now I understand client-centered therapy" because he saw tears in my eyes as I worked with her. (Brodley, 1999b; cited in Fairhurst, pp. 85–92)

Commentary

This interview illustrates, in concrete form, several principles of the process of client-centered therapy. The client's first statement, "You are my first woman therapist" precedes her direct question "Did you know that?" Barbara responds immediately, "I didn't know." Clearly, the client is implying that interacting with her first woman therapist is significant to her. Whereas some therapists might have immediately answered the question with another question, such as "Why is that significant?" client-centered therapists, in keeping with the nondirective attitude, do not prompt or lead their clients. The client here is free to pursue why it is significant or not to do so. She does say that Barbara's being a woman is important "because it sort of relates to what I'm going to talk about" but does not explain it more fully until later in the interview. And even then, she has a new awareness that she cannot really put into words. In C25, she states, "I said at the beginning that you were my first woman therapist. I was avoiding women therapists like hell. All the therapists I had were men so far and *now I know why*. I can't put why to words but I know why."

Commitment to nondirectiveness should not be understood as a tense, conscious inhibiting of what one might wish to say to a client. As therapists mature in the approach, the nondirective attitude is often described as involving an experience of relief. The therapist who has formerly felt responsible for the interaction trusts the client to decide how much to disclose and when to disclose it. In this interview, the client clearly directs the conversation toward a concern of great moment to her—the trip she will be making in a matter of weeks to see her parents, whom she had promised herself never to see again. She explains that she has been in the United States for the preceding 2 years as she studied for a master's degree and had not returned to her home country or her family. She explains that she had left home in a state of intense anger toward her parents—and now is wondering how it will be to see them after this absence that was more a voluntary exile than simply a peaceful time away.

During this part of the interview, the therapist makes several empathic following responses to check her understanding of the content of the story and also the client's immediate meaning. It is not until the therapist tentatively grasps the point of the client's narrative that it becomes possible to *experience empathic understanding*. In T5, the therapist says "You're making it [the return trip] gradual and yet at a certain point you will be there and what will that be . . . you have an anticipation or fear or something like that." This response is accepted, and the client moves on to tell of the encounter she had 3 days ago in which her attention was captured by an older woman in the streets of Budapest. Although it is unclear to the client why she associated this older woman with her own mother, she reports being strongly affected by the spontaneous perception of her mother in the future as old and weak. "So she was not this power-ful, domineering person that she used to be in [her country] who I was so much afraid of." The therapist's response in which she says "old and weakened and diminished" is an example of an accurate empathic response that exactly captures the client's im-mediate experiencing. This is an important difference between recounting an emotion (as the client had earlier when she recalled how angry she had been upon leaving her home and her parents) and the direct experiencing of the emotion. After the therapist's response, she replies, "diminished. That's the word. That's the word." At this moment she has access to deeply sensed though unidentified emotions.

Client-centered therapy, in this way, spontaneously stimulates the unfolding of the inner experiencing of the client. In experiential terms, the "felt sense" has been symbol-ized and is carried forward, allowing a new gestalt of experiencing to arise (Gendlin, 1961). But unlike process-directive and emotion-focused therapists' aims, the therapist was not aiming to produce focusing, nor was she trying to "deepen the felt sense" or to do anything except understand what the client was communicating. In this way, the pow-erful focusing effects that frequently occur in client-centered therapy are serendipitous and unintended. The stance of the nondirective therapist is expressive, not instrumental (Brodley, 2000). Barbara's use of the term *diminished* captures the client's perception of her mother in the future, and the client begins to weep.

As she moves further into the experience of her perception of the older woman, the client tells Barbara that what she saw in the woman's eyes was fear—a fear that she now realizes had been present in her own mother's eyes, although at the time she had seen it without being aware of having seen it, an instance of what Rogers has termed "subception." Barbara checks her understanding of this event, which occurred only days ago and involved a stranger in the present but someone who, for the client, rep-resented her mother in the future, noting that the client's perception of fear in the woman's eyes "had some great impact on you." The client responds with immediacy and deep feeling: "Yeah, because I felt that this woman needed me" and she continues to cry. With her immediate experiencing openly available to her, she notes, "It feels good that I am crying now. I'm feeling very well that I am crying." A moment later she places her hand over her abdomen saying "it feels right here," letting the therapist know that she is having a direct, bodily awareness of her experiencing and that it feels good to her to allow herself to cry.

We infer that the therapist's embodiment of the therapeutic conditions has facili-tated the deeply felt expression of this experience. It is also possible to infer, although we can't be sure, that the fact that the client has been to several male therapists indicates that Rogers's second condition (that the person be vulnerable and anxious) may apply to the client because of the risk she is taking to work with a woman for the first time, even though this is a single therapy session. She may be vulnerable regarding this experience, but she is actively seeking an opportunity for personal growth in the possibly intimidat-ing setting of a public workshop.

Another way to look at this experience is in terms of its complexity. The client is feeling and expressing both sorrow and pity for her mother in the future and, at the same moment, is aware of a sense of well-being or fullness in the expression of the pain. Clients can be trusted to relate what is meaningful to them, moving toward the points they wish to bring out that embody meaning. At the same time as they are giving "content," they are experiencing themselves expressing meaning, and so there is a self-reflexive as-pect of the communication that may remain implicit. In this instance, the client makes her relation to her own experiencing and expression explicit. The aim of empathic understanding is not so much to catch the underlying, implicit feeling as much as to fully grasp both the narrative and the client's inner relation to what is being expressed. The agency or intentions of the person are to be understood simultaneously with the explicit content (Brodley, 2000; Zimring, 2000).

In the next part of the interview, the client reveals that as she stood looking at the Hungarian woman, and as she felt like taking the woman in and preparing herself, she recognized that her anger toward her parents had dissipated entirely. She says, "suddenly I realized that all this anger I had was gone. There was nothing left. It was gone." In this instance, she is recounting a powerful experience she had had a few days prior to the interview. And shortly she relates that she felt sorry for her mother in the midst of this perception—a feeling she did not welcome and one that, previously in her life, she had been unable to discriminate from love. In C20, there is what Rogers calls a moment of movement in which the client says, "I don't know if the woman did really resemble my mother or if it was my wish to make her resemble my mother. Maybe I'm ready . . . (pause) . . . ready to get there. I'm ready to see my mother as a person . . . I had never perceived her as a woman in the street, just a woman, just another woman in the street vulnerable and anxious and needy and scared."

The chance encounter with the Hungarian woman stimulated the client's recognition that her perception of her mother has shifted from someone she had resisted and feared and had seen as a figure of authority to someone whom she is perhaps ready to encounter as a human being who is "just a woman, just another woman in the street." The result of this shift is enhancing to her sense of herself as a person. In C26 she says, "But at this point, I'm perceiving everybody as another person, and *that makes me feel more of a person as well.*" One way to look at this interview is that there is movement from not being sure she is ready to see her mother's need to "maybe I'm ready . . . (pause) . . . ready to get there." It is possible that as she interacts with the therapist in this climate of acceptance and empathic understanding, she begins to feel more of her own strength and coping capacity.

Another aspect of this situation is the client's fear of women therapists, which is clearly related to her fear of and anger toward her mother. Again, it is possible that in her immediate interaction with a woman therapist onto whom she has projected negative feelings in the past, she experiences quite different emotions and reactions: the warm acceptance and presence of a real woman therapist. This allows a restoration of personal congruence in that we infer she is not reacting with anxiety and fear in the interview. This integrative experience may directly interact with the reorganization she experiences toward the feared mother from the past to the vulnerable, human mother in the future who will need her. Thus she may be experiencing a greater sense of autonomy; she is no longer in the grip of anger, and she is now ready or almost ready to encounter her mother as a vulnerable person. As Ryan and Deci point out, autonomy may be thought of in terms of volition as well as in terms of independence (Ryan & Deci, 2000, p. 74). The client's increasing sense of her freedom and her emerging sense of readiness to return leads to an increase in personal authority or power, as well as to an increased sense of her own humanity as someone who is at last perceiving other persons not as "figures" but simply as individual human beings. The client appears to have greater access to her own inner subjective context and, within the psychologically facilitative environment of the client-centered core conditions, to have become more of an authentic person in her own right.

When the client-centered therapy process persists over time, clients are likely to experience a deepening sense of self-authority and personal power. They become more capable of resistance to external authority, particularly when it is unjust, and more capable of deep connections with others. These changes in self-concept lead to more effective learning and problem solving and to enhanced openness to life.

SUMMARY

The central hypothesis of the person-centered approach postulates that individuals have within themselves vast resources for self-understanding and for altering their self-concepts, behavior, and attitudes toward others. These resources are mobilized and released in a definable, facilitative, psychological climate. Such a climate is created by a psychotherapist who is empathic, caring, and genuine.

Empathy, as practiced in the person-centered approach, consists of a consistent, unflagging appreciation for the experience of the client. It involves a continuous process of checking with the client to see whether understanding is complete and accurate. It is carried out in a manner that is personal, natural, and free-flowing; it is not a mechanical kind of reflection or mirroring. *Caring* is characterized by a profound respect for the individuality of the client and by nonpossessive, warm, acceptant caring or unconditional positive regard. *Genuineness* is marked by congruence between what the therapist feels and says and by the therapist's willingness to relate on a person-to-person basis, rather than through a professionally distant role.

The impetus given to psychotherapy research by the person-centered approach has resulted in substantial evidence demonstrating that changes in personality and behavior occur when a therapeutic climate is provided and utilized by an active, generative client. Two frequent results of successful client-centered therapy are increased self-esteem and greater openness to experience. Trust in the perceptions and the self-directive capacities of clients expanded client-centered therapy into a person-centered approach to education, group process, organizational development, and conflict resolution.

When Carl Rogers began his journey in 1940, psychotherapy was dominated by individuals who practiced in a manner that encouraged a view of themselves as experts. Rogers created a way of helping in which the therapist was a facilitator of a process that was directed by the client. More than half a century later, the person-centered approach remains unique in the magnitude of its trust in the client and in its unwavering commitment to the sovereignty of the human person.

ANNOTATED BIBLIOGRAPHY AND WEB RESOURCES

Barrett-Lennard, G. T. (1998). *Carl Rogers's helping system: Journey and substance.* London: Sage Publications.
A comprehensive and scholarly presentation of the person-centered approach to psychotherapy and human relations. It starts with the beginnings of client-centered therapy and the social–political–economic milieu of the 1920s and 1930s and continues with a description of early practice and theory, detailed examinations of the helping interview and the course of therapy, applications to work with children and families, and use with groups, education, conflict resolution and the building of community, and research and training. It concludes with a retrospective and prospective look at this system of helping.

Bozarth, J. (1998). *Person-centered therapy: A revolutionary paradigm.* Ross-on-Wye, UK: PCCS Books.
A collection of 20 revised and new papers by one of the movement's outstanding teachers and theoreticians. This book is divided into sections: Theory and Philosophy, The Basics of Practice, Applications of Practice, Research, and Implications. It reflects on Carl Rogers's theoretical foundations, emphasizes the revolutionary nature of these foundations, and offers extended frames for understanding this radical approach to therapy.

Raskin, N. J. (2004). *Contributions to client-centered therapy and the person-centered approach.* Ross-on-Wye, UK: PCCS Books.
This collection of Raskin's articles includes empirical studies, historical accounts of theoretical developments in the person-centered approach, and a personal description of Raskin's own growth as a person and therapist. It is a broad, incisively written compendium of articles by one of the founders of the approach.

Rogers, C. R. (1951). *Client-centered therapy.* Boston: Houghton Mifflin.
This book describes the orientation of the therapist, the therapeutic relationship as experienced by the client, and the process of therapy. It expands and develops the ideas expressed in the earlier book *Counseling and psychotherapy* (1942).

Rogers, C. R. (1961). *On becoming a person.* Boston: Houghton Mifflin.
Perhaps Rogers's best-known work, this book helped to make his personal style and positive philosophy known globally. The book includes an autobiographical chapter and sections on the helping relationship; the ways

in which people grow in therapy; the fully functioning person; the place of research; the implications of client-centered principles for education, family life, communication, and creativity; and the impact on the individual of the growing power of the behavioral sciences.

Rogers, C. R. (1980). *A way of being.* Boston: Houghton Mifflin.

As the book jacket states, this volume "encompasses the changes that have occurred in Dr. Rogers's life and thought during the decade of the seventies in much the same way *On becoming a person* covered an earlier period of his life. The style is direct, personal, clear—the style that attracted so many readers to the earlier book." In addition to important chapters on theory, there is a large personal section, including chapters on what it means to Rogers to listen and to be heard and one on his experience of growing as he becomes older (he was 78 when the book was published). An appendix contains a chronological bibliography of Rogers's publications from 1930 to 1980.

Web Sites

Association for the Person-Centered Approach (ADPCA), www.adpca.org

British Association for the Person-Centered Approach, www.bapca.co.uk

Center for the Studies of the Person, www.centerfortheperson.org/

World Association for Person Centered & Experiential Psychotherapy & Counseling (WAPCEPC), www.pce-world.org

CASE READINGS

Ellis, J., & Zimring, F. (1994). Two therapists and a client. *Person-Centered Journal, 1*(2), 77–92.

This article contains the transcripts of short interviews by two therapists with the same client. Because 8 years intervened between the interviews, these typescripts permit a glimpse of the changes in the client over the period, as well as allowing for comparison of the style and effect of two client-centered therapists.

Knight, T. A. (2007). Showing clients the doors: Active problem-solving in person-centered psychotherapy. *Journal of Psychotherapy Integration, 17*(1), 111–124. [Reprinted in D. Wedding & R. J. Corsini (Eds.) (2011). *Case studies in psychotherapy* (6th ed.). Belmont, CA: Cengage.]

This case illustrates the ways in which a therapist can maintain a nondirective and person-centered approach while still responding to the expressed needs of clients who present with circumscribed problems they expect to solve.

Raskin, N. J. (1996). The case of Loretta: A psychiatric inpatient. In B. A. Farber, D. C. Brink, & P. M. Raskin, *The psychotherapy of Carl Rogers: Cases and commentary* (pp. 33–56). New York: Guilford.

This is one of the few verbatim recordings of a therapy interview with a psychotic patient, and it provides a concrete example of the application of client-centered therapy to a psychiatric inpatient diagnosed as paranoid schizophrenic. The interview shows a deeply disturbed individual responding positively to the therapist-offered conditions of empathy, congruence, and unconditional positive regard. It is especially dramatic because another patient can be heard screaming in the background while the interview is taking place.

Rogers, C. R. (1942). The case of Herbert Bryan. In C. R. Rogers, *Counseling and psychotherapy* (pp. 261–437). Boston: Houghton Mifflin.

This may be the first publication of a completely recorded and transcribed case of individual psychotherapy that illustrates the new nondirective approach. After each interview, Rogers provides a summary of the client's feelings and additional commentary.

Rogers, C. R. (1961). The case of Mrs. Oak. In C. Rogers, *On becoming a person.* Boston: Houghton Mifflin.

This classic case study documents a client's personal growth during a series of therapy sessions with Carl Rogers.

Rogers, C. R. (1967). A silent young man. In C. R. Rogers, G. T. Gendlin, D. V. Kiesler, & C. Truax (Eds.), *The therapeutic relationship and its impact: A study of psychotherapy with schizophrenics* (pp. 401–406). Madison: University of Wisconsin Press.

This case study consists of two transcribed interviews that were conducted by Rogers as part of a year-long treatment of a very withdrawn hospitalized schizophrenic patient who was part of a client-centered research project on client-centered therapy with a schizophrenic population.

REFERENCES

American Psychological Association Division of Humanistic Psychology. Recommended Principles and Practices For The Provision of Humanistic Psychosocial Services: Alternative To Mandated Practice and Treatment Guidelines [Web posting]. Retrieved from http://www.apa.org/divisions/div32/draft.html.

Ansbacher, H. L. (1977). Individual psychology. In R. J. Corsini (Ed.), *Current psychotherapies.* Itasca, IL: F. E. Peacock.

Asay, T. P., & Lambert, M. J. (1999). The empirical case for the common factors in therapy: Quantitative findings. In M. A. Hubble, B. L. Duncan, & S. D. Miller (Eds.), *The heart and soul of change: What works in therapy* (pp. 23–55). Washington, DC: American Psychological Association.

Axline, V. M. (1947). *Play therapy.* Boston: Houghton Mifflin.

Baldwin, M. (1987). Interview with Carl Rogers on the use of the self in therapy. In M. Baldwin & V. Satir (Eds.), *The use of self* (pp. 45–52). New York: The Haworth Press.

Barrett-Lennard, G. T. (1962). Dimensions of therapist response as causal factors in therapeutic change. *Psychological Monographs, 76,* 1–33.

Bergin, A. E., & Garfield, S. L. (Eds.). (1971). *Handbook of psychotherapy and behavior change: An empirical analysis.* New York: Wiley.

Bohart, A. C. (2002). A passionate critique of empirically supported treatments and the provision of an alternative paradigm. In J. C. Watson, R. N. Goldman, & M. S. Warner (Eds.), *Client-centered and experiential psychotherapy in the 21st century: Advances in theory, research and practice* (pp. 258–277). Ross-on-Wye, UK: PCCS Books.

Bohart, A. C. (2004). *How do clients make empathy work? Person-Centered and Experiential Psychotherapies, 3*(2), 102–116.

Bohart, A. C. (2006). The active client. In J. C. Norcross, L. E. Beutler, & R. F. Levant (Eds.). *Evidence-based practices in mental health: Debate and dialogue on the fundamental questions* (pp. 218–226). Washington, DC: American Psychological Association.

Bohart, A. C., Elliott, R., Greenberg, L. S., & Watson, J. C. (2002). Empathy. In J. C. Norcross (Ed.), *Psychotherapy relationships that work: Therapist contributions and responsiveness to patients* (pp. 89–108). New York: Oxford University Press.

Bohart, A. C., & Tallman, K. (1999). *How clients make therapy work: The process of active self-healing.* Washington, DC: American Psychological Association.

Bozarth, J. D. (1998). *Client-centered therapy: A revolutionary paradigm.* Ross-on-Wye, UK: PCCS Books.

Bozarth, J. D. (2002). Empirically supported treatment: Epitome of the "specificity myth." In J. C. Watson, R. N. Goldman, & M. S. Warner (Eds.), *Client-centered and experiential psychotherapy in the 21st century: Advances in theory, research and practice* (pp. 168–181). Ross-on-Wye, UK: PCCS Books.

Brodley, B. T. (1974). *Ethics in psychotherapy.* Unpublished paper.

Brodley, B. T. (1994). Some observations of Carl Rogers's behavior in therapy interviews. *Person-Centered Journal, 1*(2), 37–47.

Brodley, B. T. (1997). The nondirective attitude in client-centered therapy. *Person-Centered Journal, 4*(1), 18–30.

Brodley, B. T. (1999a). Reasons for responses expressing the therapist's frame of reference in client-centered therapy. *Person-Centered Journal, 6*(1), 4–27.

Brodley, B. T. (1999b). A client-centered demonstration in Hungary. In I. Fairhurst, *Women writing in the person-centered approach* (pp. 85–92). Ross-on-Wye, UK: PCCS Books.

Brodley, B. T. (1999c). The actualizing concept in client-centered theory. *Person-Centered Journal, 6,* 108–120.

Brodley, B. T. (2000). Client-centered: An expressive therapy. In J. Marques-Teixeira & S. Antunes (Eds.), *Client centered and experiential psychotherapy* (pp. 133–147). Linda a Velha, Portugal: Vale & Vale.

Brodley, B. T. (2001). Congruence and its relation to communication in client-centered therapy. In G. Wyatt (Ed.), *Rogers' therapeutic conditions: Evolution, theory and practice, Vol. I, Congruence* (pp. 55–78). Ross-on-Wye, UK: PCCS Books.

Butler, J. M., & Haigh, G. V. (1954). Changes in the relation between self-concepts and ideal concepts consequent upon client-centered counseling. In C. R. Rogers & R. F. Dymond (Eds.), *Psychotherapy and personality change* (pp. 55–75). Chicago: University of Chicago Press.

Cartwright, D. S. (1957). Annotated bibliography of research and theory construction in client-centered therapy. *Journal of Counseling Psychology, 4,* 82–100.

Deci, E. L., & Ryan, R. M. (1985). *Intrinsic motivation and self-determination in human behavior.* New York: Plenum.

Deci, E. L., & Ryan, R. M. (1991). A motivational approach to self: Integration in personality. In R. Dienstbier (Ed.), *Nebraska Symposium on Motivation: Perspectives on Motivation, 38,* 237–288. Lincoln: University of Nebraska Press.

Eckert, J., Hoger, D., & Schwab, R. (2003). Development and current state of the research on client-centered therapy in the German-language region. *Person-Centered and Experiential Psychotherapies, 2*(2), 3–18.

Ellinwood, C. G., & Raskin, N. J. (1993). Client centered/humanistic psychotherapy. In T. R. Kratochwill & R. J. Morris (Eds.), *Handbook of psychotherapy with children and adolescents* (pp. 258–287). Boston: Allyn & Bacon.

Elliott, R. (1996). Are client-centered/experiential therapies effective? A meta-analysis of outcome research. In U. Esser, H. Pabst, & G. W. Speierer (Eds.), *The power of the person-centered approach* (pp. 125–138). Koln, Germany: GwG Verlag.

Elliott, R. (1998). Editor's introduction: A guide to the empirically supported treatments controversy. *Psychotherapy Research, 8*(2), 115–125.

Elliott, R. (2002). The effectiveness of humanistic therapies: A meta-analysis. In D. J. Cain & J. Seeman (Eds.), *Humanistic psychotherapies: Handbook of research and practice* (pp. 57–81). Washington, DC: American Psychological Association.

Elliott, R. & Freire, E. (2008). Person-centred and experiential therapies are highly effective: Summary of the 2008 meta-analysis. *Person-Centred Quarterly,* Nov., 1–3.

Elliot, R., Greenberg, L. S., & Lietaer, G. (2004). Research on experiential psychotherapies. In M. J. Lambert (Ed.), *Bergin and Garfield's handbook of psychotherapy and behavior change* (5th ed., pp. 493–539). New York: Wiley.

Fairhurst, I. (Ed.). (1999). *Women writing in the person-centered approach.* Ross-on-Wye, UK: PCCS Books.

Farber, B. A., & Lane, J. S. (2002). Positive regard. In J. C. Norcross (Ed.), *Psychotherapy relationships that work: Therapist contributions and responsiveness to patients* (pp. 175–194). New York: Oxford University Press.

Gendlin, E. T. (1961). Experiencing: A variable in the process of therapeutic change. *American Journal of Psychotherapy, 15,* 233–245.

Goldstein, K. (1934/1959). *The organism: A holistic approach to biology derived from psychological data in man.* New York: American Book. (Originally published in 1934.)

Grant, B. (1995). Perfecting the therapeutic attitudes: Client-centered therapy as a spiritual discipline. *Person-Centered Journal, 2*(2), 72–77.

Greenberg, L. S., & Watson, J. (1998). Experiential therapy of depression: Differential effects of client-centered relationship conditions and process experiential interventions. *Psychotherapy Research, 8*(2), 210–224.

Holdstock, T. L., & Rogers, C. R. (1983). Person-centered theory. In R. J. Corsini & A. J. Marsella (Eds.), *Personality theories, research and assessment.* Itasca, IL: F. E. Peacock.

Kirschenbaum, H., & Henderson, V. L. (Eds.). (1989). *The Carl Rogers reader.* Boston: Houghton Mifflin.

Kirschenbaum, H., & Jourdan, A. (2005). The current status of Carl Rogers and the Person-Centered Approach. *Psychotherapy: Theory, Research, Practice, Training, 42*(1), 37–51.

Kitwood, T. (1990). Psychotherapy, postmodernism and morality. *Journal of Moral Education, 19*(1), 3–13.

Lambert, M. J. (Ed.). (2004). *Bergin and Garfield's handbook of psychotherapy and behavior change* (5th ed.). New York: Wiley.

Levitt, B. E. (Ed.). (2005). *Embracing non-directivity: Reassessing person-centered theory and practice in the 21st century.* Ross-on-Wye, UK: PCCS Books.

Luborsky, L., Singer, B., & Luborsky, L. (1975). Comparative studies of psychotherapies: Is it true that "everyone has won and all must have prizes"? *Archives of General Psychiatry, 32,* 995–1008.

Maslow, A. H. (1968). *Toward a psychology of being* (2nd ed.). Princeton, NJ: Van Nostrand.

Matson, F. W. (1969). Whatever became of the Third Force? *American Association of Humanistic Psychology Newsletter, 6*(1), 1, 14–15.

McGaw, W. H., Farson, R. E., & Rogers, C. R. (Producers). (1968). *Journey into self* [Film]. Berkeley: University of California Extension Media Center.

Meador, B. D., & Rogers, C. R. (1984). Client-centered therapy. In R. J. Corsini (Ed.), *Current psychotherapies* (3rd ed., pp. 142–195). Itasca, IL: F. E. Peacock.

Mearns, D. (2003). Problem-centered is not person-centered. *Person-Centered and Experiential Psychotherapies, 3*(2), 88–101.

Mearns, D., & McLeod, J. (1984). A person-centered approach to research. In R. F. Levant & J. M. Shlien (Eds.), *Client-centered therapy and the person-centered approach: New directions in theory, research, and practice* (pp. 370–389). New York: Praeger.

Mier, S., & Witty, M. (2004). Considerations of race and culture in the practice of non-directive client-centered therapy. In R. Moodley, C. Lago, & A. Talahite (Eds.), *Carl Rogers counsels a Black client* (pp. 85–104). Ross-on-Wye, UK: PCCS Books.

Moodley, R., Lago, C., & Talahite, A. (2004). *Carl Rogers counsels a Black client.* Ross-on-Wye, UK: PCCS Books.

Moon, K. (2002). Nondirective client-centered work with children. In J. C. Watson, R. N. Goldman, & M. S. Warner (Eds.), *Client-centered and experiential psychotherapy in the 21st century: Advances in theory, research and practice* (pp. 485–492), Ross-on-Wye, UK: PCCS Books.

Natiello, P. (1994). The collaborative relationship in psychotherapy. *The Person-Centered Journal, 1*(2), 11–17.

Natiello, P. (2001). *The person-centered approach: A passionate presence.* Ross-on-Wye, UK: PCCS Books.

Norcross, J. C., Beutler, L. E., & Levant, R. F. (Eds.). (2006). *Evidence-based practices in mental health: Debate and dialogue on the fundamental questions.* Washington DC: American Psychological Association.

Orlinsky, D. E., & Howard, K. L. (1978). The relation of process to outcome in psychotherapy. In S. L. Garfield & A. E. Bergin (Eds.), *Handbook of psychotherapy and behavior change: An empirical analysis* (2nd ed., pp. 283–329). New York: Wiley.

Orlinsky, D. E., & Howard, K. L. (1986). A generic model of psychotherapy. *Journal of Integrative and Eclectic Psychotherapy, 6,* 6–28.

Orlinsky, D. E., Grawe, K., & Parks, B. K. (1994). Process and outcome in psychotherapy: *Noch einmal.* In S. L. Garfield & A. E. Bergin (Eds.), *Handbook of psychotherapy and behavior change* (4th ed., pp. 270–376). New York: Wiley.

Patterson, C. H. (1984). Empathy, warmth, and genuineness in psychotherapy: A review of reviews. *Psychotherapy, 21,* 431–438.

Patterson, C. H. (1996). Multicultural counseling: From diversity to universality. *Journal of Counseling and Development, January/February, 74.*

Porter, E. H., Jr. (1943). The development and evaluation of a measure of counseling interview procedures. *Educational and Psychological Measurement, 3,* 105–126, 215–238.

Proctor, G., & Napier, M. (2004). *Encountering feminism: Intersections between feminism and the person-centered approach.* Ross-on-Wye, UK: PCCS Books.

Prouty, G. (1994). *Theoretical evolutions in person-centered/ experiential therapy: Applications to schizophrenic and retarded psychoses.* Westport, CT: Praeger.

Raimy, V. C. (1948). Self-reference in counseling interviews. *Journal of Consulting Psychology, 12,* 153–163.

Rank, O. (1945). *Will therapy, truth and reality.* New York: Knopf.

Raskin, N. J. (1947). *The nondirective attitude.* Unpublished paper.

Raskin, N. J. (1948). The development of nondirective therapy. *Journal of Consulting Psychology, 12,* 92–110.

Raskin, N. J. (1952). An objective study of the locus-of-evaluation factor in psychotherapy. In W. Wolfe & J. A. Precker (Eds.), *Success in psychotherapy* (pp. 143–162). New York: Grune & Stratton.

Raskin, N. J. (1974). *Studies of psychotherapeutic orientation: Ideology and practice.* Research Monograph No. 1. Orlando, FL: American Academy of Psychotherapists.

Raskin, N. J. (1996). Person-centered psychotherapy: Twenty historical steps. In W. Dryden (Ed.), *Developments in psychotherapy: Historical perspectives.* London: Sage Publications.

Raskin, N. J. (2005). The nondirective attitude. *Person-Centered Journal, 12*(1–2), 5–22.

Raskin, N. J., & Zucconi, A. (1984). *Peace, conflict resolution, and the person-centered approach.* Program presented at the annual convention of the American Psychological Association, Toronto.

Rogers, C. R. (1931). *Measuring personality adjustment in children nine to thirteen.* New York: Teachers College, Columbia University, Bureau of Publications.

Rogers, C. R. (1939). *The clinical treatment of the problem child.* Boston: Houghton Mifflin.

Rogers, C. R. (1940). The process of therapy. *Journal of Consulting Psychology, 4,* 161–164.

Rogers, C. R. (1942). *Counseling and psychotherapy.* Boston: Houghton Mifflin.

Rogers, C. R. (1951). *Client-centered therapy.* Boston: Houghton Mifflin.

Rogers, C. R. (1957). The necessary and sufficient conditions of therapeutic personality change. *Journal of Consulting Psychology, 21,* 95–103.

Rogers, C. R. (1959a). The essence of psychotherapy: A client-centered view. *Annals of Psychotherapy, 1,* 51–57.

Rogers, C. R. (1959b). A theory of therapy, personality and interpersonal relationships as developed in the client-centered framework. In S. Koch (Ed.), *Psychology: A study of science, Vol. 3. Formulations of the person and the social context* (pp. 184–256). New York: McGraw-Hill.

Rogers, C. R. (1977). *Carl Rogers on personal power.* New York: Delacorte Press.

Rogers, C. R. (1980). *A way of being.* Boston: Houghton Mifflin.

Rogers, C. R. (1983). *Freedom to learn for the 80s.* Columbus, OH: Charles E. Merrill.

Rogers, C. R. (1986a). Client-centered therapy. In I. L. Kutash & A. Wolf (Eds.), *Psychotherapist's casebook: Therapy and technique in practice* (pp. 197–208). San Francisco: Jossey-Bass.

Rogers, C. R. (1986b). The dilemmas of a South African white. *Person-Centered Review, 1,* 15–35.

Rogers, C. R. (1986d). The Rust workshop: A personal overview. *Journal of Humanistic Psychology, 26,* 23–45.

Rogers, C. R. (1987). Inside the world of the Soviet professional. *Journal of Humanistic Psychology, 27,* 277–304.

Rogers, C. R., & Dymond, R. F. (Eds.). (1954). *Psychotherapy and personality change.* Chicago: University of Chicago Press.

Rogers, C. R., Gendlin, G. T., Kiesler, D. V., & Truax, C. (Eds.). (1967). *The therapeutic relationship and its impact: A study of psychotherapy with schizophrenics.* Madison: University of Wisconsin Press.

Rogers, C. R., & Haigh, G. (1983). I walk softly through life. *Voices: The Art and Science of Psychotherapy, 18,* 6–14.

Rogers, C. R., & Ryback, D. (1984). One alternative to nuclear planetary suicide. In R. F. Levant & J. M. Shlien (Eds.), *Client-centered therapy and the person-centered approach: New directions in theory, research, and practice* (pp. 400–422). New York: Praeger.

Rogers, C. R., & Sanford, R. C. (1985). Client-centered psychotherapy. In H. I. Kaplan, B. J. Sadock, & A. M. Friedman (Eds.), *Comprehensive textbook of psychiatry* (4th ed., pp. 1374–1388). Baltimore: William & Wilkins.

Rosenberg, M. B. (1999). *Non-violent communication: A language of compassion.* Del Mar, CA: Puddledancer Press.

Rosenzweig, S. (1936). Some implicit common factors in diverse methods of psychotherapy. *American Journal of Orthopsychiatry, 6,* 412–415.

Ryan, R. M., & Deci, E. L. (2000). Self-determination theory and the facilitation of intrinsic motivation, social development, and well-being. *American Psychologist, 55*(1), 68–78.

Schmid, P. F. (2003). The characteristics of a person-centered approach to therapy and counseling: Criteria for identity and coherence. *Person-Centered and Experiential Psychotherapies, 2*(2), 104–120.

Seeman, J. (1959). Toward a concept of personality integration. *American Psychologist, 14,* 794–797.

Seeman, J. (1984). The fully functioning person: Theory and research. In R. F. Levant & J. M. Shlien (Eds.), *Client-centered therapy and the person-centered approach: New directions in theory, research, and practice* (pp. 131–152). New York: Praeger.

Sheerer, E. T. (1949). An analysis of the relationship between acceptance of and respect for others in ten counseling cases. *Journal of Consulting Psychology, 13,* 169–175.

Shlien, J. M. (1964). Comparison of results with different forms of psychotherapy. *American Journal of Psychotherapy, 28,* 15–22.

Smith, M. L., & Glass, G. V. (1977). Meta-analysis of psychotherapy outcome studies. *American Psychologist, 32,* 752–760.

Sommerbeck, L. (2003). *The client-centered therapist in psychiatric contexts: A therapist's guide to the psychiatric landscape and its inhabitants.* Ross-on-Wye, UK: PCCS Books.

Standal, S. (1954). *The need for positive regard: A contribution to client-centered theory.* Unpublished Ph.D. dissertation, University of Chicago.

Stephenson, W. V. (1953). *The study of behavior.* Chicago: University of Chicago Press.

Truax, C. B., & Mitchell, K. M. (1971). Research on certain therapist interpersonal skills in relation to process and outcome. In A. E. Bergin & S. L. Garfield (Eds.), *Handbook of psychotherapy and behavior change: An empirical analysis* (pp. 299–344). New York: Wiley.

Wampold, B. E. (2001). *The great psychotherapy debate: Models, methods, and findings.* Mahwah, NJ: Lawrence Erlbaum Associates.

Wampold, B. E. (2006). Not a scintilla of evidence to support empirically supported treatments as more effective than other treatments. In J. C. Norcross, L. E. Beutler, & R. F. Levant (Eds.), *Evidence-based practices in mental health: Debate and dialogue on the fundamental questions* (pp. 299–307). Washington, DC: American Psychological Association.

Watson, N. (1984). The empirical status of Rogers's hypotheses of the necessary and sufficient conditions for effective psychotherapy. In R. F. Levant & J. M. Shlien (Eds), *Client-centered therapy and the person-centered approach: New directions in theory, research, and practice* (pp. 17–40). New York: Praeger.

Westen, D., Novotny, C. M., & Thompson-Brenner, H. (2004). The empirical status of empirically supported psychotherapies: Assumptions, findings, and reporting in controlled clinical trials. *Psychological Bulletin, 130*(4), 631–663.

Witty, M. C. (2004). The difference directiveness makes: The ethics and consequences of guidance in psychotherapy. *The Person-Centered Journal, 11,* 22–32.

Wolter-Gustafson, C. (2004). Towards convergence: Client-centered and feminist assumptions about epistemology and power. In G. Proctor & M. B. Napier (Eds.), *Encountering feminism: Intersections between feminism and the person-centered approach* (pp. 97–115), Ross-on-Wye, UK: PCCS Books.

Zimring, F. M. (1995). A new explanation for the beneficial results of client-centered therapy: The possibility of a new paradigm. *Person-Centered Journal, 2*(2), 36–48.

Zimring, F. M. (2000). Empathic understanding grows the person. *Person-Centered Journal, 7*(2), 101–113.

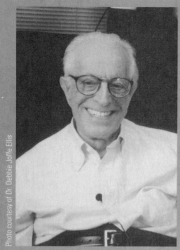

Photo courtesy of Dr. Debbie Joffe Ellis

Albert Ellis (1913–2007)

6 | RATIONAL EMOTIVE BEHAVIOR THERAPY

Albert Ellis[1]

OVERVIEW

Rational emotive behavior therapy (REBT), a theory of personality and a method of psychotherapy developed in the 1950s by clinical psychologist Albert Ellis, holds that when a highly charged emotional consequence (C) follows a significant activating event (A), event A may seem to, but actually does not, cause C. Instead, emotional consequences are largely created by B—the individual's *belief system.* When an undesirable emotional consequence occurs, such as severe anxiety, this usually involves the person's irrational beliefs, and when these beliefs are effectively disputed (at point D), by challenging them rationally and behaviorally, the disturbed consequences are reduced. From its inception, REBT has viewed cognition and emotion integratively, with thought, feeling, desires, and action interacting with each other. It is therefore a comprehensive cognitive–affective–behavioral theory and practice of psychotherapy (Ellis, 1962, 1994; Ellis & Dryden, 1997; Ellis & MacLaren, 1998).

[1] Albert Ellis worked on revising this chapter during the last months before his death. The changes to the chapter were finalized and approved by his wife, Debbie Joffe Ellis. This chapter represents the culmination of a lifetime spent practicing, writing about, and thinking about how to help people change self-defeating thoughts and behaviors so that they could create lives with less emotional suffering and experience greater joy. DW

Formerly known as rational emotive therapy (RET), this approach is more accurately referred to as rational emotive behavior therapy (REBT). From the beginning, REBT considered the importance of both mind and body or of thinking/feeling/wanting (contents of the mind according to psychology) and of behavior (the operations of the body). It has stressed that personality change can occur in both directions: therapists can talk with people and attempt to change their minds so that they will behave differently, or they can help clients to change their behaviors and thus modify their thinking. As stated in several early writings on REBT that are reprinted in *The Albert Ellis Reader* (Ellis & Blau, 1998), REBT theory states that humans rarely change a profound self-defeating belief unless they act against it. Thus, it is most accurately called rational emotive behavior therapy.

Basic Concepts

The main propositions of REBT can be described as follows:

1. *People are born with a potential to be rational (self-constructive) as well as irrational (self-defeating).* They have predispositions to be self-preserving, to think about their thinking, to be creative, to be sensuous, to be interested in other people, to learn from their mistakes, and to actualize their potential for life and growth. They also tend to be self-destructive, to be short-range hedonists, to avoid thinking things through, to procrastinate, to repeat the same mistakes, to be superstitious, to be intolerant, to be perfectionistic and grandiose, and to avoid actualizing their potential for growth.

2. *People's tendency to irrational thinking, self-damaging habituations, wishful thinking, and intolerance is frequently exacerbated by their culture and their family group.* Their suggestibility (or conditionability) is greatest during their early years because they are dependent on, and highly influenced by, family and social pressures.

3. *Humans perceive, think, emote, and behave simultaneously.* They are, therefore, at one and the same time cognitive, conative (purposive), and motoric. They rarely act without implicit thinking. Their sensations and actions are viewed in a framework of prior experiences, memories, and conclusions. People seldom emote without thinking because their feelings include and are usually triggered by an appraisal of a given situation and its importance. People rarely act without simultaneously perceiving, thinking, and emoting because these processes provide reasons for acting. For this reason, it is usually desirable to use a variety of perceptual–cognitive, emotive–evocative, and behavioralistic–reeducative methods (Bernard & Wolfe, 1993; Ellis, 1962, 1994, 2001a, 2001b, 2002, 2003a; Walen, DiGiuseppe, & Dryden, 1992).

4. *Even though all the major psychotherapies employ a variety of cognitive, emotive, and behavioral techniques, and even though all (including unscientific methods such as witch doctoring) may help individuals who have faith in them, they are probably not all equally effective or efficient.* Highly cognitive, active–directive, homework-assigning, and discipline-oriented therapies such as REBT are likely to be more effective, usually in briefer periods and with fewer sessions.

5. *REBT emphasizes the philosophy of unconditional acceptance: specifically unconditional self-acceptance (USA), unconditional other acceptance (UOA), and unconditional life acceptance (ULA).* This is explained in *The Myth of Self-Esteem* (Ellis, 2005). The humanistic principle of unconditional acceptance holds this assumption regarding human worth: I exist, I deserve to exist, I am a fallible human and I can choose to accept myself unconditionally with my flaws and mistakes, with or without great achievements—simply because I am alive, simply because I exist. It says that conditional self-esteem is one of the greatest of all human disturbances, as it leads to people praising themselves when they do well and are approved by others and damning themselves if they don't do well and

others disapprove of them. Rating traits and behaviors can be beneficial, as it allows one to learn from mistakes and to improve and grow, but to overgeneralize and rate one's whole worth, being, and totality as "good" or "bad" is inaccurate and harmful. A person's totality is too complex and ephemeral to define and measure. Hence, USA, not self-esteem, is recommended in REBT.

UOA holds that people condemn others' iniquitous thoughts, feelings, and actions but accept the others as fallible humans—just as they are. ULA encourages acceptance of adversities that we neither create nor can change—such as death of loved ones, physical disabilities, hurricanes, and floods.

REBT recognizes that life contains inevitable suffering as well as pleasure and that accepting the unpleasant circumstances that can't be changed can lead to emotional stability, self-actualization, and great fulfillment.

6. *Rational emotive behavior therapists do not believe a warm relationship between client and counselor is a necessary or a sufficient condition for effective personality change, although it is quite desirable.* They stress unconditional acceptance of and close collaboration with clients, but they also actively encourage clients to unconditionally accept themselves with their inevitable fallibility. In addition, therapists may use a variety of practical methods, including didactic discussion, behavior modification, bibliotherapy, audiovisual aids, and activity-oriented homework assignments. To discourage clients from becoming unduly dependent, therapists often use hardheaded methods of convincing them that they had better resort to self-discipline and self-direction.

7. *Rational emotive behavior therapy uses role playing, assertion training, desensitization, humor, operant conditioning, suggestion, support, and a whole bag of other "tricks."* As Arnold Lazarus points out in his "multimodal" therapy, such wide-ranging methods are effective in helping clients achieve deep-seated cognitive change. REBT is not just oriented toward symptom removal, except when it seems that this is the only kind of change likely to be accomplished. It is designed to help people examine and change some of their basic values—particularly those that keep them disturbed. If clients seriously fear failing on the job, REBT does not merely help them give up this particular symptom; it also tries to show them how to minimize their basic "awfulizing" tendencies.

The usual goal of REBT is to help people reduce their underlying symptom-creating propensities. There are two basic forms of rational emotive behavior therapy: general REBT, which is almost synonymous with cognitive–behavior therapy, and preferential REBT, which includes general REBT but also emphasizes a profound philosophical change. General REBT tends to teach clients rational or healthful behaviors. Preferential REBT teaches them how to dispute irrational ideas and unhealthful behaviors and to become more creative, scientific, and skeptical thinkers.

8. *REBT holds that most neurotic problems involve unrealistic, illogical, self-defeating thinking and that if disturbance-creating ideas are vigorously disputed by logico-empirical and pragmatic thinking, they can be minimized.* No matter how defective people's heredity may be, and no matter what trauma they may have experienced, the main reason why they usually now overreact or underreact to adversities (at point A) is that they *now* have some dogmatic, irrational, unexamined beliefs (at point B). Because these beliefs are unrealistic, they will not withstand rational scrutiny. They are often deifications and devilifications of themselves and others, and they tend to wane when empirically checked, logically disputed, and shown to be impractical. Thus, a woman with severe emotional difficulties does not merely believe it is undesirable if her lover rejects her. She tends to believe, also, that (a) it is awful; (b) she cannot stand it; (c) she should not, *must* not be rejected; (d) she will never be accepted by a desirable partner; (e) she is a worthless person because one lover has rejected her; and (f) she deserves to be rejected for being so worthless. Such common covert hypotheses are illogical, unrealistic, and destructive. They can

be revealed and disputed by a rational emotive behavior therapist who shows clients how to think more flexibly and scientifically, and the rational emotive therapist is partly that: an exposing and skeptical scientist.

9. *REBT shows how activating events or adversities (A) in people's lives contribute to but do not directly cause emotional consequences (C); these consequences stem from people's interpretations of the activating events or adversities—that is, from their unrealistic and overgeneralized beliefs (B) about those events.* The "real" cause of upsets, therefore, lies mainly in people, not in what happens to them (even though gruesome experiences obviously have considerable influence over what people think and feel). REBT provides clients with several powerful insights. Insight number one is that a person's self-defeating behavior usually follows from the interaction of A (adversity) and B (belief about A). Disturbed consequences (C) therefore usually follow the formula A–B–C.

Insight number two is the understanding that although people have become emotionally disturbed (or have *made* themselves disturbed) in the past, they are *now* upset because they keep indoctrinating themselves with similar constructed beliefs. These beliefs do not continue because people were once "conditioned" and so now hold them "automatically." No! People still, here and now, actively reinforce them, and their present active self-propagandizations and constructions keep those constructed beliefs alive. Unless people fully admit and face their own responsibilities for the continuation of their dysfunctional beliefs, it is unlikely that they will be able to uproot them.

Insight number three acknowledges that *only hard work and practice* will correct irrational beliefs—and keep them corrected. Insights 1 and 2 are not enough! Commitment to repeated rethinking of irrational beliefs and repeated actions designed to undo them will likely extinguish or minimize them.

10. *Historically, psychology was considered an S–R science, where S means "stimulus" and R means "response."* Later, it became evident that similar stimuli produce different responses in different people. This was presumed to mean that something between the S and the R is responsible for such variations.

An analogy may be helpful. If you hit the same billiard ball from the same spot with exactly the same force and let it bounce off the side of the billiard table, that ball will always come back to exactly the same spot. Otherwise, no one would play billiards. Therefore, hitting the billiard ball is the S (stimulus) and the movement of the ball is the R (response). However, suppose there were a tiny person inside a billiard ball who could control, to some degree, the direction and velocity of the ball after it was hit. Then the ball could move to different locations because the tiny person inside could guide it to a certain extent.

An analogous concept was introduced into psychology in the late 1800s by James McKeen Cattell, an American psychologist studying with Wilhelm Wundt in Leipzig, Germany. In so doing, he launched an entirely different kind of psychology known as *idiographic psychology,* in contrast to the *nomothetic psychology* that Wundt and his students were working on. Wundt and his followers were looking for average behavior, or S–R behavior, and were discounting individual variations. The truth was, according to them, the average. Cattell disagreed, and he introduced a psychology that acknowledged the importance of recognizing *individual differences.* As a result, the S–R concept changed to S–O–R. The O stood for "organism," but what it really meant was that the ball (or the person) had a mind of its own and that it did not go precisely where a ball with no mind of its own would go, because O had some degree of independence.

REBT includes precisely the same concept. RE represents the contents of the mind: rationality and emotions. REBT therapists attempt to change people's thinking and feelings (let's call the combination the *philosophy* of a person), with the goal of enabling them to change their behavior via a new understanding (rationality) and a new set of feelings (emotions) about self and others. By showing their clients how to combine thinking and feeling, REBT therapists have given the little man in the billiard ball the ability to change directions. When the ball is hit (confronted with particular stimuli) again, it no longer goes where it used to go.

In REBT, we want to empower individuals, by changing their thinking and feelings, to act differently—in a manner desired by the client, by the therapist, and by society. At the same time, REBT encourages people to act differently—this is where the B (for "behavior") comes in—and thereby to think and feel differently. The interaction goes both ways! Thinking, feeling, and behaving seem to be separate human processes, but as Ellis said in his first paper on REBT in 1956, they actually go together holistically and inevitably influence each other. When you think, you feel and act; when you feel, you think and act; and when you act, you think and feel. That is why REBT uses many cognitive, emotive, and behavioral methods to help clients change their disturbances.

Other Systems

REBT differs from psychoanalytic schools of psychotherapy by eschewing free association, compulsive gathering of material about the client's history, and most dream analysis. It is not concerned with the presumed sexual origins of disturbance or with the Oedipus complex. When transference does occur in therapy, the rational therapist is likely to attack it, showing clients that transference phenomena tend to arise from the irrational belief that they must be loved by the therapist (and others). Although REBT practitioners are much closer to modern neoanalytic schools, such as those of Karen Horney, Erich Fromm, Harry Stack Sullivan, and Franz Alexander, than to the Freudian school, they employ considerably more persuasion, philosophical analysis, homework activity assignments, and other directive techniques than practitioners of these schools.

REBT overlaps significantly with Adlerian theory, but it departs from the Adlerian practices of stressing early childhood memories and insisting that social interest is the heart of therapeutic effectiveness. REBT is more specific than Adler's Individual Psychology in disclosing, analyzing, and disputing clients' concrete internalized beliefs and is closer in this respect to general semantic theory and philosophical analysis than to Individual Psychology. It is also much more behavioral than Adlerian therapy.

Adler (1931, 1964) contended that people have basic fictional premises and goals and that they generally proceed quite logically on the basis of these false hypotheses. REBT, on the other hand, holds that people, when disturbed, may have both irrational premises and illogical deductions from these premises. Thus, in Individual Psychology, a male who has the unrealistic premise that he *should* be the king of the universe but actually has only mediocre abilities is shown that he is "logically" concluding that he is an utterly inferior person. But in REBT this same individual, with the same irrational premise, is shown that in addition to his "logical" deduction, he may be making several other illogical conclusions. For example, he may be concluding that (1) he should be king of the universe because he was once king of his own family; (2) his parents will be impressed by him only if he is outstandingly achieving and *therefore* he must achieve outstandingly; (3) if he cannot be king of the universe, he might as well do nothing and get nowhere in life; and (4) he deserves to suffer for not being the noble king that he should be.

REBT has much in common with parts of the Jungian therapeutic outlook, especially in that it views clients holistically, holds that the goals of therapy include growth and achievement of potential as well as relief of disturbed symptoms, and emphasizes enlightened individuality. However, REBT deviates radically from Jungian treatment because Jungians are preoccupied with dreams, fantasies, symbol productions, and the mythological or archetypal contents of their clients' thinking—most of which the REBT practitioner deems a waste of time.

REBT is in close agreement with person-centered or relationship therapy in some ways: they both emphasize what Carl Rogers (1961) calls *unconditional positive regard* and what in rational emotive psychology is called *full acceptance, unconditional acceptance,* or *tolerance.* Rational therapists differ from Rogerian therapists in that they actively *teach* (1) that blaming is the core of much emotional disturbance; (2) that it leads to dreadful results; (3) that it is possible, though difficult, for humans to learn to avoid rating themselves even while continuing to rate their performances; and (4) that they can give up self-rating by challenging their grandiose (*must*urbatory), self-evaluating assumptions and by deliberately risking (through homework activity assignments) possible failures and rejections. The REBT practitioner is more active–directive and more emotive–evocative than the person-centered practitioner (Ellis, 1962, 2001a, 2001b; Hauck, 1992).

REBT is in many respects an existential, phenomenologically oriented therapy because its goals overlap with the usual existentialist goals of helping clients to define their own freedom, cultivate individuality, live in dialogue with others, accept their experiencing as highly important, be fully present in the immediacy of the moment, and learn to accept limits in life (Ellis, 2001b, 2002). Many who call themselves existential therapists, however, are rather anti-intellectual, prejudiced against the technology of therapy, and confusingly nondirective, whereas REBT makes much use of incisive logical analysis, clear-cut techniques (including behavior modification procedures), and directiveness and teaching by the therapist.

REBT has much in common with behavior modification. Many behavior therapists, however, are mainly concerned with symptom removal and ignore the cognitive aspects of conditioning and deconditioning. REBT is therefore closer to cognitive and multimodal modifiers such as Aaron Beck, Arnold Lazarus, and Donald Meichenbaum.

HISTORY

Precursors

The philosophical origins of rational emotive behavior therapy go back to some of the Asian philosophers, such as Confucius, Lao-Tsu, and Buddha, and especially to Epicurus and the Stoic philosophers Epictetus and Marcus Aurelius. Although most early Stoic writings have been lost, their essence has come down to us through Epictetus, who in the 1st century AD wrote in *The Enchiridion,* "People are disturbed not by things, but by the view which they take of them."

The modern psychotherapist who was the main precursor of REBT was Alfred Adler. "I am convinced," he stated, "that *a person's behavior springs from his ideas*" (1964, italics in original). According to Adler (1964),

> The individual . . . does not relate himself to the outside world in a predetermined manner, as is often assumed. He relates himself always according to his own interpretation of himself and of his present problem. . . . It is his attitude toward life which determines his relationship to the outside world.

Adler (1931) put the A–B–C or S–O–R (stimulus–organism–response) theory of human disturbance neatly: No experience is a cause of success or failure. We do not suffer from the shock of our experiences—the so-called *trauma*—but we make out of them just what suits our purposes. We are self-determined by the meaning we give to our experiences, and it is almost a mistake to view particular experiences as the basis of our future life. Meanings are not determined by situations, but we determine ourselves by the meanings we give to situations. In his first book on Individual Psychology, Adler's motto was *Omnia ex opinione suspensa sunt* ("Everything depends on opinion").

Another important precursor of REBT was Paul DuBois, who used persuasive forms of psychotherapy. Alexander Herzberg was one of the inventors of homework assignments. Hippolyte Bernheim, Andrew Salter, and a host of other therapists have employed hypnosis and suggestion in a highly active–directive manner. Frederick Thorne created what he called directive therapy. Franz Alexander, Thomas French, John Dollard, Neal Miller, Wilhelm Stekel, and Lewis Wolberg all practiced forms of psychoanalytic psychotherapy that diverged so far from the Freudian therapy that they resemble active–directive therapy more closely and are in many ways precursors of REBT.

In addition, a large number of individuals during the 1950s, when REBT was first being formulated, independently began to arrive at some theories and methodologies that significantly overlap with the methods outlined by Ellis (1962). These theorists include Eric Berne, Jerome Frank, George Kelly, Abraham Low, E. Lakin Phillips, Julian Rotter, and Joseph Wolpe.

Beginnings

After practicing psychoanalysis for several years during the late 1940s and early 1950s, Ellis discovered that no matter how much insight his clients gained or how well they seemed to understand events from their early childhood, they rarely lost their symptoms and still retained tendencies to create new ones. He realized that this was because they were not merely indoctrinated with irrational, mistaken ideas of their own worthlessness when they were young, but also *constructed* dysfunctional demands on themselves and others and kept *reindoctrinating* themselves with these commands (Ellis, 1962, 2001b, 2002, 2003a, 2004a; Ellis & MacLaren, 1998).

Ellis also discovered that as he pressed his clients to surrender their basic irrational premises, they often tended to resist giving up these ideas. This was not, as the Freudians hypothesized, because they hated the therapist or wanted to destroy themselves or were still resisting parent images but because they *naturally,* one might say *normally,* tended to *must*urbate. They insisted (a) that they *must* do well and win others' approval, (b) that other people *must* act considerately and fairly, and (c) that environmental conditions *must* be gratifying and free of frustration. Ellis concluded that humans are *self-talking, self-evaluating,* and *self-construing.* They frequently take strong preferences, such as desires for love, approval, success, and pleasure, and misleadingly *define* them as needs. They thereby create many of their "emotional" difficulties.

People are not exclusively the products of social learning. Their so-called pathological symptoms are the result of *bio*social processes. *Because they are human,* they tend to have strong, irrational, empirically misleading ideas; and as long as they hold on to these ideas, they tend to be what is commonly called "neurotic." These irrational ideologies are not infinitely varied or hard to discover. They can be listed under a few major headings and, once understood, quickly uncovered by REBT analysis.

Ellis also discovered that people's irrational assumptions were so biosocially deep rooted that weak methods were unlikely to budge them. Passive, nondirective methodologies (such as reflection of feeling and free association) rarely changed them. Warmth and support often helped clients live more "happily" with unrealistic notions. Suggestion or "positive thinking" sometimes enabled them to cover up and live more "successfully" with underlying negative self-evaluations. Abreaction and catharsis frequently helped them to feel better but tended to reinforce rather than eliminate their demands. Classic desensitizing sometimes relieved clients of anxieties and phobias but did not undermine their anxiety-arousing, phobia-creating fundamental meanings and philosophies.

What *did* work effectively, Ellis found, was an active–directive, cognitive–emotive behavioral attack on major self-defeating "musts" and commands. The essence of effective psychotherapy, according to REBT, is full tolerance (i.e., unconditional acceptance) of oneself and of others as *persons,* combined with a campaign against one's self-defeating *ideas, traits,* and *performances.*

As Ellis abandoned his previous psychoanalytic approaches, he obtained better results (Ellis, 1962). Other therapists who began to employ REBT also found that when they switched to its procedures, more progress was made in a few weeks than had been made in months or years of prior treatment (Ellis, 2002; Lyons & Woods, 1991; Walen et al., 1992).

Current Status

When members of the Society of Clinical Psychology were asked to name the most influential person in the history of psychotherapy, the individuals most often listed were Carl Rogers, Albert Ellis, and Sigmund Freud, in that order (Corsini, 2005). This survey gives some indication of the stature of Albert Ellis in the eyes of his colleagues. In the 1980s, a similar survey done in Canada rated Albert Ellis as the number one influential figure.

The Albert Ellis Institute, a nonprofit scientific and educational organization, was founded by Albert Ellis in 1959 to teach the principles of healthy living. With headquarters in New York City and affiliates in several cities in the United States and other countries, it disseminated the rational emotive behavioral approach through (1) adult education courses and workshops in the principles of rational living, (2) postgraduate training programs, (3) moderately priced clinics for individual and group therapy, and (4) special books, monographs, pamphlets, audiovisual materials, and the *Journal of Rational-Emotive and Cognitive-Behavior Therapy.*

Ironically, Albert Ellis had a strained relationship with the Albert Ellis Institute from 2004. In 2005, the Board of Trustees of the Albert Ellis Institute removed Ellis from the board and dismissed him from all duties at the institute. From that time until May 2006, Ellis continued to give workshops in a rented space next door to the institute. Nothing but severe illness and ultimately death could stop him from working and helping others. In January 2006, the State Supreme Court in Manhattan ruled that the board was wrong in ousting Ellis at a meeting from which Ellis was excluded. The judge's decision reinstated him to the board. The judge called the institute's position regarding Dr. Ellis "disingenuous," citing case law saying that such a "dismissal, accomplished without notice of any kind or the right of confrontation, is offensive and contrary to our fundamental process of democratic and legal procedure, fair play and the spirit of the law."

Only hours after giving an inspiring Friday Night Workshop (he had been presenting these famous workshops for over four decades) in May, 2006, Ellis was hospitalized with aspiration pneumonia. For the next 14-plus months, he made every effort to recover with remarkable determination and courage. He conducted workshops with students from his hospital bed and within his rehabilitation facility and also gave interviews, worked on his writings, updated his chapter in this book, and helped others. He was often experiencing great pain and increasing health complications, and despite his incredible and heroic battle to continue, he died, peacefully, in the arms of his wife, on July 24, 2007.

The REBT Network was established in 2006 to promote rational emotive behavior therapy and the works of Dr. Albert Ellis. It was created to ensure that Dr. Ellis's life works were protected and promoted and to advocate for the legal and human rights of Dr. Ellis in his elder years.

The REBT Network provides information on the theory and practice of rational emotive therapy to mental health professionals, paraprofessionals, and the public through its Web site, publications, affiliations, and training. The REBT Network is in no way associated with the Albert Ellis Institute. In 2006, Ellis stated that the Albert Ellis Institute was following a program that was in many ways inconsistent with the theory and practice of REBT.

The REBT network has a register of numerous psychotherapists who have received training in REBT. In addition, thousands of other therapists primarily follow REBT principles, and a still greater number use some major aspects of REBT in their work. Cognitive restructuring, employed by almost all cognitive–behavior therapists today, stems mainly from REBT. But REBT also includes many other emotive and behavioral methods.

In 2004, Albert Ellis married Australian psychologist Debbie Joffe, whom he called "the greatest love of my life." She worked closely with Dr. Ellis in every aspect of his work up until his death and continues to write and give presentations and workshops on REBT. She also works with clients in private practice and is dedicated to continuing the work of her husband. Anyone interested in learning more about the life of Albert Ellis and the history of REBT will benefit from reading *Rational Emotive Behavior Therapy—It Works for Me—It Can Work for You* (Ellis, 2004a) and his autobiography, *All Out!* (Ellis, 2010).

Research Studies

Many researchers have tested the main hypotheses of REBT, and the majority of their findings support central REBT contentions (Hajzler & Bernard, 1991; Lyons & Woods, 1991; McGovern & Silverman, 1984; Silverman, McCarthy, & McGovern, 1992). These research studies show that (1) clients tend to receive more effective help from a highly active–directive approach than from a more passive one; (2) efficient therapy includes activity-oriented homework assignments; (3) people largely choose to disturb themselves and can choose to surrender these disturbances; (4) helping clients modify their beliefs helps them to make significant behavioral changes; and (5) many effective methods of cognitive therapy exist, including modeling, role playing, skill training, and problem solving.

REBT in conjunction with medication is more effective than medication alone in certain conditions. This has been shown for conditions such as major depression (Macaskill & Macaskill, 1996) and dysthymic disorder (Wang, Jia, Fang, Zhu & Huang, 1999). REBT has been shown to be an effective adjunct with inpatients with schizophrenia (Shelley, Battaglia, Lucely, Ellis & Opler, 2001), and has also been shown superior to control conditions in the treatment of obsessive–compulsive disorder, social phobia, and social anxiety (Dryden & David, 2008).

Since REBT was the first of the cognitive–behavioral psychotherapies (CBTs), all of which incorporate aspects of REBT, the research programs of CBT—especially those of Aaron T. Beck's Cognitive Therapy (CT)—serve to also support the efficacy of REBT's clinical applications. A comprehensive survey of meta-analyses that offer empirical validation for CBT in different clinical applications is found in Butler, Chapman, Forman, and Beck (2005).

Although it was the forerunner of all current cognitive–behavioral psychotherapies, REBT still offers a unique theory of emotional disturbance, one that is not completely shared by the other CBT psychotherapies. The uniqueness of REBT's model stems first of all from its claim that emotional disturbance arises from the human propensity to turn "preferences" into "demands." REBT hypothesizes that human "musts" precede Beck's (1976) "automatic thoughts" (Ellis & Whiteley, 1979).

In addition, hundreds of clinical and research papers present empirical evidence supporting REBT's main theories of personality. Many of these studies are reviewed in Ellis and Whiteley (1979). These studies tend to substantiate the following hypotheses:

1. Human thinking and emotion do not constitute two disparate or different processes but, instead, significantly overlap.

2. Although activating events or adversities (A) significantly contribute to emotional and behavioral consequences (C), people's beliefs (B) about A more importantly and more directly cause C.

3. The kinds of things people say to themselves, as well as the form in which they say these things, affect their emotions and behavior and often disturb them.

4. Humans not only think and think about their thinking but also think about thinking about their thinking. Whenever they have disturbances at C (consequence) after something unfortunate has happened in their lives at A (adversity), they tend to make C into a new A—to perceive and think about their emotional disturbances and thereby often create new ones.

5. People think about what happens to them not only in words, phrases, and sentences but also via images, fantasies, and dreams. Nonverbal cognitions contribute to their emotions and behaviors and can be used to change such behaviors.

6. Just as cognitions contribute to emotions and actions, emotions also contribute to or cause cognitions and actions, and actions contribute to or cause cognitions and emotions. When people change one of these three modalities of behaving, they concomitantly tend to change the other two (Ellis, 1994, 1998; Ellis & Dryden, 1997; Ellis & MacLaren, 1998).

7. REBT, uniquely among the schools of CBT, uses a philosophical approach that attempts to promote an overall change in the client's belief system and philosophy of life, especially in regard to demandingness and nonacceptance (Ellis, 2005), and to improve his or her functioning outside of psychotherapy (Ellis, 2004a). Furthermore, research has shown that REBT can be effectively done outside the therapeutic setting, e.g., in public presentations, to the benefit of participating volunteers and their audience members (Ellis & Joffe, 2002). Various nonpsychotherapeutic applications of REBT have been summarized by Ellis and Blau (1998). Froh, Fives, Fuller, Jacofsky, Terjesen, and Yurkewicz (2007) documented that irrationality predicted lower levels of life satisfaction, but this relationship was at least partially mediated by interpersonal relations.

PERSONALITY

Theories of Personality

Physiological Basis of Personality

REBT emphasizes the biological aspects of human personality. Obliquely, some other systems do this, too, saying something like this: "Humans are easily influenced by their parents during early childhood and thereafter remain similarly influenced for the rest of their lives unless some intervention, such as years of psychotherapy, occurs to enable them to give up this early suggestibility and to start thinking much more independently." These psychotherapeutic systems implicitly posit an "environmentalist's" position, which is actually physiologically and genetically based, because only a *special, innately predisposed* kind of person would be so prone to be "environmentally determined."

Although REBT holds that people are born constructivists and have considerable resources for human growth, and that they are in many important ways able to change their social and personal destinies, it also holds that they have powerful innate tendencies to think irrationally and to defeat themselves (Ellis, 1976, 2001b, 2003a, 2004b).

Most such human tendencies may be summarized by stating that humans are born with a tendency to want, to "need," and to condemn (1) themselves, (2) others, and (3) the world when they do not immediately get what they supposedly "need." They consequently tend to think "childishly" (or "humanly") all their lives and are able only with real effort to achieve and maintain "mature" or realistic behavior. This is not to deny, as Abraham Maslow and Carl Rogers have pointed out, that humans have impressive self-actualizing capacities. They do, and these are strong inborn propensities, too. But, alas, people frequently defeat themselves by their inborn and acquired self-sabotaging ways.

There is a great deal of evidence that people's basic personality or temperament has strong biological, as well as environmental, influences. People are born, as well as reared, with greater or lesser degrees of demandingness, and therefore they can change from demanding to *desiring* only with great difficulty. If their demandingness is largely acquired rather than innate, they still seem to have difficulty in ameliorating this tendency toward disturbance. REBT emphasizes that people nonetheless have the *choice* of changing their dysfunctional behaviors and specifically shows them many ways of doing so. It particularly stresses flexible thinking and behaving that help them remove the rigidities to which they often easily fall victim.

Social Aspects of Personality

Humans are reared in social groups and spend much of their lives trying to impress, live up to the expectations of, and outdo the performances of other people. On the surface, they are "ego-oriented," "identity-seeking," or "self-centered." Even more important, however, they usually define their "selves" as "good" or "worthwhile" when they believe that others accept and approve of them. It is realistic and sensible for people to find or fulfill themselves in their interpersonal relations and to have a good amount of what Adler calls "social interest." For, as John Donne beautifully expressed it, no one is an island unto himself or herself. The healthy individual finds it enjoyable to love and be loved by significant others and to relate to almost everyone he or she encounters. In fact, the better one's interpersonal relations are, the happier one is likely to be.

However, what is called *emotional disturbance* is frequently associated with caring *too much* about what others think. This stems from people's belief that they can accept themselves *only* if others think well of them. When disturbed, they escalate their desire for others' approval, and the practical advantages that normally go with such approval, into an absolutistic *dire need* to be liked, and in so doing they become anxious and prone to depression. Given that we have our being-in-the-world, as the existentialists point out, it is quite *important* that others to some degree value us. But it is our tendency to exaggerate the importance of others' acceptance in a way that often leads to self-denigration (Ellis, 1962, 2001a, 2002, 2005; Ellis & Harper, 1997; Hauck, 1992).

Psychological Aspects of Personality

How, specifically, do people become psychologically disordered? According to REBT, they usually needlessly upset themselves as follows: When individuals feel upset at point C after experiencing an obnoxious adversity at point A, they almost always convince themselves of irrational beliefs (B), such as "I *can't stand* adversity! It is *awful* that it exists! It *shouldn't exist!* I am a *worthless person* for not being able to get rid of it!" This set of beliefs is irrational for several reasons:

1. People *can* stand obnoxious adversities, even though they may never like them.

2. Adversities are hardly awful, because *awful* is an essentially indefinable term, with surplus meaning and little empirical referent. By calling the noxious events awful, the disturbed individual means they are (a) highly inconvenient and (b) totally inconvenient, disadvantageous, and unbeneficial. But what noxious stimuli can, in point of fact, be totally inconvenient, disadvantageous, and unbeneficial? Or as bad as it could be?

3. By holding that the unfortunate happenings in their lives *absolutely should not* exist, people really imply that they have godly power and that whatever they *want* not to exist *must* not. This hypothesis is, to say the least, highly dubious!

4. By contending that they are *worthless persons* because they have not been able to ward off unfortunate events, people hold that they should be able to control the universe and that because they are not succeeding in doing what they cannot do, they are obviously worthless. (What drivel!)

The basic tenet of REBT is that emotional *upsets,* as distinguished from feelings of sorrow, regret, annoyance, and frustration, largely stem from irrational beliefs. These beliefs are irrational because they magically insist that something in the universe *should, ought,* or *must* be different from the way it is. Although these irrational beliefs are ostensibly connected with reality (the adversity at point A), they are dogmatic ideas beyond the realm of empiricism. They generally take the form of the statement "Because I want something, it is not only desirable and preferable that it exist, but it absolutely should, and it is awful when it doesn't!" No such proposition, obviously, can be substantiated. Yet such propositions are devoutly held, every day, by literally billions of humans. That is how incredibly disturbance prone most people are!

Once people become emotionally upset—or, rather, upset themselves!—a peculiar thing frequently occurs. Most of the time, they know they feel anxious, depressed, or otherwise agitated, and they also know their symptoms are undesirable and (in our culture) socially disapproved. For who approves or respects highly agitated or "crazy" people? They therefore make their emotional consequence (C) or symptom into another activating event or adversity (A) and create a secondary symptom (C2) about this new A!

Thus, if you originally start with something like (A): "I did poorly on my job today" and (B): "Isn't that horrible!" you may wind up with (C): feelings of anxiety, worthlessness, and depression. You may now start all over with (A2): "I feel anxious and depressed, and worthless!" Then you proceed to (B2): "Isn't *that* horrible!" Now you end up with (C2): even greater feelings of anxiety, worthlessness, and depression. In other words, once you become anxious, you frequently make yourself anxious about *being* anxious; once you become depressed, you make yourself depressed about *being* depressed; and so on. You now have two consequences or symptoms for the price of one, and you often go around and around, in a vicious cycle of (1) condemning yourself for doing poorly at some task, (2) feeling guilty or depressed because of this self-condemnation, (3) condemning yourself for your feelings of guilt and depression, (4) condemning yourself for condemning yourself, (5) condemning yourself for seeing your disturbances and still not eliminating them, (6) condemning yourself for going for psychotherapeutic help and still not getting better, (7) condemning yourself for being more disturbed than other individuals, (8) concluding that you are without question hopelessly disturbed and that nothing can be done about it; and so on, in an endless spiral.

No matter what your original self-condemnation is about—and it hardly matters what it was, because your adversity (A) is often not that important—you eventually tend to end up with a chain of disturbed reactions only obliquely related to the original "traumatic events" of your life. That is why dramatic psychotherapies are often misleading—they overemphasize "traumatic events" rather than self-condemnatory attitudes *about* these events—and that is why these therapies fail to help with any secondary disturbance, such as being anxious about being anxious. Most major psychotherapies also concentrate either on A, the adversities, or on C, the emotional consequences, and rarely consider B, the belief system, which is a vital factor in creating self-disturbance.

Even assuming, moreover, that adversities and emotional consequences are important, as in posttraumatic stress disorder (PTSD), for instance, there is not too much we can do by concentrating our therapeutic attention on them. The adversities belong to the past. There is nothing that anyone can do to *change* the past.

As for clients' present feelings, the more we focus on them, the worse they are likely to feel. If we keep talking about their anxiety and getting clients to reexperience this feeling, they can become still more anxious. The best way to interrupt their disturbed process is usually to help them to focus on their anxiety-creating belief system—point B—because that is the main (though not the only) cause of their disturbance.

If, for example, say a male client feels anxious during a therapy session and the therapist reassures him that there is nothing for him to be anxious about, he may achieve a palliative "solution" to his problem by thinking, "I am afraid that I will act foolishly right here and now, and wouldn't that be awful! No, it really wouldn't be awful, because *this* therapist will accept me, anyway." He may thereby temporarily decrease his anxiety.

Or the therapist can concentrate on the past adversities in the client's life that are presumably making him anxious—by, for instance, showing him that his mother used to point out his deficiencies, that he was always afraid of speaking to authority figures who might disapprove of him, and that, *therefore,* because of all his prior and present fears, in situations A1, A2, A3 . . . A11, he is *now* anxious with the therapist. Whereupon the client might convince himself, "Ah! Now I see that I am generally anxious when I am faced with authority figures. No wonder I am anxious even with my own therapist!" In which case, he might feel better and temporarily lose his anxiety.

It would be better, however, for the therapist to show this client that he was anxious as a child and is still anxious with authority figures because he has always believed, and still believes, that he *must* be approved, that it is *awful* when an authority figure disapproves of him. Then the anxious client would tend to become diverted from concentrating on A (criticism by an authority figure) and from C (his feelings of anxiety) to a consideration of B (his irrational belief system). This diversion would help him become immediately nonanxious—for when he is focusing on "What am I telling myself (at B) to *make myself* anxious?" he cannot focus on the self-defeating, useless thought "Wouldn't it be terrible if I said something stupid to my therapist and if even he disapproved of me!" He would begin actively to dispute (at point D) his irrational beliefs, and not only could he then temporarily change them (by convincing himself, "It would be *unfortunate* if I said something stupid to my therapist and he disapproved of me, but it would hardly be *terrible* or *catastrophic!*"), but he would also tend to have a much weaker allegiance to these self-defeating beliefs the next time. Thus he would obtain, by the therapist's helping him to focus primarily on B rather than on A and C, curative and preventive, rather than merely palliative, results in connection with his anxiety.

This is the basic personality theory of REBT: Humans largely create their own emotional consequences. They appear to be born with a distinct proneness to do so, and they learn, through social conditioning, to exaggerate (rather than to minimize) that proneness. They nonetheless have considerable ability to understand what they foolishly believe to cause their distress (because they have a unique talent for thinking about their thinking) and to train themselves to change their self-sabotaging beliefs (because they also have a unique capacity for self-discipline or self-reconditioning). If they *think* and *work* hard at understanding and contradicting their *must*urbatory belief systems, they can make amazing curative and preventive changes. And if they are helped to zero in on their crooked thinking and unhealthy emoting and behaving by a highly active–directive homework-assigning therapist, they are more likely to change their beliefs than if they work with a dynamically oriented, client-centered, conventional existential therapist or with a classical therapist who emphasizes behavior modification.

Although REBT is mainly a theory of personality change, it is also a personality theory in its own right (Ellis, 1994, 2001b, 2002).

Variety of Concepts

Ellis largely agrees with Sigmund Freud that the pleasure principle (or short-range hedonism) tends to run most people's lives; with Karen Horney and Erich Fromm that cultural influences as well as early family influences tend to play a significant part in bolstering people's irrational thinking; with Alfred Adler that fictitious goals tend to order and run human lives; with Gordon Allport that when individuals begin to think and act in a certain manner, they find it very difficult to think or act differently, even when they want very much to do so; with Ivan Pavlov that our species's large cerebral cortex provides humans with a secondary signaling system through which they often become cognitively conditioned; with Jerome Frank that people are exceptionally prone to the influence of suggestion; with Jean Piaget that active learning is much more effective than passive learning; with Anna Freud that people frequently refuse to acknowledge their mistakes and resort to defenses and rationalizations to cover up underlying feelings of shame and self-deprecation; and with Abraham Maslow and Carl Rogers that humans, however disturbed they may be, have great untapped capacity for growth.

On the other hand, REBT has serious differences with certain aspects of many popular personality theories.

1. It opposes the Freudian concept that people have clear-cut libidinous instincts, which if thwarted must lead to emotional disturbances. It also objects to the view of William Glasser and many other therapists that all humans *need* to be approved and to succeed—and that if these needs are blocked, they cannot possibly accept themselves or be happy. REBT, instead, posits strong human *desires,* which become needs or necessities only when people foolishly define them as such.

2. REBT places the Oedipus complex as a relatively minor subheading under people's major irrational belief that they absolutely have to receive the approval of their parents (and others), that they *must not* fail (at lusting or almost anything else), and that when they are disapproved of and when they fail, they are worthless. Many so-called sexual problems—such as sexual inadequacy, severe inhibition, and obsessive–compulsive behavior—partly result from people's irrational beliefs that they *need* approval, success, and immediate gratification.

3. REBT holds that people's environment, particularly their childhood parental environment, *reaffirms* but does not always *create* strong tendencies to think irrationally and to be disturbed. Parents and culture teach children standards and values, but they do not always teach them "musts" about these values. People naturally and *easily* add rigid commands to socially inhibited standards.

4. REBT looks skeptically at anything mystical, devout, transpersonal, or magical when these terms are used in the strict sense. It maintains that reason itself is limited, ungodlike, and absolute (Ellis, 1962, 1994). It holds that humans may in some ways transcend themselves or experience altered states of consciousness—for example, hypnosis—that

may enhance their ability to know themselves and the world and to solve some of their problems; but it does not believe that people can transcend their humanness and become superhuman. They can become more adept and competent, but they still remain fallible and in no way godly. REBT holds that minimal disturbance goes with people's surrendering all pretensions to superhumanness and accepting, while still disliking, their own and the world's limitations.

5. For REBT, no part of a human is to be reified into an entity called the unconscious, although it holds that people have many thoughts, feelings, and even acts of which they are unaware. These "unconscious" or tacit thoughts and feelings are, for the most part, slightly below the level of consciousness, are not often deeply repressed, and can usually be brought to consciousness by brief, incisive probing. Thus, suppose a wife is angrier with her husband than she is aware of and that her anger is motivated by the unconscious grandiose thought, "After all I've done for him he *absolutely should* be having sex with me more frequently!" A rational emotive behavior therapist (who suspects that she has these unconscious feelings and thoughts) can usually induce her to (a) hypothesize that she is angry with her husband and look for some evidence with which to test that hypothesis and (b) check herself for grandiose thinking whenever she feels angry. In the majority of instances, without resorting to free association, dream analysis, analyzing the transference relationship, hypnosis, or other presumably "depth-centered" techniques for revealing unconscious thoughts and feelings, REBT practitioners can reveal these in short order—sometimes in a matter of minutes. They show the client her unconsciously held attitudes, beliefs, and values and, in addition, teach the client how to bring her self-defeating, hidden ideas to consciousness and actively dispute them.

People often see how REBT differs significantly from psychoanalysis, Rogerianism, gestalt therapy, and orthodox behavior therapy but have difficulty seeing how it differs from more closely related schools, such as Adler's Individual Psychology. REBT agrees with nearly all of Adlerian theory but has a more hardheaded and behavior-oriented practice (Ellis, 1994; Ellis & Dryden, 1997; Ellis & MacLaren, 1998). It also ignores most of the Adlerian emphasis on early-childhood memories and the importance of birth order. But the basic mistakes that Adlerians emphasize are similar to the irrational beliefs of REBT.

REBT overlaps with Beck's cognitive therapy (CT) in several ways, but it also differs in significant ways: (1) It usually disputes clients' irrational beliefs more actively, directly, quickly, and forcefully than does CT. (2) It emphasizes absolutist *musts* more than CT and holds that most major irrationalities implicitly stem from dogmatic *shoulds* and *musts*. (3) It uses psychoeducational approaches—such as books, pamphlets, audiovisual materials, talks, and workshops—as intrinsic elements and stresses their use more than CT does. (4) It clearly distinguishes between healthy negative feelings (e.g., sadness and frustration) and unhealthy negative feelings (e.g., depression and hostility). (5) REBT emphasizes several emotive-evocative methods—such as shame-attacking exercises, rational emotive imagery, and *strong* self-statements and self-dialogues—that CT often neglects. (6) REBT favors *in vivo* desensitization, preferably done implosively, more than CT does. (7) REBT often uses penalties as well as reinforcements to help people do their homework (Ellis, 2001b, 2002, 2003a). (8) It emphasizes profound philosophical and *unconditional* acceptance of oneself, other people, and the world more than CT does (Ellis, 2005).

REBT is humanistic and to some degree existentialist. It first tries to help people minimize their emotional and behavioral disturbances, but it also encourages them to make themselves happier than they normally are and to strive for more self-actualization and human growth (Ellis, 1994). It is closer in some respects to Rogers's (1961) person-centered approach than to other therapies in that it mainly emphasizes unconditional self-acceptance (USA) as well as unconditional other-acceptance (UOA) no matter how well or how badly people may perform (Ellis, 2001a, 2002, 2003a, 2005; Ellis & Blau, 1998; Ellis & Harper, 1997; Hauck, 1992).

PSYCHOTHERAPY

Theory of Psychotherapy

According to the theory of REBT, neurotic disturbance occurs when individuals demand that their wishes be satisfied, that they succeed and be approved, that others treat them fairly, and that the universe be more pleasant. When people's demandingness (and not their desirousness) gets them into emotional trouble, they tend to alleviate their pain in both inelegant and elegant ways.

Distraction

Just as a whining child can be temporarily diverted by receiving a piece of candy, so can adult demanders be transitorily sidetracked by distraction. Thus, a therapist who sees someone who is afraid of being rejected (that is, one who demands that significant others accept him) can try to divert him into activities such as sports, aesthetic creation, a political cause, yoga exercises, meditation, or preoccupation with the events of his childhood. While the individual is so diverted, he will not be so inclined to demand acceptance by others and to make himself anxious. Distraction techniques are mainly palliative, given that distracted people are still demanders and that, as soon as they are not diverted, they will probably return to their destructive commanding.

Satisfaction of Demands

If a client's insistences are always catered to, she or he will tend to feel better (but will not necessarily get better). To arrange this kind of "solution," a therapist can give her or his love and approval, provide pleasurable sensations (for example, put the client in an encounter group to be hugged or massaged), teach methods of having demands met, or give reassurance that the client eventually will be gratified. Many clients will feel immensely better when accorded this kind of treatment, but they may well have their demandingness reinforced rather than minimized.

Magic and Mysticism

A boy who demands may be assuaged by magic—for example, by his parents saying that a fairy godmother will soon satisfy his demands. Similarly, adolescent and adult demanders can be led to believe (by a therapist or someone else) that their therapist is a kind of magician who will take away their troubles merely by listening to what bothers them. These magical solutions sometimes work beautifully by getting true believers to feel better and give up disturbed symptoms, but they rarely work for any length of time and frequently lead to eventual disillusionment.

Minimization of Demandingness

The most elegant solution to the problems resulting from irrational demandingness is to help individuals to become less demanding. As children mature, they normally become less childish and less insistent that their desires be immediately gratified. REBT encourages clients to achieve minimal demandingness and maximum tolerance.

REBT practitioners may, at times, use temporary "solutions," such as distraction, satisfying the client's "needs," and even (on rare occasions) "magic." But they realize that these are low-level, inelegant, palliative solutions, mainly to be used with clients who refuse to accept a more elegant and permanent resolution. The therapist prefers to strive for the highest-order solution: minimizing *must*urbation, perfectionism, grandiosity, and low frustration tolerance.

In REBT, therapists help clients to minimize their absolutistic core philosophies by using cognitive, emotive, and behavioristic procedures.

1. REBT cognitively attempts to show clients that giving up perfectionism can help them lead happier, less anxiety-ridden lives. It teaches them how to recognize their *shoulds, oughts,* and *musts;* how to separate rational (preferential) from irrational (absolutistic) beliefs; how to be logical and pragmatic about their own problems; and how to accept reality, even when it is pretty grim. REBT is oriented toward helping disturbed people philosophize more effectively and thereby uncreate the needless problems they have constructed. Not only does it employ a one-to-one Socratic-type dialogue between the client and the therapist, but it also, in group therapy, encourages other members of the group to discuss, explain, and reason with other ineffectually thinking clients. It teaches logical and semantic precision—that a man's being rejected does not mean that he will always be rejected and that a woman's failure does not mean she cannot succeed. It helps clients to keep asking themselves whether the worst things that could happen would really be as bad as they melodramatically fantasize they would be.

2. REBT emotively employs various means of dramatizing preferences and *musts* so that clients can clearly distinguish between the two. Thus, the therapist may employ *role playing* to show clients how to adopt different ideas; *humor* to reduce disturbance-creating ideas to absurdity; *unconditional acceptance* to demonstrate that clients are acceptable, even with their unfortunate traits; and *strong disputing* to persuade people to give up some of their "crazy thinking" and replace it with more efficient notions. The therapist may also encourage clients, either in individual or group counseling, to take risks (for example, telling another group member what they really think of him or her) that will prove to be not that risky; to reveal themselves (for example, by sharing the details of their sexual problems); to convince themselves that others can accept them with their failings; and to get in touch with their "shameful" feelings (such as hostility) so that they can zero in on exactly what they are telling themselves to create these feelings. Experiential exercises are used to help clients overcome denial of their feelings and then work at REBT's ABCDs (the D refers to disputation) to change their self-defeating emotions. The therapist may also use pleasure-giving techniques, not merely to satisfy clients' unreasonable demands for immediate gratification but also to show them they are capable of doing many pleasant acts that they think, wrongly, they cannot do, and that they can seek pleasure for its own sake, even though others may frown upon them for doing so.

3. *Behavior therapy* is employed in REBT not only to help clients to become habituated to more effective ways of performing but also to help change their cognitions. Thus, their demandingness that they perform beautifully may be whittled away by their agreeing to do risk-taking assignments, such as asking a desired person for a date, deliberately failing at some task (for example, making a real attempt to speak badly in public), imagining themselves in failing situations, and throwing themselves into unusual activities that they consider especially dangerous. Clients' demandingness that others treat them fairly and that the world be kind may be challenged by the therapist's encouraging them to stay in poor circumstances and teach themselves, at least temporarily, to accept them; to take

on hard tasks (such as enrolling in college); to imagine themselves having a rough time at something and making themselves not feel terribly upset or having to "cop out" of it; to allow themselves to do a pleasant thing, such as go to a movie or see their friends, only after they have done unpleasant but desirable tasks, such as studying French or finishing a report for their boss; and so on. REBT often employs operant conditioning to reinforce people's efforts to change undesirable behavior (e.g., smoking or overeating) or to change irrational thinking (e.g., condemning themselves when they smoke or overeat).

REBT accepts that there are many kinds of psychological treatment and that most of them work to some degree. An elegant system of therapy includes (a) economy of time and effort, (b) rapid symptom reduction, (c) effectiveness with a large percentage of different kinds of clients, (d) depth of solution of the presenting problems, and (e) lastingness of the therapeutic results. Philosophically, REBT combats absoluteness and ruthlessly persists at undermining childish demandingness—the main element of much neurotic disturbance (Ellis, 1962, 1994, 2002). It theorizes that if people learn to only strongly prefer, instead of grandiosely insisting, that their desires be fulfilled, they can make themselves remarkably less disturbed and less disturb*able* (Ellis, 1999, 2001a, 2001b, 2002).

Process of Psychotherapy

REBT helps clients acquire a more realistic, tolerant philosophy of life. Because some of its methods are similar to methods used by other therapists, they are not detailed in this section. Most of the space here is devoted to the cognitive–persuasive aspects of REBT, one of its most distinguishing characteristics.

REBT practitioners generally do not spend a great deal of time listening to the client's history, encouraging long tales of woe, sympathetically getting in tune with emotionalizing, or carefully and incisively reflecting feelings. They may use all these methods, but they generally keep them short because they consider most long-winded dialogues a form of indulgence therapy, in which the client may be helped to *feel* better but rarely to *get* better. Even when these methods work, they are often inefficient and sidetracking (Ellis, 2001a).

Similarly, the rational emotive behavior therapist makes little use of free association, dream analysis, interpretations of the transference relationship, explanations of the client's present symptoms in terms of past experiences, disclosure, analysis of the so-called Oedipus complex, and other dynamically directed interpretations or explanations. When they are employed at all, they are used to help clients see some of their basic irrational ideas.

Thus, if a male therapist notes that a female client rebels against him just as she previously rebelled against her father during childhood, he will not interpret the present rebelliousness as stemming from the prior pattern but, instead, will probably say something like this:

> It looks like you frequently hated your father because he kept forcing you to follow certain rules you considered arbitrary and because you kept convincing yourself, "My father isn't being considerate of me and he *ought* to be! I'll get even with him!" I think you are now telling yourself approximately the same thing about me. But your angry rebelliousness against your father was senseless because (a) he was not a *total bastard* for perpetrating a bastardly act; (b) there was no reason why he *ought* to have been considerate of you (although there were several reasons why it *would have been preferable* if he had been); and (c) your getting angry at him and trying to "get even with him" would not, probably, encourage him to act more kindly but would actually induce him to be more cruel.

You consequently confused—as most children will—being displeased with your father's behavior with being "righteously" angry at him, and you needlessly made yourself upset about his real or imagined unfair treatment of you. In my case, too, you may be doing much the same thing. You may be taking the risks that I encourage you to take and insisting that they are too onerous (when in fact, they are only onerous), and after assuming that I am wrong in suggesting them (which I indeed may be), you are condemning me for my supposedly wrong deeds. Moreover, you are quite possibly assuming that I am "wrong" and a "louse" for being wrong because I resemble, in some ways, your "wrong" and "lousy" father.

But this is another illogical conclusion (that I resemble him in all ways) and an irrational premise (that I, like your father, am a *bad person* if I do a wrong act). So you are not only *inventing* a false connection between me and your father, but you are creating today, as you have done for many years now, a renewed *demand* that the world be an easy place for you and that everyone *ought* to treat you fairly. Now, how can you challenge these irrational premises and illogical deductions?

REBT practitioners often employ a rapid-fire active–directive–persuasive–philosophical methodology. In most instances, they quickly pin clients down to a few basic dysfunctional beliefs. They challenge them to try to defend these ideas; show that they contain illogical premises that cannot be substantiated logically; analyze these ideas and actively dispute them; vigorously show why they cannot work and why they will almost inevitably lead to more disturbance; reduce these ideas to absurdity, sometimes in a humorous manner; explain how they can be replaced with more rational philosophies; and teach clients how to think scientifically so that they can observe, logically parse, and minimize any subsequent irrational ideas and illogical deductions that lead to self-defeating feelings and behaviors.

When working with certain clients who have suffered extreme traumas (such as incest, rape, child abuse, or other violent situations), REBT practitioners may well be quite empathic and go more slowly before doing any vigorous disputing of clients' dysfunctional beliefs about these traumatic events or about anything else in their lives.

To show how REBT is sometimes, but hardly always, actively–directively done, here is a verbatim transcript of a session with a 25-year-old single woman, Sara, who worked as the head of a computer programming section of a firm and who, without any traumatic or violent history, was very insecure and self-denigrating.

T-1:   What would you want to start on first?
C-1:   I don't know. I'm petrified at the moment!
T-2:   You're petrified—of what?
C-2:   Of you!
T-3:   No, surely not of me—perhaps of yourself!
C-3:   [Laughs nervously.]
T-4:   Because of what I am going to do to you?
C-4:   Right! You are threatening me, I guess.
T-5:   But how? What am I doing? Obviously, I'm not going to take a knife and stab you. Now, in what way am I threatening you?
C-5:   I guess I'm afraid, perhaps, of what I'm going to find out—about me.
T-6:   Well, so let's suppose you find out something dreadful about you—that you're thinking foolishly or something. Now why would that be awful?
C-6:   Because I, I guess I'm the most important thing to me at the moment.

T-7:   No, I don't think that's the answer. It's, I believe, the opposite! You're really the least important thing to you. You are prepared to beat yourself over the head if I tell you that you're acting foolishly. If you were not a self-blamer, then you wouldn't care what I said. It would be important to you—but you'd just go around correcting it. But if I tell you something really negative about you, you're going to beat yourself mercilessly. Aren't you?

C-7:   Yes, I generally do.

T-8:   All right. So perhaps that's what you're really afraid of. You're not afraid of me. You're afraid of your own self-criticism.

C-8:   [Sighs.] All right.

T-9:   So why do you have to criticize yourself? Suppose I find you're the worst person I ever met? Let's just suppose that. All right, now *why* would you have to criticize yourself?

C-9:   [Pause.] I'd have to. I don't know any other behavior pattern, I guess, in this point of time. I always do. I guess I think I'm just a shit.

T-10:   Yeah. But that, that isn't so. If you don't know how to ski or swim, you could learn. You can also learn not to condemn yourself, no matter what you do.

C-10:   I don't know.

T-11:   Well, the answer is: You don't know how.

C-11:   Perhaps.

T-12:   I get the impression you're saying, "I *have* to berate myself if I do something wrong." Because isn't that where your depression comes from?

C-12:   Yes, I guess so. [Silence.]

T-13:   Now, what are you *mainly* putting yourself down for right now?

C-13:   I don't seem quite able, in this point of time, to break it down very neatly. The form [that our clinic gets clients to fill out before their sessions] gave me a great deal of trouble. Because my tendency is to say *everything*, I want to change everything; I'm depressed about everything, etc.

T-14:   Give me a couple of things, for example.

C-14:   What I'm depressed about? I, uh, don't know that I have any purpose in life. I don't know what I—what I am. And I don't know in what direction I'm going.

T-15:   Yeah, but that's—so you're saying, "I'm ignorant!" [Client nods.] Well, what's so awful about being ignorant? It's too bad you're ignorant. It would be nicer if you weren't—if you *had* a purpose and *knew* where you were going. But just let's suppose the worst: for the rest of your life you didn't have a purpose and you stayed this way. Let's suppose that. Now, why would *you* be so bad?

C-15:   Because everyone *should* have a purpose!

T-16:   Where did you get the *should?*

C-16:   'Cause it's what I believe in. [Silence.]

T-17:   I know. But think about it for a minute. You're obviously a bright woman. Now, where did that *should* come from?

C-17:   I, I don't know! I'm not thinking clearly at the moment. I'm too nervous! I'm sorry.

T-18:   Well, but you *can* think clearly. Are you now saying, "Oh, it's hopeless! I can't think clearly. What a shit I am for not thinking clearly!" You see: you're blaming yourself for *that*.

[From C-18 to C-26 the client upsets herself about not reacting well to the session, but the therapist shows her that this is not overly important and calms her down.]

C-27: I can't imagine existing, uh, or that there would be any reason for existing without a purpose!

T-28: No, but the vast majority of human beings don't have much purpose.

C-28: [Angrily.] All right, then, I should not feel bad about it.

T-29: No, no, no! Wait a minute, now. You just *jumped.* [Laughs.] You jumped from one extreme to another! You see, you said a sane sentence and an *insane* sentence. Now, if we could get you to separate the two—which you're perfectly able to do—you would solve the problem. What you really mean is "It *would be better* if I had a purpose. Because I'd be happier." Right?

C-29: Yes.

T-30: But then you magically jump to "Therefore I *should!*" Now do you see the difference between "It *would be better* if I had a purpose" and "I *should, I must,* I've *got to*"?

C-30: Yes, I do.

T-31: Well, what's the difference?

C-31: [Laughs.] I just said that to agree with you!

T-32: Yes! See, that won't be any good. We could go on that way forever, and you'll agree with me, and I'll say, "Oh, what a great woman! She agrees with me." And then you'll go out of here as nutty as you were before!

C-32: [Laughs, this time with genuine appreciation and good humor.]

T-33: You're perfectly able, as I said, to think—to stop giving up. That's what you've done most of your life. That's why you're disturbed. Because you refuse to think. And let's go over it again: "It would be better if I had a purpose in life; if I weren't depressed, etc., etc. If I had a good, nice, enjoyable purpose." We could give reasons why it would be better. "It's fairly obvious why it would be better!" Now, why is that a magical statement, that "I *should* do what would be better"?

C-33: You mean, why do I feel that way?

T-34: No, no. It's a belief. You feel that way because you believe that way.

C-34: Yes.

T-35: If you believed you were a kangaroo, you'd be hopping around and you'd *feel* like a kangaroo. Whatever you *believe,* you feel. Feelings largely come from your beliefs. Now, I'm temporarily forgetting about your feelings, because we really can't change feelings without changing beliefs. So I'm showing you; you have two beliefs—or two feelings, if you want to call them that. One, "It would be better if I had a purpose in life." Do you agree? [Client nods.] Now that's perfectly reasonable. That's quite true. We could prove it. Two, "Therefore I *should* do what would be better." Now those are two different statements. They may seem the same, but they're vastly different. Now, the first one, as I said, is sane. Because we could prove it. It's related to reality. We can list the advantages of having a purpose—for almost anybody, not just for you.

C-35: [Calm now, and listening intently to T's explanation.] Uh-huh.

T-36: But the second one, "Therefore I *should* do what would be better," is crazy. Now, why is it crazy?

C-36: I can't accept it as a crazy statement.

T-37: Because who said you *should?*

C-37: I don't know where it all began! Somebody said it.

T-38: I know, but I say whoever said it was screwy!

C-38: [Laughs.] All right.

T-39: How could the world possibly have a *should?*

C-39: Well, it does.

T-40:   But it *doesn't!* You see, that's what emotional disturbance is: believing in *shoulds, oughts,* and *musts* instead of *it would be betters.* That's exactly what makes people neurotic! Suppose you said to yourself, "I wish I had a dollar in my pocket right now," and you had only 90 cents. How would you feel?

C-40:   Not particularly upset.

T-41:   Yes, you'd be a little disappointed. It would be better to have a dollar. But now suppose you said, "I should, I must have a dollar in my pocket at all times," and you found you had only 90 cents. Now, how would you feel?

C-41:   Then I would be terribly upset, following your line of reasoning.

T-42:   But not because you had only 90 cents.

C-42:   Because I thought I should have a dollar.

T-43:   THAT'S RIGHT! The should. And what's more, let's just go one step further. Suppose you said, "I must have a dollar in my pocket at all times." And you found you had a dollar and 10 cents. Now how would you feel?

C-43:   Superb, I guess!

T-44:   No—anxious!

C-44:   [Laughs.] You mean I'd be guilty: "What was I doing with the extra money?"

T-45:   No.

C-45:   I'm sorry, I'm not following you. I—

T-46:   Because you're not thinking. Think for a minute. Why, if you said, "I must have a dollar, I should have a dollar," and you had a dollar and 10 cents, would you still be anxious? Anybody would be. Now why would anybody be anxious if they were saying, "I've got to have a dollar!" and they found they had a dollar and 10 cents?

C-46:   Because it violated their should. It violated their rule of what they thought was right, I guess.

T-47:   Well, not at the moment. But they could easily lose 20 cents.

C-47:   Oh! Well.

T-48:   Yeah! They'd still be anxious. You see, because must means, "At all times I must—"

C-48:   Oh, I see what you mean! All right. I see what you mean. They could easily lose some of the money and would therefore feel insecure.

T-49:   Yeah. Most anxiety comes from musts.

C-49:   [Long silence.] Why do you create such an anxiety-ridden situation initially for someone?

T-50:   I don't think I do. I see hundreds of people and you're one of the few who makes this so anxiety-provoking for yourself. The others may do it mildly, but you're making it very anxiety-provoking. Which just shows that you may carry must into everything, including this situation. Most people come in here very relieved. They finally get to talk to somebody who knows how to help them, and they're very happy that I stop the horseshit, and stop asking about their childhood, and don't talk about the weather, etc. And I get *right away* to what bothers them. I tell them in 5 minutes. I've just explained to you the secret of most emotional disturbance. If you really followed what I said, and used it, you'd never be disturbed about practically anything for the rest of your life!

C-50:   Uh-huh.

T-51:   Because practically every time you're disturbed, you're changing it would be better to a must! That's all neurosis is! Very, very simple. Now, why should I waste your time and not explain this—and talk about irrelevant things?

C-51:   Because perhaps I would have followed your explanation a little better if I hadn't been so threatened initially.

T-52:   But then, if I pat you on the head and hold back, etc., then you'll think for the rest of your life you have to be patted on the head! You're a bright woman!

C-52:   All right—

T-53:   That's another should. "He should pat me on the head and take it slowly—then a shit like me can understand! But if he goes fast and makes me think, oh my God I'll make an error—and that is awful!" More horseshit! You don't have to believe that horseshit! You're perfectly able to follow what I say—if you stop worrying, "I should do perfectly well!" For that's what you're basically thinking, sitting there. Well, why should you do perfectly well? Suppose we had to go over it 20 times before you got it?

C-53:   I don't *like* to appear stupid!

T-54:   No. See. Now you're lying to yourself! Because again you said a sane thing—and then you added an insane thing. The sane thing was, "I don't like to appear stupid, because it's *better* to appear bright." But then you immediately jumped over to the insane thing: "And it's *awful* if I appear stupid—"

C-54:   [Laughs appreciatively, almost joyously.]

T-55:   "—I *should* appear bright!" You see?

C-55:   [With conviction.] Yes.

T-56:   The same crap! It's always the same crap. Now if you would look at the crap—instead of "Oh, how stupid I am! He hates me! I think I'll kill myself!"—then you'd be on the road to getting better fairly quickly.

C-56:   You've been listening! [Laughs.]

T-57:   Listening to what?

C-57:   [Laughs.] Those wild statements in my mind, like that, that I make.

T-58:   That's right! Because I know that you have to make those statements—because I have a good *theory*. And according to my theory, people wouldn't usually get upset *unless* they made those nutty statements to themselves.

C-58:   I haven't the faintest idea why I've been so upset—

T-59:   But you *do* have the faintest idea. I just told you.

C-59:   All right, I know!

T-60:   Why are you upset? Report it to me.

C-60:   I'm upset because I know, I—the role that I envisioned myself being in when I walked in here and what I [Laughs, almost joyously] and what I would do and should do—

T-61:   Yeah?

C-61:   And therefore you forced me to violate that. And I don't like it.

T-62:   "And isn't it *awful* that I didn't come out greatly! If I had violated that needed role *beautifully,* and I gave him the *right* answers immediately, and he beamed, and said, 'Boy, what a bright woman, this!' then it would have been all right."

C-62:   [Laughing good-humoredly.] Certainly!

T-63:   Horseshit! You would have been exactly as disturbed as you are now! It wouldn't have helped you a bit! In fact, you would have gotten nuttier! Because then you would have gone out of here with the same philosophy you came in here with: "That when I act well and people pat me on the head and say, 'What a great woman I am!' then everything is rosy!" It's a nutty philosophy! Because even if I loved you madly, the next person you talk to is likely to hate you. So I like brown eyes and he likes blue eyes or something else. So you're then dead! Because you really think: "I've got to be *accepted!* I've got to act intelligently!" Well, why?

C-63:   [Very soberly and reflectively.] True.

T-64: You see?

C-64: Yes.

T-65: Now, if you will learn that lesson, then you've had a very valuable session. Because you *don't* have to upset yourself. As I said before, if I thought you were the worst shit who ever existed, well, that's my *opinion*. And I'm entitled to it. But does it make you a turd?

C-65: [Reflective silence.]

T-66: *Does* it?

C-66: No.

T-67: *What* makes you a turd?

C-67: *Thinking* that you are.

T-68: That's right! Your *belief* that you are. That's the only thing that could ever do it. And you never have to believe that. See? You control your thinking. I control *my* thinking—my belief about you. But you don't have to be affected by that. You *always* control what you think. And you believe you don't. So let's get back to that depression. The depression, as I said before, stems from self-castigation. That's where it comes from. Now what are you castigating yourself for?

C-68: Because I can't live up to it—there's a basic conflict in what people appear to think I am and what I think I am.

T-69: Right.

C-69: And perhaps it's not fair to blame other people. Perhaps I thrust myself into a leader's role. But, anyway, my feeling right now is that all my life I've been forced to be something that I'm not, and the older I get, the more difficult this *façade,* huh, this *appearance,* uh—that the veneer is becoming thinner and thinner and thinner, until I just can't do it anymore.

T-70: Well, but really, yeah, I'm afraid you're a little wrong. Because oddly enough, almost the opposite is happening. You are thrust into this role. That's right: the role of something of a leader. Is that correct?

C-70: Yes.

T-71: And *they* think you're filling it.

C-71: Everyone usually does.

T-72: And it just so happens they're *right.*

C-72: But it's taking more and more out of me.

T-73: Because you're not doing something else. You see, you are fulfilling *their* expectations of you. Because, obviously, they wouldn't think you are a leader, they'd think you were nothing if you *were* acting like a nonleader. So you are fulfilling their expectations. But you're not fulfilling your own idealistic and impractical expectations of leadership.

C-73: [Verging on tears.] No, I guess I'm not.

T-74: You see, that's the issue. So therefore you *are* doing O.K. by them—by your job. But you're not being an angel, you're not being *perfect!* And you *should* be, to be a real *leader.* And therefore you're a *sham!* You see? Now, if you give up those nutty expectations of yourself and go back to their expectations, you're in no trouble at all. Because obviously you're doing all right by them and *their* expectations.

C-74: Well, I haven't been. I had to, to give up one very successful situation. And, uh, when I left, they thought it was still successful. But I just couldn't go on—

T-75: "Because I must, I must *really* be a leader in *my* eyes, be pretty *perfect.*" You see, "If I satisfy the world, but I know I did badly, or less than I *should,* then I'm a slob! And they haven't found me out, so that makes me a *double* slob. Because I'm pretending to them to be a nonslob when I really am one!"

C-75: [Laughs in agreement, then grows sober.] True.

T-76:   But it's all your silly *expectations.* It's not *them.* And oddly enough, you are—even with your *handicap,* which is depression, self-deprecation, etc.—you're doing remarkably well. Imagine what you might do *without* this nutty handicap! You see, you're satisfying them while you're spending most of your time and energy flagellating yourself. Imagine what you might do *without* the self-flagellation! Can you see that?

C-76:   [Stopped in her self-blaming tracks, at least temporarily convinced, speaks very meaningfully.] Yes.

Mechanisms of Psychotherapy

From the foregoing partial protocol (which consumed about 15 minutes of the first session with the client), it can be seen that the therapist tries to do several things:

1. No matter what *feelings* the client brings out, the therapist tries to get back to her main irrational *ideas* that probably lie behind these feelings—especially her ideas that it would be *awful* if someone, including him, disliked her.

2. The therapist does not hesitate to contradict the client, using evidence from the client's own life and from his knowledge of people in general.

3. He usually is one step *ahead* of her—tells her, for example, that she is a self-blamer before she has said that she is. Knowing, on the basis of REBT theory, that she has *shoulds, oughts,* and *musts* in her thinking if she becomes anxious, depressed, and guilty, he helps her to admit these *shoulds* and then dispute them (T-16, T-17).

4. He uses the strongest philosophical approach he can think of: "Suppose," he keeps saying to her, "the *worst* thing happened and you really did do badly and others hated you, would you *still* be so bad?" (T-15). He assumes that if he can convince her that *none* of her behavior, no matter how execrable, denigrates *her,* he has helped her to make a *deep* attitudinal change.

5. He is not thrown by her distress (C-17), is not too sympathetic about these feelings, but *uses* them to try to prove to her that, right now, she still believes in foolish ideas and thereby upsets herself. He does not dwell on her "transference" feelings. He interprets the *ideas* behind these feelings, shows her why they are self-defeating, and indicates why his acting sympathetically would probably reinforce her demanding philosophy instead of helping her change it.

6. He is fairly stern with her but also shows full acceptance and demonstrates confidence in her abilities, especially her constructive ability to change herself.

7. Instead of merely *telling* her that her ideas are irrational, he keeps trying to get her to see this for herself (T-36). He wants her not merely to accept or parrot *his* rational philosophies but to think them through. He does, however, explain some relevant psychological processes, such as the way the client's feelings largely derive from her thinking (T-35, T-68).

8. He deliberately, on several occasions, uses strong language (T-18, T-50). This is done (a) to help loosen up the client, (b) to show that he, the therapist, is a down-to-earth human being, and (c) to give her an emotive jolt or shock so his words may have a more dramatic effect. Note that in this case, the client first calls herself a "shit" (C-9).

9. Although hardly sympathetic to her ideas, he is really quite empathic. Rational emotive behavior therapists are usually attuned to the client's unexpressed thoughts (her negative ideas about herself and the world), rather than to her superficial feelings (her perceptions that she is doing poorly or that others are abusing her). They empathize with the client's *feelings* and with the *beliefs* that underlie these feelings. This is a two-pronged form of empathy that many therapies miss out on.

10. The therapist keeps checking the client's ostensible understanding of what he is teaching her (T-65, T-66, T-67).

11. The therapist—as is common in early sessions of REBT—does most of the talking and explaining. He gives the client plenty of opportunity to express herself but uses her responses as points of departure for further teaching. He tries to make each "lecture" brief and trenchant and to relate it specifically to her problems and feelings. Also, at times he stops to let ideas sink in.

As can be seen from the first part of this initial REBT session, the client does not receive feelings of love and warmth from the therapist. Transference and countertransference spontaneously occur, but they are quickly analyzed, the philosophies behind them are revealed, and they tend to evaporate in the process. The client's deep feelings (shame, self-pity, weeping, anger) clearly exist, but the client is not given too much chance to revel in these feelings or to abreact strongly about them. As the therapist points out and attacks the ideologies that underlie these feelings, they swiftly change and are sometimes almost miraculously transformed into other, contradictory feelings (such as humor, joy, and reflective contemplation). The therapist's "coolness," philosophizing, and encouraging insistence that the client can feel something besides anxiety and depression help change her destructiveness into constructive feelings. That is why REBT is a constructivist rather than a purely rationalist kind of therapy (Ellis, 1994, 1999, 2001a, 2001b, 2002).

What the client does seem to experience, as the session proceeds, is (1) full acceptance of herself, in spite of her poor behavior; (2) renewed confidence that she can do certain things, such as think for herself; (3) the belief that it is her own perfectionistic *shoulds* that are upsetting her and not the attitudes of others (including the therapist); (4) reality testing, in her starting to see that even though she performs inefficiently (with the therapist and with some of the people she works with), she can still recover, try again, and probably do better in the future; and (5) reduction of some of her defenses, in that she can stop blaming others (such as her therapist) for her anxiety and can start to admit that she is doing something herself to cause it.

In these 15 minutes the client is getting only *glimmerings* of these constructive thoughts and feelings. The REBT intent, however, is that she will *keep* getting insights—that is, *philosophical* rather than merely *psychodynamic* insights—into the self-causation of her disturbed symptoms; that she will use these insights to change some of her most enduring and deep-seated ways of thinking about herself, about others, and about the world; and that she will thereby eventually become ideationally, emotionally, and behaviorally less self-defeating. Unless she finally makes an *attitudinal* (as well as symptom-reducing) change, although she may be helped to some degree, she will still be far from the ideal REBT goal of making a basic and lasting personality change.

APPLICATIONS

Who Can We Help?

It is easier to state what kinds of problems are *not* handled than what kinds *are* handled in REBT. Individuals who are out of contact with reality, in a highly manic state, seriously autistic or brain-injured, or in the lower ranges of mental deficiency are not normally treated by REBT therapists (or by most other practitioners). They are referred for medical treatment, for custodial or institutional care, or for behavior therapy along operant conditioning lines.

Most other individuals with difficulties are treated with REBT. These include (1) clients with maladjustment, moderate anxiety, or marital problems; (2) those with sexual difficulties; (3) run-of-the-mill "neurotics"; (4) individuals with character disorders; (5) truants, juvenile delinquents, and adult criminals; (6) borderline personalities and others with personality disorders; (7) overt psychotics, including those with delusions and hallucinations, when they are under medication and somewhat in contact with reality; (8) individuals with higher-grade mental deficiency; and (9) clients with psychosomatic problems.

Although varying types of problems are treated with REBT, no claim is made that they are treated with equal effectiveness. As is the case with virtually all psychotherapies, the REBT approach is more effective with clients who have a single major symptom (such as sexual inadequacy) than with seriously disordered clients (Ellis, 2001b, 2002). This is consistent with several hypotheses of REBT theory: that the tendency toward emotional distress is partly inborn and not merely acquired, that individuals with serious aberrations are more innately predisposed to have rigid and crooked thinking than are those with lesser aberrations, and that these clients consequently are less likely to make major advances. Moreover, REBT emphasizes commitment to changing one's thinking and to doing homework activity assignments, and it is clinically observable that many of the most dramatically symptom-ridden individuals (such as those who are severely depressed) tend to do considerably less work and more shirking (including shirking at therapy) than those with milder symptoms. Nevertheless, seasoned REBT practitioners claim they get better results with a wide variety of clients than do therapists from other schools of psychological thought (Ellis, 1994; Lyons & Woods, 1991; McGovern & Silverman, 1984; Silverman et al., 1992).

REBT is applicable for preventive purposes. Rational–emotive procedures are closely connected to the field of education and have enormous implications for emotional prophylaxis (Ellis, 2003b). A number of clinicians have shown how they have helped prevent normal children from eventually becoming seriously disturbed. Evidence shows that when nondisturbed grade school pupils are given, along with regular elements of an academic education, a steady process of REBT education, they can learn to understand themselves and others and to live more rationally and happily in this difficult world (Hajzler & Bernard, 1991; Vernon, 2001).

Treatment

REBT employs virtually all forms of individual and group psychotherapy. Some of the main methods are described in this section.

Individual Therapy

Most clients with whom REBT is practiced are seen for individual sessions, usually on a weekly basis, for from 5 to 50 sessions. They generally begin their sessions by telling the most upsetting feelings or consequences (C) that they have experienced during the week. REBT therapists then discover what adversities (A) occurred before clients felt so badly and help them to see what rational beliefs and what irrational beliefs (B) they hold in connection with these adversities. They teach clients to dispute (D) their irrational beliefs and often agree on concrete homework activity assignments to help with this disputing. They then check up in the following session, sometimes with the help of an REBT Self-Help Report Form, to see how the clients have tried to use the REBT approach during the week. If clients work at REBT, they arrive at an effective new philosophy (E)—which they reach through *effort* and *exercise*.

In particular, REBT therapists try to show clients how to (1) minimize anxiety, guilt, and depression by unconditionally accepting themselves, (2) alleviate their anger, hostility, and violence by unconditionally accepting other people, and (3) reduce their low frustration tolerance and inertia by learning to accept life unconditionally even when it is grim (Ellis, 2001a; Ellis & Blau, 1998; Ellis & Dryden, 1997; Ellis & MacLaren, 1998).

Group Therapy

REBT is particularly applicable to group therapy. Because group members are taught to apply REBT procedures to one another, they can help others learn the procedures and get practice (under the direct supervision of the group leader) in applying them. In group work, moreover, there is usually more opportunity for the members to agree on homework assignments (some of which are to be carried out in the group itself), to get assertiveness training, to engage in role playing, to interact with other people, to take verbal and nonverbal risks, to learn from the experiences of others, to interact therapeutically and socially with each other in after-group sessions and to have their behavior directly observed by the therapist and other group members (Ellis, 2001b; Ellis & Dryden, 1997).

REBT Workshops, Rational Encounter Marathons and Intensives

REBT has successfully used marathon encounter groups and large-scale one-day intensive workshops that include many verbal and nonverbal exercises, dramatic risk-taking procedures, evocative lectures, personal encounters, homework assignments, and other emotive and behavioral methods. Research studies have shown that these workshops, marathons, and intensive workshops have beneficial, immediate, and lasting effects (Ellis & Dryden, 1997; Ellis & Joffe, 2002).

Brief Therapy

REBT is naturally designed for brief therapy. It is preferable that individuals with severe disturbances come to individual and/or group sessions for at least 6 months. But for individuals who are going to stay in therapy for only a short while, REBT can teach them, in 1 to 10 sessions, the A–B–C method of understanding emotional problems, seeing their main philosophical source, and beginning to change fundamental disturbance-creating attitudes (Ellis, 2001b).

This is particularly true for the person who has a specific problem—such as hostility toward a boss or sexual inadequacy—and who is not too *generally* disturbed. Such an individual can, with the help of REBT, be almost completely "cured" in a few sessions. But even clients with long-standing difficulties may be significantly helped as a result of brief therapy.

Two special devices often employed in REBT can help speed the therapeutic process. The first is to tape the entire session. These recordings are then listened to, usually several times, by the clients in their own home, car, or office, so that they can more clearly see their problems and the rational emotive behavioral way of handling them. Many clients who have difficulty "hearing" what goes on during the face-to-face sessions (because they are too intent on talking themselves, are easily distracted, or are too anxious) are able to get more from listening to a recording of these sessions than from the original encounter.

Second, an REBT Self-Help Form is frequently used with clients to help teach them how to use the method when they encounter emotional problems between therapy sessions or after therapy has ended. This form is reproduced on pages 226–227.

Marriage and Family Therapy

From its beginning, REBT has been used extensively in marriage and family counseling (Ellis, 1962, 2001b; Ellis & Dryden, 1997; Ellis & Harper, 1997, 2003). Usually, marital or love partners are seen together. REBT therapists listen to their complaints about each other and then try to show that even if the complaints are justified, making themselves unduly upset is not. Work is done with either or both participants to minimize anxiety, depression, guilt, and (especially) hostility. As they begin to learn and apply the REBT principles, they usually become much less disturbed, often within a few sessions, and then are much better able to minimize their incompatibilities and maximize their compatibilities.

Sometimes, of course, they decide that they would be better off separated or divorced, but usually they decide to work at their problems to achieve a happier marital arrangement. They are frequently taught contracting, compromising, communication, and other relating skills. The therapist is concerned with both of them as individuals who can be helped emotionally, whether or not they decide to stay together. But the more they work at helping themselves, the better their relationship tends to become (Ellis, 2001b; Ellis & Crawford, 2000; Ellis & Harper, 2003).

In family therapy, REBT practitioners sometimes see all members of the same family together, see the children in one session and the parents in another, or see them all individually. Several joint sessions are usually held to observe the interactions among family members. Whether together or separately, parents are frequently shown how to accept their children and to stop condemning them, and children are similarly shown that they can accept their parents and their siblings. The general REBT principles of unconditionally accepting oneself and others are repeatedly taught. As is common with other REBT procedures, bibliotherapy supplements counseling with REBT materials such as *A Guide to Rational Living* (Ellis & Harper, 1997), *A Rational Counseling Primer* (Young, 1974), *How to Make Yourself Happy and Remarkably Less Disturbable* (Ellis, 1999), and *Feeling Better, Getting Better, Staying Better* (Ellis, 2001a), and *The Myth of Self-Esteem* (Ellis, 2005).

The *setting* of REBT sessions is much like that for other types of therapy. Most individual sessions take place in an office, but there may well be no desk between the therapist and the client, and REBT therapists tend to be informally dressed and to use simple language. They tend to be more open, authentic, and less "professional" than the average therapist. The main special equipment used is a tape recorder. The client is likely to be encouraged to make a recording of the session to take home for replaying.

REBT therapists are highly active, give their own views without hesitation, usually answer direct questions about their personal lives, are quite energetic and often directive in group therapy, and do a good deal of speaking, particularly during early sessions. At the same time, they unconditionally accept clients. They may engage in considerable explaining, interpreting, and "lecturing" and may easily work with clients they personally do not like. Because they tend to have complete tolerance for all individuals, REBT therapists are often seen as warm and caring by their clients.

Resistance is usually handled by showing clients that they resist changing because they would like to find a magical, easy solution rather than work at changing themselves. Resistance is not usually interpreted as their particular feelings about the therapist. If a client tries to seduce a therapist, this is usually explained not in terms of "transference" but in terms of (1) the client's need for love, (2) normal attraction to a helpful person, and (3) the natural sex urges of two people who have intimate mental–emotional contact. If the therapist is attracted to the client, he or she usually admits the attraction but explains why it is unethical to have sexual or personal relations with a client (Ellis, 2002).

Evidence

REBT has directly or indirectly inspired scores of experiments to test its theories, and there are now hundreds of research studies that tend to validate its major theoretical hypotheses (Ellis & Whiteley, 1979). More than 200 outcome studies have been published showing that REBT is effective in changing the thoughts, feelings, and behaviors of groups of individuals with various kinds of disturbances (DiGiuseppe, Terjesen, Rose, Doyle, & Vadalakis, 1998). These studies tend to show that REBT disputing and other methods usually work better than no therapy and are often more effective than other forms of psychotherapy (DiGiuseppe, Miller, & Trexler, 1979; Engels, Garnefski, & Diekstra, 1993; Haaga & Davison, 1993; Hajzler & Bernard, 1991; Jorn, 1989; Lyons & Woods, 1991; McGovern & Silverman, 1984; Silverman et al., 1992).

Applications of REBT to special kinds of clients have also been shown to be effective. It has yielded particularly good results with individuals who have anger disorders (Ellis, 2003a), with religious clients (Nielsen, Johnson, & Ellis, 2001), and with school-children (Seligman, Revich, Jaycox, & Gillham, 1995).

In addition, hundreds of other outcome studies done by cognitive therapists—particularly by Aaron Beck (Alford & Beck, 1997) and his associates—also support the clinical hypothesis of REBT. Finally, more than 1,000 other investigations have shown that the irrationality scales derived from Ellis's original list of irrational beliefs significantly correlate with the diagnostic disorders with which these scales have been tested (Hollon & Beck, 1994; Woods, 1992). Although much has yet to be learned about the effectiveness of REBT and other cognitive–behavior therapies, the research results so far are impressive.

Individual Evaluations

REBT therapists may use various diagnostic instruments and psychological tests, and they especially employ tests of irrationality, such as the Jones Irrational Beliefs Test, the Beck Depression Inventory, and the Dysfunctional Attitude Scale. Many of these tests have been shown to have considerable reliability and validity in controlled experiments.

Psychotherapy in a Multicultural World

It is important for all therapists to appreciate the multicultural aspects of psychotherapy, since this is a vital issue (Sue & Sue, 2003). REBT has always taken a multicultural position and promotes flexibility and open-mindedness so that practitioners who use it can deal with clients who follow different family, religious, and cultural customs. This is because it practically never gets people to dispute or discard their cultural goals, values, and ideals but only their grandiose insistences that these goals *absolutely must* be achieved.

Suppose a client lives in an American city populated largely by middle-class white Protestant citizens, and she is a relatively poor, dark-skinned, Pakistani-born Muslim. She will naturally have some real differences with her neighbors and coworkers and may upset herself about these differences. Her REBT therapist would give her unconditional acceptance, even though the therapist was a member of the majority group in the client's region and viewed some of her views and leanings as "peculiar." Her cultural and religious values would be respected as being legitimate and good for her, in spite of her differences with her community's values.

This client would be supported in following her goals and purposes—as long as she was willing to accept the consequences of displeasing some of the townspeople by sticking to them. She could be shown, with REBT, how to refuse to put herself down

REBT Self-Help Form

A (ACTIVATING EVENTS OR ADVERSITIES)

- Briefly summarize the situation you are disturbed about (what would a camera see?)
- An A can be *internal* or *external, real* or *imagined.*
- An A can be an event in the *past, present,* or *future.*

IBs (IRRATIONAL BELIEFS)

D (DISPUTING IBs)

To identify IBs, look for

- Dogmatic Demands
  (musts, absolutes, shoulds)

- Awfulizing
  (It's awful, terrible, horrible)

- Low Frustration Tolerance
  (I can't stand it)

- Self/Other Rating
  (I'm/he is/she is bad, worthless)

To dispute, ask yourself:

- Where is holding this belief getting me? Is it *helpful* or *self-defeating?*

- Where is the evidence to support the existence of my irrational belief? Is it *consistent with social reality?*

- Is my belief *logical?* Does it follow from my preferences?

- Is it really *awful* (as bad as it could be)?

- Can I really not *stand* it?

REBT Self-Help Form (*continued*)

C (CONSEQUENCES)

Major unhealthy negative **emotions:**

Major self-defeating **behaviors:**

Unhealthy negative emotions include

- Anxiety
- Depression
- Rage
- Low Frustration Tolerance
- Shame/Embarrassment
- Hurt
- Jealousy
- Guilt

E (EFFECTIVE NEW PHILOSOPHIES)

E (EFFECTIVE EMOTIONS & BEHAVIORS)

New healthy
negative emotions:

New constructive
behaviors:

To think more rationally, strive for:

- Non-Dogmatic Preferences
  (wishes, wants, desires)

- Evaluating Badness
  (it's bad, unfortunate)

- High Frustration Tolerance
  (I don't like it, but I can stand it)

- Not Globally Rating Self or Others
  (I—and others—are fallible human
  beings)

Healthy negative emotions include:

- Disappointment
- Concern
- Annoyance
- Sadness
- Regret
- Frustration

if she suffered from community criticism, and her "peculiar" cultural and religious ways would be questioned only if they were so rigidly held that they interfered with her basic aims.

Thus, if she flouted the social–sexual mores of her own religion and culture and concluded that she was worthless for not following them perfectly, she would be shown that it was her rigid demand that she *absolutely must* inflexibly adhere to them that was leading to her feelings of worthlessness and depression. If she changed her *must* to a *preference,* she could choose to follow or not to follow these cultural rules and not feel worthless and depressed.

REBT, then, has three main principles relevant to cross-cultural psychotherapy:

(1) Clients can unconditionally accept themselves and other individuals and can achieve high frustration tolerance when faced with life adversities. (2) If the therapist follows these rules and encourages her or his clients to follow them and to lead a flexible life, multicultural problems may sometimes exist but can be resolved with minimum intercultural and intracultural prejudice. (3) Most multicultural issues involve bias and intolerance, which REBT particularly works against (see *The Road to Tolerance*, Ellis, 2004).

Client Problems

No matter what the presenting problem may be, REBT therapists first help clients to express their disturbed emotional and behavioral reactions to their practical difficulties and to see and tackle the basic ideas or philosophies that underlie these reactions. This is apparent in the course of workshops for executives. In these workshops, the executives constantly bring up business, management, organizational, personal, and other problems. But they are shown that these practical problems often are tied to their self-defeating belief systems, and it is *this* problem that REBT mainly helps them resolve (Ellis, Gordon, Neenan, & Palmer, 1998).

Some individuals, however, may be so inhibited or defensive that they do not permit themselves to feel and therefore may not even be aware of some of their underlying emotional problems. Thus, the successful executive who comes for psychological help only because his wife insists they have a poor relationship and who claims that nothing really bothers him other than his wife's complaints may have to be jolted out of his complacency by direct confrontation. REBT group therapy may be particularly helpful for such an individual so that he finally expresses underlying anxieties and resentments and begins to acknowledge that he has emotional problems.

Extreme emotionalism in the course of REBT sessions—such as crying, psychotic behavior, and violent expressions of suicidal or homicidal intent—are naturally difficult to handle. But therapists handle these problems by their own, presumably rational philosophy of life and therapy, which includes these ideas: (1) Client outbursts make things difficult, but they are hardly *awful, terrible,* or *catastrophic.* (2) Behind each outburst is some irrational idea. Now, what is this idea? How can it be brought to the client's attention and what can be done to help change it? (3) No therapist can possibly help every client all the time. If this particular client cannot be helped and has to be referred elsewhere or lost to therapy, this is unfortunate. But it does not mean that the therapist is a failure.

REBT therapists usually handle clients' profound depressions by showing them, as quickly, directly, and vigorously as possible, that they are probably creating or exacerbating their depression by (1) blaming themselves for what they have done or not done, (2) castigating themselves for being depressed and inert, and (3) bemoaning their fate because of the hassles and harshness of environmental conditions. Their self-condemnation is not only revealed but firmly disputed, and in the meantime, the therapist may give clients reassurance and support, may refer them for supplementary medication, may speak to their relatives or friends to enlist their aid, and may recommend temporary withdrawal from some activities. Through an immediate and direct disputing of clients' extreme self-deprecation and self-pity, the therapist often helps deeply depressed and suicidal people in a short period.

The most difficult clients are usually the chronic avoiders or shirkers who keep looking for magical solutions. These individuals are shown that no such magic exists; that if they do not want to work hard to get better, it is their privilege to keep suffering; and that they are not *terrible persons* for goofing off but could live much more enjoyably if they worked at helping themselves. To help them get going, a form of people-involved therapy, such as group therapy, is frequently a method of choice. Results with unresponsive clients are still relatively poor in REBT (and in virtually all other therapies), but persistence and vigor on the part of the therapist often eventually overcome this kind of resistance (Ellis, 1994, 2002; Ellis & Tafrate, 1998).

CASE EXAMPLE

This section is relatively brief because it concerns the 25-year-old computer programmer whose initial session was presented in this chapter (pp. 214–220). Other case material on this client follows.

Background

Sara came from an Orthodox Jewish family. Her mother died in childbirth when Sara was 2 years of age, so Sara was raised by a loving but strict and somewhat remote father and a dominating paternal grandmother. She did well in school but had few friends up to and through college. Although fairly attractive, she was always ashamed of her body, did little dating, and occupied herself mainly with her work. At the age of 25, she was head of a section in a data processing firm. She was highly sexed and masturbated several times a week, but she had had intercourse with a man only once, when she was too drunk to know what she was doing. She had been overeating and overdrinking steadily since her college days. She had had 3 years of classical psychoanalysis. She thought her analyst was "a very kind and helpful man," but she had not really been helped by the process. She was quite disillusioned about therapy as a result of this experience and returned to it only because the president of her company, who liked her a great deal, told her that he would no longer put up with her constant drinking and insisted that she come to see the author of this chapter.

Treatment

Treatment continued for six sessions along the same lines indicated in the transcript included previously in this chapter. This was followed by 24 weeks of REBT group therapy and a weekend-long rational encounter marathon.

Cognitively, the client was shown repeatedly that her central problem was that she devoutly believed she *had* to be almost perfect and that she *must not* be criticized in any major way by significant others. She was persistently shown, instead, how to refrain from rating her *self* but only to measure her *performances;* to see that she could never be, except by arbitrary definition, a "worm" even if she never succeeded in overcoming her overeating, compulsive drinking, and foolish symptoms; to see that it was highly desirable but not necessary that she relate intimately to a man and win the approval of her peers and her bosses at work; and first to accept herself *with* her hostility and then to give up her childish *demands* on others that led her to be so hostile to them. Although she devoutly believed in the "fact" that she and others *should* be extremely efficient and follow strict disciplinary rules, and although time and again she resisted the therapist's and the group members' assaults against her moralistic *shoulds,* she was finally induced to replace them, in her vocabulary as well as in her internalized beliefs, with *it would be betters.* She claimed to have completely overthrown her original religious orthodoxy, but she was shown that she had merely replaced it with an inordinate demand for certainty in her personal life and in world affairs, and she was finally induced to give this up, too (Ellis, 2003b).

Emotively, Sara was fully accepted by the therapist *as a person,* even though he strongly assailed many of her *ideas* and sometimes humorously reduced them to absurdity. She was assertively confronted by some of the group members, who helped her see how she was angrily condemning other group members for their stupidities and their shirking, and she was encouraged to accept these "bad" group members (as well as people outside the group) in spite of their inadequacies. The therapist, and some of the others in her group and in the marathon weekend of rational encounter in which she participated, used vigorous, down-to-earth language with her. This initially horrified Sara, but she later began to loosen up and to use similar language. When she went on a drinking bout for a few weeks and felt utterly depressed and hopeless, two group members brought out their own previous difficulties with alcohol and drugs and showed how they had managed to get through that almost impossible period in their lives. Another member gave her steady support through many phone calls and visits. At times when she clammed up and sulked, the therapist and other group members pushed her to open up and voice her real feelings. Then they went after her defenses, revealed her foolish ideas (especially the idea that she had to be terribly hurt if others rejected her), and showed how these could be uprooted. During the marathon, she was able, for the first time in her life, to let herself be really touched emotionally by a man who, up to that time, was a perfect stranger to her, and this showed her that she could afford to let down her long-held barriers to intimacy and allow herself to love.

Behaviorally, Sara was given homework assignments that included talking to attractive men in public places and thereby overcoming her fears of being rejected. She was shown how to stay on a long-term diet (which she had never done before) by allowing herself rewarding experiences (such as listening to classical music) only when she had first maintained her diet for a certain number of hours. Through role playing with the therapist and other group members, she was given training in being assertive with people at work and in her social life without being aggressive (Ellis, 2003a; Wolfe, 1992).

Resolution

Sara progressed in several ways: (1) She stopped drinking completely, lost 25 pounds, and appeared to be maintaining both her sobriety and her weight loss. (2) She became considerably less condemnatory of both herself and others and began to make some close friends. (3) She had satisfactory sexual relations with three different men and began to date one of them steadily. (4) She only rarely made herself guilty or depressed, accepted herself with her failings, and began to focus much more on enjoying than on rating herself.

Follow-Up

Sara had REBT individual and group sessions for 6 months and occasional follow-up sessions the next year. She married her steady boyfriend about a year after she had originally begun treatment, after having two premarital counseling sessions with him following their engagement. Two and a half years after the close of therapy, she and her husband reported that everything was going well in their marriage, at her job, and in their social life. Her husband seemed particularly appreciative of the use she was making of REBT principles and noted, "she still works hard at what she learned with you and the group and, frankly, I think that she keeps improving, because of this work, all the time." She smilingly and enthusiastically agreed.

SUMMARY

Rational emotive behavior therapy (REBT) is a comprehensive system of personality change that incorporates cognitive, emotive, and behavior therapy methods. It is based on a clear-cut theory of emotional health and disturbance, and the many techniques it employs are usually related to that theory. Its major hypotheses also apply to childrearing, education, social and political affairs, the extension of people's intellectual and emotional frontiers, and support of their unique potential for growth. REBT psychology is hardheaded, empirically oriented, rational, and nonmagical. It fosters the use of reason, science, and technology. It is humanistic, existentialist, and hedonistic. It aims for reduced emotional disturbance as well as increased growth and self-actualization in people's intrapersonal and interpersonal lives.

REBT theory holds that people are biologically and culturally predisposed to choose, create, and enjoy, but that they are also strongly predisposed to overconform, be suggestible, hate, and foolishly block their enjoying. Although they have remarkable capacities to observe, reason, imaginatively enhance their experiencing, and transcend some of their own essential limitations, they also have strong tendencies to ignore social reality, misuse reason, and invent absolutist *musts* that frequently sabotage their health and happiness. Because of their refusals to accept social reality, their continual *must*urbation, and their absorption in deifying and devilifying themselves and others, people frequently wind up with emotional disturbances.

When noxious stimuli occur in people's lives at point A (their adversities), they usually observe these events objectively and conclude, at point rB (their rational belief), that this event is unfortunate, inconvenient, and disadvantageous and that they wish it would change. Then they healthily feel, at point C (the consequence), sad, regretful, frustrated, or annoyed. These healthy negative feelings usually help them to try to do something about their adversities to improve or change them. Their inborn and acquired hedonism and constructivism encourage them to have, in regard to adversities, rational thoughts ("I don't like this; let's see what I can do to change it") and healthy negative feelings (sorrow and annoyance) that enable them to reorder their environment and to live more enjoyably.

Very often, however, when similar adversities occur in people's lives, they observe these events intolerantly and grandiosely and conclude, at point iB (their irrational beliefs), that these events are awful, horrible, and catastrophic; that they *must* not exist; and that they absolutely cannot stand them. They then self-defeatingly feel the consequence, at point C, of worthlessness, guilt, anxiety, depression, rage, and inertia. Their disturbed feelings usually interfere with their doing something constructive about the adversities, and they tend to condemn themselves for their unconstructiveness and to experience more feelings of shame, inferiority, and hopelessness. Their inborn and acquired self-critical, antihumanistic, and deifying and devilifying philosophies encourage them to have, in regard to unfortunate activating events, foolish thoughts ("How awful this is and I am! There's nothing I can do about it!") and dysfunctional feelings (hatred of themselves, of others, and of the world) that encourage them to whine and rant and live less enjoyably.

REBT is a cognitive–emotive–behavioristic method of psychotherapy uniquely designed to enable people to observe, understand, and persistently dispute their irrational, grandiose, perfectionistic *shoulds, oughts,* and *musts* and their *awfulizing.* It employs the logico-empirical method of science to encourage people to surrender magic, absolutes, and damnation; to acknowledge that nothing is sacred or all-important (although many things are exceptionally unpleasant and inconvenient); and to gradually teach themselves and to practice the philosophy of desiring rather than demanding and of working at changing what they can change and gracefully accepting what they cannot change about themselves, about others, and about the world (Ellis, 1994, 2002; Ellis & Blau, 1998; Ellis & Dryden, 1997; Ellis & MacLaren, 1998).

In conclusion, rational emotive behavior therapy is a method of personality change that quickly and efficiently helps people resist their tendencies to be too conforming, suggestible, and anhedonic. It actively and didactically, as well as emotively and behaviorally, shows people how to abet and enhance one side of their humanness while simultaneously changing and living more happily with (and not repressing or squelching) another side. It is thus realistic and practical as well as idealistic and future oriented. It helps individuals to more fully actualize, experience, and enjoy the here and now, but it also espouses long-range hedonism, which includes planning for their own (and others') future. It is what its name implies: rational *and* emotive *and* behavioral, realistic *and* visionary, empirical *and* humanistic. As, in all their complexity, are humans.

ANNOTATED BIBLIOGRAPHY

Web sites

Dr. Debbie Joffe Ellis, www.debbiejoffeellis.com
Friends of Albert Ellis, www.albert-ellis-friends.net
REBT Network, www.rebtnetwork.org

Books

Ellis, A. (2004). *Rational emotive behavior therapy—it works for me—it can work for you.* Amherst, NY: Prometheus Books. This autobiographical book presents an excellent overview of the life and work of Albert Ellis.

Ellis, A. (2004). *The road to tolerance: The philosophy of rational emotive behavior therapy.* Amherst, NY: Prometheus Books. This book reviews the theoretical underpinnings of REBT and advocates tolerance for and patience with the all-too-common shortcomings of human beings.

Ellis, A. (2005). *The myth of self-esteem.* New York: Prometheus Books.
The book provides an overview of Ellis's approach to life and psychotherapy and REBT's emphasis on unconditional acceptance, and it gives some insight into the breadth of his intellect. Separate chapters deal with Jean-Paul Sartre, Martin Heidegger, Martin Buber, D. T. Suzuki, and Zen Buddhism.

Ellis, A. (2010). *All out! An autobiography.* Amherst, NY: Prometheus Books.
Albert Ellis's last work, this fascinating, candid, and substantial autobiography includes memorable episodes, descriptions of the important people in his life, the way he coped with difficulties, his developing of REBT, his love life, and personal reflections.

Ellis, A., & Dryden, W. (1997). *The practice of rational emotive behavior therapy.* New York: Springer.
This book presents the general theory and basic practice of rational emotive behavior therapy (REBT), with special chapters on how it is used in individual, couples, family, group, and sex therapy. It brings the original seminal book on REBT, *Reason and Emotion in Psychotherapy* (Ellis, 1962) up to date and gives many details about REBT therapy procedures.

Ellis, A., & Harper, R. A. (1997). *A guide to rational living.* North Hollywood, CA: Wilshire Books.
This completely revised and rewritten version of the REBT self-help classic is one of the most widely read self-help books ever published, and it is often recommended by cognitive–behavior therapists to their clients. It is a succinct, straightforward approach to REBT based on self-questioning and homework and shows how readers can help themselves with various emotional problems.

CASE READINGS

Ellis, A. (1971). A twenty-three-year-old woman, guilty about not following her parents' rules. In A. Ellis, *Growth through reason: Verbatim cases in rational-emotive therapy* (pp. 223–286). Hollywood: Wilshire Books. [Reprinted in D. Wedding & R. J. Corsini (Eds.). (2011). *Case studies in psychotherapy.* Belmont, CA: Brooks/Cole.]

> Ellis presents a verbatim protocol of the first, second, and fourth sessions with a woman who comes for help because she is self-punishing, impulsive and compulsive, and afraid of males, has no goals in life, and is guilty about her relations with her parents. The therapist quickly zeroes in on her main problems and shows her that she need not feel guilty about doing what she wants to do in life, even if her parents keep upsetting themselves about her beliefs and actions.

Ellis, A. (1977). Verbatim psychotherapy session with a procrastinator. In A. Ellis & W. J. Knaus, *Overcoming procrastination* (pp. 152–167). New York: New American Library.

Ellis presents a single verbatim session with a procrastinator who was failing to finish her doctoral thesis in sociology. He deals with her problems in a direct, no-nonsense manner typical of rational emotive behavior therapy, and she later reports that as a result of a single session, she finished her thesis, although she had previously been procrastinating on it for a number of years.

Ellis, A., & Dryden, W. (1996). Transcript of a demonstration session, with comments on the session by Windy Dryden and Albert Ellis. In W. Dryden, *Practical skills in rational emotive behavior therapy* (pp. 91–117). London: Whurr.

Ellis presents a verbatim protocol with a therapist who volunteers to bring up problems of feeling inadequate as a therapist and as a person. Albert Ellis shows her some core beliefs leading to her self-downing and how to actively dispute and surrender these beliefs. Ellis and Windy Dryden then review the protocol to analyze its REBT aspects.

REFERENCES

Adler, A. (1931). *What life should mean to you.* New York: Blue Ribbon Books.

Adler, A. (1964). *Social interest: A challenge to mankind.* New York: Capricorn.

Alford, B. A., & Beck, A. T. (1997). *The integrative power of cognitive therapy.* New York: Guilford Press.

Beck, A.T. (1976). *Cognitive therapy and the emotional disorders.* New York: International Universities Press.

Bernard, M. E., & Wolfe, J. W. (Eds.). (1993). *The RET resource book for practitioners.* New York: Institute for Rational-Emotive Therapy.

Butler, A. C., Chapman, J. E., Forman, E. M., & Beck. A. T. (2005). The empirical status of cognitive–behavioral therapy: A review of meta-analyses. *Clinical Psychology Review, 26*(1), 17–31.

Corsini, R. J. (2005, January 5). The incredible Albert Ellis. [Review of the book *Rational emotive behavior therapy—It works for me—It can work for you.*] *PsycCRITIQUES: Contemporary Psychology—APA Review of Books, 50,* Article 2. Retrieved September 9, 2006, from the *PsycCRITIQUES* database.

DiGiuseppe, R. A., Miller, N. K., & Trexler, L. D. (1979). A review of rational-emotive psychotherapy outcome studies. In A. Ellis & J. M. Whiteley (Eds.), *Theoretical and empirical foundations of rational-emotive therapy* (pp. 218–235). Monterey, CA: Brooks/Cole.

DiGiuseppe, R. A., Terjesen, M., Rose, R., Doyle, K., & Vadalakis, N. (1998, August). *Selective abstractions errors in reviewing REBT outcome studies: A review of reviews.* Poster presented at the 106th Annual Convention of the American Psychological Association, San Francisco, CA.

Dryden, W., & David, D. (2008). Rational emotive behavior therapy: Current status. *Journal of Cognitive Psychotherapy: An International Quarterly, 22*(3), 195–209.

Ellis, A. (1962). *Reason and emotion in psychotherapy.* Secaucus, NJ: Citadel.

Ellis, A. (1976). The biological basis of human irrationality. *Journal of Individual Psychology, 32,* 145–168.

Ellis, A. (1994). *Reason and emotion in psychotherapy* (rev. ed.). New York: Citadel.

Ellis, A. (1998). *How to control your anxiety before it controls you.* New York: Citadel.

Ellis, A. (1999). *How to make yourself happy and remarkably less disturbable.* San Luis Obispo, CA: Impact Publishers.

Ellis, A. (2001a). *Feeling better, getting better, staying better.* Atascadero, CA: Impact Publishers.

Ellis, A. (2001b). *Overcoming destructive beliefs, feelings, and behaviors.* Amherst, NY: Prometheus Books.

Ellis, A. (2002). *Overcoming resistance: A rational emotive behavior therapy integrative approach.* New York: Springer.

Ellis, A. (2003a). *Anger: How to live with it and without it* (rev. ed.). New York: Citadel Press.

Ellis, A. (2003b). *Sex without guilt in the twenty-first century.* Teaneck, NJ: Battleside Books.

Ellis, A. (2004a). *Rational emotive behavior therapy: It works for me, it can work for you.* Amherst, NY: Prometheus Books.

Ellis, A. (2004b). *The road to tolerance: The philosophy of rational emotive behavior therapy.* Amherst, NY: Prometheus Books.

Ellis, A. (2005). *The myth of self-esteem.* Amherst, NY: Prometheus Books.

Ellis, A. (2002). *All out! An autobiography.* Amherst, NY: Prometheus Books.

Ellis, A., & Blau, S. (1998). (Eds.). *The Albert Ellis reader.* Secaucus, NJ: Carol Publishing Group.

Ellis, A., & Crawford, T. (2000). *Making intimate connections.* Atascadero, CA: Impact Publishers.

Ellis, A., & Dryden, W. (1996). Transcript of demonstration session. Commentary on Albert Ellis' demonstration session by Windy Dryden and Albert Ellis. In W. Dryden, *Practical skills in rational emotive behavior therapy* (pp. 91–117). London: Whurr.

Ellis, A., & Dryden, W. (1997). *The practice of rational emotive behavior therapy.* New York: Springer.

Ellis, A., Gordon, J., Neenan, M., & Palmer, S. (1998). *Stress counseling.* New York: Springer.

Ellis, A., & Harper, R. A. (1997). *A guide to rational living.* North Hollywood, CA: Melvin Powers.

Ellis, A., & Harper, R. A. (2003). *Dating, mating, and relating.* New York: Citadel.

Ellis, A., & Joffe, D. (2002). A study of volunteer clients who experience live sessions of rational emotive behavior therapy in front of a public audience. *Journal of Rational-Emotive and Cognitive-Behavior Therapy, 20,* 151–158.

Ellis, A., & MacLaren, C. (1998). *Rational emotive behavior therapy: A therapist's guide.* Atascadero, CA: Impact Publishers.

Ellis, A., & Tafrate, R. C. (1998). *How to control your anger before it controls you.* Secaucus, NJ: Birch Lane Press.

Ellis, A., & Whiteley, J. (1979). *Theoretical and empirical foundations of rational-emotive therapy.* Pacific Grove, CA: Brooks/Cole.

Engels, G. I., Garnefski, N., & Diekstra, R. F. W. (1993). Efficacy of rational-emotive therapy: A quantitative analysis. *Journal of Consulting & Clinical Psychology, 61,* 1083–1090.

Froh, J. J., Fives, C. K., Fuller, J. R., Jacofsky, M. D., Terjesen, M. D., & Yurkewicz, C. (2007). Interpersonal relationships and irrationality as predictors of life satisfaction. *Journal of Positive Psychology, 2*(1), 29–39.

Haaga, D. A. F., & Davison, G. C. (1993). An appraisal of rational-emotive therapy. *Journal of Consulting & Clinical Psychology, 61,* 215–220.

Hajzler, D., & Bernard, M. E. (1991). A review of rational emotive outcome studies. *School Psychology Studies, 6*(1), 27–49.

Hauck, P. A. (1992). *Overcoming the rating game: Beyond self-love—Beyond self-esteem.* Louisville, KY: Westminster/John Knox.

Hollon, S. D., & Beck, A. T. (1994). Cognitive and cognitive-behavioral therapies. In A. E. Bergin & S. L. Garfield (Eds.), *Handbook of psychotherapy and behavior change* (4th ed., pp. 428–466). New York: Wiley.

Jorn, A. F. (1989). Modifiability and neuroticism: A meta-analysis of the literature. *Australian and New Zealand Journal of Psychiatry, 23,* 21–29.

Lyons, L. C., & Woods, P. J. (1991). The efficacy of rational-emotive therapy: A quantitative review of the outcome research. *Clinical Psychology Review, 11,* 357–369.

Macaskill, N. D., & Macaskill, A. (1996). Rational-emotive therapy plus pharmacotherapy versus pharmacotherapy alone in the treatment of high cognitive dysfunction depression. *Cognitive Therapy and Research, 20,* 575–592.

McGovern, T. E., & Silverman, M. S. (1984). A review of outcome studies of rational-emotive therapy from 1977 to 1982. *Journal of Rational-Emotive Therapy, 2*(1), 7–18.

Nielsen, S., Johnson, W. B., & Ellis, A. (2001). *Counseling and psychotherapy with religious persons.* Mahwah, NJ: Erlbaum.

Rogers, C. R. (1961). *On becoming a person.* Boston: Houghton Mifflin.

Seligman, M. E. P., Revich, K., Jaycox, L., & Gillham, J. (1995). *The optimistic child.* Boston: Houghton Mifflin.

Shelley, A. M., Battaglia, J., Lucely, J., Ellis, A., & Opler, A. (2001). Symptom-specific group therapy for inpatients with schizophrenia. *Einstein Quarterly Journal of Biology and Medicine, 18,* 21–28.

Silverman, M. S., McCarthy, M., & McGovern, T. (1992). A review of outcome studies of rational-emotive therapy from 1982–1989. *Journal of Rational-Emotive and Cognitive-Behavior Therapy, 10*(3), 111–186.

Sue, D. W., & Sue, D. (2003). *Counseling with the culturally diverse.* New York: Wiley.

Vernon, A. (2001). *The passport program.* 3 vols. Champaign, IL: Research Press.

Walen, S. R., DiGiuseppe, R., & Dryden, W. (1992). *A practitioner's guide to rational-emotive therapy* (2nd ed.). New York: Oxford.

Wang, C., Jia, F., Fang, R., Zhu, Y., & Huang, Y. (1999). Comparative study of rational-emotive therapy for 95 patients with dysthymic disorder. *Chinese Mental Health Journal, 13,* 172–183.

Wolfe, J. L. (1992). *What to do when he has a headache.* New York: Hyperion.

Woods, P. J. (1992). A study of belief and non-belief items from the Jones Irrational Beliefs Test with implications for the theory of RET. *Journal of Rational-Emotive and Cognitive-Behavior Therapy, 10,* 41–52.

Young, H. S. (1974). *A rational counseling primer.* New York: Albert Ellis Institute.

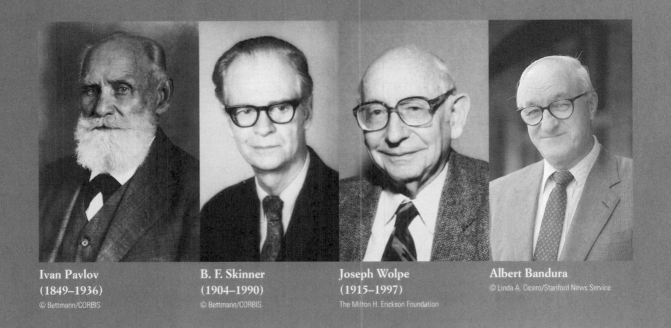

Ivan Pavlov
(1849–1936)
© Bettmann/CORBIS

B. F. Skinner
(1904–1990)
© Bettmann/CORBIS

Joseph Wolpe
(1915–1997)
The Milton H. Erickson Foundation

Albert Bandura
© Linda A. Cicero/Stanford News Service

7 | BEHAVIOR THERAPY

G. Terence Wilson

OVERVIEW

Behavior therapy is a relative newcomer on the psychotherapy scene. Not until the late 1950s did it emerge as a systematic approach to the assessment and treatment of psychological disorders. In its early stages, behavior therapy was defined as the application of modern learning theory to the treatment of clinical problems. The phrase *modern learning theory* referred to the principles and procedures of classical and operant conditioning. Behavior therapy was seen as the logical extension of behaviorism to complex forms of human activities.

Behavior therapy has undergone significant changes in both nature and scope, and it has been responsive to advances in experimental psychology and innovations in clinical practice. It has grown more complex and sophisticated. Behavior therapy can no longer be defined simply as the clinical application of classical and operant conditioning theory.

Behavior therapy today is marked by a diversity of views. It now comprises a broad range of heterogeneous procedures with different theoretical rationales and open debate about conceptual bases, methodological requirements, and evidence of efficacy. As behavior therapy expands, it increasingly overlaps with other psychotherapeutic approaches. Nevertheless, the basic concepts characteristic of the behavioral approach are clear and its commonalities with and differences from nonbehavioral therapeutic systems can be readily identified.

Basic Concepts

Traditionally, three main approaches in contemporary behavior therapy have been identified: (1) *applied behavior analysis,* (2) a *neobehavioristic mediational stimulus–response model,* and (3) *social–cognitive theory.* These three approaches differ in the extent to which they use cognitive concepts and procedures. At one end of this continuum is *applied behavior analysis,* which focuses exclusively on observable behavior and rejects all cognitive mediating processes. At the other end is *social–cognitive theory,* which relies heavily on cognitive theories.

Applied Behavior Analysis

This approach is a direct extension of Skinner's (1953) radical behaviorism. It relies on operant conditioning, the fundamental assumption being that behavior is a function of its consequences. Accordingly, treatment procedures are based on altering relationships between overt behaviors and their consequences. Applied behavior analysis makes use of reinforcement, punishment, extinction, stimulus control, and other procedures derived from laboratory research. Cognitive processes are considered private events and are not regarded as proper subjects of scientific analysis.

The Neobehavioristic Mediational Stimulus–Response (S–R) Model

This approach features the application of the principles of classical conditioning, and it derives from the learning theories of Ivan Pavlov, E. R. Guthrie, Clark Hull, O. H. Mowrer, and N. E. Miller. Unlike the operant approach, the S–R model is mediational, with intervening variables and hypothetical constructs prominently featured. S–R theorists have been particularly interested in the study of anxiety; the techniques of systematic desensitization and flooding, both closely associated with this model, are directed toward the extinction of the underlying anxiety assumed to maintain phobic disorders.

Private events, especially imagery, have been an integral part of this approach, including systematic desensitization. The rationale is that covert processes follow the laws of learning that govern overt behaviors.

Social–Cognitive Theory

The social–cognitive approach depends on the theory that behavior is based on three separate but interacting regulatory systems (Bandura, 1986). They are (1) external stimulus events, (2) external reinforcement, and (3) cognitive mediational processes.

In the social–cognitive approach, the influence of environmental events on behavior is largely determined by cognitive processes governing how environmental influences are perceived and how the individual interprets them. Psychological functioning, according to this view, involves a reciprocal interaction among three interlocking sets of influences: behavior, cognitive processes, and environmental factors. Bandura put it as follows:

> Personal and environmental factors do not function as independent determinants; rather, they determine each other. Nor can "persons" be considered causes independent of their behavior. It is largely through their actions that people produce the environmental conditions that affect their behavior in a reciprocal fashion. The experiences generated by behavior also partly determine what individuals think, expect, and can do, which in turn affect their subsequent behavior. (1977, p. 345)

In social–cognitive theory, the person is the agent of change. The theory emphasizes the human capacity for self-directed behavior change. Strongly influenced by the social–cognitive model, the clinical practice of behavior therapy has increasingly included cognitive methods, especially those described by Aaron Beck (see Chapter 8). A primary focus of both cognitive and behavioral techniques is to change the cognitive processes viewed as essential to therapeutic success. The basic assumption is that it is not so much experience itself but rather the person's interpretation of that experience that produces psychological disturbance. This position is also reflected in the work of Albert Ellis (see Chapter 6). Both cognitive and behavioral methods are used to modify faulty perceptions and interpretations of important life events. For these reasons, it is now common to refer to "cognitive behavior therapy" (CBT) instead of "behavior therapy." As Jacobson (1987) pointed out, "incorporation of cognitive theory and therapy into behavior therapy has been so total that it is difficult to find pure behavior therapists working with outpatients" (pp. 4–5). The term "behavior therapy" is used throughout this chapter, although it could just as easily be replaced with "CBT." Behavior therapy, in a broad sense, refers to practice based primarily on social–cognitive theory and encompassing a range of cognitive principles and procedures.

Common Characteristics

Although the three preceding behavior therapy approaches involve conceptual differences, behavior therapists subscribe to a common core of basic concepts. The two foundations of behavior therapy are (1) a psychological model of human behavior that differs fundamentally from the traditional psychodynamic model, and (2) a commitment to the scientific method.

The emphasis on a psychological model of abnormal behavior and the commitment to a scientific approach have the following consequences:

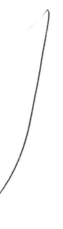

1. Many types of abnormal behavior formerly regarded as illnesses or as signs and symptoms of illness are better construed as nonpathological "problems of living" (key examples include anxiety reactions, as well as sexual and conduct disorders). This position is similar to that of Alfred Adler.

2. Most abnormal behavior is assumed to be acquired and maintained in the same manner as normal behavior. It can be treated through the application of behavioral procedures.

3. Behavioral assessment focuses on the current determinants of behavior rather than on the analysis of possible historical antecedents. Specificity is the hallmark of behavioral assessment and treatment, and it is assumed that the person is best understood and described by what the person does in a particular situation.

4. Treatment requires a prior analysis of the problem into components or subparts. Procedures are then systematically targeted at specific components.

5. Treatment strategies are individually tailored to different problems in different individuals.

6. Understanding the origins of a psychological problem is not essential for producing behavior change. Conversely, success in changing a problem behavior does not imply knowledge about its etiology.

7. Behavior therapy involves a commitment to the scientific method. This includes an explicit, testable conceptual framework; treatment derived from or at least consistent with the content and method of experimental–clinical psychology; therapeutic techniques that have measurable outcomes and can be replicated; the experimental evaluation of treatment methods and concepts; and emphasis on innovative research strategies that allow rigorous evaluation of specific methods applied to particular problems instead of global assessment of ill-defined procedures applied to heterogeneous problems.

The "Third Wave" of Behavior Therapy

Behavior therapy continues to evolve. The most recent developments, emerging in the 1990s and gathering momentum in the new century, have been labeled the "third wave" of behavior therapy by Hayes, Follette, and Linehan (2004). According to this view, the first wave of behavior therapy focused primarily on modifying overt behavior. The second wave was the emphasis on cognitive factors, resulting in what is known as cognitive behavior therapy (CBT). Hayes et al. (2004) and others, however, have argued that the cognitive revolution in behavior therapy did not adequately address the problems of people's private experience—their thoughts and feelings. Hayes has argued that cognitive theories in CBT have owed more to common-sense notions than to scientific analyses. The third wave comprises a group of therapeutic approaches with overlapping conceptual and technical foundations. The two most prominent forms of these developments are dialectical behavior therapy (DBT) (Linehan, 1993) and acceptance and commitment therapy (ACT) (Hayes, Luoma, Bond, Masuda, & Lillis, 2006).

Dialectical Behavior Therapy (DBT)

Acceptance and Change.   A defining feature of DBT is the focus on balancing the traditional emphasis on behavior change with the value of acceptance and the importance of the relationship between the two—which Linehan sees as the central dialectic of therapy. The following clinical example may clarify this point. Patients with an eating disorder typically define their self-worth in terms of body shape and weight in part because appearance and weight seem more controllable to them than other aspects of life. In reality, however, they have less control over changing body shape and weight than they wish. Nevertheless, these individuals resort to extreme and self-destructive behaviors in an effort to lose more weight than is healthy or even possible, such as starving themselves and self-inducing vomiting. The result is that they develop an eating disorder. By trying to change what cannot be changed, or what cannot be changed except by extreme measures that undermine health and psychological well-being, these individuals avoid making other important life changes. The solution would be to make nutritionally sound and psychologically adaptive lifestyle changes and then accept whatever shape and weight results. It is more feasible for these patients to make other changes in their lives, such as improving interpersonal relationships and coping more effectively with negative emotions.

Wilson (2004) likened this balancing of acceptance with change to the practical wisdom of the Serenity Prayer: "God, give me the serenity to accept the things I cannot change, the courage to change the things I can, and the wisdom to know the difference." It is important to understand that the concept of acceptance does not mean giving up or resigning yourself to life's problems. Rather, Linehan emphasizes that it is an active process of self-affirmation. Similarly, Hayes and Smith (2005) explain that acceptance can be viewed as a willingness to choose to experience negative thoughts or feelings without defense.

Mindfulness.   DBT makes use of typical behavior therapy techniques and strategies as summarized above. But a distinctive and seminal therapeutic strategy in DBT is mindfulness training. Mindfulness consists of five core skills:

1. *Observe or attend to emotions without trying to terminate them when painful.* "What the client learns here is to allow herself to experience with awareness, in the moment, whatever is happening, rather than leaving a situation or trying to terminate an emotion. Generally, the ability to attend to events requires a corresponding ability to step back from the event. Observing an event is separate or different from the event itself" (Linehan, 1993, p. 63).

2. *Describe a thought or emotion.* "Learning to describe requires that a person learn not to take emotions and thoughts literally—that is, as literal reflections of environmental events. For example, feeling afraid does not necessarily mean that a situation is threatening . . . thoughts are often taken literally; that is, thoughts ("I feel unloved") are confused with facts ("I am unloved")" (Linehan, 1993, p. 64).

3. *Be nonjudgmental.* The goal here is to take a nonjudgmental stance when observing, describing, and being aware of feelings and events. Judging is evaluating oneself or some experience as good or bad, as worthy or worthless.

4. *Stay in the present.* The principle here is to be aware of and stay in contact with immediate experience while at the same time achieving distance from it. Wiser and Telch (1999) give the example of watching "clouds moving across a sky; they are fully present with experience, but are also outside observing it" (p. 759).

5. *Focus on one thing at a time (one-mindfully).* For example, when eating, attend to the act and experience of eating without distractions such as watching TV or reading a book.

Linehan (1993) developed DBT primarily for treating borderline personality disorder. However, the basic concepts of DBT, such as acceptance and mindfulness, are now being applied to the treatment of a wide range of clinical problems including anxiety disorders, depression, and eating disorders (Hayes, Follette, & Linehan, 2004). Lynch & Cozza (2009) recently examined nonsuicidal self-injury (NSSI) from a behavioral perspective that regards negative emotions as the proximal cause of NSSI. The authors demonstrate how to conduct a functional analysis of NSSI and describe the utility of DBT in the treatment of this recalcitrant disorder.

Acceptance and Commitment Therapy (ACT)

ACT combines grounding in behaviorism with an innovative, post-Skinnerian account of language and cognition and how they are involved in psychopathology (Hayes et al., 2006). The details of the specific theory of language that is behind ACT, called relational frame theory, are beyond the scope of the present chapter. The focus here is on core therapeutic principles.

Experiential Avoidance. Experiential avoidance refers to the process of trying to avoid negative or distressing private experiences, such as thoughts, feelings, memories, and sensations. The basic principle is that experiential avoidance ultimately does not work—in fact, it is more likely to make matters worse. For example, there is evidence showing that attempts to suppress negative or unwanted thoughts will, in due course, produce an increase in the very thoughts you want to avoid. In one study, patients with anxiety and mood disorders were shown a brief, emotion-provoking film (Campbell-Sills, Barlow, Brown, & Hofmann, 2006). One group was instructed to suppress their emotional reactions to the film. The other group were asked to experience their emotions fully and not to struggle to control them in any way. The results showed that the suppression group suffered from greater distress after the film and also showed greater physiological arousal than the acceptance group during the film.

Experiential avoidance is seen to be pervasive across different clinical disorders (Harvey, Watkins, Mansell, & Shafran, 2004). According to Hayes et al. (2006), there are two main reasons. First, in the outside world (outside of the body), it makes sense to avoid or change what is bad. For example, if you are trapped in a dysfunctional relationship, the effective course of action is to end the relationship or to work actively on repairing it. Rational problem solving and thoughtful action are the most effective ways of solving this problem. Second, techniques like distraction or suppression of thoughts or feelings often do work in the short term. The trouble is that these are maladaptive coping strategies in the long term. For a young person plagued by self-doubt and low self-esteem, alcohol or drug use might well provide a quick fix, but these methods only add to her problems over time.

Acceptance.   ACT is designed to help patients learn that experiential avoidance does not work, and that it is part of the problem rather than the solution. Patients need to learn how to accept the thoughts and feelings they have been trying to get rid of. The goal of acceptance in ACT is essentially the same as in DBT, and mindfulness is taught in both systems. Treatment employs various experiential exercises during therapy sessions and, as with behavior therapy in general, uses homework assignments designed to help patients discover the benefits of acceptance over avoidance.

Cognitive Defusion.   This concept refers to separating thoughts from their referents and differentiating the thinker from the thoughts. It means not taking thoughts as inherent aspects of self or as necessarily valid reflections of reality. For example, the thought "I am so fat" is very different from the thought "I am not fat, but a normal-weight person who experiences thoughts/feelings that she is fat." The latter is more defused than the former, and much less distressing. This is similar to the practice of describing feelings in mindfulness training in DBT. The assumption is that learning how to defuse language promotes acceptance and being in the present, and thus helps clients overcome psychological problems. Defusion is basically the same concept as that of distancing, which is described in Aaron Beck's chapter on cognitive therapy (Chapter 8).

Commitment.   ACT focuses on action. Commitment in this context refers to making mindful decisions about what is important in your life and what you are going to do in order to live a valued life. Therapy involves helping patients choose the values they hold dear, setting specific goals, and taking concrete steps to achieve these goals.

ACT is increasingly being adapted to a wide range of clinical problems. One of the reasons for its popularity among clinicians is its foundation in core therapeutic principles that are linked to psychological science and have broad applicability to different disorders. It emphasizes common processes across clinical disorders, making it easier to teach fundamental treatment skills. Clinicians are then free to implement these basic principles in diverse and creative ways.

Other Systems

Behavior therapy has much in common with other psychological therapies, particularly those that tend to be brief and directive. In some cases, behavior therapy has borrowed concepts and methods from other systems. For example, cognitive behavioral treatment strategies have incorporated some of the concepts of Albert Ellis's rational emotive behavior therapy and especially Beck's cognitive therapy (O'Leary & Wilson, 1987). CBT is closer to Beck's cognitive therapy than Ellis's approach because Beck emphasizes the importance of behavioral procedures in correcting the dysfunctional beliefs assumed to cause emotional distress. Ellis's REBT, despite the later inclusion of *behavior* in the name, is mainly a semantic treatment in which the goal is to alter the person's basic philosophy of life through reason and logic. The overlap between BT and Beck's cognitive therapy is extensive. Both systems include cognitive and behavioral components but may differ in how these components are combined and especially in their theories about mechanisms of therapeutic change (Hollon & Beck, 1994).

Despite substantial overlap between behavior therapy and Beck's cognitive therapy, there are important theoretical and practical differences between certain forms of BT and cognitive therapy. For example, the emphasis on acceptance in DBT and ACT is inconsistent with the major cognitive therapy technique of challenging or disputing specific thoughts and beliefs. In addition, the focus in more behaviorally oriented treatments is on the function of cognitions rather than their content as in cognitive therapy. Consider the following illustration. A common belief for someone who is depressed would be "I am worthless and incompetent at everything I do." As opposed to questioning the accuracy or validity of this belief as in cognitive therapy, the behavioral activation approach to treating depression (see below) would focus on its impact on behavior. A functional analysis would be conducted to identify the conditions under which the thought occurred and what happened as a result of the thought. The person would then be helped to act differently in those situations (Martell, Addis, & Jacobson, 2001).

In terms of clinical practice, behavior therapy and multimodal therapy are similar. The majority of the techniques that Arnold Lazarus (1981) lists as the most frequently used in multimodal therapy (see Chapter 11) are standard behavior therapy strategies. This is not surprising, given that Lazarus (1971) was one of the pioneers of clinical behavior therapy.

Therapists are guided in their formulations and treatment of different problems either by clearly stated principles or by their personal experience and intuition. Behavior therapy represents an attempt to move beyond idiosyncratic practices and to base clinical practice on secure scientific foundations. This does not mean that clinical practice by behavior therapists is always based on solid empirical evidence. Behavior therapists, not unlike therapists from other approaches, have developed their own clinical lore, much of which is not based on experimental research. Lacking sufficient information and guidelines from research, behavior therapists often adopt a trial-and-error approach. Nonetheless, behavior therapy is clearly linked to a specifiable and testable conceptual framework.

Behavior therapy differs fundamentally from psychodynamic approaches to treatment. Based on a learning or educational model of human development, it rejects the psychoanalytic model, in which abnormal behavior is viewed as a symptom of underlying unconscious conflicts. Psychoanalytic therapy has difficulty explaining the successes of behavior therapy that contradict basic concepts that psychoanalysts claim are crucial for therapeutic change. Some psychodynamic therapists state that behavioral treatments result in symptom substitution because behavioral treatment allegedly overlooks the "real" cause of the problem. Yet the evidence is clear that symptom substitution does not occur in successful behavior therapy (e.g., Sloane, Staples, Cristol, Yorkston, & Whipple, 1975). Both behavioral and psychodynamic treatments attempt to modify underlying causes of behavior. The difference is what proponents of each approach regard as causes. Behavior analysts look for current variables and conditions that control behavior. Some psychodynamic approaches (e.g., psychoanalysis) ask, "How did the client become this kind of person?" Others (e.g., Adlerian psychotherapy) ask, "What is this person trying to achieve?" Behavioral approaches ask, "What is causing this person to behave in this way right now, and what can we do right now to change that behavior?"

Family and systems therapists assert that individuals can best be understood and treated by changing the interpersonal system within a family. Behavior therapy has increasingly emphasized the importance of including family members in treatment. However, behavior therapists reject the assumption that every problem requires a broad-scale intervention in the family system. The findings of outcome studies show that this is not always necessary (Mathews, Gelder, & Johnston, 1981). For example, not only does individual behavior therapy for agoraphobics produce long-term improvement in phobic avoidance, it often also results in increases in marital satisfaction and improvements in other aspects of interpersonal functioning. Data such as these discredit the claims of some family systems theorists.

The focus on the problems of experiential avoidance, which is such a key aspect of ACT, clearly overlaps with some experiential and humanistic therapies such as Gestalt therapy and Rogers's person-centered treatment.

Most forms of psychotherapy are limited to specific populations. Traditional psychoanalytic therapy, for instance, has focused predominantly on white, well-educated, socially and economically advantaged clients. Behavior therapy is more broadly applicable to the full range of psychological disorders than is traditional psychotherapy (Kazdin & Wilson, 1978). It has also been shown to be effective with diverse patient populations, including disadvantaged minority groups (Miranda, Bernal, Kohn, Hwang, & La Fromboise, 2005).

Overall evaluation of the comparative efficacy of behavior therapy versus other psychotherapies is uncertain. As described below, behavioral treatments have been reliably shown to be more effective than no treatment or placebo treatments. However, there are few well-designed head-to-head comparisons with other psychological therapies. With rare exceptions, alternative psychological treatments have not been submitted to rigorous empirical evaluations. The evidence, unsatisfactory as it is, indicates that behavior therapy is more effective than psychoanalytic and other verbal psychotherapies (Hollon & Beck, 1994; O'Leary & Wilson, 1987).

HISTORY

Precursors

Two historical events stand out as foundations for behavior therapy. The first was the rise of behaviorism in the early 1900s. The key figure in the United States was J. B. Watson, who criticized the subjectivity and mentalism of the psychology of the time and advocated behaviorism as the basis for the objective study of behavior. Watson's emphasis on the importance of environmental events, his rejection of covert aspects of the individual, and his claim that all behavior could be understood as a result of learning became the formal bases of behaviorism.

Watson's position has been widely rejected by behavior therapists, and more refined versions of behaviorism have been developed by theorists such as B. F. Skinner, whose radical behaviorism has had a significant impact not only on behavior therapy but also on psychology in general. Like Watson, Skinner insisted that overt behavior is the only acceptable subject of scientific investigation.

The second event was experimental research on the psychology of learning. In Russia, around the turn of the 20th century, Ivan Pavlov, a Nobel laureate in physiology, established the foundations of classical conditioning. At about the same time in the United States, pioneering research on animal learning by E. L. Thorndike showed the influence of consequences (rewarding and punishing events) on behavior.

Research on conditioning and learning principles, conducted largely in the animal laboratory, became a dominant part of experimental psychology in the United States following World War II. Workers in this area, in the traditions of Pavlov and Skinner, were committed to the scientific analysis of behavior using the laboratory rat and pigeon as their prototypic subjects. Among the early applications of conditioning principles to the treatment of clinical problems were two particularly notable studies. In 1924, Mary Cover Jones described different behavioral procedures for overcoming children's fears. In 1938, O. Hobart Mowrer and E. Mowrer extended conditioning principles to the treatment of enuresis. The treatment they developed is now an effective and widely used approach (Ross, 1981). These isolated and sporadic efforts had scant impact on psychotherapy at the time, partly because conditioning principles, demonstrated with animals, were rejected as too simplistic for treating complex human problems. Conditioning treatments were rejected as superficial, mechanistic, and naive. In addition, a schism existed between academic–experimental and clinical psychologists. The former were trained in scientific methods, with an emphasis on controlled experimentation and quantitative measurement. The latter concerned themselves with the "soft" side of psychology, including uncontrolled case studies, speculative hypotheses, and psycho-dynamic hypotheses. Some efforts were made to integrate conditioning principles with psychodynamic theories of abnormal behavior, but these formulations only obscured crucial differences between behavioral and psychodynamic approaches.

The advent of behavior therapy was marked by its challenge of the status quo through the presentation of a systematic and explicitly formulated clinical alternative that attempted to bridge the gap between the laboratory and the clinic.

Beginnings

The formal beginnings of behavior therapy can be traced to separate but related developments in the 1950s in three countries.

Joseph Wolpe, in South Africa, presented procedural details and results of his application of learning principles to adult neurotic disorders in his book *Psychotherapy by Reciprocal Inhibition* (1958). Wolpe introduced several therapeutic techniques based on Pavlov's conditioning principles, Hull's S–R learning theory, and his own experimental research on fear reduction in laboratory animals. Wolpe regarded anxiety as the causal agent in all neurotic reactions. It was defined as a persistent response of the autonomic nervous system acquired through classical conditioning. Wolpe developed specific techniques designed to extinguish these conditioned autonomic reactions, including systematic desensitization, one of the most widely used methods of behavior therapy. Wolpe made the controversial claim that 90% of his patients were either "cured" or "markedly improved." Moreover, this unprecedented success rate was apparently accomplished within a few months, or even weeks. Wolpe influenced Arnold Lazarus and Stanley Rachman, both of whom became leading figures in the development of behavior therapy. Wolpe's conditioning techniques in therapy were consistent with similar proposals that had been put forward by Andrew Salter (1949) in New York.

Another landmark in the development of behavior therapy was the research and writings of Hans J. Eysenck and his students at the Institute of Psychiatry of London University. In a seminal paper published in 1959, Eysenck defined behavior therapy as the application of modern learning theory to the treatment of behavioral and emotional disorders. Eysenck emphasized the principles and procedures of Pavlov and Hull, as well as learning theorists such as Mowrer (1947) and Miller (1948). In Eysenck's formulation, behavior therapy was an applied science, the defining feature of which was that it was testable and falsifiable. In 1963, Eysenck and Rachman established the first journal devoted exclusively to behavior therapy—*Behaviour Research and Therapy.*

A third force in the emergence of behavior therapy was the publication in 1953 of Skinner's book *Science and Human Behavior,* in which he criticized psychodynamic concepts and reformulated psychotherapy in behavioral terms. The most important initial clinical application of operant conditioning was with children, work carried out under the direction of Sidney Bijou at the University of Washington. The broad application of operant conditioning to the whole range of psychiatric disorders reached full expression in the 1965 publication of Leonard Ullmann and Leonard Krasner's *Case Studies in Behavior Modification.* In 1968, the first issue of the *Journal of Applied Behavior Analysis* was published. This journal provided the premier outlet for research on the modification of socially significant problems through the use of operant conditioning.

Toward the end of the 1960s, the theoretical and research bases of behavior therapy began to expand. Increasingly, behavior therapists turned to social, personality, and developmental psychology as sources of innovative therapeutic strategies. Particularly noteworthy in this regard was Bandura's (1969) social learning theory, with its emphases on vicarious learning (modeling), symbolic processes, and self-regulatory mechanisms. The 1970s witnessed an increased emphasis on cognitive processes and procedures in behavior therapy.

The 1980s and 1990s were marked by an even broader focus on developments in other areas of psychology. Particular attention has been paid to the role of affect in therapeutic change. The 1990s and turn of the century have also witnessed the evolution of newer forms of behavior therapy, such as DBT and ACT, described earlier in this chapter.

The experimental analysis of the complex interactions among cognition, affect, and behavior is one of the more important areas of theory and research in contemporary behavior therapy. There is also increasing recognition of the importance of biological factors and brain mechanisms in many of the disorders commonly treated with behavioral methods (e.g., anxiety disorders and obesity). The study of biobehavioral interactions is an increasingly significant part of behavior therapy. For example, research on brain mechanisms has identified the specific receptors in the amygdala of the brain that are involved in the extinction of learned fear responses. Behavior therapy treatments such as exposure are designed to promote extinction of phobic (fear) responses. D-cycloserine is a drug that facilitates extinction because it is an agonist at these receptor sites in the brain. Combining exposure (extinction) treatment with this drug results in significantly more rapid reduction in fear responses in laboratory animals as well as in patients with specific phobias (Davis, Myers, Ressler, & Rothbaum, 2005).

Current Status

Behavior therapy has had a profound impact on the field of psychotherapy. An important measure of the influence of behavior therapy is the degree to which psychotherapists use cognitive–behavioral principles and procedures in their clinical practice. Based on his survey of the theoretical orientations of clinical psychologists in the United States, Darrell Smith (1982) concluded that "No single theme dominates the present development of professional psychotherapy. Our findings suggest, however, that cognitive behavioral options represent one of the strongest, if not the strongest, theoretical emphases today" (p. 310). It seems likely that behavior therapy techniques will be increasingly used to treat a broad range of psychological problems.

In the 1990s, a panel of 75 expert psychotherapists comprising representatives of a wide range of different theoretical orientations in the United States was asked to predict what would happen to the practice of psychotherapy in the future (regardless of their personal preferences) (Norcross, Alford, & DeMichele, 1992). The panel largely agreed in ranking CBT techniques as those most likely to be used in the future. The reason? As health care policy in the United States is changing to contain costs and provide coverage to more people, the emphasis is switching to problem-focused, time-limited psychological treatment. Moreover, future third-party reimbursement for mental health services will not only emphasize cost containment but also demand that treatments be demonstrably effective in producing specified goals. Behavior therapy will be an important part of those interventions.

In its formative years in the 1950s and 1960s, behavior therapy was a radical minority movement that challenged the then-dominant psychoanalytic establishment. Today behavior therapy is part of the psychotherapeutic establishment. Beginning in the 1960s in the United States, several graduate clinical programs in some of the country's most distinguished universities placed primary emphasis on a behavioral orientation in their training of predoctoral students. Many others began to include behavior therapy as part of an eclectic approach to clinical training. In their analysis of the orientations of faculty in doctoral programs accredited by the American Psychological Association, Sayette and Mayne (1990) found that 14% could be described as having an applied behavioral or radical behavioral approach, while an additional 42% emphasized cognitive behavioral or social learning approaches.

In contrast to the impact on the training and practice of clinical psychologists, behavior therapy has had little influence on that of other mental health professionals in the United States (Glass & Arnkoff, 1992). The minimal impact on psychiatry is ironic, given the seminal contributions of some psychiatrists to the development of cognitive behavior therapy (e.g., Joseph Wolpe and Aaron Beck). This is probably due to the total dominance of psychoanalysis in American psychiatry for more than 40 years. More recently, biological psychiatry has often supplanted the psychoanalytic model in training programs. As a result, psychological treatment has been deemphasized in the training of psychiatrists.

The first behavior therapy journal, *Behaviour Research and Therapy,* was published in 1963 in part because the psychodynamically inclined editors of existing clinical journals were unreceptive to behavior therapy. Today there are numerous journals devoted to behavior therapy in different countries. Moreover, behavior therapists have been editors and editorial board members of major all-purpose clinical psychology journals, such as the *Journal of Consulting and Clinical Psychology* in the United States.

The increasing tendency of behavior therapists to identify themselves as cognitive behavior therapists is reflected in the decision in 2005 to change the name of the Association for Advancement of Behavioral Therapy (AABT) to the Association for Behavioral and Cognitive Therapies (ABCT). It is unclear if behavior therapy will continue to be practiced as a pure approach to therapy or if it will eventually simply become subsumed under the general rubric of cognitive behavior therapy.

PERSONALITY

Theory of Personality

There are specific theoretical differences within the broad framework of contemporary behavior therapy. These differences are most noticeable in the personality theories on which the respective approaches are based. For example, Eysenck (1967) has developed an elaborate trait theory of personality. Briefly, Eysenck classifies people on two major personality dimensions. The first, *introversion–extraversion,* refers to characteristics usually associated with the words *introverted* and *extraverted.* The second dimension is *neuroticism–emotional stability,* ranging from moody and touchy at one extreme to stable and even-tempered at the other. Eysenck believed these personality dimensions are genetically determined and that introverts are more responsive to conditioning procedures than extraverts. In general, however, personality theory appears to have had little impact on clinical behavior therapy, and most behavior therapists have rejected trait theories of personality.

Applied behavior analysis, derived directly from Skinner's radical behaviorism, restricts itself to the study of overt behavior and environmental conditions that presumably regulate behavior. Covert, unobservable elements, such as needs, drives, motives, traits, and conflicts, are disregarded. Skinner's analyses of behavior, for example, are couched in terms of conditioning processes, such as reinforcement, discrimination, and generalization.

Radical behaviorism has been criticized for losing sight of the importance of the person and for lacking a theory of personality. Humanistic psychologists believe applied behavior analysts treat people as though they were controlled only by external, situational forces. A solution to this clash between two extreme viewpoints is to recognize that the characteristics of the environment *interact* with the nature of the people in it. Both commonsense and experimental findings demonstrate the folly of ignoring either side of this crucial interaction. A social learning framework of personality development and change provides a detailed and sophisticated analysis of this interaction between person and situation (Bandura, 1969; Mischel, 1968, 1981).

Many people have debated whether the person or the situation is more important in predicting behavior. However, this question is unanswerable. The relative importance of individual differences and situations will depend on the situation selected, the type of behavior assessed, the particular individual differences sampled, and the purpose of the assessment (Mischel, 1973).

Evidence clearly shows that an individual's behavioral patterns are generally stable and consistent over time. However, the specificity of behavior in different situations poses a problem for trait theories of personality. The central assumption of such theories is that stable and generalized personality traits determine behavioral consistency in a wide variety of different situations. Yet, as Mischel (1968) has pointed out, the correlations between different measures of the same trait are usually very low, and there is little consistency in behavior patterns across different situations.

Psychodynamic conceptualizations of personality assume that the underlying personality structure is stable across situations. Overt behavior is of interest to psychodynamic theorists only to the extent that the behavior provides signs of deep-seated personality traits. Psychodynamic theorists believe that behavior cannot be taken at face value but must be interpreted symbolically because the personality's defense mechanisms disguise and distort the "real" motivations being expressed. However,

> the accumulated findings give little support for the utility of clinical judgments. . . . Clinicians guided by concepts about underlying genotypic dispositions have not been able to predict behavior better than have the person's own direct self-report, simple indices of directly relevant past behavior, or demographic variables. (Mischel, 1973, p. 254)

Social–cognitive theory readily accounts for the discriminatory nature of human behavior. A person would be predicted to act consistently in different situations only to the extent that similar behavior leads, or is expected to lead, to similar consequences. An illustration from Mischel helps clarify this key concept:

> Consider a woman who seems hostile and fiercely independent some of the time but passive, dependent, and feminine on other occasions. What is she really like? Which one of these two patterns reflects the woman that she really is? Is one pattern in the service of the other, or might both be in the service of a third motive? Must she be a really aggressive person with a facade of passivity—or is she a warm, passive dependent woman with a surface defense of aggressiveness? Social learning theory suggests that it is possible for her to be all of these—a hostile, fiercely independent, passive, dependent, feminine, aggressive, warm person all in one. Of course, which of these she is at any particular moment would not be random and capricious; it would depend on discriminative stimuli—who she is with, when, how, and much, much more. But each of these aspects of herself may be a quite genuine and real aspect of her total being. (1976, p. 86)

The difference between the behavioral and psychodynamic approaches in explaining the development of abnormal behavior can be illustrated by Freud's case of Little Hans. This child developed a phobia of horses, which Freud attributed to castration anxiety and oedipal conflict. In their reinterpretation of this case, Wolpe and Rachman (1960) point out that Little Hans had recently experienced four incidents in which horses were associated with frightening events that could have created a classically conditioned phobic reaction. For example, Hans was terrified when he saw a horse that was pulling a loaded cart knocked down and apparently killed. From a psychodynamic viewpoint, the external stimuli (what Little Hans saw) had little effect on the phobia; the fear of horses per se was less significant than the underlying conflict. As Freud put it, "the anxiety originally had no reference to horses but was transposed onto them secondarily." This interpretation does not account for the discriminative pattern of the boy's reactions. For example, he was fearful of a single horse pulling a loaded cart (viewed by Freud as a symbol of pregnancy) but not of two horses, of large horses but not small ones, and of rapidly moving horse-drawn carts but not slowly moving ones. How is this pattern predicted by a global, internal construct such as an oedipal conflict? In the accident that the boy witnessed, a single, large horse, moving rapidly, was believed to have been killed. A conditioning explanation emphasizes that specific stimulus elements elicit particular responses and therefore accounts plausibly for the discriminative fear responses of Little Hans.

Trait theories emphasize differences among people on dimensions selected by the clinician. For some purposes, such as gross screening (e.g., administering the Minnesota Multiphasic Personality Inventory [MMPI] to a client) or group comparisons, a trait approach is useful. But it does not aid the therapist in making treatment decisions about a particular individual. For example, consider the trait of introversion–extraversion. According to Eysenck's theory, particular treatments will have different effects on clients who vary along these dimensions. In a well-controlled study, Paul (1966) correlated performance on paper-and-pencil personality tests measuring extraversion, emotionality, and anxiety, among other traits, with the therapeutic success obtained by treating public speaking anxiety with systematic desensitization. His results revealed no relationship whatsoever between global personality measures and therapeutic outcome. This result is typical of other outcome studies.

Variety of Concepts

Learning Principles

The use of learning principles in behavior therapy is summarized in Agras and Wilson (2005). The case of Little Hans illustrates the role of classical conditioning. When a previously neutral stimulus is paired with a frightening event (the unconditioned stimulus, or US), it can become a *conditioned stimulus* (CS) that elicits a *conditioned response* (CR) such as anxiety. Current analyses of classical conditioning have moved away from the once popular notion that what was learned consisted of simple S–R bonds. Rather, people learn that there are correlational or contingent relationships between the CS and US. This learning defines the conditioning process. Classical conditioning is no longer seen as the simple pairing of a single CS with a single US. Instead, correlations between entire classes of stimulus events can be learned. People may be exposed to traumatic events (contiguity), but not develop phobic reactions unless a correlational or contingent relationship is formed between the situation and the traumatic event.

Operant conditioning emphasizes that behavior is a function of its environmental consequences. Behavior is strengthened by positive and negative reinforcement; it is weakened by punishment. *Positive reinforcement* refers to an increase in the frequency of a response followed by a favorable event. An example would be a teacher or parent praising a child for obtaining a good report card. *Negative reinforcement* refers to an increase in behavior as a result of avoiding or escaping from an aversive event that one would have expected to occur. For example, an agoraphobic, fearing loss of control and panic in a crowded shopping mall, will escape this aversive prospect by staying at home. This individual then experiences relief from anxiety by having avoided this panic and finds it increasingly difficult to leave the house.

In *punishment,* an aversive event is contingent on a response; the result is a decrease in the frequency of that response. If a child is criticized or punished by his parents for speaking up, he is likely to become an inhibited and unassertive adult.

Extinction refers to the cessation or removal of a response. For example, the family of an obsessive–compulsive client might be instructed to ignore requests for reassurance from the client that he has not done something wrong. The reinforcer that is no longer presented is inappropriate attention.

Discrimination learning occurs when a response is rewarded (or punished) in one situation but not in another. Behavior is then under specific *stimulus control.* This process is particularly important in explaining the flexibility of human behavior. For example, an obese client who goes on eating binges may show good self-control under some circumstances but lose control in predictable situations (e.g., when alone and feeling frustrated or depressed).

Generalization refers to the occurrence of behavior in situations other than that in which it was acquired. A therapist might help a client to become more assertive and expressive during treatment sessions. But the ultimate goal of therapy is to have the client act more assertively in real-life situations.

Social–cognitive theory recognizes both the importance of awareness in learning and the person's active cognitive appraisal of environmental events. Learning is facilitated when people are aware of the rules and contingencies governing the consequences of their actions. Reinforcement does not involve an automatic strengthening of behavior. Learning is a consequence of the informative and incentive functions of rewards. By observing the consequences of behavior, a person learns what action is appropriate in what situation. By symbolic representation of anticipated future outcomes of behavior, one generates the motivation to initiate and sustain current actions (Bandura, 1977). Often, people's expectations and hypotheses about what is happening to them may affect their behavior more than the objective reality.

The importance social–cognitive theory attaches to *vicarious learning (modeling)* is consistent with its emphasis on cognitive processes. In this form of learning, people acquire new knowledge and behavior by observing other people and events, without engaging in the behavior and without any direct consequences to themselves. Vicarious learning may occur when people watch what others do. The influence of vicarious learning on human behavior is pervasive, and this concept greatly expands the power of social–cognitive theory.

Person Variables

People do not passively interact with situations with empty heads or an absence of feelings. Rather, they actively attend to environmental stimuli, interpret them, encode them, and selectively remember them. Mischel (1973) has spelled out a series of *person variables* that explain the interchange between person and situation. These person variables are the products of each person's social experience and cognitive development that, in turn, determine how future experiences influence him or her. Briefly, they include the individual's *competencies* to construct diverse behaviors under appropriate conditions. In addition, there is the person's *categorization* of events and people, including the self. To understand how a person will perform in particular situations also requires attention to his or her *expectancies,* the *subjective values* of any expected outcomes, and the individual's *self-regulatory systems and plans.*

A full discussion of these person variables is beyond the scope of the present chapter, but some illustrative examples may be given. For example, consider the role of *personal constructs.* It is common in clinical practice to find clients who constantly put themselves down, even though it is clear to the objective onlooker that they are competent and that they are distorting reality. In cases like these, behavior is mainly under the control of internal stimuli rather than environmental events. Different people might respond differently to the same objective stimulus situation, depending on how they interpret what is happening to them. Therapy concentrates on correcting such faulty cognitive perceptions. But the behavior therapist must also assess a client's cognitive and behavioral *competencies* to ascertain whether he or she really can respond in a particular way. A client may be depressed not because he misperceives the situation but because he actually lacks the appropriate skills to secure rewards. A case in point would be a shy, underassertive college freshman who is motivated to date but who realizes he does not have the social skills needed to establish relationships with women. Therapy would be geared to overcoming his behavioral deficit, helping the student acquire the requisite interpersonal skills.

Self-efficacy refers to one's belief about being able to perform certain tasks or achieve certain goals (Bandura, 1998). Self-efficacy is assessed simply by asking a person to indicate the degree of confidence that he or she can do a particular task.

Such person variables differ from traits in that they do not assume broad cross-situational consistency but depend on specific contexts. Constructs such as generalized expectancies have not proved fruitful in predicting behavior. However, specific evaluations of individuals' efficacy expectations with respect to particular tasks are useful.

Applied behavior analysts reject cognitive mediating processes and have little use for person variables. They agree that the environment interacts with the person but contend that the role of the person is best explained in terms of *past history of reinforcement*. To illustrate the differences between the social–cognitive approach and the radical behaviorist position, imagine a client who is phobic about flying. This client typically becomes highly anxious when he hears the plane's landing gear retracting. A therapist with a social–cognitive view might attribute this anxiety reaction to the client's perception that something is wrong. The radical behaviorist would suggest that the client is reacting not only to the present environment (the sudden noise) but also to stories he has heard in the past about engines falling off and planes crashing. This example makes it clear that radical behaviorism is not free from inferential reasoning. The question is not whether inferences will be made in trying to account for human behavior, but what sort of inference is the most useful. There is now evidence to demonstrate that taking person variables into account improves prediction about behavior and enhances therapeutic efficacy (O'Leary & Wilson, 1987).

PSYCHOTHERAPY

Theory of Psychotherapy

Learning

Behavior therapy emphasizes corrective learning experiences in which clients acquire new coping skills, improve communication, or learn to break maladaptive habits and overcome self-defeating emotional conflicts. These corrective learning experiences involve broad changes in cognitive, affective, and behavioral functioning: They are not limited to modifications of narrow response patterns in overt behavior.

The learning that characterizes behavior therapy is carefully structured. Perhaps more than any other form of treatment, behavior therapy involves asking a patient to do something such as practice relaxation training, self-monitor daily caloric intake, engage in assertive acts, confront anxiety-eliciting situations, and refrain from carrying out compulsive rituals. The high degree to which behavior therapists emphasize the client's activities in the real world between therapy sessions is one of the distinctive features of the behavioral approach. However, behavior therapy is not a one-sided influence process by the therapist to effect changes in a client's beliefs and behavior. It involves both dynamic interaction between therapist and client and directed work on the part of the client. A crucial factor in all forms of therapy is the client's motivation, the willingness to cooperate in the arduous and challenging task of making significant changes in real-life behavior. Resistance to change and lack of motivation are common reasons for treatment failures in behavior therapy. Much of the art in therapy involves coping with these issues (Lazarus & Fay, 1982).

The Therapeutic Relationship

Behavior therapy demands skill, sensitivity, and clinical acumen. Brady et al. (1980) underscore the importance of the therapeutic relationship as follows:

> There is no question that qualitative aspects of the therapist–patient relationship can greatly influence the course of therapy for good or bad. In general, if the patient's relationship to the therapist is characterized by belief in the therapist's competence

(knowledge, sophistication, and training) and if the patient regards the therapist as an honest, trustworthy, and decent human being with good social and ethical values (in his own scheme of things), the patient is more apt to invest himself in the therapy. Equally important is the quality and tone of the relationship he has with the therapist. That is, if he feels trusting and warm toward the therapist, this generally will facilitate following the treatment regimen, will be associated with higher expectations of improvement, and other generally favorable factors. The feelings of the therapist toward the patient are also important. If the therapist feels that his patient is not a desirable person or a decent human being or simply does not like the patient for whatever reasons, he may not succeed in concealing these attitudes toward the patient, and in general they will have a deleterious effect. (1980, pp. 285–286)

As opposed to the neutral and detached role that the psychoanalytically oriented therapist is taught to assume, the behavior therapist is directive and concerned—a problem solver and a coping model. In their comparative study of behavior therapy and psychoanalytically oriented psychotherapy, Staples, Sloane, Whipple, Cristol, and Yorkston concluded:

Differences between behavior therapy and analytically-oriented psychotherapy . . . involved the basic patterns of interactions between patient and therapist and the type of relationship formed. Behavior therapy is not psychotherapy with special "scientific techniques" superimposed on the traditional therapeutic paradigm; rather, the two appear to represent quite different styles of treatment although they share common elements. (1975, p. 1521)

The behavior therapists in this study were rated as more directive, more open, more genuine, and more disclosing than their psychoanalytically oriented counterparts.

A strong therapeutic alliance is essential for effective behavior therapy, including manual-based treatment. It is a misconception that manual-based treatment undermines the therapeutic relationship because the therapist is focused on administering a somewhat standardized treatment protocol. For example, it is important in engaging the patient in treatment process, enhancing motivation to change, and facilitating adherence to homework assignments. Nonetheless, the therapeutic alliance does not mediate treatment outcome in behavior therapy (DeRubeis et al., 2005). It is necessary but not sufficient. Treatment method accounts for more variance than measures of therapeutic alliance (Loeb et al., 2005). It is a misconception that manual-based treatment undermines the therapeutic relationship because the therapist is focused on administering a somewhat standardized treatment protocol. Studies show that competently conducted manual-based CBT results in highly positive therapeutic alliance as in earlier forms of behavior therapy as noted above.

Ethical Issues

In behavior therapy the client is encouraged to participate actively. Consider, for example, the important issue of who determines the goals of therapy. Because it is fundamental to behavior therapy that the client should have the major say in setting treatment goals, it is important that the client is fully informed and consents to and participates in setting goals. A distinction is drawn between how behavior is to be changed—in which the therapist is presumably expert—and the objectives of therapy. The latter ultimately must be determined by the client. The client controls what; the therapist controls how. The major contribution of the therapist is to assist clients by helping them to generate alternative courses of action and to analyze the consequences of pursuing various goals. Because this process involves an expression of the therapist's own values, the therapist should identify them and explain how they might affect his or her analysis of therapeutic goals.

Selecting goals is far more complicated in the case of disturbed clients (such as institutionalized patients who are struggling with psychosis) who are unable to participate meaningfully in deciding treatment objectives. To ensure that treatment is in the client's best interests, it is important to monitor program goals and procedures through conferences with other professionals (Risley & Sheldon-Wildgen, 1982).

All forms of therapy involve social influence. The critical ethical question is whether therapists are aware of this influence. Behavior therapy entails an explicit recognition of the influence process and emphasizes specific, client-oriented behavioral objectives. Behavior therapists have formulated procedures to guarantee the protection of human rights and personal dignity of all clients (Stolz, 1978; Wilson & O'Leary, 1980).

Process of Psychotherapy

Problem Identification and Assessment

The initial task of a behavior therapist is to identify and understand the client's presenting problem(s). The therapist seeks detailed information about the specific dimensions of problems, such as initial occurrence, severity, and frequency. What has the client done to cope with the problems? What does the client think about his or her problem and any previous therapeutic contacts? Obtaining answers to such searching questions is facilitated by a relationship of trust and mutual understanding. To achieve this, the therapist is attentive, trying to be objective and empathic. The therapist then proceeds to make a functional analysis of the client's problem, attempting to identify specific environmental and person variables that are thought to be maintaining maladaptive thoughts, feelings, or behavior. The emphasis on variables currently maintaining the problem does not mean that the client's past history is ignored. However, past experiences are important only to the degree that they directly contribute to the client's present distress.

Assessment Methods

In the behaviorally oriented interview, the therapist seldom asks the client *why* questions, e.g., "Why do you become anxious in crowded places?" Questions starting with *how, when, where,* and *what* are more useful. The therapist does not necessarily take everything the client says at face value and is constantly looking for inconsistencies, evasiveness, or apparent distortions. Nevertheless, the therapist relies heavily on clients' self-reports, particularly in assessing thoughts, fantasies, and feelings. Self-report has often proved to be a superior predictor of behavior when compared to clinicians' judgments or scores on personality tests (Mischel, 1981). Of course, therapists must ask the right questions if they are to get meaningful answers. Given the tendency of most people to describe themselves with broad personality labels, therapists may have to help clients to identify specific behavioral referents for global subjective impressions.

Guided Imagery

A useful method for assessing clients reactions to particular situations is to have them symbolically recreate a problematic life situation. Instead of asking clients simply to talk about an event, the therapist has them imagine the event actually happening to them. When clients have conjured up an image of a situation, they are then asked to verbalize any thoughts that come to mind, an especially useful way of uncovering the specific thoughts associated with particular events.

Role-Playing

Another option is to ask clients to role-play a situation. This method lends itself to the assessment of interpersonal problems, with the therapist adopting the role of the person with whom the client reports problems. Role-playing provides the therapist with a sample of the problem behavior, albeit under somewhat artificial circumstances. If the therapist is assessing a client couple, the two partners are asked to discuss chosen issues that enable the therapist to observe first-hand the extent of their interpersonal skills and their ability to resolve conflict.

Physiological Recording

Technological progress in monitoring different psychophysiological reactions has made it possible to objectively measure a number of problems. Monitoring a client's sexual arousal in response to specific stimuli that cause changes in penile or vaginal blood flow (Rosen & Keefe, 1978) is an example of the use of physiological recording instruments in behavioral assessment and treatment strategies.

Self-Monitoring

Clients are typically instructed to keep detailed, daily records of particular events or psychological reactions. Obese clients, for example, are asked to self-monitor daily caloric intake, the degree to which they engage in planned physical activities, the conditions under which they eat, and so on. In this way it is possible to detect behavioral patterns in clients' lives functionally related to their problems.

Behavioral Observation

Assessment of overt problem behavior, ideally, is based on actual observation of the client's behavior in the natural environment. Accordingly, behavior therapists have developed sophisticated behavioral observation rating procedures. These procedures most often have been used with children and hospitalized patients. Parents, teachers, nurses, and hospital aides have been trained as behavioral observers. Once these individuals have learned to observe behavior, they can be taught to make a behavioral analysis of a problem and then instructed to alter their own behavior to influence the problem behavior of another person.

Psychological Tests and Questionnaires

In general, behavior therapists do not use standardized psychodiagnostic tests. Tests such as the MMPI may be useful for providing an overall picture of the client's personality profile, but they do not yield the kind of information necessary for a functional analysis or for the development of therapeutic interventions. Projective tests are widely rejected because of a lack of acceptable evidence for their validity or utility (Lilienfeld, Lynn, & Lohr, 2003). Behavior therapists do use checklists and questionnaires, such as the Marks and Mathews Fear Questionnaire (1979), self-report scales of depression like the Beck Depression Inventory (Beck, Rush, Shaw, & Emery, 1979), assertion inventories like the Rathus (1973) questionnaire, and paper-and-pencil measures of marital satisfaction such as the Locke and Wallace (1959) inventory of marital adjustment. These assessment devices are not sufficient for carrying out a functional analysis of the determinants of a problem, but are useful in establishing the initial severity of the problem and charting therapeutic efficacy over the course of treatment.

Treatment Techniques

Behavior therapy offers a wide range of different treatment methods and attempts to tailor the principles of social–cognitive theory to each individual's unique problem. In selecting treatment techniques, the behavior therapist relies heavily on empirical evidence about the efficacy of that technique applied to the particular problem. In many cases, the empirical evidence is unclear or largely nonexistent. Here the therapist is influenced by accepted clinical practice and the basic logic and philosophy of a social–cognitive approach to human behavior and its modification. In the process, the therapist must often use intuitive skill and clinical judgment to select appropriate treatment methods and determine the best time to implement specific techniques. Both science and art influence clinical practice, and the most effective therapists are aware of the advantages and limitations of each.

The following are some selective illustrations of the varied methods the typical behavior therapist is likely to employ in clinical practice.

Imagery-Based Techniques.   In systematic desensitization, after isolating specific events that trigger unrealistic anxiety, the therapist constructs a stimulus hierarchy in which different situations that the client fears are ordered along a continuum from mildly stressful to very threatening. The client is instructed to imagine each event while he or she is deeply relaxed. Wolpe (1958) adapted Jacobson's (1938) method of progressive relaxation training as a means of producing a response incompatible with anxiety. Briefly, this consists of training clients to concentrate on systematically relaxing different muscle groups. When any item produces excessive anxiety, the client is instructed to cease visualizing the particular item and to restore feelings of relaxation. The item is then repeated, or the hierarchy adjusted, until the client can visualize the scene without experiencing anxiety. Only then does the therapist present the next item of the hierarchy. Real-life exposure, where possible, is even more powerful than using imagination and is the technique of choice for treating anxiety disorders. An example of exposure treatment for an agoraphobic client is described in the "Applications" section.

Symbolically generated aversive reactions are used to treat diverse problems such as alcoholism and sexual disorders (e.g., exhibitionism). In this procedure, the client is asked to imagine aversive consequences associated with the problem behavior. An alcoholic might be asked to imagine experiencing nausea at the thought of a drink; an exhibitionist might be asked to imagine being apprehended by the police. This method is often referred to as covert sensitization (Cautela, 1967). A hierarchy of scenes that reliably elicit the problem urge or behavior is developed, and each scene is systematically presented until the client gains control over the problem.

Cognitive Restructuring.   The treatment techniques in this category are based on the assumption that emotional disorders result, at least in part, from dysfunctional thinking. The task of therapy is to alter this maladaptive thinking. Although there is some overlap with Ellis's REBT, the cognitive restructuring method most commonly used by behavior therapists is derived from Beck's cognitive therapy. An example of this method is illustrated in the following excerpt from a therapy session. Notice how the therapist prompts the patient to examine his dysfunctional assumptions and how behavioral tasks are used to help the patient to alter his assumption (P = Patient; T = Therapist):

P: In the middle of a panic attack, I usually think I am going to faint or collapse . . .
T: Have you ever fainted in an attack?
P: No.
T: What is it then that makes you think you might faint?
P: I feel faint, and the feeling can be very strong.

T: So, to summarize, your evidence that you are going to faint is the fact that you feel faint?

P: Yes.

T: How can you then account for the fact that you have felt faint many hundreds of times and have not yet fainted?

P: So far, the attacks have always stopped just in time or I have managed to hold onto something to stop myself from collapsing.

T: Right. So one explanation of the fact that you have frequently felt faint, had the thought that you would faint, but have not actually fainted, is that you have always done something to save yourself just in time. However, an alternative explanation is that the feeling of faintness that you get in a panic attack will never lead to you collapsing, even if you don't control it.

P: Yes, I suppose.

T: In order to decide which of these two possibilities is correct, we need to know what has to happen to your body for you to actually faint. Do you know?

P: No.

T: Your blood pressure needs to drop. Do you know what happens to your blood pressure during a panic attack?

P: Well, my pulse is racing. I guess my blood pressure must be up.

T: That's right. In anxiety, heart rate and blood pressure tend to go together. So, you are actually less likely to faint when you are anxious than when you are not.

P: That's very interesting and helpful to know. However, if it's true, why do I feel so faint?

T: Your feeling of faintness is a sign that your body is reacting in a normal way to the perception of danger. Most of the bodily reactions you are experiencing when anxious were probably designed to deal with the threats experienced by primitive people, such as being approached by a hungry tiger. What would be the best thing to do in that situation?

P: Run away as fast as you can.

T: That's right. And in order to help you run, you need the maximum amount of energy in your muscles. This is achieved by sending more of your blood to your muscles and relatively less to the brain. This means that there is a small drop in oxygen to the brain and that is why you feel faint. However, this feeling is misleading because your overall blood pressure is up, not down.

P: That's very clear. So next time I feel faint, I can check out whether I am going to faint by taking my pulse. If it is normal, or quicker than normal, I know I won't faint. (Clark, 1989, pp. 76–77)

Assertiveness and Social Skills Training.   Unassertive clients often fail to express their emotions or to stand up for their rights. They are often exploited by others, feel anxious in social situations, and lack self-esteem. In behavior rehearsal, the therapist may model the appropriate assertive behavior and may ask the client to engage repeatedly in a graduated sequence of similar actions (Alberti & Emmons, 2001). Initially, the therapist focuses on expressive behavior (e.g., body posture, voice training, and eye contact). The therapist then encourages the client to carry out assertive actions in the real world to ensure generalization. Behavior therapy is frequently conducted in a group as well as on an individual basis. Behavior rehearsal for assertiveness training is well suited to group therapy, because group members can provide more varied sources of educational feedback and can also offer a diversified range of modeling influences.

The instructional, modeling, and feedback components of behavior rehearsal facilitate a broad range of communication competencies, including active listening, giving personal feedback, and building trust through self-disclosure. These communication principles, drawn from nonbehavioral approaches to counseling but integrated within a behavioral framework, are an important ingredient of behavioral marital therapy (Margolin, 1987).

Self-Control Procedures.   Behavior therapists use a number of self-control procedures (Bandura, 1977; Kanfer, 1977). Fundamental to successful self-regulation of behavior is self-monitoring, which requires helping the client set goals or standards that guide behavior. In the treatment of obesity, for example, daily caloric goals are mutually selected. Behavioral research has identified certain properties of goals that increase the probability of successful self-control. For example, one should set highly specific, unambiguous, and short-term goals, such as consumption of no more than 1,200 calories each day. Compare this to the goal of "cutting back" on eating for the "next week." Failure to achieve such vague goals elicits negative self-evaluative reactions by clients, whereas successful accomplishment of goals produces self-reinforcement that increases the likelihood of maintaining the new behavior.

Self-instructional training, described above, is often used as a self-control method for coping with impulsivity, stress, excessive anger, and pain. Similarly, progressive relaxation training is widely applied as a self-control method for reducing different forms of stress, including insomnia, tension headaches, and hypertension (O'Leary & Wilson, 1987). Biofeedback methods used to treat a variety of psychophysiological disorders also fall under the category of self-control procedures (Yates, 1980).

Real-Life Performance-Based Techniques.   The foregoing techniques are applied during treatment sessions, and most are routinely coupled with instructions to clients to complete homework assignments in their natural environment.

The diversity of behavioral treatment methods is seen in the application of operant conditioning principles in settings ranging from classrooms to institutions for people affected by retardation or mental illness. An excellent illustration is the use of a *token economy.* The main elements of a token reinforcement program can be summarized as follows: (a) carefully specified and operationally defined target behaviors, (b) backup reinforcers, (c) tokens that represent the backup reinforcers, and (d) rules of exchange that specify the number of tokens required to obtain backup reinforcers.

A token economy in a classroom might consist of the teacher, at regular intervals, making ratings indicating how well a student had behaved, both academically and socially. At the end of the day, good ratings could be exchanged for various small prizes. These procedures reduce disruptive social behavior in the classroom and can improve academic performance (O'Leary & O'Leary, 1977). In the case of psychiatric inpatients, the staff might make tokens contingent upon improvements in self-care activities, reductions in belligerent acts, and cooperative problem-solving behavior (Kazdin, 1977). The behavior therapist designs the token economy and monitors its implementation and efficacy. The procedures themselves are implemented in real-life settings by teachers, parents, nurses, and psychiatric aides—whoever has most direct contact with the patient. Ensuring that these psychological assistants are well trained and supervised is the responsibility of the behavior therapist.

Length of Treatment.   There are no established guidelines for deciding on the length of therapy. Much of behavior therapy is short-term treatment, but therapy lasting from 25 to 50 sessions is commonplace, and still longer treatment is not unusual. Therapy in excess of 100 sessions is relatively rare. The usual approach in clinical practice is to carry out a detailed behavioral assessment of a client's problem(s) and to embark upon interventions as rapidly as possible. Assessment is an ongoing process, as the consequences of initial treatment interventions are evaluated against therapeutic goals. Unless treatment time is explicitly limited from the start, the length of therapy and the scheduling of the treatment sessions are contingent upon the patient's progress.

Typically, a behavior therapist might contract with a patient to pursue a treatment plan for two to three months (approximately 8 to 12 sessions) and reevaluate progress at the end of this period. The relative absence of any discernible improvement is cause for the therapist to reevaluate whether he or she conceptualized the problem accurately, whether he or she is using the appropriate techniques or needs to switch tactics, whether there is some personal problem with him or her as the therapist, or whether a referral to another therapist or another form of treatment might be necessary.

In terminating a successful case, the behavior therapist usually avoids abruptness. A typical procedure is to lengthen gradually the time between successive therapy sessions, from weekly to fortnightly to monthly and so on. These concluding sessions may be shorter than earlier ones, with occasional telephone contact.

Manual-Based Treatments

The use of standardized, manual-based treatments in clinical practice represents a new and controversial development with far-reaching implications for clinical practice. Cognitive behavioral therapists have been at the forefront of this development (Wilson, 1998), and there are now evidence-based CBT treatment manuals for a variety of clinical disorders, including different anxiety disorders, depressions, and eating disorders.

A treatment manual describes a limited and set number of techniques for treating a specific clinical disorder. These techniques are implemented in the same sequence over a more or less fixed number of treatment sessions, and all patients diagnosed with the disorder in question are treated with the same manual-based approach. For example, all patients with the eating disorder of bulimia nervosa would be treated in essentially the same fashion using the cognitive behavior therapy manual developed specifically for this disorder by Fairburn and his colleagues (Fairburn, Marcus, & Wilson, 1993).

A particular strength of these manuals is that they describe treatment programs that have been evaluated in controlled clinical trials. Treatment manuals make psychological therapy, whatever its particular form, more consistent and more widely available. They make it easier for therapists to learn specific treatment strategies and to acquire skill in using them. They not only facilitate the training of therapists but also make it easier for supervisors to monitor their trainees' expertise. The structured and time-limited nature of treatment manuals results in more highly focused treatment than might otherwise be the case.

Nonetheless, manual-based treatments have been criticized by practitioners, including some behavior therapists, because the standardized approach limits the role of the therapist's clinical judgment in tailoring specific interventions to the individual patient's needs (Davison & Lazarus, 1995). In response, proponents of manual-based treatments argue that therapists' clinical judgments are often highly subjective, relying more on intuition than empirical evidence.

The limitations of clinical judgment have been well documented. Clinical judgment as a form of human inference is no better, and is worse in some situations, than actuarial prediction in which patients' behavior is predicted by viewing them as members of an aggregate (e.g., a diagnostic category) and by determining what variables generally predict for that aggregate or diagnostic category (Dawes, 1994). Empirically supported, manual-based treatments are consistent with the actuarial approach. The relative effectiveness of manual-based behavior therapy versus reliance on the therapist's clinical judgment is the subject of ongoing clinical investigation.

Mechanisms of Psychotherapy

Research on behavior therapy has demonstrated that particular treatment methods are effective and has identified what components of multifaceted treatment methods and programs are responsible for therapeutic success. For example, empirical evidence has established that the changes produced by token reinforcement programs are due to the learning principles of operant conditioning on which they are based (Kazdin, 1977).

Learning Processes

Ayllon and Azrin (1965) described a pioneering token reinforcement program with predominantly schizophrenic patients on a psychiatric hospital ward. The target behaviors in this investigation were self-care and improved capacity for productive work. Rewards were made contingent on improvement in these two areas. Following a period during which the job assignments of all 44 patients on the entire ward were rewarded contingently (phase A), tokens were administered on a noncontingent basis (phase B). In phase B, patients were given tokens each day regardless of their performance, which broke the contingency between reinforcer and response. This ensured that the amount of social interaction between the attendants and ward staff who administered the tokens and the patients remained unchanged. Any deterioration in performance was then directly attributable to the precise functional relationship between behavior and reinforcement.

Phase C marked a return to contingent reinforcement as in phase A. The results showed that "free" reinforcement (phase B) was totally ineffective. Similarly, the complete withdrawal of all tokens resulted in performance decreasing to less than one-fourth the rate at which it had previously been maintained by contingently rewarding the patients with tokens.

No single, monolithic theory encompasses the diverse methods and applications of the different behavior therapies. Although operant conditioning principles explain the efficacy of a broad range of behavioral procedures, they do not account for the success of a number of other methods. Classical conditioning and different cognitive processes all play a part in determining the effects of the various cognitive behavioral treatment methods described in this chapter. In many cases, the mechanisms responsible for the therapeutic success of a method remain unclear. Consider exposure treatment for phobic and obsessive–compulsive disorders. The effectiveness of this method has been well established, but its explanation is still a matter of some controversy. Originally, the explanation was based on Mowrer's (1947) two-factor theory of learning, according to which repeated exposure to anxiety-eliciting situations, as in systematic desensitization, resulted in the extinction of the classically conditioned anxiety that mediates phobic avoidance behavior. However, other research (Bandura, 1986) casts doubt on the validity of this explanation.

Cognitive Mechanisms

In terms of social–cognitive theory, exposure leads not to the extinction of any underlying anxiety drive state, but rather to modification of the client's expectations of self-efficacy (Bandura, 1982). Self-efficacy refers to clients' beliefs that they can cope with formerly feared situations. For efficacy expectations to change, the client must make a self-attribution of behavioral change. For example, it is not uncommon for an agoraphobic client to approach situations she has avoided without increases in self-efficacy or reductions in fear. The explanation seems to be that some clients do not credit themselves for the behavioral change. The agoraphobic might say that she was "lucky" that she did not have a panic attack or that she just happened to have one of those rare "good days." The therapist must be prepared to help the client use cognitive methods to attribute changes to herself so that her sense of personal efficacy increases.

Initial studies with phobic subjects have generally provided empirical support for self-efficacy theory, although the findings are mixed. Experiments by Bandura and his associates have shown that efficacy expectations accurately predicted reductions in phobic avoidance regardless of whether they were created by real-life exposure or symbolic modeling, covert modeling, or systematic desensitization. Moreover, measures of personal efficacy predicted differences in coping behavior by different individuals receiving the same treatment and even specific performance by subjects in different tasks. Consistent with the theory, participant modeling, a performance-based treatment, produced greater increases in level and strength of efficacy expectations and in related behavior change (Bandura, 1986).

APPLICATIONS

Who Can We Help?

Behavior therapy can be used to treat a full range of psychological disorders in different populations (Kazdin & Wilson, 1978). It also has broad applicability to problems in education, medicine, and community living. The following are selected examples of problems for which behavior therapy is an effective treatment.

Anxiety Disorders

Several well-controlled studies have established that behavior therapy is an effective form of treatment for anxiety disorders. Simple phobias are successfully eliminated within a short number of sessions by using guided exposure treatment in which patients are helped to gradually approach and confront the objects or situations they fear and avoid. For example, Tom Ollendick and his colleagues (2009) demonstrated that even a one-session in vivo graduated exposure treatment of up to three hours was superior to an education support treatment and treatment effects were maintained at follow-up. Behavior therapy also is the treatment of choice for more complex and debilitating disorders such as panic disorder and obsessive–compulsive disorder.

Panic Disorder.   Panic disorder is defined by a discrete period of intense fear that develops suddenly and involves physiological symptoms such as a pounding heart, shortness of breath, sweating, dizziness, and fear of going crazy. Effective treatment typically combines both behavioral and cognitive components. At Oxford University in England, David Clark and his colleagues tested the effects of a treatment that focused mainly on changing panic patients' catastrophic interpretation of bodily sensations. This cognitive behavioral treatment proved to be superior to pharmacological therapy with imipramine, an antidepressant often assumed to be the therapy of choice for panic disorder. Patients treated with cognitive–behavioral therapy maintained their improvement over a one-year follow-up period, whereas patients treated with imipramine tended to relapse when the drug was discontinued (Clark, Salkovskis, Hackmann, Middleton, & Gelder, 1994).

In the United States, studies by David Barlow and his colleagues have evaluated the effects of a panic control treatment (PCT) that includes both behavioral and cognitive components. The two main behavioral components are (1) progressive relaxation training designed to help patients cope with their anxiety and (2) exposure (extinction) treatment in which patients are systematically exposed to cues (mainly internal bodily sensations) that typically trigger panic attacks. The treatment eliminates the panic reactions via the process of extinction. PCT was more effective than a wait list control condition (in which patients were assessed but their treatment delayed) or relaxation training alone. A two-year follow-up showed that 81% of patients treated with PCT were panic-free (Craske, Brown, & Barlow, 1991). A subsequent large, controlled study of panic disorder showed that both CBT and imipramine were effective treatments in the short term. Again, the therapeutic effects of CBT were maintained over follow-up, whereas patients withdrawn from their medication tended to relapse (Barlow, Gorman, Shear, & Woods, 2000). Most recently, Craske and her colleagues have shown that this form of cognitive behavior therapy can be successfully implemented to treat panic disorder in primary-care medical settings where the customary therapy has been antidepressant medication. Adding cognitive behavioral treatment to the medication results in significantly superior results than medication alone (Craske et al., 2005).

Obsessive—Compulsive Disorders.   Traditional psychotherapy is ineffective in treating obsessive–compulsive disorder (OCD). A significant advance was made in the 1970s with the development of specific behavioral methods. The most effective treatment is exposure and response prevention, which can be illustrated with compulsive hand washers. The different objects or activities leading the patient to wash his or her hands are first identified through behavioral assessment. Then, following a thorough explanation of the technique and its rationale, and with the patient's fully informed consent, touching objects that trigger hand washing is systematically encouraged. This is the exposure part of treatment. Once the patient has touched what is unrealistically viewed as contaminated, he or she refrains from washing. This is the response prevention part of treatment. The patient's anxiety typically rises after initially touching the object and then decreases over the course of the session. Focusing the patient's attention on fear of contamination assists the treatment. The goal of treatment is to break the negative reinforcing value of the compulsion, extinguish the anxiety elicited by the contaminated object, and enhance the patient's self-efficacy in coping with this kind of situation. Imaginal exposure is used in cases when in vivo exposure is impractical or impossible. Patients are instructed to conjure up detailed imagery of compulsive activities and stay with these images until their anxiety decreases.

Research has shown that roughly 65 to 75% of patients with OCD show marked improvement following behavioral treatment (Barlow, 2002). This therapeutic success is maintained during follow-ups as long as two years after treatment. Of particular interest is the finding that exposure treatment influences the biological basis of OCD. Successfully treated patients show significant changes in glucose metabolism in the caudate nucleus, a specific region of the brain that is known to be connected with anxiety. These changes are identical to those produced by successful pharmacological treatment (Baxter et al., 1992).

Posttraumatic stress disorder (PTSD).   PTSD develops following an intensely stressful event that is likely to cause significant distress in most people. Common examples are traumatic experiences in military combat and rape-related trauma. The major symptoms of PTSD include: (1) re-experiencing symptoms, flashbacks, feeling as if the event were re-occurring, nightmares, and distressing intrusive images; (2) avoidance, in which people try to suppress memories of the event; (3) hyperarousal, including hypervigilance for threat, irritability, difficulty concentrating, and sleep difficulties; and (4) emotional numbing, including the lack of ability to experience feelings and amnesia for significant aspects of the event. Associated difficulties, such as depression, substance abuse, and interpersonal problems, are commonplace.

Different combinations of both cognitive and behavioral techniques have been used to treat PTSD, but the strongest evidence supports exposure therapy (Foa, Hembree, Cahill, Rauch, & Riggs, 2005). In this treatment, following detailed assessment and education about the nature of trauma the therapist and patient develop a hierarchy of threatening situations. Homework exercises are designed to have the patient confront these situations in a graded fashion. In addition, using imaginal exposure, therapy sessions are devoted to having the patient re-experience the trauma itself, for example, being raped by a stranger. The patient's reactions to these imaginal exposure sessions are discussed and progress carefully monitored. In a large treatment study of rape survivors,

Foa et al. (2005) showed that 12 sessions of this therapy not only produced significant improvement in PTSD, but also associated depression, work, and social functioning.

Depression

Beck's cognitive therapy (CT) for depression is described in Chapter 8. CT is a mix of cognitive and behavioral strategies. Several well-controlled treatment outcome studies have shown that CT is an effective treatment for depression, including severe depression among adults. What is especially significant is that CT appears to be as effective as antidepressant medication (DeRubeis, Brotman, & Gibbons, 2005). Moreover, CT may be even more effective over the long term because when medication is discontinued, patients often relapse rapidly. In short, patients would have to continue taking medication over a period of years in order to equal the enduring effects of several months of CT (Hollon, Stewart, & Strunk, 2006). Importantly, CT is effective not just in research conducted at major universities, but also in routine clinical practice and with minority groups who are typically underserved (Miranda et al., 2005).

CT comprises the following overlapping series of different strategies: Systematic self-observation (self-monitoring); behavioral activation; monitoring thoughts; challenging accuracy of thoughts; exploring underlying core beliefs or what are called schemas; and relapse prevention (Hollon, 1999). Notice that the strategies begin with behavioral techniques (self-monitoring and behavioral activation) and become progressively more cognitive in nature as the therapy develops. An important theoretical and practical question is which of these strategies accounts for the success of the approach? Jacobson and his colleagues (1996) conducted a component analysis of CT in order to determine the necessary and sufficient treatment elements of this approach. They compared the full CT treatment package, which by definition focused on modifying dysfunctional cognitions, to the behavioral component that they labeled behavioral activation (BA). The focus in BA is helping patients to become more active. They learn to self-monitor their daily activities, assess pleasure from engaging in different activities, complete increasingly difficult tasks designed to promote a sense of mastery, and overcome deficits in social skills. The results showed that BA was as effective as the full CT package in decreasing depression both at the end of therapy and at 6-month and 2-year follow-ups (Gortner, Gollan, Dobson, & Jacobson, 1998). Furthermore, BA was equally effective in altering negative thinking in these depressed patients. Jacobson et al. (1996) concluded that CT is no more effective than the behavioral component of the full treatment package.

The results of the Jacobson et al. (1996) study have been replicated by Dimidjian et al. (in press). These investigators found no difference between a behavioral activation treatment and the full CT approach. However, when the results from only the most severely depressed patients were analyzed, behavioral activation proved more effective than CT. Finally, the apparent efficacy of behavioral activation is consistent with the finding that most of the improvement in CT occurs early in treatment (Ilardi & Craighead, 1994). As noted above, the behavioral component is especially prominent during the early part of CT, and these findings collectively call into question the added value of specific cognitive procedures for treating depression.

Another innovative treatment for depression is mindfulness-based cognitive behavior therapy, or MBCT (Segal, Teasdale, & Williams, 2004). This therapy has many features of Beck's CT, with two important differences. First, instead of encouraging patients to actively challenge the validity of their beliefs, MBCT teaches patients to use mindfulness skills in reacting to negative thoughts or bad feelings. The focus is on what Segal et al. (2004) call meta-cognitive awareness—this is essentially the same concept as defusion or distancing as described earlier in this chapter in the section of DBT and ACT. Second, and consistent with behavioral activation and ACT, the focus is on dealing with the functional consequences of thoughts and beliefs rather than on analyzing their content or truth value. Preliminary findings indicate that MBCT is effective in reducing relapse.

Two additional forms of behavior therapy have been used successfully to treat depression. One, developed by Peter Lewinsohn, combines many of the cognitive strategies of Beck's approach with a more traditional behavioral emphasis on increasing the range of patients' positive reinforcers. This approach has been shown to be effective in overcoming depression in adolescents (Lewinsohn, Clarke, Hops, & Andrews, 1990). The other is a form of behavioral marital therapy. The goal in this treatment is to modify the interpersonal influences on unipolar depression by reducing marital conflict and facilitating increased feelings of closeness and open sharing of thoughts and feelings (O'Leary & Beach, 1990). This treatment seems especially effective with depressed women who also have marital problems.

Dobson et al. (2008) conducted a randomized controlled trial that compared the effectiveness of cognitive therapy, behavioral activation, and antidepressant medication. These researchers found no significant difference between behavioral activation and cognitive therapy, but each treatment was at least as efficacious as continued treatment with antidepressant medication, and the psychological treatments were longer lasting and actually cost less than continued treatment with antidepressant medications.

Eating and Weight Disorders

Binge Eating and Bulimia Nervosa.   Bulimia nervosa (BN) is an eating disorder that occurs mainly in adolescent and young adult women. It is characterized by a severe disturbance of eating in which determined attempts to restrict food intake are punctuated by binge eating, namely, episodes of uncontrolled consumption of very large amounts of food. Binges are commonly followed by purging (self-induced vomiting or the misuse of laxatives). BN patients have dysfunctional concerns about body shape and weight and judge their self-worth in terms of shape and weight. Other psychiatric disorders, such as depression, substance abuse, and personality disorders, are commonly associated with BN. Binge eating disorder (BED) is diagnosed if patients show recurrent binge eating in the absence of extreme attempts at weight control such as purging. Whereas BN patients are typically of normal weight, BED patients are usually overweight or obese.

Manual-based CBT for BN (Fairburn et al., 1993) is designed to eliminate binge eating and purging, replace rigid dieting with more normal and flexible eating patterns, and modify dysfunctional thoughts and feelings about the personal significance of body weight and shape. Patients are helped to achieve enhanced self-acceptance instead of struggling to conform to unrealistic societal ideals of feminine beauty. In addition, cognitive and behavioral strategies are used to help patients cope more adaptively with stressful events instead of resorting to binge eating.

Numerous controlled studies in the United States and Europe have demonstrated the effectiveness of CBT in treating BN (Wilson & Fairburn, 2002). CBT has proved to be more effective than several other psychological treatments, including supportive psychotherapy, supportive–expressive psychotherapy, stress management therapy, and a form of behavior therapy that did not address the cognitive features of bulimia nervosa. The exception is interpersonal psychotherapy (IPT). A major comparative outcome study found that at the end of treatment, IPT was less effective than CBT, but during a one-year follow-up, the difference between the two treatments disappeared due to continuing improvement among the patients who received IPT (Fairburn et al., 1995).

Antidepressant medication has also been shown to be an effective treatment for BN. Research studies evaluating the relative and combined effectiveness of CBT and antidepressant drug treatment have, as a whole, shown that CBT is superior to medication alone. Combining CBT with medication is significantly more effective than medication alone. Combining the two has produced few benefits over CBT alone on the reduction of the core features of bulimia nervosa. In contrast to the data on CBT, there is virtually no evidence of the long-term effect of pharmacological treatment on BN (Wilson, 1997).

CBT is also effective in treating binge eating and associated psychopathology in BED patients, but does not produce significant weight loss (Wilson, Grilo, & Vitousek, 2007).

Obesity.   A comprehensive behavioral weight control program, comprising components of improved eating habits, lifestyle change, sound nutrition, and increased exercise, is widely viewed as the treatment of choice for mild to moderate cases of obesity. Short-term results are good. Following 5 months of treatment, behavioral treatment combined with moderate dietary restriction (1,200 calories of self-selected foods daily) results in a mean weight loss of roughly 20 pounds, together with significant decreases in depression and body image dissatisfaction. The problem is that these treatment effects are not maintained over time (Wadden, Butryn, & Byrne, 2004).

The pattern of weight loss and regain in behavioral treatment is consistent. The rate of initial weight loss is rapid but then slowly declines. The low point is reached after approximately 6 months. Weight regain then begins and continues gradually until weight stabilizes near baseline levels. Obesity is a chronic condition that may require treatment of indefinite duration. Continuing therapist contact appears to be a key element in successful maintenance programs (Perri, 1998).

Schizophrenia

In the early days of behavior therapy, the treatment of schizophrenic patients consisted of token economy programs in mental hospitals. The most prominent example of this approach was a study by Paul and Lentz (1977). They treated chronic mental patients, all of whom were diagnosed as process schizophrenic and were of low socioeconomic status. These patients had been confined to a mental hospital for an average of 17 years and had been treated previously with drugs and other methods without success. Approximately 90% were taking medication at the onset of the study. Their level of self-care was too low and the severity of their bizarre behavior too great to permit community placement. According to Paul and Lentz, these subjects were "the most severely debilitated chronically institutionalized adults ever subjected to systematic study" (p. v). In the most detailed, comprehensive, and well-controlled evaluation of the treatment of chronic mental hospital patients ever conducted, Paul and Lentz produced a wealth of objective data, including evidence of cost effectiveness, showing that behavioral procedures (predominantly a sophisticated token reinforcement program) were effective.

In the 1980s, research began to show that family environment was decisive in determining whether schizophrenic patients discharged from hospital relapsed or maintained their improvement. As a result, family interventions were developed for preventing relapse, and some of these were strongly behavioral in nature (Tarrier & Wykes, 2004). Given the success of cognitive behavioral treatment for anxiety and other disorders, the same strategies began to be applied to schizophrenic patients. The treatments were designed to modify schizophrenic symptoms that proved resistant to medication as well as acute psychotic episodes. Overall, the evidence that these treatments are effective is promising, but not definitive. Tarrier and Wykes (2004) note that there has been a tendency for more behavioral interventions to be more effective than those relying on cognitive methods.

Childhood Disorders

Children have been treated from the earliest days of behavior therapy. Treatment programs have addressed problems ranging from circumscribed habit disorders in children to multiple responses of children who suffer all-encompassing excesses, deficits, or bizarre behavior patterns. These problems include conduct disorders, aggression, and delinquency. Hyperactivity is widely treated by behavioral methods, such as token reinforcement programs. The documented success of the behavioral approach, particularly in improving the academic performance of these children, suggests that it can sometimes be used as an alternative to drug treatment (O'Leary, 1980).

Autism is a particularly severe early childhood disorder with a very poor prognosis. Traditional psychological and medical treatments have proved ineffective. Behavioral methods, however, have achieved notable success. Lovaas (1987) has reported that intensive, long-term behavioral treatment of autistic children resulted in 47% achieving normal intellectual and educational functioning. Another 40% were mildly retarded and assigned to special classes for the language delayed. Of a control group of autistic children, only 2% achieved normal functioning. These findings are the most positive ever obtained with autistic children and illustrate the efficacy of behavioral methods with serious childhood disorders.

Childhood psychoses have also been treated with behavioral techniques. Self-stimulatory and self-destructive behavior such as biting and head banging have been eliminated with aversive procedures. Positive behaviors have been developed to improve language and speech, play, social interaction and responsiveness, and basic academic skills (O'Leary & Carr, 1982).

One of the most effectively treated childhood problems has been enuresis. The bell-and-pad method has produced improvement rates greater than 80% in many reports. Toileting accidents have been effectively altered with other behavioral procedures (Ross, 1981).

Behavioral Medicine

Behavioral medicine has been defined as the "interdisciplinary field concerned with the development and integration of behavioral and biomedical science knowledge and techniques relevant to health and illness and application of this knowledge and these techniques to prevention, diagnosis, treatment and rehabilitation" (Schwartz & Weiss, 1978, p. 250). Behavior therapy has helped to catalyze the rapid growth of this field.

Prevention and Treatment of Cardiovascular Disease

Specific behavior patterns appear to increase the risk of needless or premature cardiovascular disease. Modification of these behavior patterns is likely to produce significant reductions in cardiovascular disease. Among the risk factors that have been the target of behavioral treatment programs are cigarette smoking, obesity, lack of exercise, stress, hypertension, and excessive alcohol consumption. Substance abuse is typically treated with a combination of the self-control procedures. Stress and hypertension have been successfully treated using methods such as relaxation training. Behavior intervention methods have been applied not only to identified clients in both individual and group therapy sessions but also to essentially healthy individuals in the workplace and the community in programs designed to prevent cardiovascular disease.

Other Applications

Behavioral techniques have been successfully applied to such diverse health-related problems as tension headaches, different forms of pain, asthma, epilepsy, sleep disorders, nausea reactions in cancer patients (resulting from radiation therapy), and children's fears about being hospitalized and undergoing surgery (Melamed & Siegel, 1980). Behavior therapy has also been applied successfully to the treatment of alcoholism (McCrady, Epstein, Cook, Jensen, & Hildebrandt, 2009), suicidal adults with borderline personality and substance dependence disorders (Harned et al., 2008), and suicidal adolescents (Miller, Rathus, & Linehan, 2007). Finally, cognitive–behavioral principles show promise in increasing compliance with medical treatments (Meichenbaum & Turk, 1987).

Treatment

Some clinical details of a cognitive–behavioral approach to therapy may be illustrated by the treatment of agoraphobia, a complex anxiety disorder. Initially, the therapist carries out a careful assessment of the nature of the problem and the variables that seem to be maintaining it. Subsequent treatment may vary, but it is probable that some form of real-life exposure will be a central part of therapy. Together, therapist and client work out a hierarchy of increasingly fear-eliciting situations that the client has been avoiding. Repeated and systematic exposure to these situations occurs until avoidance is eliminated and fear is decreased.

The therapist is careful to distinguish systematic exposure from the unsystematic and ill-considered attempts clients have typically made to enter feared situations too quickly. Preparation for each exposure experience involves anticipating the inevitable fearful reactions and teaching clients appropriate coping skills. This includes recognizing and accepting feelings of fear, identifying cognitive distortions that elicit or exacerbate fear, and counteracting cognitive distortions.

The therapist might accompany the client during real-life exposure sessions, providing encouragement, support, and social reinforcement. Although empathic, the therapist remains firm about the necessity for systematic exposure. Once the client enters the feared situation, it is important for the client not to leave until his or her anxiety has decreased.

Following exposure, therapist and client analyze what happened. This provides the therapist an opportunity to see how the client interprets his or her experience and to uncover any faulty cognitive processing. For example, people coping with agoraphobia tend to discount positive accomplishments, do not always attribute success experiences to their own coping ability, and therefore do not develop greater self-efficacy.

Clients are given specific instructions about exposure homework assignments between therapy sessions and are asked to keep detailed daily records of what they attempted, how they felt, and what problems they encountered. These self-recordings are reviewed by the therapist at the beginning of each session. In addition to providing the therapist with information on clients' progress (or lack of progress), these daily records facilitate the process of changing clients' cognitive sets about their problems. By directing their attention to the records of their own experience, the therapist helps clients to gain a more objective and balanced view of their problems and progress.

Homework assignments typically require the active cooperation of the client's spouse (or some other family member). The therapist invites the spouse to one or more therapy sessions to assess his or her willingness and ability to provide the necessary support and to explain what is required. It is common practice to use treatment manuals for both the client and the spouse in which they detail each step of real-life exposure treatment and describe mutual responsibilities. In many cases, these manuals can greatly reduce the number of sessions the couple spends with the therapist.

Clients often fail to complete homework assignments. There are several possible reasons for lack of compliance, ranging from poorly chosen homework assignments to resistance to change. Another possibility is that the spouse is uncooperative or tries to sabotage therapy. One of the advantages of including the spouse in treatment is that this resistance to progress is rapidly uncovered and can be addressed directly in therapy sessions.

To supplement real-life exposure, some clients need assertiveness training, whereas others need to acquire ways of coping with suppressed anger. Before terminating successful treatment, the therapist works on relapse prevention training with clients. Briefly, clients are told that it is possible that they might experience an unexpected return of some fear at unpredictable points in the future. Using imagery to project ahead to such a recurrence of fear, clients learn to cope with their feelings by reinstituting previously successful coping responses. They are reassured that these feelings are quite normal and time-limited and do not necessarily signal a relapse. Clients learn that it is primarily the way they interpret these feelings that determines whether or not they experience a relapse. Specifically, the therapist tries to inoculate them against such anxiety-inducing cognitive errors as catastrophizing or selective focus on an isolated anxiety symptom.

Evidence

Behavior therapy consists of a broad range of different strategies and techniques, some of which are differentially effective for different problems. Hence, it is difficult to evaluate some global entity called "behavior therapy." Instead, evaluation must be directed at specific methods applied to particular problems.

Research Strategies

Behavior therapists have developed various research strategies for evaluating therapy outcome. Single-case experimental designs are important because they enable cause–effect relationships to be drawn between treatments and outcome in the individual case. The ABA, or reversal, design was illustrated in the Ayllon and Azrin (1965) study previously described. In the multiple-baseline design, different responses are continuously measured. Treatment is then applied successively to each response. If the desired behavior changes maximally only when treated, then a cause–effect relationship can be inferred. Limitations of single-subject methodology include the inability to examine the interaction of subject variables with specific treatment effects and difficulty in generalizing findings to other cases.

Laboratory-based studies permit the evaluation of specific techniques applied to particular problems under tightly controlled conditions; for example, evaluating fear reduction methods with snake-phobic subjects (Bandura, 1986). The advantages of this methodology include the use of multiple objective measures of outcome, the selection of homogeneous subject samples and therapists, and the freedom to assign subjects to experimental and control groups. Limitations include the possibility that findings with only mildly disturbed subjects might not be generalizable to more severely disturbed clients.

The treatment package strategy evaluates the effect of a multifaceted treatment program. If the package proves to be successful, its effective components are analyzed in subsequent research. One way of doing this is to use the dismantling strategy, in which components of the treatment package are systematically eliminated and the associated decrement in treatment outcome is measured.

The comparative research strategy is directed toward determining whether some therapeutic techniques are superior to others. Comparative studies are most appropriate after specific techniques have been shown to be effective in single-subject or laboratory-based research. Different group designs require different control groups, depending on the research question addressed. The no-treatment control group controls for the possible therapeutic effects of assessment of outcome, maturation, and other changes in clients' behavior that occur independently of formal treatment. Attention–placebo control groups are used to parcel out the contribution to treatment effects of factors that are common to most forms of therapy and often called *nonspecific factors*. These factors include the relationship between therapist and client, expectations of therapeutic progress, and suggestion. For example, behavior therapy has been increasingly compared with antidepressant medication in the treatment of anxiety, mood, and eating disorders (as mentioned earlier in this chapter) in what are called randomized controlled trials (RCTs). In the basic design, the antidepressant medication and the behavioral treatment are compared with each other and with a pill–placebo. If the medication or behavioral treatment is significantly more effective than the pill–placebo condition, the treatment has been shown to have a specific therapeutic effect above and beyond so-called "nonspecific" factors.

In research on the effects of both pharmacological and psychological treatments, a distinction is made between efficacy and effectiveness studies. An *efficacy study* is tightly controlled, with random assignment of patients to different treatments, the use of manual-based treatments, the inclusion of therapists who have been carefully trained in the use of the specific treatments, and rigorous assessment of outcome by independent evaluators. They are typically conducted in specialty university and medical school settings. In contrast, *effectiveness studies* are usually less well-controlled: Formal therapy manuals are not used, there is no specific training or supervision of therapists for the purposes of the study, and the study is conducted under conditions of routine clinical practice (e.g., in a community mental health center). The goal of effectiveness research is to evaluate the "clinical representativeness" of efficacy outcome research. We need to assess how well the results of controlled research generalize to diverse patient populations, clinical settings, and different therapists.

Research Findings

The efficacy and effectiveness of behavior therapy has been studied more intensively than in any other form of psychological treatment. In addition to traditional qualitative reviews of the evidence for different disorders, numerous meta-analyses exist that provide comprehensive and quantitative evaluations of the findings of large numbers of different treatment outcome studies (Nathan & Gorman, in press). The most rigorous and complete evaluations of both psychological and pharmacological treatment of different clinical disorders are those of the National Institute for Clinical Excellence (NICE) in the United Kingdom (NICE, 2004). NICE issues treatment guidelines that are a product of a multidisciplinary process in which the standard is consistent across all of medicine. The guidelines are based on data and are graded from A (strong empirical support from well-controlled RCTs) to C (expert opinion with strong empirical data).

Behavior therapy has fared well in the NICE evaluations of the evidence for the various clinical disorders. The level of empirical support for behavioral treatments is typically rated as A. These treatments are recommended as the psychological treatment of choice for specific mood and anxiety disorders and evaluated as equally effective as pharmacological therapy. In the case of eating disorders, behavior therapy has been evaluated as even more effective than medication (Fairburn, Cooper, & Shafran, 2008; Wilson & Shafran, 2005). Examples of individual research studies documenting the efficacy of behavior therapy have been summarized in the earlier section on Applications.

In another evaluation of the evidence for different psychological treatments, Division 12 of the American Psychological Association established criteria for judging treatments as "empirically supported." For example, a treatment had to have at least two well-controlled studies, conducted by different investigators, that showed the treatment to be significantly more effective than a pill, psychological placebo, or other form of treatment. They then identified those treatments that met these standards of evidence (Woody, Weisz, & McLean, 2005). Behavioral treatments dominate the list of what have been called empirically supported therapies.

The treatments that have been evaluated in the NICE guidelines and by Woody et al. (2005) have been traditional behavioral and cognitive behavioral interventions. Evidence on third-wave forms of behavior therapy is gradually emerging. DBT for borderline personality disorder clearly enjoys empirical support, as summarized earlier (Lieb et al., 2004; Linehan et al., 2006). The evidence on ACT is promising albeit still at a rudimentary stage (Hayes et al., 2006).

Most of the evidence in support of behavior therapy treatments for different clinical disorders is based on well-controlled efficacy research. It is important to point out, however, that effectiveness studies are beginning to show that the results of the efficacy studies do generalize to routine clinical practice (Wilson, 2007). For example, there is now evidence that cognitive and behavioral treatments for anxiety disorders and depression are effective in helping minority group members in community-based treatment settings (e.g., Foa et al., 2005; Miranda et al., 2005). Demonstrating the relevance of evidence-based psychological therapy for members of minority groups is a research priority given that these individuals tend to be underrepresented in RCTs in specialized university and medical school settings.

Psychotherapy in a Multicultural World

Junko Tanaka-Matsumi (2008) has examined the interface between two growing domains in psychotherapy: multiculturalism and the demand for empirically supported psychotherapy. She noted the importance of providing culturally responsive cognitive–behavioral therapy to people of diverse cultural backgrounds and points out that the minority population in the United States grew 11 times as rapidly as the non-Hispanic population between 1980 and 2000. This rapid growth of the minority population in the United States shows no sign of abating. However, Tanaka-Matsumi also notes that the well-documented effectiveness of behavioral therapy is largely based on evidence derived from Caucasian groups from North America or with European cultural backgrounds, and there is a pressing need to develop evidence from diverse populations around the globe. She writes:

> globalization will encourage training of multicultural mental health professionals who can apply universally applicable principles of behavior change and implement culturally specific treatment. Functional analysis is a flexible and individualized method that can identify culture-relevant content in cognitive–behavior therapy for diverse clients. (p. 191)

CASE EXAMPLE[1]

Melissa was a 22-year-old graduate student who sought treatment at the counseling center of her university because of her eating disorder. Her body mass index was 23, which is in the middle of the normal (healthy) range.

During the first session Dr. Jones, the female clinical psychologist to whom she had been assigned, asked a number of questions to learn as much as possible about Melissa's problems, such as when the eating disorder had started and how it had developed. Dr. Jones also inquired about any other associated problems (e.g., substance abuse, depression, and anxiety), as well as Melissa's social interactions with family and friends. Melissa's score on the Beck Depression Inventory (BDI) was 25, indicating a high probability of clinical depression.

As she talked about her problems, Melissa became teary and mentioned how ashamed she felt about her behavior. Dr. Jones expressed empathy, saying that she knew how upset Melissa was and how hard it must have been the last few months struggling with the eating disorder without confiding in anyone, including her boyfriend. She praised Melissa for having the courage to seek treatment and reassured her that they could work together to help her overcome the problem. Dr. Jones explained that Melissa's pattern

---

[1] This case example consists of a composite of features from more than one patient in order to fully ensure confidentiality. The therapeutic strategies summarized in this case study are described in detail in Fairburn et al. (1993) and Wilson (2004).

of regular binge eating followed by self-induced vomiting, together with her attempts to diet to lose more weight, were consistent with bulimia nervosa (BN). She gave Melissa a copy of *Overcoming Binge Eating*, an evidence-based self-help book written by Chris Fairburn (see Fairburn, 1995), one of the world's leading authorities on eating disorders. She asked Melissa to read the first half of the book that described the nature of eating disorders like BN. Dr. Jones also asked Melissa to keep a daily written record of everything she ate and drank, when, and under what circumstances—i.e., she was asked to practice self-monitoring. Dr. Jones took care to explain why this was important—it would provide valuable information for her as the therapist but would also immediately begin to help Melissa understand and begin to take control of her eating behavior. After explaining self-monitoring, Dr. Jones asked Melissa what she thought about it. Did it make sense to her? Could she anticipate any obstacles that would interfere with self-monitoring? Melissa answered that she understood the purpose of the assignment and expressed her willingness to work on the task. When leaving, she thanked Dr. Jones and said that she felt a great sense of relief in finally having confided in someone, especially someone who was caring and seemed to understand the problem.

At the beginning of the second session, Dr. Jones and Melissa jointly reviewed her self-monitoring records. She had kept excellent records for 5 of the 7 days, although over the weekend her recording was very spotty. Melissa ruefully stated that the week had been a bad one, although she had not binged or vomited on two of the days. Dr. Jones made a point of praising Melissa's self-monitoring while at the same time encouraging her to keep accurate daily records. She also checked to see if Melissa had read the self-help book. She had and was encouraged to learn that other young women like her had successfully overcome the problem. As she would do every session, Dr. Jones then set the agenda for the rest of the session. She explained that she wanted to go over the reasons Melissa was binge eating and vomiting and to explore what was different between the two days that Melissa had not binged and the rest of the past week. Dr. Jones invited Melissa's feedback on the agenda and asked if she wanted to cover any other issue so as to reinforce the concept of collaboration between therapist and patient.

Dr. Jones then presented the cognitive behavioral model of the factors that maintain BN. The core of the model is that extreme concerns about the importance of body shape and weight lead individuals to diet in dysfunctional and unhealthy ways. This leads to binge eating for both biological (hunger) and psychological (setting rules for eating that are too rigid and unrealistic) reasons. Finally, vomiting and laxative abuse are attempts to compensate for the binge eating to avoid weight gain. The vomiting induces shame and only leads to more unhealthy attempts to diet—thereby perpetuating the problem.

Melissa agreed that the model accurately described what was happening to her and understood that she would have to deal with her over-concern about body shape and weight and change her unhealthy dieting to overcome BN. But she expressed her reluctance to give up dieting. She worried that this would lead to weight gain—the thing she feared most. In response to Dr. Jones's gentle questioning, Melissa made clear her ambivalence about change—she wanted to stop binge eating and vomiting, but she feared the potential consequences associated with these changes. Dr. Jones empathized with Melissa's conflict and asked her to complete the following homework assignment. Melissa was to write down (1) the advantages and disadvantages of continuing to diet; and (2) the corresponding advantages and disadvantages of stopping dysfunctional dieting (see Wilson [2004] for details of this strategy for overcoming ambivalence).

In the third session, Dr. Jones reviewed Melissa's self-monitoring and homework. She had concluded that, on the whole, it was worth changing her dysfunctional behavior—the advantages were greater than the disadvantages. Dr. Jones then explained what needed to be done to change dysfunctional dieting into healthy eating patterns. The first step would be to eat regular meals—breakfast, lunch, and dinner, with planned snacks in the morning and afternoon. Melissa could still choose "safe" foods but needed to change her pattern of skipping meals. Dr. Jones also asked Melissa to weigh herself no more than once a week instead of weighing multiple times each day. Melissa expressed her concern that without frequent daily weighing she would gain weight. Dr. Jones suggested that Melissa think of this task as an experiment—she was encouraged to try it for the next 2 weeks and see what would happen to her weight. Melissa liked this idea and agreed to give it a try.

In the next two sessions the focus remained on Melissa self-monitoring, adopting a regular eating pattern, and weighing herself weekly. She was able to accomplish each of these goals. Her binge eating stopped and her depression score on the BDI that Dr. Jones administered each session dropped significantly (BDI = 16). However, Melissa was still eating in a very restrictive fashion. She avoided so-called "forbidden" foods out of fear that they would trigger binge eating. Dr. Jones encouraged her to try another experiment—one in which she planned to eat a "forbidden food" such as ice cream. She was to do this one afternoon when she had not skipped breakfast or lunch, and when she felt good about herself. Melissa was amazed to discover that she did not experience an urge to binge and felt in control. The goal of this behavioral experiment was to show Melissa that she could eat a wider range of foods than she previously believed without losing control.

The focus in Sessions #6 and #7 remained on overcoming dysfunctional dieting. Melissa was no longer binge eating, but she still occasionally resorted to vomiting as a means of coping with negative feelings about herself. Based on her self-monitoring records, it was clear that these occasions were typically triggered by conflicts with her boyfriend.

In Sessions #8 through 10, therapy focused on helping Melissa to become more assertive (see Alberti & Emmons, 2001) and not allow herself to be treated badly by her boyfriend. She learned to express her feelings and to insist on being treated with respect. This led to her leaving her boyfriend and dating someone else with whom she developed a close and caring relationship. Her self-esteem increased, her mood improved (BDI = 6), and she stopped vomiting.

Despite her good progress, Melissa remained over-concerned about the importance of her body shape and weight. She continued to "feel fat" even though, objectively, she was of normal weight. She constantly worried about her appearance and how people would judge her. As is typical in BN, she constantly "body-checked," such as pinching parts of her body to see how fat she was and checking herself out in mirrors. She also avoided some situations that would expose her body, such as wearing form-fitting clothes or a bikini at the shore.

Dr. Jones explained how important it was to stop this pathological body-checking and body-avoidance. Over the course of Sessions #11 through 14, she encouraged Melissa to try another behavioral experiment, namely, stopping all body-checking and seeing what effect it would have. Melissa was afraid that by being less vigilant she would gain weight, just as she was previously worried about giving up weighing herself multiple times a day. To her surprise, she found that her weight remained stable and her preoccupation with body weight diminished. Dr. Jones also encouraged her to combat body-avoidance by wearing clothes she liked and by participating in fun social events.

In Sessions #13 and #14, Dr. Jones used a mindfulness-based procedure in which she asked Melissa to stand in front of a full-size mirror. Her task was to observe and describe her body, from her head to her toes, in a nonjudgmental fashion while staying in the present (see Wilson, 2004). Initially Melissa found this task very upsetting—she was very judgmental and focused exclusively on her stomach and thighs, the areas she always worried about. With practice, however, she was able to describe her whole body and "let go" of negative feelings without reacting to them. She learned to "distance" herself from thoughts and feelings that she was fat and to say to herself that she was a normal-weight woman who was often beset by thoughts that she was fat. She complemented this in-session mirror exposure with homework assignments in which she tried to adopt a mindful approach to looking at herself in a mirror. She used a mirror only for an agreed-upon purpose and time, and never in response to an urge to check her body because she "felt fat." Melissa became more accepting of her body shape and weight and happier with her life.

Melissa's last two sessions focused on relapse prevention. With the help of Dr. Jones, Melissa wrote up her own personal maintenance manual in which she summarized the improvements she had made, what she needed to focus on in the future, and what she would do if she ever slipped and binged or vomited again. Therapy terminated with Melissa confident and prepared to maintain the improvement she had made in working with Dr. Jones.

SUMMARY

Behavior therapy helped to change the face of psychotherapy in the latter half of the 20th century by generating innovative treatment strategies and influencing how we conduct research on psychological treatment. In turn, behavior therapy itself has changed and continues to evolve. Its theoretical foundations have broadened and its treatment techniques have become more diverse. In the process, its overlaps with other systems of psychotherapy have become more apparent. Nonetheless, it remains a distinctive approach to assessment and treatment.

Methodological rigor and innovation have been major contributions of behavior therapy to the field of psychotherapy. Behavioral treatments have been subjected to more rigorous evaluation than any other psychological therapy.

Behavior therapy faces two immediate challenges in the 21st century. One is the need to improve the dissemination and adoption of demonstrably effective behavioral treatments for a number of common disorders. Although behavior therapy has become an accepted part of the psychotherapeutic establishment, its methods are not being used as widely as the evidence would warrant (Persons, 1997). As noted earlier in this chapter, the growing demand for accountability in health care will provide an impetus for more widespread application of behavioral methods.

The evidence supporting behavior therapy comes mainly from well-controlled research studies conducted at universities where therapists are carefully selected and highly trained and patients are recruited specifically for the treatment studies. However, many practitioners question the relevance of this type of research to actual clinical practice in which they are confronted with a diverse mix of patients and varying clinical problems. Encouragingly, an increasing emphasis on clinical research focused on evaluating the generalizability of the findings from tightly controlled, university-based research to different service settings such as mental health clinics and independent practice is showing that the research findings are holding up in routine clinical practice.

Another likely trend will be the use of a stepped-care approach to treatment services. In a stepped-care framework, which is widely used in medicine, treatments are provided sequentially according to need. Initially, all patients receive the lowest step—the simplest, least intrusive, and most cost-effective treatment. More complex or intensive interventions are administered to patients who do not respond to these initial efforts. To date, most behavior therapy treatments have been designed for use within specialist settings and require professional training. Relatively few therapists are sufficiently well trained in these specialized, manual-based treatments (Wilson, 1998). Moreover, there are unlikely ever to be sufficient specialist treatment resources for all patients. Briefer and simpler methods that can be used by a wide range of different mental health professionals are needed. It will be challenging but critical to identify reliable predictors of patients for whom these cost-effective methods are appropriate.

The second major challenge confronting behavior therapy is the need to develop more effective treatments for a broader range of problems. At present, even the most effective treatments are often not good enough. Clinical researchers and practitioners need to cooperate in devising innovative and improved methods for treating patients who do not respond to the best available treatments.

Whereas considerable progress has been made in developing effective treatments, the field has lagged behind in understanding how these treatments achieve their therapeutic effects. We need to learn more about the mechanisms of therapeutic change. Understanding the mechanisms through which behavior therapy methods operate is vital to the development of innovative and more potent interventions. With respect to current manual-based treatments, active therapeutic procedures could be enhanced and inactive elements discarded. Theory-driven, experimental analysis of therapy outcome and its mechanisms of action is a priority for future research.

Finally, to fulfill its original promise of linking clinical practice to advances in scientific research, behavior therapy must be responsive to developments both in experimental psychology and in biology. Dramatic breakthroughs in genetics and neuroscience have already revolutionized the biological sciences. Progress will continue in unlocking the secrets of the brain. A better understanding of the role of brain mechanisms in the development and maintenance of clinical disorders will lead to better theories and therapies for behavior change.

ANNOTATED BIBLIOGRAPHY

Barlow, D. H. (Ed.). (2008). *Clinical handbook of psychological disorders* (4th ed.). New York: Guilford Press.
This edited volume provides detailed clinical descriptions of the cognitive–behavioral treatment of several adult clinical disorders. A particularly informative feature is the extensive use of transcripts from actual therapy sessions with individual patients.

Linehan, M. M., & Dexter-Mazza, E. T. (2008). Dialectical behavior therapy for borderline personality disorder. In Barlow, D. H. (Ed.), *Clinical handbook of psychological disorders: A step-by-step treatment manual* (4th ed.). (pp. 365–420). New York: Guilford Press.
This chapter is an excellent introduction to the practice of dialectical behavior therapy (DBT).

Luoma, J. B., Hayes, S. C., & Walser, R. D. (2007). *Learning ACT: An acceptance and commitment therapy skills-training manual for therapists.* Oakland, CA: New Harbinger Publications.
This skills manual is a good introduction to acceptance and commitment therapy that will introduce you to the

theory and practice of ACT; an accompanying DVD offers role-played examples of core ACT methods.

Martell, C., Addis, M., & Jacobson, N. S. (2001). *Depression in context.* New York: Norton.
This volume provides a detailed and very practical description of the clinical application of behavioral activation (BA) treatment for depression. Informative clinical illustrations are used to highlight differences between BA and cognitive therapy.

Roemer, L., & Orsillo, S. M. (2009). *Mindfulness- and acceptance-based behavioral therapies in practice.* New York: Guilford.
This book present a synthesis of several of the mindfulness- and acceptance-based behavioral therapies, including acceptance and commitment therapy, mindfulness-based cognitive therapy, mindfulness-based relapse prevention, integrative behavioral couple therapy, and dialectical behavior therapy. The authors propose a general model that involves three related mechanisms: a maladaptive relationship to internal experience (such as fusion, judgment, and/or lack of awareness), experiential avoidance, and behavioral constriction.

CASE READINGS

Barlow, D. (1993). Covert sensitization for paraphilia. In J. R. Cautela, A. J. Kearney, L. Ascher, A. Kearney, & M. Kleinman (Eds.), *Covert conditioning casebook* (pp. 188–197). Pacific Grove, CA: Cengage Learning. [Reprinted in D. Wedding & R. J. Corsini (Eds.). (2011). *Case studies in psychotherapy.* Belmont, CA: Brooks/Cole.]

This is a detailed case that demonstrates the use of covert sensitization in the treatment of a deeply troubled minister.

Bond, F. W. (2004). *ACT for stress.* In S. C. Hayes and K. Strosahl (Eds.), *A practical guide to acceptance and commitment therapy* (pp. 275–294). New York: Springer.

This chapter provides a detailed account of clinical case conceptualization and application of techniques in the use of ACT for common stress-related problems.

Craske, M. G., & Barlow, D. H. (2001). Panic disorder and agoraphobia. In D. H. Barlow (Ed.), *Clinical handbook of psychological disorders* (3rd ed., pp. 1–59). New York: Guilford Press.

> This chapter provides a detailed clinical case illustration, with therapist–patient dialogue, of DBT in the treatment of panic disorder.

Foa, E. B., & Franklin, M. E. (2001). Obsessive–compulsive disorder. In D. H. Barlow (Ed.), *Clinical handbook of psychological disorders* (3rd ed., pp. 209–263). New York: Guilford Press.

> This chapter provides a detailed clinical case illustration, with therapist–patient dialogue, of DBT in the treatment of obsessive-compulsive disorder.

Linehan, M. M., Cochran, B. N., & Kehrer, C. A. (2001). Dialectical behavior therapy for Borderline Personality Disorder. In D. H. Barlow (Ed.), *Clinical handbook of psychological disorders: A step-by-step treatment manual* (3rd ed., pp. 470–522). New York: Guilford Press.

> This chapter provides a detailed clinical case illustration, with therapist–patient dialogue, of DBT in the treatment of borderline–personality disorder.

Martell, C. R., Addis, M. E., & Jacobson, N. S. (2001). *Depression in context*. New York: Norton.

> Chapter 8 provides explicit clinical examples of the application of behavioral activation treatment for depression.

Wilson, G. T., & Pike, K. (2001). *Eating disorders*. In D. H. Barlow (Ed.), *Clinical handbook of psychological disorders* (3rd ed.). New York: Guilford Press.

> This chapter provides an in-depth illustration of the treatment of a female patient with bulimia nervosa, an eating disorder that is common among college-aged and young adult women.

Wolf, M. M., Risley, T., & Mees, H. (1965). Application of operant conditioning procedures to the behavior problems of an autistic child. In L. P. Ullmann & L. Krasner (Eds.), *Case studies in behavior modification* (pp. 138–145). New York: Holt, Rinehart and Winston.

> This classic case study illustrates the application of operant principles and procedures to the treatment of an autistic child. The assessment and treatment approach described here provide a model for the use of behavioral methods with a wide range of problems among the developmentally disabled.

Wolpe, J. (1991). *A complex case. The practice of behavior therapy* (4th ed.). New York: Pergamon. [Reprinted in D. Wedding & R. J. Corsini (Eds.). (1995). *Case studies in psychotherapy.* Itasca, IL: F. E. Peacock.]

> This case study describes the way one of the founders of behavior therapy treated a 31-year-old man who presented with symptoms of anxiety and an obsession about his wife's premarital loss of virginity.

REFERENCES

Agras, W. S., & Wilson, G. T. (2005). Learning theory. In B. J. Sadock & V. A. Sadock (Eds.), *Comprehensive textbook of psychiatry* (8th ed., pp. 541–552). Baltimore, MD: Williams & Wilkins.

Alberti, R., & Emmons, M. (2001). *Your perfect right* (8th ed.). Atascadero, CA: Impact.

Ayllon, T., & Azrin, N. H. (1965). The measurement and reinforcement of behavior of psychotics. *Journal of the Experimental Analysis of Behavior, 8,* 357–383.

Bandura, A. (1969). *Principles of behavior modification.* New York: Holt, Rinehart and Winston.

Bandura, A. (1977). *Social learning theory.* Englewood Cliffs, NJ: Prentice-Hall.

Bandura, A. (1982). Self-efficacy mechanism in human agency. *American Psychologist, 37,* 122–147.

Bandura, A. (1986). *Social foundations of thought and action: A social cognitive theory.* Englewood Cliffs, NJ: Prentice-Hall.

Bandura, A. (1998). Personal and collective efficacy in human adaptation and change. In J. G. Adair, D. Belanger, & K. L. Dion (Eds.), *Advances in psychological science* (pp. 51–72). East Sussex, UK: Psychology Press.

Barlow, D. H. (2002). *Anxiety and its disorders* (2nd ed.). New York: Guilford Press.

Barlow, D. H., Gorman, J. M., Shear, M. K., & Woods, S. W. (2000). Cognitive behavioral therapy, imipramine, or their combination for panic disorder. *Journal of the American Medical Association, 283,* 2529–2536.

Baxter, L. R., Schwartz, J. M., Bergman, K. S., Szuba, M. P., Guze, B. H., Mazziotata, J. C., et al. (1992). Caudate glucose metabolic rate changes with both drug and behavior therapy for obsessive–compulsive disorder. *Archives of General Psychiatry, 49,* 681–689.

Beck, A. T., Rush, A. J., Shaw, B. E., & Emery, G. (1979). *Cognitive therapy of depression.* New York: Guilford Press.

Brady, J., Davison, G., Dewald, P., Egan, G., Fadiman, J., Frank, J., et al. (1980). Some views on effective principles of psychotherapy, *Cognitive Therapy and Research, 4,* 271–306.

Campbell-Sills, L., Barlow, D. H., Brown, T. A., & Hoffmann, S. G. (2006). Effects of suppression and acceptance on emotional responses of individuals with anxiety and mood disorders. *Behaviour Research and Therapy, 44,* 1251–1263.

Cautela, J. (1967). Covert sensitization. *Psychological Reports, 20,* 459–468.

Clark, D.M. (1989). Anxiety states. In K. Hawton, P. M. Salkovskis, J. Kirk, & D. M. Clark (Eds.). *Cognitive behaviour therapy for psychiatric problems: A practical guide.* Oxford: Oxford University Press.

Clark, D. M., Salkovskis, P. M., Hackmann, A., Middleton, H., & Gelder, M. (1994). A comparison of cognitive therapy, applied relaxation and imipramine in the treatment of panic disorder. *British Journal of Psychiatry, 164,* 759–769.

Craske, M. G., Brown, T. A., & Barlow, D. H. (1991). Behavioral treatment of panic disorder: A two-year follow-up. *Behavior Therapy, 22,* 289–304.

Craske, M. G., Golinelli, D., Stein, M. B., Roy-Byrne, P., Bystritsky, A., & Sherbourne, C. (2005). Does the addition of cognitive behavioral therapy improve panic disorder treatment outcome relative to medication alone in the primary-care setting? *Psychological Medicine, 35,* 1–10.

Davis, M., Myers, K. M., Ressler, K. J., & Rothbaum, B. O. (2005). Facilitation of extinction of conditioned fear by d-cycloserine: Implications for psychotherapy. *Current Directions in Psychological Science, 14,* 214–219.

Davison, G. C., & Lazarus, A. A. (1995). The dialectics of science and practice. In S. C. Hayes, V. M. Follette, R. M. Dawes, & K. E. Grady (Eds.), *Scientific standards of psychological practice: Issues and recommendations* (pp. 95–120). Reno, NV: Context Press.

Dawes, R. M. (1994). *House of cards.* New York: Free Press.

DeRubeis, R. J., Hollon, S. D., Amsterdam, J. D., Shelton, R. C., Young, P. R., Salomon, R. M., O'Reardon, J. P., Lovett, M. L., Gladis, M. M., Brown, L. L., & Gallop, R. (2005). Cognitive therapy vs. medications in the treatment of moderate to severe depression. *Archives of General Psychiatry, 62,* 409–416.

DeRubeis, R. J., Brotman, M. A., & Gibbons, C. J. (2005). A conceptual and methodological analysis of the nonspecifics argument. *Clinical Psychology: Science and Practice, 12,* 174–183.

Dimidjian, S., Hollon, S. D., Dobson, K. S., Schmaling, K. B., Kohlenberg, R. J., Addis, M. E., Gallop, R., McGlinchey, J. B., Markley, D. K., Gollan, J. K., Atkins. D. C., Dunner, D. L., & Jacobson, N. S. (in press). Behavioral activation, cognitive therapy and antidepressant medication in the acute treatment of major depression. *Journal of Consulting and Clinical Psychology.*

Dobson, K. S., Hollon, S. D., Dimidjian, S., Schmaling, K. B., Kohlenberg, R. J., Gallop, R. J., Rizvi, S. L., Gollan, J. K., Dunner, D. L., & Jacobson, N. S. (2008). Randomized trial of behavioral activation, cognitive therapy, and antidepressant medication in the prevention of relapse and recurrence in major depression. *Journal of Consulting and Clinical Psychology, 76,* 468–477.

Eysenck, H. J. (1959). Learning theory and behavior therapy. *British Journal of Medical Science, 105,* 61–75.

Eysenck, H. J. (1967). *The biological basis of personality.* Springfield, IL: Charles C. Thomas.

Fairburn, C. G. (1995). *Overcoming binge eating.* New York: Guilford Press.

Fairburn, C. G., Cooper, Z., & Shafran, R. (2008). Enhanced cognitive behavior therapy for eating disorders ("CBT-E"): An overview. In Fairburn, C. G., *Cognitive behavior therapy and eating disorders* (pp. 23–34). New York: Guilford Press.

Fairburn, C. G., Marcus, M. D., & Wilson, G. T. (1993). Cognitive behaviour therapy for binge eating and bulimia nervosa: A comprehensive treatment manual. In C. G. Fairburn & G. T. Wilson (Eds.), *Binge eating: Nature, assessment and treatment* (pp. 361–404). New York: Guilford Press.

Foa, E. B., Hembree, E. A., Cahill, S. P., Rauch, S. A. M., & Riggs, D. S., et al. (2005). Randomized trial of prolonged exposure for posttraumatic stress disorder with and without cognitive restructuring: Outcome at academic and community clinics. *Journal of Consulting and Clinical Psychology, 73,* 953–964.

Glass, C. R., & Arnkoff, D. B. (1992). Behavior therapy. In D. K. Freedheim, H. J. Freudenberger, J. W. Kessler, S. B. Messer, D. R. Peterson, H. H. Strupp, et al. (Eds.), *History of psychotherapy: A century of change* (pp. 587–628). Washington, DC: American Psychological Association.

Gortner, E. T., Gollan, J. K., Dobson, K. S., & Jacobson, N. S. (1998). Cognitive–behavioral treatment for depression: Relapse prevention. *Journal of Consulting and Clinical Psychology, 66,* 377–384.

Harned, M. S., Chapman, A. L., Dexter-Mazza, E. T., Murray, A., Comtois, K. A., & Linehan, M. M. (2008). Treating co-occurring Axis I disorders in recurrently suicidal women with borderline personality disorder: A 2-year randomized trial of dialectical behavior therapy versus community treatment by experts. *Journal of Consulting and Clinical Psychology, 76,* 1068–1075.

Harvey, A., Watkins, E., Mansell, W., & Shafran, R. (2004). *Cognitive behavioural processes across psychological disorders: A transdiagnostic approach to research and treatment.* New York: Oxford University Press.

Hayes, S. C., Follette, V. M., & Linehan, M. M. (2004). *Mindfulness and acceptance.* New York: Guilford Press.

Hayes, S. C., Luoma, J. B., Bond, F. W., Masuda, A., & Lillis, J. (2006). Acceptance and commitment therapy: Model, processes and outcomes. *Behaviour Research and Therapy, 44,* 1–25.

Hayes, S., & Smith, S. (2005). *Get out of your mind and into your life.* Oakland, CA: New Harbinger Publications.

Hollon, S.H. (1999). Rapid early response in cognitive behavior therapy. *Clinical Psychology: Science and Practice, 6,* 305–309.

Hollon, S. D., & Beck, A. (1994). Cognitive and cognitive behavioral therapies. In S. L. Garfield & A. E. Bergin (Eds.), *Handbook of psychotherapy and behavior change: An empirical analysis* (4th ed.). New York: Wiley.

Hollon, S. D., Stewart, M. O., & Strunk, D. (2006). Enduring effects for cognitive behavior therapy in the treatment of depression and anxiety. *Annual Review of Psychology, 57,* 11.1–11.31.

Ilardi, S. S., & Craighead, W. E. (1994). The role of nonspecific factors in cognitive–behavior therapy for depression. *Clinical Psychology, 1,* 138–156.

Jacobson, E. (1938). *Progressive relaxation.* Chicago: University of Chicago Press.

Jacobson, N. S. (Ed.). (1987). *Psychotherapists in clinical practice: Cognitive and behavioral perspectives.* New York: Guilford Press.

Jacobson, N. S., Dobson, K. S., Truax, P. A., Addis, M. E., Koerner, K., Gollan, J. K., et al. (1996). A component analysis of cognitive–behavioral treatment for depression. *Journal of Consulting and Clinical Psychology, 64,* 295–304.

Jones, M. C. (1924). The elimination of children's fears. *Journal of Experimental Psychology, 7,* 382–390.

Kanfer, F. H. (1977). The many faces of self-control, or behavior modification changes its focus. In R. B. Stuart (Ed.), *Behavioral self-management* (pp. 1–48). New York: Brunner/Mazel.

Kazdin, A. E. (1977). *The token economy.* New York: Plenum.

Kazdin, A. E., & Wilson, G. T. (1978). *Evaluation of behavior therapy: Issues, evidence and research strategies.* Cambridge, MA: Ballinger.

Lazarus, A. A. (1971). *Behavior therapy and beyond.* New York: McGraw-Hill.

Lazarus, A. A. (1981). *The practice of multimodal therapy.* New York: McGraw-Hill.

Lazarus, A. A., & Fay, A. (1982). Resistance or rationalization? A cognitive-behavioral perspective. In P. L. Wachtel (Ed.), *Resistance: Psychodynamic and behavioral approaches* (pp. 94–107). New York: Plenum.

Lewinsohn, P. M., Clarke, G. N., Hops, H., & Andrews, J. (1990). Cognitive–behavioral treatment for depressed adolescents. *Behavior Therapy, 21,* 385–401.

Lieb, K., Zanarini, M.C., Schmahl, C., Linehan, M., & Bohus, M (2004). Borderline personality disorder. *Lancet, 364,* 453–461.

Lilienfeld, S. O., Lynn, S. J., & Lohr, J. M. (Eds.) (2003). *Science and pseudoscience in clinical psychology.* New York: Guilford Press.

Linehan, M. M. (1993). *Skills training manual for treating borderline personality disorder.* New York: Guilford Press.

Linehan, M. M., Comtois, K. A., Murray, A. M., Brown, M. Z., Gallop, R. J. et al. (2006). Two-year randomized trial + follow-up of dialectical behavior therapy vs. therapy by experts for suicidal behaviors and borderline personality disorder. *Archives of General Psychiatry, 63,* 757–766.

Locke, H. J., & Wallace, K. M. (1959). Short marital adjustment and prediction tests: Their reliability and validity. *Marriage and Family Living, 21,* 251–255.

Loeb, K. L., Wilson, G. T., Labouvie, E., Pratt, E. M., Hayaki, J., Walsh, B. T., Agras, W. S., & Fairburn, C. G. (2005). Therapeutic alliance and treatment adherence in two interventions for bulimia nervosa: A study of process and outcome. *Journal of Consulting and Clinical Psychology, 73,* 1097–1106.

Lovaas, O. I. (1987). Behavioral treatment and normal educational and intellectual functioning in young autistic children. *Journal of Consulting and Clinical Psychology, 55,* 3–9.

Lynch, T. R., & Cozza, C. (2009). Behavior therapy for nonsuicidal self-injury. In M. K. Nock, (Ed.), *Understanding nonsuicidal self-injury: Origins, assessment, and treatment* (pp. 211–250). Washington, DC: American Psychological Association.

Marks, I., & Mathews, A. (1979). Brief standard self-rating for phobic patients. *Behaviour Research and Therapy, 17,* 263–267.

Margolin, G. (1987). Marital therapy: A cognitive–behavioral–affective approach. In N. S. Jacobson (Ed.), *Psychotherapists in clinical practice* (pp. 232–285). New York: Guilford.

Martell, C., Addis, M., & Jacobson, N. S. (2001). *Depression in context.* New York: Norton.

Mathews, A. M., Gelder, M. G., & Johnston, D. W. (1981). *Agoraphobia: Nature and treatment.* New York: Guilford Press.

Melamed, B., & Siegel, L. (1980). *Behavioral medicine.* New York: Springer.

McCrady, B. S., Epstein, E. E., Cook, S., Jensen, N., & Hildebrandt, T. (2009). A randomized trial of individual and couple behavioral alcohol treatment for women. *Journal of Consulting and Clinical Psychology, 77,* 243–256.

Meichenbaum, D., & Turk, D. (1987). *Facilitating treatment adherence.* New York: Plenum.

Miller, A. L., Rathus, J. H., & Linehan, M. M. (2007). *Dialectical behavior therapy with suicidal adolescents.* New York: Guilford.

Miller, N. E. (1948). Studies of fear as an acquirable drive. Fear as motivation and fear reduction as reinforcement in the learning of new responses. *Journal of Experimental Psychology, 38,* 89–101.

Miranda, J., Bernal, G., Kohn, A., Hwang, Wei-Chin, & La Fromboise, T. (2005). Psychosocial treatment of minority groups. In S. Nolen-Hoeksema (Ed.), *Annual review of clinical psychology*, Vol. 1 (pp. 113–142). Palo Alto: Annual Reviews Inc.

Mischel, W. (1968). *Personality and assessment.* New York: Wiley.

Mischel, W. (1973). Toward a cognitive social learning reconceptualization of personality. *Psychological Review, 80,* 252–283.

Mischel, W. (1976). *Introduction to personality.* New York: Holt, Rinehart and Winston.

Mischel, W. (1981). A cognitive social learning approach to assessment. In T. V. Merluzzi, C. R. Glass, & M. Genest (Eds.), *Cognitive assessment* (pp. 479–500). New York: Guilford Press.

Mowrer, O. H. (1947). On the dual nature of learning—A reinterpretation of "conditioning" and "problem solving." *Harvard Educational Review, 17,* 102–148.

Mowrer, O. H., & Mowrer, E. (1938). Enuresis: A method for its study and treatment. *American Journal of Orthopsychiatry, 4,* 436–459.

Nathan, P. E. & Gorman, J. M. (Eds.). (in press). *A guide to treatments that work* (3rd ed.). New York: Oxford University Press.

National Institute for Clinical Excellence. (2004). *Eating disorders—Core interventions in the treatment and management of anorexia nervosa, bulimia nervosa, and related eating disorders.* NICE Clinical Guideline No. 9. London: NICE.

Norcross, J. C., Alford, B. A., & DeMichele, J. T. (1992). The future of psychotherapy: Delphi data and concluding observations. *Psychotherapy, 29,* 150–158.

O'Leary, K. D. (1980). Pills or skills for hyperactive children. *Journal of Applied Behavior Analysis, 13,* 191–204.

O'Leary, K. D., & Beach, S. R. H. (1990). Marital therapy: A viable treatment for depression. *American Journal of Psychiatry, 147,* 183–186.

O'Leary, K. D., & Carr, E. G. (1982). Childhood disorders. In G. T. Wilson & C. M. Franks (Eds.), *Contemporary behavior therapy: Conceptual and empirical foundations* (pp. 495–496). New York: Guilford.

O'Leary, K. D., & O'Leary, S. (1977). *Classroom management: The successful use of behavior modification* (2nd ed.). New York: Pergamon Press.

O'Leary, K. D., & Wilson, G. T. (1987). *Behavior therapy: Application and outcome* (2nd ed.). Englewood Cliffs, NJ: Prentice-Hall.

Ollendick, T. H., Öst, L., Reuterskiöld, L., Costa, N., Cederlund, R., Sirbu, C., Davis III, T. E., & Jarrett, M. A. (2009). One-session treatment of specific phobias in youth: A randomized clinical trial in the United States and Sweden. *Journal of Consulting and Clinical Psychology, 77,* 504–516.

Paul, G. L. (1966). *Insight versus desensitization in psychotherapy.* Stanford, CA: Stanford University Press.

Paul, G. L., & Lentz, R. J. (1977). *Psychological treatment of chronic mental patients.* Cambridge, MA: Harvard University Press.

Perri, M. G. (1998). The maintenance of treatment effects in the long-term management of obesity. *Clinical Psychology: Theory and Practice, 5,* 526–543.

Persons, J. B. (1997). Dissemination of effective methods: Behavior therapy's next challenge. *Behavior Therapy, 28,* 465–471.

Rathus, S. A. (1973). A 30-item schedule for assessing assertive behavior. *Behavior Therapy, 4,* 398–406.

Risley, T., & Sheldon-Wildgen, J. (1982). Invited peer review: The AABT experience. *Professional Psychology, 13,* 125–131.

Roemer, L., & Orsillo, S. M. (2009). *Mindfulness- and acceptance-based behavioral therapies in practice.* New York: Guilford.

Rosen, R. C., & Keefe, F. J. (1978). The measurement of human penile tumescence. *Psychophysiology, 15,* 366–376.

Ross, A. (1981). *Child behavior therapy.* New York: Wiley.

Salter, A. (1949). *Conditioned reflex therapy.* New York: Farrar, Straus.

Sayette, M., & Mayne, T. (1990). Survey of current clinical and research trends in clinical psychology. *American Psychologist, 45,* 1263–1266.

Schwartz, G. E., & Weiss, S. M. (1978). Behavioral medicine revisited: An amended definition. *Journal of Behavioral Medicine, 1,* 249–252.

Segal, Z. V., Teasdale, J. D., & Williams, M. (2004). Mindfulness-based cognitive therapy: Theoretical rationale and empirical status. In S. C. Hayes, V. M. Follette, & M. M. Linehan (Eds.), *Mindfulness and acceptance: Expanding the cognitive-behavioral tradition* (pp. 45–65). New York: Guilford Press.

Skinner, B. F. (1953). *Science and human behavior.* New York: Macmillan.

Sloane, R. B., Staples, F. R., Cristol, A. H., Yorkston, J. J., & Whipple, K. (1975). *Psychotherapy versus behavior therapy.* Cambridge, MA: Harvard University Press.

Smith, D. (1982). Trends in counseling and psychotherapy. *American Psychologist, 37,* 802–809.

Staples, F. R., Sloane, R. B., Whipple, K., Cristol, A. H., & Yorkston, N. (1975). Differences between behavior therapists and psychotherapists. *Archives of General Psychiatry, 32,* 1517–1522.

Stolz, S. G. (1978). *Ethical issues in behavior modification.* San Francisco: Jossey-Bass.

Tarrier, N., & Wykes, T. (2004). Is there evidence that cognitive behaviour therapy is an effective treatment for schizophrenia? A cautious or cautionary tale? *Behaviour Research and Therapy, 42,* 1377–1401.

Tanaka-Matsumi, J. (2008). Functional approaches to evidence-based practice in multicultural counseling and therapy. In U. P. Gielen, J. G. Draguns, & J. M. Fish (Eds.). *Principles of multicultural counseling and therapy* (pp. 169–198). New York: Routledge/Taylor & Francis Group.

Ullmann, L. P., & Krasner, L. (1965). *Case studies in behavior modification.* New York: Holt, Rinehart and Winston.

Wadden, T. A., Butryn, M. L., & Byrne, K. J. (2004). Efficacy of lifestyle modification for long-term weight control. *Obesity Research, 12,* 151S–162S.

Wilson, G. T. (1997). Cognitive behavioral treatment of bulimia nervosa. *The Clinical Psychologist, 50*(2), 10–12.

Wilson, G. T. (1998). Manual-based treatment and clinical practice. *Clinical Psychology: Science and Practice, 5,* 363–375.

Wilson, G. T. (2004). Acceptance and change in the treatment of eating disorders: The evolution of manual-based cognitive behavioral therapy (CBT). In S. C. Hayes, V. M. Follette, & M. Linehan (Eds.), *Acceptance, mindfulness, and behavior change.* New York: Guilford Press.

Wilson, G. T. (2007). Manual-based treatment: Evolution and evaluation. In T. A. Treat, R. R. Bootzin, & T. B. Baker (Eds.), *Psychological clinical science: Papers in honor of Richard M. McFall.* Mahwah, NJ: Lawrence Erlbaum.

Wilson, G. T., & Fairburn, C. G. (2002). Eating disorders. In P. E. Nathan & J. M. Gorman (Eds.), *A guide to treatments that work* (2nd ed., pp. 559–592). New York: Oxford University Press.

Wilson, G.T., Grilo, C., & Vitousek, K. (2007). Psychological treatment of eating disorders. *American Psychologist, 62,* 199–216.

Wilson, G. T., & O'Leary, K. D. (1980). *Principles of behavior therapy.* Englewood Cliffs, NJ: Prentice-Hall.

Wilson, G. T., & Shafran, R. (2005). Eating disorders guidelines from NICE. *The Lancet, 365,* 79–81.

Wiser, S., & Telch, C. F. (1999). Dialectical behavior therapy for binge-eating disorder. *Journal of Clinical Psychology, 55,* 755–768.

Wolpe, J. (1958). *Psychotherapy by reciprocal inhibition.* Stanford, CA: Stanford University Press.

Wolpe, J., & Rachman, S. (1960). Psychoanalytic evidence: A critique based on Freud's case of Little Hans. *Journal of Nervous and Mental Disorders, 131,* 135–145.

Woody, S. R., Weisz, J., & McLean, C. (2005). Empirically supported treatments: 10 years later. *The Clinical Psychologist, 58,* 5–11.

Yates, A. J. (1980). *Biofeedback and the modification of behavior.* New York: Plenum.

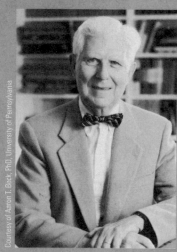

Aaron T. Beck

8 | COGNITIVE THERAPY

Aaron T. Beck and Marjorie E. Weishaar

OVERVIEW

Cognitive therapy is based on a theory of personality that maintains that people respond to life events through a combination of cognitive, affective, motivational, and behavioral responses. These responses are based in human evolution and individual learning history. The cognitive system deals with the way individuals perceive, interpret, and assign meanings to events. It interacts with the other affective, motivational, and physiological systems to process information from the physical and social environments and to respond accordingly. Sometimes responses are maladaptive because of misperceptions, misinterpretations, or dysfunctional, idiosyncratic interpretations of situations.

Cognitive therapy aims to adjust information processing and initiate positive change in all systems by acting through the cognitive system. In a collaborative process, the therapist and patient examine the patient's beliefs about himself or herself, other people, and the world. The patient's maladaptive conclusions are treated as testable hypotheses. Behavioral experiments and verbal procedures are used to examine alternative interpretations and to generate contradictory evidence that supports more adaptive beliefs and leads to therapeutic change.

Basic Concepts

Cognitive therapy can be thought of as a theory, a system of strategies, and a series of techniques. The theory is based on the idea that the processing of information is crucial

276

for the survival of any organism. If we did not have a functional apparatus for taking in relevant information from the environment, synthesizing it, and formulating a plan of action on the basis of this synthesis, we would soon die or be killed.

Each system involved in survival—cognitive, behavioral, affective, and motivational—is composed of structures known as *schemas*. Cognitive schemas contain people's perceptions of themselves and others and of their goals and expectations, memories, fantasies, and previous learning. These greatly influence, if not control, the processing of information.

In various psychopathological conditions such as anxiety disorders, depressive disorders, mania, paranoid states, obsessive–compulsive neuroses, and others, a specific bias affects how the person incorporates new information. Thus, a depressed person has a negative bias, including a negative view of self, world, and future. In anxiety, there is a systematic bias or *cognitive shift* toward selectively interpreting themes of danger. In paranoid conditions, the dominant shift is toward indiscriminate attributions of abuse or interference, and in mania the shift is toward exaggerated interpretations of personal gain.

Contributing to these shifts are certain specific attitudes or core beliefs that predispose people under the influence of certain life situations to interpret their experiences in a biased way. These are known as *cognitive vulnerabilities*. For example, a person who has the belief that any minor loss represents a major deprivation may react catastrophically to even the smallest loss. A person who feels vulnerable to sudden death may overinterpret normal body sensations as signs of impending death and have a panic attack.

Previously, cognitive theory emphasized a linear relationship between the activation of cognitive schemas and changes in the other systems; that is, cognitions (beliefs and assumptions) triggered affect, motivation, and behavior. Current cognitive theory, benefiting from recent developments in clinical, evolutionary, and cognitive psychology, views all systems as acting together as a mode. *Modes* are networks of cognitive, affective, motivational, and behavioral schemas that compose personality and interpret ongoing situations. Some modes, such as the anxiety mode, are *primal,* meaning they are universal and tied to survival. Other modes, such as conversing or studying, are minor and under conscious control. Although primal modes are thought to have been adaptive in an evolutionary sense, individuals may find them maladaptive in everyday life when they are triggered by misperceptions or overreactions. Even personality disorders may be viewed as exaggerated versions of formerly adaptive strategies. In personality disorders, primal modes are operational almost continuously.

Primal modes include primal thinking, which is rigid, absolute, automatic, and biased. Nevertheless, conscious intentions can override primal thinking and make it more flexible. Automatic and reflexive responses can be replaced by deliberate thinking, conscious goals, problem solving, and long-term planning. In cognitive therapy, a thorough understanding of the mode and all its integral systems is part of the case conceptualization. This approach to therapy teaches patients to use conscious control to recognize and override maladaptive responses.

Strategies

The overall strategies of cognitive therapy involve primarily a collaborative enterprise between the patient and the therapist to explore dysfunctional interpretations and try to modify them. This *collaborative empiricism* views the patient as a practical scientist who lives by interpreting stimuli but who has been temporarily thwarted by his or her own information-gathering and integrating apparatus (cf. Kelly, 1955).

The second strategy, *guided discovery,* is directed toward discovering what threads run through the patient's present misperceptions and beliefs and linking them to analogous experiences in the past. Thus, the therapist and patient collaboratively weave a tapestry that tells the story of the development of the patient's disorder.

Both these strategies are implemented using *Socratic dialogue*, a style of questioning that helps uncover the patient's views and examines his or her adaptive and maladaptive features.

The therapy attempts to improve reality testing through continuous evaluation of personal conclusions. The immediate goal is to shift the information-processing apparatus to a more "neutral" condition so that events will be evaluated in a more balanced way.

There are three major approaches to treating dysfunctional modes: (1) deactivating them, (2) modifying their content and structure, and (3) constructing more adaptive modes to neutralize them. In therapy, the first and third approaches are often accomplished simultaneously, for the particular belief may be demonstrated to be dysfunctional and a new belief to be more accurate or adaptive. The deactivation of a dysfunctional mode can occur through distraction or reassurance, but lasting change is unlikely unless a person's underlying, core beliefs are modified.

Techniques

Techniques used in cognitive therapy are directed primarily at correcting errors and biases in information processing and at modifying the core beliefs that promote faulty conclusions. The purely cognitive techniques focus on identifying and testing the patient's beliefs, exploring their origins and basis, correcting them if they fail an empirical or logical test, or problem solving. For example, some beliefs are tied to one's culture, gender role, religion, or socioeconomic status. Therapy may be directed toward problem solving with an understanding of how these beliefs influence the patient.

Core beliefs are explored in a similar manner and are tested for their accuracy and adaptiveness. The patient who discovers that these beliefs are not accurate is encouraged to try out a different set of beliefs to determine whether the new beliefs are more accurate and functional.

Cognitive therapy also uses behavioral techniques such as skills training (e.g., relaxation, assertiveness training, social skills training), role playing, behavioral rehearsal, and exposure therapy.

Other Systems

Procedures used in cognitive therapy, such as identifying common themes in a patient's emotional reactions, narratives, and imagery, are similar to the *psychoanalytic method*. However, in cognitive therapy the common thread is a meaning readily accessible to conscious interpretation, whereas in psychoanalysis the meaning is unconscious (or repressed) and must be inferred.

Both psychodynamic psychotherapy and cognitive therapy assume that behavior can be influenced by beliefs of which one is not immediately aware. However, cognitive therapy maintains that the thoughts contributing to a patient's distress are not deeply buried in the unconscious. Moreover, the cognitive therapist does not regard the patient's self-report as a screen for more deeply concealed ideas. Cognitive therapy focuses on the linkages among symptoms, conscious beliefs, and current experiences. Psychoanalytic approaches are oriented toward repressed childhood memories and motivational constructs, such as libidinal needs and infantile sexuality.

Cognitive therapy is highly structured and usually short term, typically lasting from 12 to 16 weeks. The therapist is actively engaged in collaboration with the patient. Psychoanalytic therapy is long term and relatively unstructured. The analyst is largely passive. Cognitive therapy attempts to shift biased information processing through the application of logic to dysfunctional ideas and the use of behavioral experiments to test dysfunctional beliefs. Psychoanalysts rely on free association and in-depth interpretations to penetrate the encapsulated unconscious residue of unresolved childhood conflicts.

Cognitive therapy and rational emotive behavior therapy (REBT) share an emphasis on the primary importance of cognition in psychological dysfunction, and both see the task of therapy as changing maladaptive assumptions and the stance of the therapist as active and directive. There are some differences, nevertheless, between these two approaches.

Cognitive therapy, using an information-processing model, is directed toward modifying the "cognitive shift" by addressing biased selection of information and distorted interpretations. The shift to normal cognitive processing is accomplished by testing the erroneous inferences that result from biased processing. Continual disconfirmation of cognitive errors, working as a feedback system, gradually restores more adaptive functioning. However, the dysfunctional beliefs that contributed to the unbalanced cognitive processing in the first place also require further testing and invalidation.

REBT theory states that a distressed individual has irrational beliefs that contribute to irrational thoughts and that when these are modified through confrontation, they will disappear and the disorder will clear up. The cognitive therapist, operating from an inductive model, helps the patient translate interpretations and beliefs into hypotheses, which are then subjected to empirical testing. An REBT therapist is more inclined to use a deductive model to point out irrational beliefs. The cognitive therapist eschews the word *irrational* in favor of *dysfunctional* because problematic beliefs are nonadaptive rather than irrational. They contribute to psychological disorders because they interfere with normal cognitive processing, not because they are irrational.

A profound difference between these two approaches is that cognitive therapy maintains that each disorder has its own typical cognitive content or *cognitive specificity*. The *cognitive profiles* of depression, anxiety, and panic disorder are significantly different and require substantially different techniques. REBT, on the other hand, does not conceptualize disorders as having cognitive themes but, rather, focuses on the "musts," "shoulds," and other imperatives presumed to underlie all disorders.

The cognitive therapy model emphasizes the impact of cognitive deficits in psychopathology. Some clients experience problems because their cognitive deficits do not let them foresee delayed or long-range negative consequences. Others have trouble with concentration, directed thinking, or recall. These difficulties occur in severe anxiety, depression, and panic attacks. Cognitive deficits produce perceptual errors as well as faulty interpretations. Further, inadequate cognitive processing may interfere with the client's use of coping abilities or techniques and with interpersonal problem solving, as occurs in suicidal people.

Finally, REBT views patients' beliefs as philosophically incongruent with reality. Meichenbaum (1977) criticizes this perspective, stating that nonpatients have irrational beliefs as well but are able to cope with them. Cognitive therapy teaches patients to *self-correct* faulty cognitive processing and to bolster assumptions that allow them to cope. Thus, REBT views the problem as philosophical; cognitive therapy views it as functional.

Cognitive therapy shares many similarities with some forms of *behavior therapy* but is quite different from others. Within behavior therapy are numerous approaches that vary in their emphasis on cognitive processes. At one end of the behavioral spectrum is applied behavioral analysis, an approach that ignores "internal events," such as interpretations and inferences, as much as possible. As one moves in the other direction, cognitive mediating processes are given increasing attention until one arrives at a variety of cognitive–behavioral approaches. At this point, the distinction between the purely cognitive and the distinctly behavioral becomes unclear.

Cognitive therapy and behavior therapy share some features: They are empirical, present centered, and problem oriented, and they require explicit identification of problems and the situations in which they occur, as well as of the consequences resulting from them. In contrast to radical behaviorism, cognitive therapy applies the same kind of functional analysis to internal experiences—to thoughts, attitudes, and images. Cognitions, like behaviors, can be modified by active collaboration through behavioral experiments that foster new learning. Also, in contrast to behavioral approaches based on simple conditioning paradigms, cognitive therapy sees individuals as active participants in their environments, judging and evaluating stimuli, interpreting events and sensations, and judging their own responses.

Studies of some behavioral techniques, such as exposure methods for the treatment of phobias, demonstrate that cognitive and behavioral changes work together. For example, in agoraphobia, cognitive improvement has been concomitant with behavioral improvement (Williams & Rappoport, 1983). Simple exposure to agoraphobic situations while verbalizing negative automatic thoughts may lead to improvement on cognitive measures (Gournay, 1986). Bandura (1977) has demonstrated that one of the most effective ways to change cognitions is to change performance. In real-life exposure, patients confront not only the threatening situations but also their personal expectations of danger and their assumed inability to cope with their reactions. Because the experience itself is processed cognitively, exposure can be considered a cognitive procedure.

Cognitive therapy maintains that a comprehensive approach to the treatment of anxiety and other disorders includes targeting anxiety-provoking thoughts and images. Work with depressed patients (Beck, Rush, Shaw, & Emery, 1979) demonstrates that desired cognitive changes do not necessarily follow from changes in behavior. For this reason, it is vital to know the patient's expectations, interpretations, and reactions to events. Cognitive change must be demonstrated, not assumed.

HISTORY

Precursors

Cognitive therapy's theoretical underpinnings are derived from three main sources: (1) the phenomenological approach to psychology, (2) structural theory and depth psychology, and (3) cognitive psychology. The phenomenological approach posits that the individual's view of self and the personal world are central to behavior. This concept originated in Greek Stoic philosophy and can be seen in Immanuel Kant's (1798) emphasis on conscious subjective experience. This approach is also evident in the writings of Adler (1936), Alexander (1950), Horney (1950), and Sullivan (1953).

The second major influence was the structural theory and depth psychology of Kant and Freud, particularly Freud's concept of the hierarchical structuring of cognition into primary and secondary processes.

More recent developments in cognitive psychology also have had an impact. George Kelly (1955) is credited with being the first among contemporaries to describe the cognitive model through his use of "personal constructs" and his emphasis on the role of beliefs in behavior change. Cognitive theories of emotion, such as those of Magda Arnold (1960) and Richard Lazarus (1984), which give primacy to cognition in emotional and behavioral change, have also contributed to cognitive therapy.

Beginnings

Cognitive therapy began in the early 1960s as the result of Aaron Beck's research on depression (Beck, 1963, 1964, 1967). Trained in psychoanalysis, Beck attempted to validate Freud's theory of depression as having at its core "anger turned on the self."

To substantiate this formulation, Beck made clinical observations of depressed patients and investigated their treatment under traditional psychoanalysis. Rather than finding retroflected anger in their thoughts and dreams, Beck observed a negative bias in their cognitive processing. With continued clinical observations and experimental testing, Beck developed his theory of emotional disorders and a cognitive model of depression.

The work of Albert Ellis (1962) gave major impetus to the development of cognitive behavior therapies. Both Ellis and Beck believed that people can consciously adopt reason, and both viewed the patient's underlying assumptions as targets of intervention. Similarly, they both rejected their analytic training and replaced passive listening with active, direct dialogues with patients. Whereas Ellis confronted patients and persuaded them that the philosophies they lived by were unrealistic, Beck "turned the client into a colleague who researches verifiable reality" (Wessler, 1986, p. 5).

The work of a number of contemporary behaviorists influenced the development of cognitive therapy. Bandura's (1977) concepts of expectancy of reinforcement, self and outcome efficacies, the interaction between person and environment, modeling, and vicarious learning catalyzed a shift in behavior therapy toward the cognitive domain. Mahoney's (1974) early work on the cognitive control of behavior and his later theoretical contributions also influenced cognitive therapy. Along with cognitive therapy and rational emotive behavior therapy, Meichenbaum's (1977) cognitive–behavior modification is recognized as one of the three major self-control therapies (Mahoney & Arnkoff, 1978). Meichenbaum's combination of cognitive modification and skills training in a coping skills paradigm is particularly useful in treating anxiety, anger, and stress. The constructivist movement in psychology and the modern movement for psychotherapy integration have been recent influences shaping contemporary cognitive therapy.

Current Status

Research: Cognitive Model and Outcome Studies

Research has tested both the theoretical aspects of the cognitive model and the efficacy of cognitive therapy for a range of clinical disorders. In terms of the cognitive model of depression, negatively biased interpretations have been found in all forms of depression: unipolar and bipolar, reactive and endogenous (Haaga, Dyck, & Ernst, 1991). The cognitive triad, negatively biased cognitive processing of stimuli, and identifiable dysfunctional beliefs have also been found to operate in depression (Hollon, Kendall, & Lumry, 1986). The efficacy of cognitive therapy for depression has been demonstrated in numerous studies summarized by Clark, Beck and Alford (1999). Recently, Beck (2008) has traced the evolution of the cognitive model of depression from its basis in information processing to its incorporation of the effect of early traumatic experiences on the formation of dysfunctional beliefs and sensitivity to precipitating factors in depression. He is presently interested in how genetic, neurochemical, and cognitive factors interact in depression.

For the anxiety disorders, a danger-related bias has been demonstrated in all anxiety diagnoses, including the presumed danger of physical sensations in panic attacks, the distorted perception of evaluation in social anxiety, and the negative appraisals of self and the world in PTSD. Moreover, the cognitive specificity hypothesis, which states that there is a distinct cognitive profile for each psychiatric disorder, has been supported for a range of disorders (Beck, 2005).

Controlled studies have demonstrated the efficacy of cognitive therapy in the treatment of panic disorder (Beck, Sokol, Clark, Berchick, & Wright, 1992; Clark, 1996; Clark, Salkovskis, Hackmann, Middleton, & Gelder, 1992), social phobia (Clark, 1997; Eng, Roth, & Heimberg, 2001), generalized anxiety disorder (Butler, Fennell, Robson,

& Gelder, 1991), substance abuse (Woody et al., 1983), eating disorders (Bowers, 2001; Fairburn, Jones, Peveler, Hope, Carr, Solomon, et al., 1991; Garner et al., 1993; Pike, Walsh, Vitousek, Wilson, & Bauer, 2003; Vitousek, 1996), marital problems (Baucom, Sayers, & Sher, 1990), obsessive–compulsive disorder (Freeston et al., 1997), post-traumatic stress disorder (Ehlers & Clark, 2000; Gillespie, Duffy, Hackmann, & Clark, 2002; Resick, 2001), and schizophrenia (Turkington, Dudley, Warman, & Beck, 2004; Zimmerman, Favrod, Trieu, & Pomini, 2005).

In addition, cognitive therapy appears to lead to lower rates of relapse than other treatments for anxiety and depression (Clark, 1996; Eng, Roth, & Heimberg, 2001; Hollon, DeRubeis, & Evans, 1996; Hollon et al., 2005; Hollon, Stewart, & Strunk, 2006; Strunk & DeRubeis, 2001).

Suicide Research

Beck has developed key theoretical concepts regarding suicide and its prevention. Chief among his findings about suicide risk is the notion of *hopelessness.* Longitudinal studies of both inpatients and outpatients who had suicidal ideation have found that a cutoff score of 9 or more on the Beck Hopelessness Scale is predictive of eventual suicide (Beck, Brown, Berchick, Stewart, & Steer, 1990; Beck, Steer, Kovacs, & Garrison, 1985). Hopelessness has been confirmed as a predictor of eventual suicide in subsequent studies.

A recent randomized controlled trial investigated the efficacy of a brief cognitive therapy treatment for those at high risk of attempting suicide by virtue of the fact that they had previously attempted suicide and had significant psychopathology and substance abuse problems. Results indicate that cognitive therapy reduced the rate of re-attempt by 50% over an 18-month period (Brown et al., 2005).

Psychotherapy Integration

Cognitive therapy has been integrated with other modalities to yield new therapeutic approaches. Schema therapy, developed by Jeffrey Young (Young, Klosko, & Weishaar, 2003), focuses on modifying maladaptive core beliefs that are developed early in life and that can underlie chronic depression and anxiety. Another approach, mindfulness-based cognitive therapy (Segal, Williams, & Teasdale, 2002), uses acceptance and meditation strategies to promote resilience and prevent recurrence of depressive episodes.

Assessment Scales

Beck's work has generated a number of assessment scales, most notably the Beck Depression Inventory (Beck, Steer, & Brown, 1996; Beck, Ward, Mendelson, Mock, & Erbaugh, 1961), the Scale for Suicide Ideation (Beck, Kovacs, & Weissman, 1979), the Suicide Intent Scale (Beck, Schuyler, & Herman, 1974), the Beck Hopelessness Scale (Beck, Weissman, Lester, & Trexler, 1974), the Beck Anxiety Inventory (Beck & Steer, 1990), the Beck Self-concept Test (Beck, Steer, Brown, & Epstein, 1990), the Dysfunctional Attitude Scale (Weissman & Beck, 1978), the Sociotropy-Autonomy Scale (Beck, Epstein, & Harrison, 1983), the Beck Youth Inventories (Beck & Beck, 2002), the Personality Beliefs Questionnaire (Beck & Beck, 1995), and the Clark-Beck Obsessive–Compulsive Inventory (Clark & Beck, 2002). The Beck Depression Inventory is the best known of these. It has been used in hundreds of outcome studies and is routinely employed by psychologists, physicians, and social workers to monitor depression in their patients and clients.

Training

The Center for Cognitive Therapy, which is affiliated with the University of Pennsylvania Medical School, provides outpatient services and is a research institute that integrates clinical observations with empirical findings to develop theory. The Beck Institute in Bala Cynwyd, Pennsylvania, provides both outpatient services and training opportunities. In addition, clinical psychology internships and postdoctoral fellowships offer training in cognitive therapy. Research and treatment efforts in cognitive therapy are being conducted in a number of universities and hospitals in the United States and Europe. The *International Cognitive Therapy Newsletter* was launched in 1985 for the exchange of information among cognitive therapists. Therapists from five continents participate in the newsletter network. Founded in 1971, the European Association for Behavioural and Cognitive Therapies will hold its annual conference in Milan in 2010. The World Congress of Behavioural and Cognitive Therapies, composed of seven organizations from around the world, will hold its next conference in 2010. The International Association for Cognitive Psychotherapy will host the 7th International Congress of Cognitive Psychotherapy in Istanbul in 2011.

The Academy of Cognitive Therapy, a nonprofit organization, was founded in 1999 by a group of leading clinicians, educators, and researchers in the field of cognitive therapy. The academy administers an objective evaluation to identify and certify clinicians skilled in cognitive therapy. In 1999, the Accreditation Council for Graduate Medical Education mandated that psychiatry residency training programs train residents to be competent in the practice of cognitive behavior therapy.

Cognitive therapists routinely contribute to psychology, psychiatry, and behavior therapy journals. The primary journals devoted to research in cognitive therapy are *Cognitive Therapy and Research,* the *Journal of Cognitive Psychotherapy: An International Quarterly,* and *Cognitive and Behavioral Practice.*

Cognitive therapy is represented at the annual meetings of the American Psychological Association, the American Psychiatric Association, the American Association of Suicidology, and others. It has been such a major force in the Association for the Advancement of Behavior Therapy that the organization changed its name in 2005 to the Association for Behavioral and Cognitive Therapies (ABCT).

Because of its efficacy as a short-term form of psychotherapy, cognitive therapy is achieving wider use in settings that must demonstrate cost-effectiveness or that require short-term contact with patients. It has applications in both inpatient and outpatient settings.

Many talented researchers and innovative therapists have contributed to the development of cognitive therapy. Controlled outcome studies comparing cognitive therapy with other forms of treatment are conducted with anxiety disorders, panic, drug abuse, anorexia and bulimia, geriatric depression, acute depression, and dysphoric disorder. Beck's students and associates do research on the nature and treatment of depression, anxiety, loneliness, marital conflict, eating disorders, agoraphobia, pain, personality disorders, substance abuse, bipolar disorder, and schizophrenia.

PERSONALITY

Theory of Personality

Cognitive therapy emphasizes the role of information processing in human responses and adaptation. When an individual perceives that the situation requires a response, a whole set of cognitive, emotional, motivational, and behavioral schemas are mobilized. Previously, cognitive therapy viewed cognition as largely determining emotions and behaviors. Current thinking views all aspects of human functioning as acting simultaneously as a mode.

Cognitive therapy views personality as shaped by the interaction between innate disposition and environment (Beck, Freeman, & Davis, 2003). Personality attributes are seen as reflecting basic schemas, or interpersonal "strategies," developed in response to the environment.

Cognitive therapy sees psychological distress as being the consequence of a number of factors. Although people may have biochemical predispositions to illness, they respond to specific stressors because of their learning history. The phenomena of psychopathology (but not necessarily the cause) are on the same continuum as normal emotional reactions, but they are manifested in exaggerated and persistent ways. In depression, for example, sadness and loss of interest are intensified and prolonged, in mania there is heightened investment in self-aggrandizement, and in anxiety there is an extreme sense of vulnerability and danger.

Individuals experience psychological distress when they perceive a situation as threatening their vital interests. At such times, their perceptions and interpretations of events are highly selective, egocentric, and rigid. This results in a functional impairment of normal cognitive activity. There is a decreased ability to turn off idiosyncratic thinking, to concentrate, recall, or reason. Corrective functions, which allow reality testing and refinement of global conceptualizations, are attenuated.

Cognitive Vulnerability

Each individual has a set of idiosyncratic vulnerabilities and sensitivities that predispose him or her to psychological distress. These vulnerabilities appear to be related to personality structure. Personality is shaped by temperament and cognitive schemas. Cognitive schemas are structures that contain the individual's fundamental beliefs and assumptions. Schemas develop early in life from personal experience and identification with significant others. These concepts are reinforced by further learning experiences and, in turn, influence the formation of beliefs, values, and attitudes.

Cognitive schemas may be adaptive or dysfunctional. They may be general or specific in nature. A person may have competing schemas. Cognitive schemas are generally latent but become active when stimulated by specific stressors, circumstances, or stimuli. In personality disorders, they are triggered very easily and often so that the person overresponds to a wide range of situations in a stereotyped manner.

Dimensions of Personality

The idea that certain clusters of personality attributes or cognitive structures are related to certain types of emotional response has been studied by Beck, Epstein, and Harrison (1983), who found two major personality dimensions relevant to depression and possibly to other disorders: social dependence (sociotropy) and autonomy. Beck's research revealed that dependent individuals became depressed following disruption of relationships. Autonomous people became depressed after defeat or failure to attain a desired goal. The sociotropic dimension is organized around closeness, nurturance, and dependence, the autonomous dimension around independence, goal setting, self-determination, and self-imposed obligations.

Research has also established that although "pure" cases of sociotropy and autonomy do exist, most people display features of each, depending on the situation. Thus, sociotropy and autonomy are styles of behavior, not fixed personality structures. This position stands in marked contrast with psychodynamic theories of personality, which postulate fixed personality dimensions.

Thus, cognitive therapy views personality as reflecting the individual's cognitive organization and structure, which are both biologically and socially influenced. Within the constraints of one's neuroanatomy and biochemistry, personal learning experiences help determine how one develops and responds.

Variety of Concepts

Cognitive therapy emphasizes the individual's learning history, including the influence of significant life events, in the development of psychological disturbance. It is not a reductive model but recognizes that psychological distress is usually the result of many interacting factors.

Cognitive therapy's emphasis on the individual's learning history endorses social learning theory and the importance of reinforcement. The social learning perspective requires a thorough examination of the individual's developmental history and his or her own idiosyncratic meanings and interpretations of events. Cognitive therapy emphasizes the idiographic nature of cognition, because the same event may have very different meanings for two individuals.

The conceptualization of personality as reflective of schemas and underlying assumptions is also related to social learning theory. The way a person structures experience is based on consequences of past behavior, vicarious learning from significant others, and expectations about the future.

Theory of Causality

Psychological distress is ultimately caused by many innate, biological, developmental, and environmental factors interacting with one another, so there is no single "cause" of psychopathology. Depression, for instance, is characterized by predisposing factors such as hereditary susceptibility, diseases that cause persistent neurochemical abnormalities, developmental traumas leading to specific cognitive vulnerabilities, inadequate personal experiences that fail to provide appropriate coping skills, and counterproductive cognitive patterns, such as unrealistic goals, assumptions, or imperatives. Physical disease, severe and acute stress, and chronic stress are also precipitating factors.

Cognitive Distortions

Systematic errors in reasoning called *cognitive distortions* are evident during psychological distress (Beck, 1967).

Arbitrary inference: Drawing a specific conclusion without supporting evidence or even in the face of contradictory evidence. An example is the working mother who concludes, after a particularly busy day, "I'm a terrible mother."

Selective abstraction: Conceptualizing a situation on the basis of a detail taken out of context, ignoring other information. An example is the man who becomes jealous upon seeing his girlfriend tilt her head toward another man to hear him better at a noisy party.

Overgeneralization: Abstracting a general rule from one or a few isolated incidents and applying it too broadly and to unrelated situations. After a discouraging date, a woman concluded, "All men are alike. I'll always be rejected."

Magnification and minimization: Seeing something as far more significant or less significant than it actually is. A student catastrophized, "If I appear the least bit nervous in class, it will mean disaster." Another person, rather than facing the fact that his mother is terminally ill, decides that she will soon recover from her "cold."

Personalization: Attributing external events to oneself without evidence supporting a causal connection. A man waved to an acquaintance across a busy street. After not getting a greeting in return, he concluded, "I must have done something to offend him."

Dichotomous thinking: Categorizing experiences in one of two extremes; for example, as complete success or total failure. A doctoral candidate stated, "Unless I write the best exam they've ever seen, I'm a failure as a student."

Systematic Bias in Psychological Disorders

A bias in information processing characterizes most psychological disorders (see Table 8.1). This bias is generally applied to "external" information, such as communications or threats, and may start operating at early stages of information processing. A person's orienting schema identifies a situation as posing a danger or loss, for instance, and signals the appropriate mode to respond.

Cognitive Model of Depression

A *cognitive triad* characterizes depression (Beck, 1967). The depressed individual has a negative view of the self, the world, and the future and perceives the self as inadequate, deserted, and worthless. A negative view is apparent in beliefs that enormous demands exist and that immense barriers block access to goals. The world seems devoid of pleasure or gratification. The depressed person's view of the future is pessimistic, reflecting the belief that current troubles will not improve. This hopelessness may lead to suicidal ideation.

Motivational, behavioral, emotional, and physical symptoms of depression are also activated in the depressed mode. These symptoms influence a person's beliefs and assumptions, and vice versa. For example, motivational symptoms of paralysis of will are related to the belief that one lacks the ability to cope or to control an event's outcome.

TABLE 8.1   The Cognitive Profile of Psychological Disorders

Disorder	Systematic Bias in Processing Information
Depression	Negative view of self, experience, and future
Hypomania	Inflated view of self and future
Anxiety disorder	Sense of physical or psychological danger
Panic disorder	Catastrophic interpretation of bodily/mental experiences
Phobia	Sense of danger in specific, avoidable situations
Paranoid state	Attribution of bias to others
Hysteria	Concept of motor or sensory abnormality
Obsession	Repeated warning or doubts about safety
Compulsion	Rituals to ward off perceived threat
Suicidal behavior	Hopelessness and deficiencies in problem solving
Anorexia nervosa	Fear of being fat
Hypochondriasis	Attribution of serious medical disorder

Consequently, there is a reluctance to commit oneself to a goal. Suicidal wishes often reflect a desire to escape unbearable problems.

The increased dependency often observed in depressed patients reflects the view of self as incompetent, an overestimation of the difficulty of normal life tasks, the expectation of failure, and the desire for someone more capable to take over. Indecisiveness similarly reflects the belief that one is incapable of making correct decisions. The physical symptoms of depression—low energy, fatigue, and inertia—are also related to negative expectations. Work with depressed patients indicates that initiating activity actually reduces inertia and fatigue. Moreover, refuting negative expectations and demonstrating motor ability play important roles in recovery.

Cognitive Model of Anxiety Disorders

Anxiety disorders are conceptualized as excessive functioning or malfunctioning of normal survival mechanisms. Thus, the basic mechanisms for coping with threat are the same for both normal and anxious people: physiological responses prepare the body for escape or self-defense. The same physiological responses occur in the face of psychosocial threats as in the case of physical dangers. The anxious person's perception of danger is either based on false assumptions or exaggerated, whereas the normal response is based on a more accurate assessment of risk and the magnitude of danger. In addition, normal individuals can correct their misperceptions using logic and evidence. Anxious individuals have difficulty recognizing cues of safety and other evidence that would reduce the threat of danger. Thus, in cases of anxiety, cognitive content revolves around themes of danger, and the individual tends to maximize the likelihood of harm and minimize his or her ability to cope.

Mania

The manic patient's biased thinking is the reverse of the depressive's. Such individuals selectively perceive significant gains in each life experience, blocking out negative experiences or reinterpreting them as positive, and unrealistically expecting favorable results from various enterprises. Exaggerated concepts of abilities, worth, and accomplishments lead to feelings of euphoria. The continued stimulation from inflated self-evaluations and overly optimistic expectations provides vast sources of energy and drives the manic individual into continuous goal-directed activity.

Panic Disorder

Patients with panic disorder are prone to regard any unexplained symptom or sensation as a sign of some impending catastrophe. Their cognitive processing system focuses their attention on bodily or psychological experiences and shapes these sources of internal information into the conviction that disaster is imminent. Each patient has a specific "equation." For one, distress in the chest or stomach equals heart attack; for another, shortness of breath means the cessation of all breathing; and for another, lightheadedness is a sign of impending unconsciousness.

Some patients regard a sudden surge of anger as a sign that they will lose control and injure somebody. Others interpret a mental lapse, momentary confusion, or mild disorientation to mean that they are losing their mind. A crucial characteristic of people having panic attacks is the conclusion that vital systems (the cardiovascular, respiratory, or central nervous system) will collapse. Because of their fear, they tend to be overly vigilant toward internal sensations and thus to detect and magnify sensations that pass unnoticed in other people.

Patients with panic disorder show a specific cognitive deficit—an inability to view their symptoms and catastrophic interpretations realistically.

Agoraphobia

Patients who have had one or more panic attacks in a particular situation tend to avoid that situation. For example, people who have had panic attacks in supermarkets avoid going there. If they push themselves to go, they become increasingly vigilant toward their sensations and begin to anticipate having another panic attack.

The anticipation of such an attack triggers a variety of autonomic symptoms that are then misinterpreted as signs of an impending disaster (e.g., heart attack, loss of consciousness, suffocation), which can lead to a full-blown panic attack. Patients with a panic disorder that goes untreated frequently develop agoraphobia. They may eventually become housebound or so restricted in their activities that they cannot travel far from home and require a companion to venture any distance.

Phobia

In phobias, there is anticipation of physical or psychological harm in specific situations. As long as patients can avoid these situations, they do not feel threatened and may be relatively comfortable. When they enter into these situations, however, they experience the typical subjective and physiological symptoms of severe anxiety. As a result of this unpleasant reaction, their tendency to avoid the situation in the future is reinforced.

In *evaluation phobias,* there is fear of disparagement or failure in social situations, examinations, and public speaking. The behavioral and physiological reactions to the potential "danger" (rejection, devaluation, failure) may interfere with the patient's functioning to the extent that they can produce just what the patient fears will happen.

Paranoid States

The paranoid individual is biased toward attributing prejudice to others. The paranoid persists in assuming that other people are deliberately abusive, interfering, or critical. In contrast to depressed patients, who believe that supposed insults or rejections are justified, paranoid patients persevere in thinking that others treat them unjustly.

Unlike depressed patients, paranoid patients do not experience low self-esteem. They are more concerned with the *injustice* of the presumed attacks, thwarting, or intrusions than with the actual loss, and they rail against the presumed prejudice and malicious intent of others.

Obsessions and Compulsions

Patients with obsessions introduce uncertainty into the appraisal of situations that most people would consider safe. The uncertainty is generally attached to circumstances that are potentially unsafe and is manifested by continual doubts—even though there is no evidence of danger.

Obsessives continually doubt whether they have performed an act necessary for safety (for example, turning off a gas oven or locking the door at night). They may fear contamination by germs, and no amount of reassurance can alleviate the fear. A key characteristic of obsessives is this *sense of responsibility* and the belief that they are accountable for having taken an action—or having failed to take an action—that could harm them or others. Cognitive therapy views such intrusive thoughts as universal. It is the meaning assigned to the intrusive thought—that the patient has done something immoral or dangerous—that causes distress.

Compulsions are attempts to reduce excessive doubts by performing rituals designed to neutralize the anticipated disaster. A hand-washing compulsion, for instance, is based on the patients' belief that they have not removed all the dirt or contaminants from parts of their body. Some patients regard dirt as a source of danger, either as a cause of physical disease or as a source of offensive, unpleasant odors, and they are compelled to remove this source of physical or social danger.

Suicidal Behavior

The cognitive processing in suicidal individuals has two features. First, there is a high degree of hopelessness or belief that things cannot improve. A second feature is a cognitive deficit—a difficulty in solving problems. Although the hopelessness accentuates poor problem solving, and vice versa, the difficulties in coping with life situations can, by themselves, contribute to the suicidal potential. Thinking becomes more rigid, and suicide appears as the only alternative in a diminished response repertoire.

Anorexia Nervosa

Anorexia nervosa and bulimia represent a constellation of maladaptive beliefs that revolve around one central assumption: "My body weight and shape determine my worth and/or my social acceptability." Revolving around this assumption are such beliefs as "I will look ugly if I gain much more weight," "The only thing in my life that I can control is my weight," and "If I don't starve myself, I will let go completely and become enormous."

Anorexics show typical distortions in information processing. They misinterpret symptoms of fullness after meals as signs that they are getting fat. And they misperceive their image in a mirror or photograph as being much fatter than it actually is.

Schizophrenia

In schizophrenia, there is a complex interaction of predisposing neurobiological, environmental, cognitive, and behavioral factors. The impaired integrative function of the brain, along with specific cognitive deficits, increases vulnerability to stressful life events and leads to dysfunctional beliefs (e.g., "I am inferior.") and behaviors (e.g., social withdrawal). Excessive psychophysiological reactions occur in response to stress and repeated negative thinking. The release of corticosteroids activates the dopaminergic system, which contributes to the development of delusions and hallucinations. Cognitive disorganization is a result of neurocognitive deficits such as attentional problems, impaired executive function and working memory. These impairments interact with heightened rejection sensitivity to produce communication deviance and intrusive, inappropriate thoughts. Delusions stem from the interplay of cognitive biases like external attributions and the cognitive shortcut of jumping to conclusions. A tendency to perceptualize combines with negative self-schemas to generate auditory hallucinations, which are exacerbated by beliefs that the "voice" is uncontrollable, powerful, infallible, and externally generated. Engagement in social, vocational, and pleasurable activity is compromised by neurocognitive impairment that is magnified by dysfunctional attitudes such as social indifference, low expectancies for pleasure, and defeatist beliefs regarding task performance. Low expectations for performance and success further contribute to negative symptoms.

PSYCHOTHERAPY

Theory of Psychotherapy

The goals of cognitive therapy are to correct faulty information processing and to help patients modify assumptions that maintain maladaptive behaviors and emotions. Cognitive and behavioral methods are used to challenge dysfunctional beliefs and to promote more realistic adaptive thinking. Cognitive therapy initially addresses symptom relief, but its ultimate goals are to remove systematic biases in thinking and modify the core beliefs that predispose the person to future distress.

Cognitive therapy fosters change in patients' beliefs by treating beliefs as testable hypotheses to be examined through behavioral experiments jointly agreed upon by patient and therapist. The cognitive therapist does not tell the client that the beliefs are irrational or wrong or that the beliefs of the therapist should be adopted. Instead, the therapist asks questions to elicit the meaning, function, usefulness, and consequences of the patient's beliefs. The patient ultimately decides whether to reject, modify, or maintain all personal beliefs, being well aware of their emotional and behavioral consequences.

Cognitive therapy is not the substitution of positive beliefs for negative ones. It is based in reality, not in wishful thinking. Similarly, cognitive therapy does not maintain that people's problems are imaginary. Patients may have serious social, financial, or health problems as well as functional deficits. In addition to real problems, however, they have biased views of themselves, their situations, and their resources that limit their range of responses and prevent them from generating solutions.

Cognitive change can promote behavioral change by allowing the patient to take risks. In turn, experience in applying new behaviors can validate the new perspective. Emotions can be moderated by enlarging perspectives to include alternative interpretations of events. Emotions play a role in cognitive change, for learning is enhanced when emotions are triggered. Thus, the cognitive, behavioral, and emotional channels interact in therapeutic change, but cognitive therapy emphasizes the primacy of cognition in promoting and maintaining therapeutic change.

Cognitive change occurs at several levels: voluntary thoughts, continuous or automatic thoughts, underlying assumptions, and core beliefs. According to the cognitive model, cognitions are organized in a hierarchy, each level differing from the next in its accessibility and stability. The most accessible and least stable cognitions are voluntary thoughts. At the next level are automatic thoughts, which come to mind spontaneously when triggered by circumstances. They are the thoughts that intercede between an event or stimulus and the individual's emotional and behavioral reactions.

An example of an automatic thought is "Everyone will see I'm nervous," experienced by a socially anxious person before going to a party. Automatic thoughts are accompanied by emotions and at the time they are experienced seem plausible, are highly salient, and are internally consistent with individual logic. They are given credibility without ever being challenged. Although automatic thoughts are more stable and less accessible than voluntary thoughts, patients can be taught to recognize and monitor them. Cognitive distortions are evident in automatic thoughts.

Automatic thoughts are generated from underlying assumptions. For example, the belief "I am responsible for other people's happiness" produces numerous negative automatic thoughts in people who perceive themselves as causing distress to others. Assumptions shape perceptions into cognitions, determine goals, and provide interpretations and meanings to events. They may be quite stable and outside the patient's awareness.

Core beliefs are contained in cognitive schemas. Therapy aims at identifying these absolute beliefs and counteracting their effects. If the beliefs themselves can be changed, the patient is less vulnerable to future distress. In Schema therapy, these core beliefs are called Early Maladaptive Schemas (EMSs; Young, Klosko, & Weishaar. 2003).

The Therapeutic Relationship

The therapeutic relationship is collaborative. The therapist assesses sources of distress and dysfunction and helps the patient clarify goals. In cases of severe depression or anxiety, patients may need the therapist to take a directive role. In other instances, patients may take the lead in determining goals for therapy. As part of the collaboration, the patient provides the thoughts, images, and beliefs that occur in various situations, as well as the emotions and behaviors that accompany the thoughts. The patient also shares responsibility by helping to set the agenda for each session and by doing homework between sessions. Homework helps therapy to proceed more quickly and gives the patient an opportunity to practice newly learned skills and perspectives.

The therapist functions as a guide who helps the patient understand how beliefs and attitudes interact with affect and behavior. The therapist is also a catalyst who promotes corrective experiences that lead to cognitive change and skills acquisition. Thus, cognitive therapy employs a learning model of psychotherapy. The therapist has expertise in examining and modifying beliefs and behavior but does not adopt the role of a passive expert.

Cognitive therapists actively pursue the patient's point of view. By using warmth, accurate empathy, and genuineness (see Rogers, 1951), the cognitive therapist appreciates the patient's personal world view. However, these qualities alone are not sufficient for therapeutic change. The cognitive therapist specifies problems, focuses on important areas, and teaches specific cognitive and behavioral techniques.

Along with having good interpersonal skills, cognitive therapists are flexible. They are sensitive to the patient's level of comfort and use self-disclosure judiciously. They provide supportive contact, when necessary, and operate within the goals and agenda of the cognitive approach. Flexibility in the use of therapeutic techniques depends on the targeted symptoms. For example, the inertia of depression responds best to behavioral interventions, whereas the suicidal ideation and pessimism of depression respond best to cognitive techniques. A good cognitive therapist does not use techniques arbitrarily or mechanically but applies them with sound rationale and skill—and with an understanding of each individual's needs.

To maintain collaboration, the therapist elicits feedback from the patient, usually at the end of each session. Feedback focuses on what the patient found helpful or not helpful, whether the patient has concerns about the therapist, and whether the patient has questions. The therapist may summarize the session or ask the patient to do so. Another way the therapist encourages collaboration is by providing the patient with a rationale for each procedure used. This demystifies the therapy process, increases patients' participation, and reinforces a learning paradigm in which patients gradually assume more responsibility for therapeutic change.

Definitions

Three fundamental concepts in cognitive therapy are collaborative empiricism, Socratic dialogue, and guided discovery.

Collaborative Empiricism.   The therapeutic relationship is collaborative and requires jointly determining the goals for treatment, eliciting and providing feedback, and thereby demystifying how therapeutic change occurs. The therapist and patient become co-investigators, examining the evidence to support or reject the patient's cognitions. As in scientific inquiry, interpretations or assumptions are treated as testable hypotheses.

Empirical evidence is used to determine whether particular cognitions serve any useful purpose. Prior conclusions are subjected to logical analysis. Biased thinking is exposed as the patient becomes aware of alternative sources of information. This process is conducted as a partnership between patient and therapist, with either taking a more active role as needed.

Socratic Dialogue.   Questioning is a major therapeutic device in cognitive therapy, and Socratic dialogue is the preferred method. The therapist carefully designs a series of questions to promote new learning. The purposes of the therapist's questions are generally to (1) clarify or define problems, (2) assist in the identification of thoughts, images, and assumptions, (3) examine the meanings of events for the patient, and (4) assess the consequences of maintaining maladaptive thoughts and behaviors.

Socratic dialogue implies that the patient arrives at logical conclusions based on the questions posed by the therapist. Questions are not used to "trap" patients, lead them to inevitable conclusions, or attack them. Questions enable the therapist to understand the patient's point of view and are posed with sensitivity so that patients may look at their assumptions objectively and nondefensively.

Young, Rygh, Weinberger, and Beck (2008, p. 274) describe how questions change throughout the course of therapy:

> In the beginning of therapy, questions are employed to obtain a full and detailed picture of the patient's particular difficulties. They are used to obtain background and diagnostic data; to evaluate the patient's stress tolerance, capacity for introspection, coping methods and so on; to obtain information about the patient's external situation and interpersonal context; and to modify vague complaints by working with the patient to arrive at specific target problems to work on.
>
> As therapy progresses, the therapist uses questioning to explore approaches to problems, to help the patient weigh advantages and disadvantages of possible solutions, to examine the consequences of staying with particular maladaptive behaviors, to elicit automatic thoughts, and to demonstrate EMSs and their consequences. In short, the therapist uses questioning in most cognitive therapeutic techniques.

Guided Discovery.   Through guided discovery, the patient modifies maladaptive beliefs and assumptions. The therapist serves as a guide who elucidates problem behaviors and errors in logic by designing new experiences (*behavioral experiments*) that lead to the acquisition of new skills and perspectives. Guided discovery implies that the therapist does not exhort or cajole the patient to adopt a new set of beliefs. Rather, the therapist encourages the patient's use of information, facts, and probabilities to obtain a realistic perspective.

Process of Psychotherapy

Initial Sessions

The goals of the first interview are to initiate a relationship with the patient, to elicit essential information, and to produce symptom relief. Building a relationship with the patient may begin with questions about feelings and thoughts about beginning therapy. Discussing the patient's expectations helps put the patient at ease, yields information about the patient's expectations, and presents an opportunity to demonstrate the relationship between cognition and affect (Beck, Rush, et al., 1979). The therapist also uses the initial sessions to accustom the patient to cognitive therapy, establish a collaborative framework, and deal with any misconceptions about therapy. The types of information the therapist seeks in the initial session include diagnosis, past history, present life situation, psychological problems, attitudes about treatment, and motivation for treatment.

Problem definition and symptom relief begin in the first session. Although problem definition and collection of background information may take several sessions, it is often critical to focus on a very specific problem and provide rapid relief in the first session. For example, a suicidal patient needs direct intervention to undermine hopelessness immediately. Symptom relief can come from several sources: specific problem solving, clarifying vague or general complaints into workable goals, or gaining objectivity about a disorder (e.g., making it clear that a patient's symptoms represent anxiety and nothing worse, or that difficulty concentrating is a symptom of depression and not a sign of brain disease).

Problem definition entails both functional and cognitive analyses of the problem. A functional analysis identifies elements of the problem: how it is manifested; situations in which it occurs; its frequency, intensity, and duration; and its consequences. A cognitive analysis of the problem identifies the thoughts and images a person has when emotion is triggered. It also includes investigation of the extent to which the person feels in control of thoughts and images, what the person imagines will happen in a distressing situation, and the probability of such an outcome actually occurring.

In the early sessions, then, the cognitive therapist plays a more active role than the patient. The therapist gathers information, conceptualizes the patient's problems, socializes the patient to cognitive therapy, and actively intervenes to provide symptom relief. The patient is assigned homework beginning at the first session.

Homework, at this early stage, is usually directed at recognizing the connections among thoughts, feelings, and behavior. For example, patients might be asked to record their automatic thoughts when distressed. Thus, the patient is trained from the outset to self-monitor thoughts and behaviors. In later sessions, the patient plays an increasingly active role in determining homework, and assignments focus on testing very specific assumptions.

During the initial sessions, a problem list is generated. The problem list may include specific symptoms, behaviors, or pervasive problems. These problems are assigned priorities as targets for intervention. Priorities are based on the relative magnitude of distress, the likelihood of making progress, the severity of symptoms, and the pervasiveness of a particular theme or topic.

If the therapist can help the patient solve a problem early in treatment, this success can motivate the patient to make further changes. As each problem is approached, the therapist chooses the appropriate cognitive or behavioral technique to apply and provides the patient with a rationale for the technique. Throughout therapy, the therapist elicits the patient's reactions to various techniques to ascertain whether they are being applied correctly, whether they are successful, and how they can be incorporated into homework or practical experience outside the session.

Middle and Later Sessions

As cognitive therapy proceeds, the emphasis shifts from the patient's symptoms to the patient's patterns of thinking. The connections among thoughts, emotions, and behavior are chiefly demonstrated through the examination of automatic thoughts. Once the patient can challenge thoughts that interfere with functioning, he or she can consider the underlying assumptions that generate such thoughts.

There is usually a greater emphasis on cognitive than on behavioral techniques in later sessions, which focus on complex problems that involve several dysfunctional thoughts. Often these thoughts are more amenable to logical analysis than to behavioral experimentation. For example, the prophecy "I'll never get what I want in life" is not easily tested. However, one can question the logic of this generalization and look at the advantages and disadvantages of maintaining it as a belief.

Often such assumptions outside the patient's awareness are discovered as themes of automatic thoughts. When automatic thoughts are observed over time and across situations, assumptions appear or can be inferred. Once these assumptions and their power have been recognized, therapy aims at modifying them by examining their validity, adaptiveness, and utility for the patient.

In later sessions, the patient assumes more responsibility for identifying problems and solutions and for creating homework assignments. The therapist takes on the role of advisor rather than teacher as the patient becomes better able to use cognitive techniques to solve problems. The frequency of sessions decreases as the patient becomes more self-sufficient. Therapy is terminated when goals have been reached and the patient feels able to practice his or her new skills and perspectives independently.

Ending Treatment

Length of treatment depends primarily on the severity of the client's problems. The usual length for unipolar depression is 15 to 25 sessions at weekly intervals (Beck, Rush, et al., 1979). Moderately to severely depressed patients usually require sessions twice a week for 4 to 5 weeks and then weekly sessions for 10 to 15 weeks. Most cases of anxiety are treated within a comparable period of time.

Some patients find it extremely difficult to tolerate the anxiety involved in giving up old ways of thinking. For them, therapy may last several months. Still others experience early symptom relief and leave therapy early. In these cases, little structural change has occurred, and problems are likely to recur.

From the outset, the therapist and patient share the expectation that therapy is time limited. Because cognitive therapy is present centered and time limited, there tend to be fewer problems with termination than in longer forms of therapy. As the patient develops self-reliance, therapy sessions become less frequent.

Termination is planned for, even in the first session as the rationale for cognitive therapy is presented. Patients are told that a goal of the therapy is for them to learn to be their own therapists. The problem list makes explicit what is to be accomplished in treatment. Behavioral observation, self-monitoring, self-report, and sometimes questionnaires (e.g., the Beck Depression Inventory) measure progress toward the goals on the problem list. Feedback from the patient aids the therapist in designing experiences to foster cognitive change.

Some patients have concerns about relapse or about functioning autonomously. Some of these concerns include cognitive distortions, such as dichotomous thinking ("I'm either sick or 100% cured") or negative prediction ("I'll get depressed again and won't be able to help myself"). It may be necessary to review the goal of therapy: to teach the patient ways to handle problems more effectively, not to produce a "cure" or restructure core personality (Beck, Rush, et al., 1979). Education about psychological disorders, such as acknowledging the possibility of recurrent depression, is done throughout treatment so that the patient has a realistic perspective on prognosis.

During the usual course of therapy, the patient experiences both successes and setbacks. Such problems give the patient the opportunity to practice new skills. As termination approaches, the patient can be reminded that setbacks are normal and have been handled before. The therapist might ask the patient to describe how prior specific problems were handled during treatment. Therapists can also use cognitive rehearsal prior to termination by having patients imagine future difficulties and report how they would deal with them.

Termination is usually followed by one to two booster sessions, usually 1 month and 2 months after termination. Such sessions consolidate gains and assist the patient in employing new skills.

Mechanisms of Psychotherapy

Several common denominators cut across effective treatments. Three mechanisms of change common to all successful forms of psychotherapy are (1) a comprehensible framework, (2) the patient's emotional engagement in the problem situation, and (3) reality testing in that situation.

Cognitive therapy maintains that the modification of dysfunctional assumptions leads to effective cognitive, emotional, and behavioral change. Patients change by recognizing automatic thoughts, questioning the evidence used to support them, and modifying cognitions. Next, the patient behaves in ways congruent with new, more adaptive ways of thinking.

Change can occur only if the patient experiences a problematic situation as a real threat. According to cognitive therapy, core beliefs are linked to emotions, and with affective arousal, those beliefs become accessible and modifiable. One mechanism of change, then, focuses on making accessible those cognitive constellations that produced the maladaptive behavior or symptomatology. This mechanism is analogous to what psychoanalysts call "making the unconscious conscious."

Simply arousing emotions and the accompanying cognitions are not sufficient to cause lasting change. People express emotion, sometimes explosively, throughout their lives without benefit. However, the therapeutic milieu allows the patient to experience emotional arousal and reality testing simultaneously. For a variety of psychotherapies, what is therapeutic is the patient's ability to be engaged in a problem situation and yet respond to it adaptively. In terms of cognitive therapy, this means to experience the cognitions and to test them within the therapeutic framework.

APPLICATIONS

Who Can We Help?

Cognitive therapy is a present-centered, structured, active, cognitive, problem-oriented approach best suited for cases in which problems can be delineated and cognitive distortions are apparent. It was originally developed for the treatment of Axis I disorders but has been elaborated to treat Axis II disorders as well. It has wide-ranging applications to a variety of clinical and nonclinical problems. Though originally used in individual psychotherapy, it is now used with couples, families, and groups. It can be applied alone or in combination with pharmacotherapy in inpatient and outpatient settings.

Cognitive therapy is widely recognized as an effective treatment for unipolar depression. Beck, Rush, et al. (1979, p. 27) list criteria for using cognitive therapy alone or in combination with medication. It is the treatment of choice in cases where the patient refuses medication, prefers a psychological treatment, has unacceptable side effects to antidepressant medication, has a medical condition that precludes the use of antidepressants, or has proved to be refractory to adequate trials of antidepressants. Recent research by DeRubeis, Hollon, et al. (2005) indicates that cognitive therapy can be as effective as medications for the initial treatment of moderate to severe major depression.

Cognitive therapy is not recommended as the exclusive treatment in cases of bipolar affective disorder or psychotic depression. It is also not used alone for the treatment of other psychoses, such as schizophrenia. Some patients with anxiety may begin treatment on medication, but cognitive therapy teaches them to function without relying on medication.

Cognitive therapy produces the best results with patients who have adequate reality testing (i.e., no hallucinations or delusions), good concentration, and sufficient memory functions. It is ideally suited to patients who can focus on their automatic thoughts, accept the therapist–patient roles, are willing to tolerate anxiety in order to do experiments, can alter assumptions permanently, take responsibility for their problems, and are willing to postpone gratification in order to complete therapy. Although these ideals are not always met, this therapy can proceed with some adjustment of outcome expectations and flexibility of structure. For example, therapy may not permanently alter schemas but may improve the patient's daily functioning.

Cognitive therapy is effective for patients with different levels of income, education, and background (Persons, Burns, & Perloff, 1988). As long as the patient can recognize the relationships among thoughts, feelings, and behaviors and takes some responsibility for self-help, cognitive therapy can be beneficial.

Treatment

Cognitive therapy consists of highly specific learning experiences designed to teach patients (1) to monitor their negative, automatic thoughts (cognitions), (2) to recognize the connections among cognition, affect, and behavior, (3) to examine the evidence for and against distorted automatic thoughts, (4) to substitute more reality-oriented interpretations for these biased cognitions, and (5) to learn to identify and alter the beliefs that predispose them to distort their experiences (Beck, Rush, et al., 1979).

Both cognitive and behavioral techniques are used in cognitive therapy to reach these goals. The technique used at any given time depends on the patient's level of functioning and on the particular symptoms and problems presented.

Cognitive Techniques

Verbal techniques are used to elicit the patient's automatic thoughts, analyze the logic behind the thoughts, identify maladaptive assumptions, and examine the validity of those assumptions. Automatic thoughts are elicited by questioning the patient about those thoughts that occur during upsetting situations. If the patient has difficulty recalling thoughts, imagery or role playing can be used. Automatic thoughts are most accurately reported when they occur in real-life situations. Such "hot" cognitions are accessible, powerful, and habitual. The patient is taught to recognize and identify thoughts and to record them when upset.

Cognitive therapists do not interpret patients' automatic thoughts but, rather, explore their meanings, particularly when a patient reports fairly neutral thoughts yet displays strong emotions. In such cases, the therapist asks what those thoughts mean to the patient. For example, after an initial visit, an anxious patient called his therapist in great distress. He had just read an article about drug treatments for anxiety. His automatic thought was "Drug therapy is helpful for anxiety." The meaning he ascribed to this was "Cognitive therapy can't possibly help me. I am doomed to failure again."

Automatic thoughts are tested by direct evidence or by logical analysis. Evidence can be derived from past and present circumstances, but, true to scientific inquiry, it must be as close to the facts as possible. Data can also be gathered in behavioral experiments. For example, if a man believes he cannot carry on a conversation, he might try to initiate brief exchanges with three people. The empirical nature of behavioral experiments allows patients to think in a more objective way.

Examination of the patient's thoughts can also lead to cognitive change. Questioning may uncover logical inconsistencies, contradictions, and other errors in thinking. Identifying cognitive distortions is in itself helpful, for patients then have specific errors to correct.

Maladaptive assumptions are usually much less accessible to patients than automatic thoughts. Some patients are able to articulate their assumptions, but most find it difficult.

Assumptions appear as themes in automatic thoughts. The therapist may ask the patient to abstract rules underlying specific thoughts. The therapist might also infer assumptions from these data and present these assumptions to the patient for verification. A patient who had trouble identifying her assumptions broke into tears upon reading an assumption inferred by her therapist—an indication of the salience of that assumption. Patients always have the right to disagree with the therapist and find more accurate statements of their beliefs.

Once an assumption has been identified, it is open to modification. This can occur in several ways: by asking the patient whether the assumption seems reasonable, by having the patient generate reasons for and against maintaining the assumption, and by presenting evidence contrary to the assumption. Even though a particular assumption may seem reasonable in a specific situation, it may appear dysfunctional when universally applied. For example, being highly productive at work is generally reasonable, but being highly productive during recreational time may be unreasonable. A physician who believed he should work to his top capacity throughout his career may not have considered the prospect of early burnout. Thus, what may have made him successful in the short run could lead to problems in the long run. Specific cognitive techniques include decatastrophizing, reattribution, redefining, and decentering.

Decatastrophizing, also known as the "what if" technique (Beck & Emery, 1985), helps patients prepare for feared consequences. This is helpful in decreasing avoidance, particularly when combined with coping plans (Beck & Emery, 1985). If anticipated consequences are likely to happen, these techniques help to identify problem-solving strategies. Decatastrophizing is often used with a time-projection technique to widen the range of information and broaden the patient's time perspective.

Reattribution techniques test automatic thoughts and assumptions by considering alternative causes of events. This is especially helpful when patients personalize or perceive themselves as the cause of events. It is unreasonable to conclude, in the absence of evidence, that another person or single factor is the sole cause of an event. Reattribution techniques encourage reality testing and appropriate assignment of responsibility by requiring examination of all the factors that impinge on a situation.

Redefining is a way to mobilize a patient who believes a problem to be beyond personal control. Burns (1985) recommends that lonely people who think, "Nobody pays any attention to me" redefine the problem as "I need to reach out to other people and be caring." Redefining a problem may include making it more concrete and specific and stating it in terms of the patient's own behavior.

Decentering is used primarily in treating anxious patients who wrongly believe they are the focus of everyone's attention. After they examine the logic behind the conviction that others would stare at them and be able to read their minds, behavioral experiments are designed to test these particular beliefs. For example, one student who was reluctant to speak in class believed his classmates watched him constantly and noticed his anxiety. By observing them instead of focusing on his own discomfort, he saw some students taking notes, some looking at the professor, and some daydreaming. He concluded that his classmates had other concerns.

The cognitive domain comprises thoughts and images. For some patients, pictorial images are more accessible and easier to report than thoughts. This is often the case with anxious patients. Ninety percent of anxious patients in one study reported visual images before and during episodes of anxiety (Beck, Laude, & Bohnert, 1974). Gathering information about imagery, then, is another way to understand conceptual systems. Spontaneous images provide data on the patient's perceptions and interpretations of events. Other specific imagery procedures used to modify distorted cognitions are discussed by Beck and Emery (1985) and by Judith Beck (1995).

In some cases, imagery is modified for its own sake. Intrusive imagery, such as imagery related to trauma, can be directly modified to reduce its impact. Patients can change aspects of an image by "rewriting the script" of what happened, making an attacker shrink in size to the point of powerlessness or empowering themselves in the image. The point of restructuring such images is not to deny what actually happened but to reduce the ability of the image to disrupt daily functioning.

Imagery is also used in role-plays because of its ability to access emotions. Experiential techniques, such as dialogues between one's healthy self and one's negative thoughts, are used to mobilize affect and help patients both believe and feel that they have the right to be free of harmful and self-defeating patterns.

Behavioral Techniques

Cognitive therapy uses behavioral techniques to modify automatic thoughts and assumptions. It employs behavioral experiments designed to challenge specific maladaptive beliefs and promote new learning. In a behavioral experiment, for example, a patient may predict an outcome based on personal automatic thoughts, carry out the agreed-upon behavior, and then evaluate the evidence in light of the new experience.

Behavioral techniques are also used to expand patients' response repertories (skills training), to relax them (progressive relaxation) or make them active (activity scheduling), to prepare them for avoided situations (behavioral rehearsal), or to expose them to feared stimuli (exposure therapy). Because behavioral techniques are used to foster cognitive change, it is crucial to know the patient's perceptions, thoughts, and conclusions after each behavioral experiment.

Homework gives patients the opportunity to apply cognitive principles between sessions. Typical homework assignments focus on self-observation and self-monitoring, structuring time effectively, and implementing procedures for dealing with concrete situations. Self-monitoring is applied to the patient's automatic thoughts and reactions in various situations. New skills, such as challenging automatic thoughts, are also practiced as homework.

Hypothesis testing has both cognitive and behavioral components. In framing a "hypothesis," it is necessary to make it specific and concrete. A resident who insisted, "I am not a good doctor" was asked to list what was needed to arrive at that conclusion. The therapist contributed other criteria as well, for the physician had overlooked such factors as rapport with patients and the ability to make decisions under pressure. The resident then monitored his behavior and sought feedback from colleagues and supervisors to test his hypothesis, coming to the conclusion "I am a good doctor *for my level of training and experience.*"

Exposure therapy serves to provide data on the thoughts, images, physiological symptoms, and self-reported level of tension experienced by the anxious patient. Specific thoughts and images can be examined for distortions, and specific coping skills can be taught. By dealing directly with a patient's idiosyncratic thoughts, cognitive therapy is able to focus on that patient's particular needs. Patients learn that their predictions are not always accurate, and they then have the data to challenge anxious thoughts in the future.

Behavioral rehearsal and *role playing* are used to practice skills or techniques that are later applied in real life. Modeling is also used in skills training. Often role playing is videotaped so that an objective source of information is available with which to evaluate performance.

Diversion techniques, which are used to reduce strong emotions and to decrease negative thinking, include physical activity, social contact, work, play, and visual imagery.

Activity scheduling provides structure and encourages involvement. Rating (on a scale of 0 to 10) the degree of mastery and pleasure experienced during each activity of the day achieves several things: Patients who believe their depression is at a constant level see mood fluctuations; those who believe they cannot accomplish or enjoy anything are contradicted by the evidence; and those who believe they are inactive because of an inherent defect are shown that activity involves some planning and is reinforcing in itself.

Graded-task assignment calls for the patient to initiate an activity at a nonthreatening level while the therapist gradually increases the difficulty of assigned tasks. For example, someone who has difficulty socializing might begin interacting with one other person, interact with a small group of acquaintances, or socialize with people for just a brief period of time. Step by step, the patient comes to increase the time spent with others.

Cognitive therapists work in a variety of settings. Patients are referred by physicians, schools and universities, and other therapists who believe that cognitive therapy would be especially helpful. Many patients are self-referred. The Academy of Cognitive Therapy maintains an international referral list of therapists on its Web site (www.academyofct.org).

Cognitive therapists generally adhere to 45-minute sessions. Because of the structure of cognitive therapy, much can be accomplished in this time. Patients are frequently asked to complete questionnaires, such as the BDI, before the start of each session. Most sessions take place in the therapist's office. However, real-life work with anxious patients occurs outside the therapist's office. A therapist might take public transportation with an agoraphobic, go to a pet store with a rodent phobic, or travel in an airplane with someone afraid of flying.

Confidentiality is always maintained, and the therapist obtains informed consent for audiotaping and videotaping. Such recording is used in skills training or as a way to present evidence contradicting the patient's assumptions. For example, a patient who believes she looks nervous whenever she converses might be videotaped in conversation to test this assumption. Her appearance on camera may convince her that her assumption was in error or help her to identify specific behaviors to improve. Occasionally, patients take audiotaped sessions home to review content material between sessions.

Sessions are usually conducted on a weekly basis, with severely disturbed patients seen more frequently in the beginning. Cognitive therapists give their patients phone numbers at which they can be reached in the event of an emergency.

Whenever possible, and with the patient's permission, significant others, such as friends and family members, are included in a therapy session to review the treatment goals and to explore ways in which the significant others might be helpful. This is especially important when family members misunderstand the nature of the illness, are overly solicitous, or are behaving in counterproductive ways. Significant others can be of great assistance in therapy, helping to sustain behavioral improvements by encouraging homework and assisting the patient with reality testing.

Problems may arise in the practice of cognitive therapy. For example, patients may misunderstand what the therapist says, and this may result in anger, dissatisfaction, or hopelessness. When the therapist perceives such a reaction, he or she elicits the patient's thoughts, just as with any other automatic thoughts. Together the therapist and client look for alternative interpretations. The therapist who has made an error accepts responsibility and corrects the mistake.

Problems sometimes result from unrealistic expectations about how quickly behaviors should change, from the incorrect or inflexible application of a technique, or from lack of attention to central issues. Problems in therapy require that the therapist attend to his or her own automatic thoughts and look for distortions in logic that create strong affect or prevent adequate problem solving.

Beck, Rush, et al. (1979) provide guidelines for working with difficult patients and those who have histories of unsuccessful therapy: (1) avoid stereotyping the patient as *being* the problem rather than *having* the problem; (2) remain optimistic; (3) identify and deal with your own dysfunctional cognitions; (4) remain focused on the task instead of blaming the patient; and (5) maintain a problem-solving attitude. By following these guidelines, the therapist is able to be more resourceful with difficult patients. The therapist also can serve as a model for the patient, demonstrating that frustration does not automatically lead to anger and despair.

Evidence

Evidence-based practice in psychology (EBPP) advocates the application of empirically supported principles of psychological assessment, case formulation, therapeutic relationship, and intervention in the delivery of effective psychological care (APA Presidential Task Force on Evidence-Based Practice, 2006). The evidence base for any psychological treatment is evaluated in terms of its efficacy, or demonstrated causal relationship to outcome, and its utility or generalizability and feasibility—in other words, its internal and external validity. The best available research is then combined with clinical expertise in the context of patient characteristics, culture, and preferences to promote the effective practice of psychology and public health.

A fundamental component of evidence-based practice is empirically supported treatments, those demonstrated to work for a certain disorder or problem under specified circumstances. Randomized controlled trials (RCTs) in psychology, as in other health fields, are the standard for drawing causal inferences and provide the most direct and internally valid demonstration of treatment efficacy. Meta-analysis, a systematic way to synthesize results from multiple studies, is used to quantitatively measure treatment outcome and effect sizes. Other research designs, such as qualitative research and single-case experimental designs, are used to describe experiences, generate new hypotheses, and examine causal relationships for an individual, but RCTs and meta-analysis are best suited for examining whether a treatment works for a number of people.

Cognitive therapy (CT) and cognitive–behavior therapies (CBT, the atheoretical combination of cognitive and behavioral strategies) are based on empirical studies. Individual RCTs, reviews of the literature of outcome studies for a range of disorders, and meta-analyses all document the success of CT and CBT in the treatment of depression and anxiety disorders in particular (Beck, 2005; Butler, Chapman, Forman, & Beck, 2006; DeRubeis & Crits-Christoph, 1998; Gloaguen, Cottraux, Cucherat, & Blackburn, 1998; Gould, Otto, & Pollack, 1995; Wampold, Minami, Baskin, & Callen Tierney, 2002). The recent review of 16 methodologically rigorous meta-analyses by Butler et al. (2006) found large effect sizes for unipolar depression, generalized anxiety disorder, panic disorder with or without agoraphobia, social phobia, and childhood depressive and anxiety disorders. Moderate effect sizes were found for marital distress, anger, childhood somatic disorders, and chronic pain. Relatively small effect sizes were found for adjunctive CBT for schizophrenia and for bulimia nervosa. Other studies have found that CT/CBT yields lower relapse rates than antidepressant medications (Hollon, DeRubeis, Shelton, et al., 2005) and reduces the risk of symptoms returning following treatment termination for depression and anxiety disorders (Hollon, Stewart, & Strunk, 2006).

One criticism of the reliance on RCTs in psychotherapy research is that the samples studied are so carefully screened to eliminate comorbidity or other threats to experimental control that they do not represent real groups in the community, who often have multiple problems. However, a recent study by Brown et al. (2005) showed success for cognitive therapy for the prevention of suicide attempts among people at high risk for suicide. The participants in this study had more than one psychiatric diagnosis, and 68% had substance abuse problems. A study by DeRubeis et al. (2005) similarly included participants with comorbidity.

In addition to best available research, another component of evidence-based practice is clinical expertise—the advanced clinical skills to assess, diagnose, and treat disorders. The importance of clinical expertise is demonstrated in the study by DeRubeis et al. (2005), which concluded that CT can be as effective as medications for the initial treatment of depression, but the degree of effectiveness may depend on a high level of therapist experience or expertise.

The generalizability of CT/CBT has been examined in a few studies. Stirman and colleagues (Stirman, DeRubeis, Crits-Cristoph & Rothman, 2005) found that clinical characteristics of subjects in RCTs matched those of patients in clinical settings. Similarly, Persons and associates (Persons, Bostrom, & Bertagnolli, 1999) found that clinic patients treated with CT for depression improved comparably to those in RTCs. In addition, studies of schizophrenic patients at National Health Service clinics in the U.K. found improved symptoms using CT as an adjunct to pharmacotherapy (Tarrier, 2008).

Because training in evidence-based therapies has been mandated by the Accreditation Council for Graduate Medical Education, CT/CBT is being taught in psychiatry residency programs in the United States. As the number of professionals with expertise in cognitive therapy increases, research may be further directed both toward refining the therapy for more populations in need and toward exploring ways to make it cost-effective and available in community settings.

Psychotherapy in a Multicultural World

Cognitive therapy begins with an understanding of the patient's beliefs, values and attitudes. These exist within a cultural context, and the therapist must understand that context. Cognitive therapy focuses on whether these beliefs are adaptive for the patient, and whether they pose difficulties or lead to dysfunctional behavior. Cognitive therapy does not work on changing beliefs in an arbitrary way, nor is it an attempt to impose the therapist's beliefs on the patient. Rather, it helps the individual examine his or her own beliefs and whether they foster emotional well-being. Sometimes people's personal beliefs are at odds with the cultural values around them. Other times, a person's beliefs may be changing with culture change, as in rapid modernization or migration to a new country, and discrepancies may cause distress. In these cases, cognitive therapy may help patients think flexibly in order to reconcile their beliefs with environmental constraints or empower them to find solutions.

Beck's work has been translated into more than a dozen languages, and cognitive therapists are represented by organizations worldwide. Research in cognitive therapy has been conducted in many countries, primarily industrial economies. There is a need to expand cognitive therapy research further into developing nations.

CASE EXAMPLE

This case example of the course of treatment for an anxious patient illustrates the use of both behavioral and cognitive techniques.

Presenting Problem

The patient was a 21-year-old male college student who complained of sleep-onset insomnia and frequent awakenings, halting speech and stuttering, shakiness, feelings of nervousness, dizziness, and worrying. His sleep difficulties were particularly acute prior to exams or athletic competitions. He attributed his speech problems to his search for the "perfect word."

The patient was raised in a family that valued competition. As the eldest child, he was expected to win all the contests. His parents were determined that their children should surpass them in achievements and successes. They so strongly identified with the patient's achievements that he believed, "My success is their success."

The patient was taught to compete with other children outside the family as well. His father reminded him, "Never let anyone get the best of you." As a consequence of viewing others as adversaries, he developed few friends. Feeling lonely, he tried desperately to attract friends by becoming a prankster and by telling lies to enhance his image and make his family appear more attractive. Although he had acquaintances in college, he had few friends, for he was unable to self-disclose, fearing that others would discover he was not all that he would like to be.

Early Sessions

After gathering initial data regarding diagnosis, context, and history, the therapist attempted to define how the patient's cognitions contributed to his distress (T = Therapist; P = Patient).

T: What types of situations are most upsetting to you?
P: When I do poorly in sports, particularly swimming. I'm on the swim team. Also, if I make a mistake, even when I play cards with my roommates. I feel really upset if I get rejected by a girl.
T: What thoughts go through your mind, let's say, when you don't do so well at swimming?
P: I think people think much less of me if I'm not on top, a winner.
T: And how about if you make a mistake playing cards?
P: I doubt my own intelligence.
T: And if a girl rejects you?
P: It means I'm not special. I lose value as a person.
T: Do you see any connections here, among these thoughts?
P: Well, I guess my mood depends on what other people think of me. But that's important. I don't want to be lonely.
T: What would that mean to you, to be lonely?
P: It would mean there's something wrong with me, that I'm a loser.

At this point, the therapist began to hypothesize about the patient's organizing beliefs: that his worth is determined by others, that he is unattractive because there is something inherently wrong with him, that he is a loser. The therapist looked for evidence to support the centrality of these beliefs and remained open to other possibilities.

The therapist assisted the patient in generating a list of goals to work on in therapy. These goals included (1) decreasing perfectionism, (2) decreasing anxiety symptoms, (3) decreasing sleep difficulties, (4) increasing closeness in friendships, and (5) developing his own values apart from those of his parents. The first problem addressed was anxiety. An upcoming exam was chosen as a target situation. This student typically studied far beyond what was necessary, went to bed worried, finally fell asleep, woke during the night thinking about details or possible consequences of his performance, and went to exams exhausted. To reduce ruminations about his performance, the therapist asked him to name the advantages of dwelling on thoughts of the exam.

P: Well, if I don't think about the exam all the time I might forget something. If I think about the exam constantly, I think I'll do better. I'll be more prepared.
T: Have you ever gone into a situation less "prepared"?

P: Not an exam, but once I was in a big swim meet and the night before I went out with friends and didn't think about it. I came home, went to sleep, got up, and swam.

T: And how did it work out?

P: Fine. I felt great and swam pretty well.

T: Based on that experience, do you think there's any reason to try to worry less about your performance?

P: I guess so. It didn't hurt me not to worry. Actually, worrying can be pretty distracting. I end up focusing more on how I'm doing than on what I'm doing.

The patient came up with his own rationale for decreasing his ruminations. He was then ready to consider giving up his maladaptive behavior and risk trying something new. The therapist taught the patient progressive relaxation, and the patient began to use physical exercise as a way to relieve anxiety.

The patient was also instructed in how cognitions affect behavior and mood. Picking up on the patient's statement that worries can be distracting, the therapist proceeded.

T: You mentioned that when you worry about your exams, you feel anxious. What I'd like you to do now is imagine lying in your bed the night before an exam.

P: Okay, I can picture it.

T: Imagine that you are thinking about the exam and you decide that you haven't done enough to prepare.

P: Yeah, OK.

T: How are you feeling?

P: I'm feeling nervous. My heart is beginning to race. I think I need to get up and study some more

T: Good. When you think you're not prepared, you get anxious and want to get up out of bed. Now, I want you to imagine that you are in bed the night before the exam. You have prepared in your usual way and are ready. You remind yourself of what you have done. You think that you are prepared and know the material.

P: OK. Now I feel confident.

T: Can you see how your thoughts affect your feelings of anxiety?

The patient was instructed to record automatic thoughts, recognize cognitive distortions, and respond to them. For homework, he was asked to record his automatic thoughts if he had trouble falling asleep before an exam. One automatic thought he had while lying in bed was "I should be thinking about the exam." His response was "Thinking about the exam is not going to make a difference at this point. I did study." Another thought was "I must go to sleep now! I must get eight hours of sleep!" His response was "I have left leeway, so I have time. Sleep is not so crucial that I have to worry about it." He was able to shift his thinking to a positive image of himself floating in clear blue water.

By observing his automatic thoughts across a variety of situations—academic, athletic, and social—the patient identified dichotomous thinking (e.g., "I'm either a winner or a loser") as a frequent cognitive distortion. Perceiving the consequences of his behavior as either totally good or completely bad resulted in major shifts in mood. Two techniques that helped with his dichotomous thinking were reframing the problem and building a continuum between his dichotomous categories.

Here the problem is reframed:

T: Can you think of reasons for someone not to respond to you other than because you're a loser?

P: No. Unless I really convince them I'm great, they won't be attracted.

T: How would you convince them of that?

P: To tell you the truth, I'd exaggerate what I've done. I'd lie about my grade point average or tell someone I placed first in a race.

T: How does that work out?

P: Actually, not too well. I get uncomfortable and they get confused by my stories. Sometimes they don't seem to care. Other times they walk away after I've been talking a lot about myself.

T: So in some cases, they don't respond to you when you focus the conversation on yourself.

P: Right.

T: Does this have anything to do with whether you're a winner or a loser?

P: No, they don't even know who I am deep down. They're just turned off because I talk too much.

T: Right. It sounds like they're responding to your conversational style.

The therapist reframed the problem from a situation in which something was inherently wrong with the patient to one characterized by a problem of social skills. Moreover, the theme "I am a loser" appeared so powerful to the patient that he labeled it as his "main belief." This assumption was traced historically to the constant criticism from his parents for mistakes and perceived shortcomings. By reviewing his history, he was able to see that his lies prevented people from getting closer, reinforcing his belief that they didn't want to be close. In addition, he believed that his parents made him whatever success he was and that no achievement was his alone. This had made him angry and lacking in self-confidence.

Later Sessions

As therapy progressed, the patient's homework increasingly focused on social interaction. He practiced initiating conversations and asking questions in order to learn more about other people. He also practiced "biting his tongue" instead of telling small lies about himself. He monitored people's reactions to him and saw that they were varied, but generally positive. By listening to others, he found that he admired people who could openly admit shortcomings and joke about their mistakes. This experience helped him understand that it was useless to categorize people, including himself, as winners and losers.

In later sessions, the patient described his belief that his behavior reflected on his parents, and vice versa. He said, "If they look good, it says something about me and if I look good, they get the credit." One assignment required him to list the ways in which he was different from his parents. He remarked, "Realizing that my parents and I are separate made me realize I could stop telling lies." Recognizing how he was different from his parents freed him from their absolute standards and allowed him to be less self-conscious when interacting with others.

Subsequently, the patient was able to pursue interests and hobbies that had nothing to do with achievement. He was able to set moderate and realistic goals for schoolwork, and he began to date.

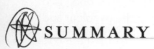 SUMMARY

Cognitive therapy has grown quickly because of its empirical basis and demonstrated efficacy. Borrowing some of its concepts from cognitive theorists and a number of techniques from behavior therapy and client-oriented psychotherapy, cognitive therapy consists of a broad theoretical structure of personality and psychopathology, a set of well-defined therapeutic strategies, and a wide variety of therapeutic techniques. Similar in many ways to rational emotive behavior therapy, which preceded but developed parallel to cognitive therapy, this system of psychotherapy has acquired strong empirical support for its theoretical foundations. A number of outcome studies have demonstrated its efficacy, especially in the treatment of depression. The related theoretical formulations of depression have been supported by more than 100 empirical studies. Other concepts, such as the cognitive triad in depression, the concept of specific cognitive profiles for specific disorders, cognitive processing, and the relationship of hopelessness to suicide, have also received strong support.

Outcome studies have investigated cognitive therapy with major depressive disorders, generalized anxiety disorder, dysthymic disorder, drug abuse, alcoholism, panic disorder, anorexia, and bulimia. In addition, cognitive therapy has been applied successfully to the treatment of obsessive–compulsive disorder, hypochondriasis, and various personality disorders. In conjunction with psychotropic medication, it has been used to treat delusional disorders and bipolar disorder.

Much of the popularity of cognitive therapy is attributable to strong empirical support for its theoretical framework and to the large number of outcome studies with clinical populations. In addition, there is no doubt that the intellectual atmosphere of the "cognitive revolution" has made the field of psychotherapy more receptive to this new therapy. A further attractive feature of cognitive therapy is that it is readily teachable. The various therapeutic strategies and techniques have been described and defined in such a way that one year's training is usually sufficient for a psychotherapist to attain a reasonable level of competence as a cognitive therapist.

Although cognitive therapy focuses on understanding the patient's problems and applying appropriate techniques, it also attends to the nonspecific therapeutic characteristics of the therapist. Consequently the basic qualities of empathy, acceptance, and personal regard are highly valued.

Because therapy is not conducted in a vacuum, cognitive therapists pay close attention to patients' interpersonal relations and confront patients continuously with problems they may be avoiding. Further, therapeutic change can take place only when patients are emotionally engaged with their problems. Therefore, the experience of emotion during therapy is a crucial feature. The patient's reactions to the therapist, and the therapist's to the patient, are also important. Excessive and distorted responses to the therapist are elicited and evaluated just like any other type of ideational material. In the presence of the therapist, patients learn to correct their misconceptions, which were often derived from early experiences.

Cognitive therapy may offer an opportunity for a rapprochement between psychodynamic therapy and behavior therapy. In many ways it provides a common ground for these two disciplines. At the present time, the number of cognitive therapists within the behavior therapy movement is growing. In fact, many behavior therapists view themselves as cognitive–behavior therapists.

Looking to the future, it is anticipated that the boundaries of the theoretical background of cognitive therapy will gradually expand to encompass or penetrate the fields of cognitive psychology and social psychology. There is already an enormous amount of interest in social psychology, which provides the theoretical background of cognitive therapy.

In an era of cost containment, this short-term approach will prove to be increasingly attractive to third-party payers as well as to patients. Future empirical studies of its processes and effectiveness will undoubtedly be conducted to determine whether cognitive therapy can fulfill its promise.

ANNOTATED BIBLIOGRAPHY

Beck, A. T., Freeman, A., Davis, D., & Associates. (2004). *Cognitive therapy of personality disorders* (2nd edition). New York: Guilford Press.
This book presents the research and theory behind the cognitive conceptualization of Axis II disorders. Specific beliefs and attitudes for each personality disorder are presented along with intervention techiniques.

Beck, A. T., Rush, A. J., Shaw, B. F., & Emery, G. (1979). *Cognitive therapy of depression.* New York: Guilford Press.
Perhaps Beck's most influential book, this work presents the cognitive model of depression and treatment interventions. This book served to codify what actually happens in cognitive therapy and thus set a standard for other psychotherapies to follow.

Beck, J. S. (1995). *Cognitive therapy: Basics and beyond.* New York: Guilford Press.
Dr. Judith Beck presents an updated manual for cognitive therapy. She begins with how to develop a cognitive case conceptualization and instructs the reader in how to identify deeper-level cognitions, prepare for termination, and anticipate problems.

Ellis, T. E., & Newman, C. F. (1996). *Choosing to live: How to defeat suicide through cognitive therapy.* Oakland, CA: New Harbinger Publications.
This book is for clients and clinicians alike. The strategies presented are well-grounded in research aimed at reducing hopelessness and increasing problem-solving. This book, in turn, has been used as a treatment manual in clinical research.

Greenberger, D., & Padesky, C. A. (1995). *Mind over mood: A cognitive therapy treatment manual for clients.* New York: Guilford Press.
This is a workbook for clients that teaches cognitive techniques. It can stand alone but is most helpful when used within therapy. It is also an excellent resource for cognitive therapists in training. The *Clinician's Guide to Mind Over Mood* is a companion volume.

Weishaar, M. E. (1993). *Aaron T. Beck.* London: Sage Publications.
This biography of Aaron Beck includes chapters on the theoretical and practical contributions of cognitive therapy to psychotherapy, as well as criticisms of cognitive therapy, rebuttals to the criticisms, and a review of the overall contributions of Beck's cognitive therapy to psychotherapy and counseling.

CASE READINGS

Beck, A. T., Rush, J., Shaw, B., & Emery, G. (1979). Interview with a depressed and suicidal patient. In *Cognitive therapy of depression* (pp. 225–243). New York: Guilford Press. [Reprinted in D. Wedding & R. J. Corsini (Eds.). (2011), *Case studies in psychotherapy.* Belmont, CA: Brooks/Cole.]
This interview with a suicidal patient features an outline of the types of assessments and interventions made by cognitive therapists in an initial session. Substantial change occurs in one session, as demonstrated in the verbatim transcript of the interview.

Young, J. E., Rygh, J. L., Weinberger, A. D., & Beck, A .T. (2008). Cognitive therapy for depression. In D. Barlow (Ed.), *Clinical handbook of psychological disorders* (4th ed., pp. 250–305). New York: Guilford Press.
This chapter presents two cases of depressed individuals. Both cases demonstrate how to elicit and test automatic thoughts and assumptions, and one case demonstrates schema-focused treatment for relapse prevention.

Freeman, A., & Dattilio, E. M. (Eds.). (1992). *Comprehensive casebook of cognitive therapy.* New York: Plenum Press.
This edited volume contains a variety of cases that illustrate the use of cognitive therapy.

Greenberger, D., & Padesky, C. A. (1995). *Mind over mood: A cognitive therapy treatment manual for clients.* New York: Guilford Press.
This treatment manual describes how to apply various cognitive therapy strategies, using cases throughout the book.

REFERENCES

Adler, A. (1936). The neurotic's picture of the world. *International Journal of Individual Psychology, 2,* 3–10.

Alexander, E. (1950). *Psychosomatic medicine: Its principles and applications.* New York: Norton.

APA Presidential Task Force on Evidence-Based Practice (2006). Evidence-based practice in psychology. *American Psychologist, 61,* 271–285.

Arnold, M. (1960). *Emotion and personality* (vol. 1). New York: Columbia University Press.

Bandura, A. (1977). *Social learning theory.* Englewood Cliffs, NJ: Prentice-Hall.

Baucom, D., Sayers, S., & Sher, T. (1990). Supplementary behavioral marital therapy with cognitive restructuring and emotional expressiveness training: An outcome investigation. *Journal of Consulting & Clinical Psychology, 58,* 636–645.

Beck, A. T. (1963). Thinking and depression. 1. Idiosyncratic content and cognitive distortions. *Archives of General Psychiatry, 9,* 324–333.

Beck, A. T. (1964). Thinking and depression. 2. Theory and therapy. *Archives of General Psychiatry, 10,* 561–571.

Beck, A. T. (1967). *Depression: Clinical, experimental, and theoretical aspects.* New York: Hoeber. [Republished as *Depression: Causes and treatment.* Philadelphia: University of Pennsylvania Press, 1972.]

Beck, A. T. (2005). The current state of cognitive therapy. *Archives of General Psychiatry, 62,* 953–959.

Beck, A. T. (2008). The evolution of the cognitive model of depression and its neurobiological correlates. *American Journal of Psychiatry, 165*(8), 969–977.

Beck, J. S. (1995). *Cognitive therapy: Basics and beyond.* New York: Guilford Press.

Beck, A. T., & Beck, J. S. (1995). *The Personality Belief Questionnaire.* Bala Cynwyd, PA: Beck Institute for Cognitive Therapy and Research.

Beck, J. S., & Beck, A. T. (2002). *Beck Youth Inventories of Emotional and Social Impairment.* San Antonio, TX: The Psychological Corporation.

Beck, A. T., Brown, G., Berchick, R. J., Stewart, B. L., & Steer, R. A. (1990). Relationship between hopelessness and ultimate suicide: A replication with psychiatric outpatients. *American Journal of Psychiatry, 147*(2), 190–195.

Beck, A. T., & Emery, G. (1985). *Anxiety disorders and phobias: A cognitive perspective.* New York: Basic Books.

Beck, A. T., Epstein, N., & Harrison, R. (1983). Cognitions, attitudes and personality dimensions in depression. *British Journal of Cognitive Psychotherapy, 1*(1), 1–16.

Beck, A. T., Freeman, A., & Davis, D. D. (2003). *Cognitive therapy of personality disorders.* New York: Plenum.

Beck, A. T., Kovacs, M., & Weissman, A. (1979). Assessment of suicidal intention: The scale for suicidal ideation. *Journal of Consulting and Clinical Psychology, 47,* 343–352.

Beck, A. T., Laude, R., & Bohnert, M. (1974). Ideational components of anxiety neurosis. *Archives of General Psychiatry, 31,* 319–325.

Beck, A. T., Rush, A. J., Shaw, B. F., & Emery, G. (1979). *Cognitive therapy of depression.* New York: Guilford Press.

Beck, A. T., Schuyler, D., & Herman, I. (1974). Development of the suicidal intent scales. In A. T. Beck, H. L. P. Resnik, & D. J. Lettieri (Eds.), *The prediction of suicide* (pp. 45–56). Bowie, MD: Charles Press.

Beck, A. T., Sokol, L., Clark, D. A., Berchick, R. J., & Wright, F. D. (1992). A crossover study of focused cognitive therapy for panic disorder. *American Journal of Psychiatry, 149,* 778–783.

Beck, A. T., & Steer, R. A. (1990). *Beck Anxiety Inventory manual.* San Antonio, TX: The Psychological Corporation.

Beck, A. T., Steer, R. A., & Brown, G. K. (1996). *The Beck Depression Inventory manual* (2nd ed.). San Antonio, TX: The Psychological Corporation.

Beck, A. T., Steer, R. A., Brown, G., & Epstein, N. (1990). The Beck Self-concept Test. *Psychological Assessment: A Journal of Consulting and Clinical Psychology, 2,* 191–197.

Beck, A. T., Steer, R. A., Kovacs, M., & Garrison, B. (1985). Hopelessness and eventual suicide: A 10-year study of patients hospitalized with suicidal ideation. *American Journal of Psychiatry, 412,* 559–563.

Beck, A. T., Ward, C. H., Mendelson, M., Mock, J. E., & Erbaugh, J. K. (1961). An inventory for measuring depression. *Archives of General Psychiatry, 4,* 561–571.

Beck, A. T., Weissman, A., Lester, D., & Trexler, L. (1974). The measurement of pessimism: The hopelessness scale. *Journal of Consulting and Clinical Psychology, 42,* 861–865.

Bowers, W. A. (2001). Cognitive model of eating disorders. *Journal of Cognitive Psychotherapy: An International Quarterly, 15,* 331–340.

Brown, G. K, Ten Have, T., Henriques, G. R, Xie, S. X., Hollander, J. E., & Beck, A. T. (2005). Cognitive therapy for the prevention of suicide attempts: A randomized controlled trial. *Journal of the American Medical Association, 294*(5), 563–570.

Burns, D. D. (1985). *Intimate connections.* New York: Morrow.

Butler, A. C., Chapman, J. E., Forman, E. M., & Beck, A. T. (2006). The empirical status of cognitive–behavioral therapy: A review of meta-analyses. *Clinical Psychology Review, 26,* 17–31.

Butler, G., Fennell, M., Robson, D., & Gelder, M. (1991). Comparison of behavior therapy and cognitive behavior therapy in the treatment of generalized anxiety disorder. *Journal of Consulting & Clinical Psychology, 59,* 167–175.

Clark, D. A., & Beck, A. T. (2002). *Clark-Beck Obsessive Compulsive Inventory.* San Antonio, TX: The Psychological Corporation.

Clark, D. A., Beck, A. T., & Alford, B. A. (1999). *Scientific foundations of cognitive theory and therapy of depression.* New York: John Wiley.

Clark, D. M. (1996). Panic disorder: From theory to therapy. In P. Salkovskis (Ed.), *Frontiers of cognitive therapy* (pp. 318–344). New York: Guilford Press.

Clark, D. M. (1997). Panic disorder and social phobia. In D. M. Clark & C. G. Fairburn (Eds.), *Science and practice of cognitive behavior therapy* (pp. 122–153). New York: Oxford University Press.

Clark, D. M., Salkovskis, P. M., Hackmann, A., Middleton, H., & Gelder, M. (1992). A comparison of cognitive therapy, applied relaxation, and imipramine in the treatment of panic disorder. *British Journal of Psychiatry, 164,* 759–769.

DeRubeis, R. J., and Crits-Cristoph, P. (1998). Empirically supported individual and group psychological treatments for adult mental disorders. *Journal of Consulting and Clinical Psychology, 66,* 37–52.

DeRubeis, R. J., Hollon, S. D., Amsterdam, J. D., Shelton, R. C., Young, P. R., Salomon, R. M., O'Reardon, J. P., Lovett, M. L., Gladis, M. M., Brown, L. L., & Gallup, R. (2005). Cognitive therapy vs. medication in the treatment of moderate to severe depression. *Archives of General Psychiatry, 62,* 409–416.

Ehlers, A., & Clark, D. M. (2000). A cognitive model of posttraumatic stress disorder. *Behaviour Research and Therapy, 38,* 319–345.

Ellis, A. (1962). *Reason and emotion in psychotherapy.* New York: Lyle Stuart.

Eng, W., Roth, D. A., & Heimberg, R. G. (2001). Cognitive behavioral therapy for social anxiety. *Journal of Cognitive Psychotherapy: An International Quarterly, 15,* 311–319.

Fairburn, C. C., Jones, R., Peveler, R. C., Hope, R. A., Carr, S. J., Solomon, R. A., et al. (1991). Three psychological treatments for bulimia nervosa: A comparative trial. *Archives of General Psychiatry, 48,* 463–469.

Freeston, M. H., Ladoucer, R., Gagnon, F., Thibodeau, N., Rheaume, J., Letarte, H., et al. (1997). Cognitive behavioral treatment of obsessive thoughts: A controlled study. *Journal of Consulting and Clinical Psychology, 65,* 405–413.

Garner, D. M., Rockert, W., Davis, R., Garner, M. V., Olmsted, M. P., & Eagle, M. (1993). Comparison of cognitive–behavioral and supportive–expressive therapy for bulimia nervosa. *American Journal of Psychiatry, 150,* 37–46.

Gillespie, K., Duffy, M., Hackmann, A., & Clark, D. M. (2002). Community-based cognitive therapy in the treatment of posttraumatic stress disorder following the Omagh bomb. *Behaviour Research and Therapy, 40,* 345–357.

Gloaguen, V., Cottraux, J., Cucherat, M., & Blackburn, I. M. (1998). A meta-analysis of the effects of cognitive therapy in depressed patients. *Journal of Affective Disorders, 49,* 59–72.

Gould, R. A., Otto, M. W., & Pollack, M. H. (1995). A meta-analysis of treatment outcome for panic disorder. *Clinical Psychology Review, 15,* 819–844.

Gournay, K. (1986, September). *Cognitive change during the behavioral treatment of agoraphobia.* Paper presented at Congress of the 16th European Association for Behavior Therapy, Lucerne, Switzerland. September 1986.

Haaga, D. A. E., Dyck, M. J., & Ernst, D. (1991). Empirical status of cognitive theory of depression. *Psychological Bulletin, 110*(2), 215–236.

Hollon, S. D., DeRubeis, R. J., & Evans, M. D. (1996). Cognitive therapy in the treatment and prevention of depression. In P. Salkovskis (Ed.), *Frontiers of cognitive therapy* (pp. 293–317). New York: Guilford.

Hollon, S. D., DeRubeis, R. J., Shelton, R. C., Amsterdam, J. D., Salomon, R. M., O'Reardon, J. P., Lovett, M. L., Young, P. R., Haman, K. L., Freeman, B. B., & Gallop, R. (2005). Prevention of relapse following cognitive therapy vs. medication in moderate to severe depression. *Archives of General Psychiatry, 62,* 417–422.

Hollon, S. D., Kendall, P. C., & Lumry, A. (1986). Specificity of depressotypic cognitions in clinical depression. *Journal of Abnormal Psychology, 95,* 52–59.

Hollon, S. D., Stewart, M. O., & Strunk, D. (2006) Enduring effects for cognitive behavior therapy in the treatment of depression and anxiety. *Annual Review of Psychology, 57,* 285–315.

Horney, K. (1950). *Neurosis and human growth: The struggle toward self-realization.* New York: Norton.

Kant, I. (1798). *The classification of mental disorders.* Konigsberg, Germany: Nicolovius.

Kelly, G. (1955). *The psychology of personal constructs.* New York: Norton.

Lazarus, R. (1984). On the primacy of cognition. *American Psychologist, 39,* 124–129.

Mahoney, M. J. (1974). *Cognition and behavior modification.* Cambridge, MA: Ballinger.

Mahoney, M. J., & Arnkoff, D. (1978). Cognitive and self-control therapies. In S. L. Garfield & A. E. Bergin (Eds.), *Handbook of psychotherapy and behavior change: An empirical analysis* (pp. 689–722). New York: Wiley.

Meichenbaum, D. (1977). *Cognitive–behavior modification: An integrative approach.* New York: Plenum.

Persons, J. B., Bostrom, A., & Bertagnolli, A. (1999). Results of randomized controlled trials of cognitive therapy for depression generalize to private practice. *Cognitive Therapy and Research, 23,* 535–548.

Persons, J. B., Burns, D. D., & Perloff, J. M. (1988). Predictors of dropout and outcome in cognitive therapy for depression in a private practice setting. *Cognitive Therapy and Research, 12,* 557–575.

Pike, K. M., Walsh, B. T., Vitousek, K., Wilson, G. T., & Bauer, J. (2003). Cognitive behavior therapy in the post hospitalization treatment of anorexia nervosa. *American Journal of Psychiatry, 160,* 2046–2049.

Resick, P. A. (2001). Cognitive therapy for posttraumatic stress disorder. *Journal of Cognitive Psychotherapy: An International Quarterly, 15,* 321–329.

Rogers, C. (1951). *Client-centered therapy.* Boston: Houghton Mifflin.

Segal, Z. V., Williams, J. M. G., & Teasdale, J. D. (2002). *Mindfulness-based cognitive therapy for depression.* New York: Guilford Press.

Stirman, S. W., DeRubeis, R. J., Crits-Cristoph, P., & Rothman, A. (2005). Can the randomized controlled trial literature generalize to nonrandomized patients? *Journal of Consulting and Clinical Psychology, 73,* 127–135.

Strunk, D. R., & DeRubeis, R. J. (2001). Cognitive therapy for depression: A review of its efficacy. *Journal of Cognitive Psychotherapy: An International Quarterly, 15,* 289–297.

Sullivan, H. S. (1953). *The interpersonal theory of psychiatry.* New York: Norton.

Tarrier, N. (2008). Schizophrenia and other psychotic disorders. In D. H. Barlow (Ed.), *Clinical handbook for psychological disorders: A step-by-step treatment manual* (4th ed., pp. 463–491). New York: Guilford Press.

Turkington, D., Dudley, R., Warman, D. M., & Beck, A. T. (2004). Cognitive–behavioral therapy for schizophrenia: A review. *Journal of Psychiatric Practice, 10,* 5–16.

Vitousek, K. M. (1996). The current status of cognitive behavioral models of anorexia nervosa and bulimia nervosa. In P. Salkovskis (Ed.), *Frontiers of cognitive therapy* (pp. 383–418). New York: Guilford.

Wampold, B. E., Minami, T., Baskin, T. W., & Callen Tierney, S. (2002), A meta-(re)analysis of the effects of cognitive therapy versus other therapies for depression. *Journal of Affective Disorders, 68,* 159–165.

Weissman, A., & Beck, A. T. (1978). *Development and validation of the Dysfunctional Attitude Scale.* Paper presented at the 12th annual meeting of the Association for Advancement of Behavior Therapy, Chicago.

Wessler, R. L. (1986). Conceptualizing cognitions in the cognitive–behavioral therapies. In W. Dryden & W. Golden (Eds.), *Cognitive–behavioural approaches to psychotherapy* (pp. 1–30). London: Harper & Row.

Williams, S. L., & Rappoport, A. (1983). Cognitive treatment in the natural environment for agoraphobics. *Behavior Therapy, 14,* 299–313.

Woody, G. E., Luborsky. L., McClellan, A. T., O'Brien, C. P., Beck, A. T., Blaine, J., et al. (1983). Psychotherapy for opiate addicts: Does it help? *Archives of General Psychiatry, 40,* 639–645.

Young, J. E., Rygh, J. L., Weinberger, A. D., & Beck, A. T. (2008). Cognitive therapy for depression. In D. H. Barlow (Ed.), *Clinical handbook of psychological disorders: A step-by-step treatment manual* (4th ed., pp. 250–305). New York: Guilford Press.

Young, J. E., Klosko, J. S., & Weishaar, M. E. (2003). *Schema therapy: A practitioner's guide.* New York: Guilford Press.

Zimmerman, G., Favrod, J., Trieu, V. H., & Pomini, V. (2005). The effect of cognitive behavioural treatment on the positive symptoms of schizophrenia spectrum disorders: A meta-analysis. *Schizophrenia Research, 77,* 1–9.

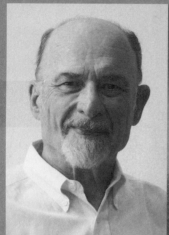
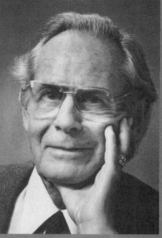

Irvin Yalom
Courtesy of Irvin Yalom

Rollo May (1909–1994)
Courtesy of Kirk Schneider

9 | EXISTENTIAL PSYCHOTHERAPY[1]

Irvin D. Yalom and Ruthellen Josselson

OVERVIEW

Existential psychotherapy is a form of therapy that can be integrated with other approaches, not an independent "school" of therapy like cognitive behaviorism or psychoanalysis. Rather than being a technical approach that offers a new set of rules for psychotherapy, it represents a way of thinking about human experience that can—or perhaps should be—a part all therapies.

Everyone must confront the timeless and intractable issues of the *ultimate concerns:* death, freedom, isolation, and meaning. An existential approach to therapy involves someone, a therapist, willing to walk unflinchingly with patients through life's deepest and most vexing problems. Existential psychotherapy is an attitude toward human suffering and has no manual. It asks deep questions about the nature of the human being and the nature of anxiety, despair, grief, loneliness, isolation, and anomie. It also deals centrally with the questions of meaning, creativity, and love. Out of reflection on these human experiences, existential psychotherapists have devised attitudes toward therapy that do not distort human beings in the very effort of trying to help them.

Many therapists in fact, practice existential psychotherapy without labeling it as such. In his seminal work, *Existential Psychotherapy,* Yalom (1980) tells of taking part

---

[1] This chapter includes material from an earlier chapter in *Current Psychotherapies* by Rollo May and Irvin Yalom.

in an Armenian cooking class where the teacher, who did not speak English well, taught mainly by demonstration. But as hard as he tried, he could never quite make his dishes taste as good as hers. He decided to observe his teacher more carefully, and in one lesson noted that when she finished her preparation she handed her dish to her assistant, who took it into the kitchen to place into the oven. He observed the assistant and was astounded, and edified, to note that that before throwing the dish in the oven, she threw in handfuls of various spices that struck her fancy. These "throw-ins" he likened to the interactions that therapists have with their patients, which, because they are not conceptualized within their theoretical "recipe," go unnoticed. Perhaps, however, these off-the-record extras are the critical ingredients. And perhaps these throw-ins refer to the shared issues of human existence—in short, to existential psychotherapy.

Basic Concepts

Existentialists regard people as meaning-making beings who are both subjects of experience and objects of self-reflection. We are mortal creatures who, because we are self-aware, know that we are mortal. Yet it is only in reflecting on our mortality that we can learn how to live. People ask themselves questions concerning their being: Who am I? Is life worth living? Does it have a meaning? How can I realize my humanity? Existentialists hold that ultimately, each of us must come to terms with these questions and each of us is responsible for who we are and what we become.

Because existentialists are sensitive to the ways in which theories may dehumanize people and render them as objects, authentic experience takes precedence over artificial explanations. When experiences are molded into some preexisting theoretical model, they lose their authenticity and become disconnected from the individual who experienced them. Existential psychotherapists, then, focus on the subjectivity of experience rather than "objective" diagnostic categories.

The Ultimate Concerns

Issues such as "choice," responsibility," "mortality," or "purpose in life" are ones that all therapists suspect are central concerns of patients. More and more, patients come to therapy with vague complaints about loss of purpose or meaning. But it is often more comfortable for the therapist to reframe these concerns into symptoms and to talk with patients about medication or to prescribe manualized exercises than to engage genuinely with them as they search for meaning in life. Many diagnosable presenting "symptoms" may mask existential crises.

The existential dilemma ensues from the existential reality that although we crave to persist in our being, we are finite creatures; that we are thrown alone into existence without a predestined life structure and destiny; that each of us must decide how to live as fully, happily, ethically, and meaningfully as possible. Yalom defines four categories of "ultimate concerns" that encompass these fundamental challenges of the human condition. These are freedom, isolation, meaning, and death.

Freedom

The term *freedom* in the existential sense does not refer to political liberty or to the greater range of possibilities in life that come from increasing one's psychological awareness. Instead, it refers to the idea that we all live in a universe without inherent design in which we are the authors of our own lives. Life is groundless, and we alone are responsible for our choices. This existential freedom carries with it terrifying responsibility and is always connected to dread. It is the kind of freedom people fear so much that they enlist dictators, masters, and gods to remove the burden from them. Erich Fromm (1941) described "the lust for submission" that accompanies the effort to escape from that freedom.

Ultimately, we are responsible for what we experience in and of the world. Responsibility is inextricably linked to freedom because we are responsible for the sense we make of our world and for all of our actions and our failures to act. An appreciation of responsibility in this sense is very unsettling. If we are, in Sartre's terms, "the uncontested author" of everything that we have experienced, then our most cherished ideas, our most noble truths, the very bedrock of our convictions are all undermined by the awareness that everything in the universe is contingent. We bear the burden of *knowing* that we are responsible for all of our experience.

The complement to responsibility is our *will.* While this concept has waned lately in the social sciences, replaced by terms such as *motivation,* people are still ultimately responsible for the decisions they make. To claim that a person's behavior is explained (i.e., caused) by a certain motivation is to deny that person's responsibility for his or her actions. To abrogate such responsibility is to live inauthentically, in what Sartre has called *bad faith*. Because of the dread of our ultimate freedom, people erect a plethora of defenses, some of which give rise to psychopathology. The work of therapy is very much about the (re)assumption of responsibility for one's experience. Indeed, the therapeutic enterprise can be conceived of as one in which the client actively increases and embraces his or her freedom: freedom from destructive habits, from self-imposed paralysis of the will, or from self-limiting beliefs, just to name a few.

Isolation

Individuals may be isolated from others (*interpersonal isolation)* or from parts of themselves (*intrapersonal isolation).* But there is a more basic form of isolation, *existential isolation,* that pertains to our aloneness in the universe, which, though assuaged by connections to other human beings, yet remains. We enter and leave the world alone and while we are alive, we must always manage the tension between our wish for contact with others and our knowledge of our aloneness. Erich Fromm believed that isolation is the primary source of anxiety.

Aloneness is different from loneliness, which is also a ubiquitous issue in therapy. Loneliness results from social, geographic, and cultural factors that support the breakdown of intimacy. Or people may lack the social skills or have personality styles inimical to intimacy. But *existential* isolation cuts even deeper; it is a more basic isolation that is riveted to existence and refers *to an unbridgeable gulf between oneself and others.* It is most commonly experienced in the recognition that one's death is always solitary, a common theme among poets and writers. But many people are in touch with their dread of existential isolation when they recognize the terror of feeling that there may be moments when no one in the world is thinking of them. Or walking alone on a deserted beach in another country, one may be struck with a dreadful thought: "Right at this moment, no one knows where I am." If one is not being thought about by someone else, is one still real?

In working with people who have lost a spouse, Yalom was struck not only by their loneliness but also by the accompanying despair at living an unobserved life—of having no one who knows what time they come home, go to bed, or wake up. Many individuals continue a highly unsatisfying relationship precisely because they crave a life witness, a buffer against the experience of existential isolation.

The professional literature regarding the therapist–patient relationship abounds with discussions of encounter, genuineness, accurate empathy, positive unconditional regard, and "I–Thou" relating. A deep sense of connection does not "solve" the problem of existential isolation, but it provides solace. Yalom recalls one of the members of his cancer group who said, "I know we are each ships passing in the dark and each of us is a lonely ship, but still it is mighty comforting to see the bobbing lights of the other nearby boats." Still, we are ultimately alone. Even a therapist cannot change that. Yalom comments that an important milestone in therapy is the patient's realization that, "there is a point beyond which [the therapist] can offer nothing more. In therapy, as in life, there is an inescapable substrate of lonely work and lonely existence" (1981, p. 137).

To the extent that one takes full responsibility for one's life, one also encounters the sense of existential isolation. To forego the sense that one is created or guarded by another is to confront the cosmic indifference of the universe and one's fundamental aloneness within it.

Meaning

All humans must find some meaning in life, although none is absolute and none is given to us. We create our own world and have to answer for ourselves why we live and how we shall live. One of our major life tasks is to invent a purpose sturdy enough to support a life; often we have a sense of discovering a meaning, and then it may seem to us that it was out there waiting for us. Our ongoing search for substantial purpose-providing life structures often throws us into a crisis. More individuals seek therapy because of concerns about purpose in life than therapists often realize. The complaints take many different forms: "I have no passion for anything." "Why am I living? Surely life must have some deeper significance." "I feel so empty—just trying to get ahead makes me feel so pointless, so useless." "Even now, at the age of 50, I still don't know what I want to do when I grow up."

In his memoir of being an existential psychotherapist, *The Listener,* Allen Wheelis (1999) tells about a moment with his dog, Monty:

> If then I bend over and pick up a stick, he is instantly before me. The great thing has now happened. He has a mission . . . It never occurs to him to evaluate the mission. His dedication is solely to its fulfillment. He runs or swims any distance, over or through any obstacle, to get that stick.
>
> And, having got it, he brings it back: for his mission is not simply to get it but to return it. Yet, as he approaches me, he moves more slowly. He wants to give it to me and give closure to his task, yet he hates to have done with his mission, to again be in the position of waiting.
>
> For him as for me, it is necessary to be in the service of something beyond the self. Until I am ready he must wait. *He is lucky to have me to throw his stick.* I am waiting for God to throw mine. Have been waiting a long time. Who knows when, if ever, he will again turn his attention to me, and allow me, as I allow Monty, my mood of mission? (as cited in http://www.yalom.com/lec/pfister)

Who among us has not had the wish, *If only someone would throw me* my *stick.* How reassuring it would be to know that somewhere there exists a true purpose in life rather than only the *sense* of purpose in life. If all purpose is self-authored, one must confront the ultimate groundlessness of existence. We throw our own sticks.

A sense of meaning emerges from plunging into an enlarging, fulfilling, self-transcending endeavor. The work of the therapist is to identify and help to remove the obstacles to such engagement. If one is authentically immersed in the river of life, then the question of meaning drifts away.

Death

Overshadowing all these ultimate concerns, the awareness of our inevitable demise is the most painful and difficult. We strive to find meaning in the context of our existential aloneness and take responsibility for the choices we make within our freedom to choose, yet one day we will cease to be. And we live our lives with that awareness in the shadow. Death is always the distant thunder at our picnic, however much we may wish to deny it.

Of course, we cannot live every moment wholly aware of death. This would be, in Yalom's phrase, like staring at the sun. Because we cannot live frozen in fear, we generate methods to soften death's terror. We assuage it by projecting ourselves into the future through our children, by trying to grow rich and famous, by developing compulsive behaviors, or by fostering an impregnable belief in an ultimate rescuer. Our fear of death is a profound dread of nonbeing, the impossibility of further possibility, as Hegel put it. And fears of death can lurk disguised behind many symptoms as well. Yet confronting death allows us to live fuller, richer, and more compassionate lives.

Everything fades. This is the sad existential truth. Life is truly linear and irreversible. This knowledge can lead us to take stock of ourselves and ask how we can live our lives as fully as possible. Existential psychotherapy emphasizes the importance of living mindfully and purposefully, aware of one's possibilities and limits in a context of absolute freedom and choice. Death, in this view, enriches life.

The Therapeutic Stance: The Fellow Traveler

Awareness of the ultimate concerns as givens of existence fundamentally changes the relationship between therapist and patient to that of *fellow travelers.* From this vantage point, even labels of patient/therapist, client/counselor, analysand/analyst become inappropriate to the nature of the relationship, for they suggest distinctions between "them" (the afflicted) and "us" (the healers). However, *we are all in this together,* and there is no therapist and no person immune to the inherent tragedies of existence. Sharing the essence of the human condition becomes the bedrock of the work of existential psychotherapy.

HISTORY

Precursors

These major existential concerns are not new, of course. An unbroken stream of philosophers, theologians, and poets since the beginning of recorded history has wrestled with these issues. Down through history, these questions have occupied many thinkers.

The Greek philosopher Epicurus anticipated the contemporary idea of the unconscious when he emphasized that death concerns may not be conscious to the individual but might be inferred by disguised manifestations. He constructed a number of arguments to alleviate death anxiety, which he taught his students. Epicurus believed that the soul was mortal and perishes with the body; hence, there is nothing to fear in the afterlife. And why fear death, he wondered, when we can never perceive it? Another argument he advanced was that of symmetry: Our state of nonbeing after death is the same as before our birth. As Vladimir Nabokov, the great Russian novelist later wrote, "our life is a crack of light between two eternities of darkness" (p. 17). St. Augustine believed that only in the face of death is a person's self born. And many philosophers since the dawn of philosophy have concluded that the idea of death enriches life.

Beginnings

The contemporary term *existentialism* is most often associated with the French philosophers Jean Paul Sartre and Gabriel Marcel, who developed this philosophy in the 1940s. Existential therapists have also been influenced by the work of such philosophers as Martin Heidegger, Edmund Husserl, Emmanuel Levinas, and Martin Buber.

The central foundational philosophers of existential psychotherapy are two 19th-century intellectual giants, Søren Kierkegaard and Friedrich Nietzsche. Both were reacting to the mechanistic dehumanization of people in a technological world, and both can be counted among the most remarkable psychologists of all time. When one reads Kierkegaard's profound analyses of anxiety and despair or Nietzsche's acute insights into the dynamics of resentment and the guilt and hostility that accompany repressed emotional powers, it is difficult to realize that one is reading works written more than 150 years ago and not a contemporary psychological analysis.

The Swiss psychiatrist Ludwig Einswanger (1881–1966), a colleague and friend of Sigmund Freud, was the first physician to combine psychotherapy with existentialism. His famous, now classic, case of Ellen West, published in 1944 (see Binswanger, 1958), in which a patient with anorexia nervosa decides to commit suicide, provoked much debate within psychotherapeutic circles. Binswanger's work was part of a broader phenomenological–existential psychotherapeutic orientation that developed in central Europe in response to dissatisfaction with the theoretical frameworks of psychiatry and psychoanalysis. The members of this movement—among them Medard Boss, Eugene Minkowski, Erwin Straus, and Roland Kuhn—thought that the effort to detail human existence by means of an objective–descriptive scientific theory distracted attention from the authentic encounter that formed the basis of therapy. In 1988, a Society for Existential Analysis was formed in the United Kingdom that publishes a journal, *Existential Analysis.*

Existential psychotherapy was introduced to the United States in 1958 with the publication of *Existence: A New Dimension in Psychiatry and Psychology,* edited by Rollo May, Ernest Angel, and Henri Ellenberger. The main presentation and summary of existential therapy were in the first two chapters, written by May: "The Origins of the Existential Movement in Psychology" and "Contributions of Existential Psychology." The remainder of the book is made up of essays and case studies by the European existentialists (Henri Ellenberger, Eugene Minkowski, Erwin Straus, V E. von Gebsattel, Ludwig Binswanger, and Ronald Kuhn).

Rollo May was trained as a psychoanalyst in the William Alanson White Institute, a neo-Freudian institute in New York, and was already a practicing analyst when he read in the early 1950s about existential therapies in Europe. His books, which sought to reconcile existential ideas with psychoanalysis, became important texts of existential psychotherapy, especially in the United States. He wrote, among other books, *Man's Search for Himself* (1953), *Freedom and Destiny (1981),* and *The Cry for Myth (1991).*

Erich Fromm, a founder (in 1946) of the William Alanson White Institute, also wrote many books that explored existential issues. *Escape from Freedom* (1941) focuses on the human tendency to submit to authority as a way of defending against the existential terrors of free choice. *The Art of Loving* (1956) addressed the dilemmas of existential isolation.

The first comprehensive textbook in existential psychotherapy was written by Irvin Yalom (1980) and titled *Existential Psychotherapy.* In this work and in his subsequent books of case studies, *Love's Executioner* (1989) and *Momma and the Meaning of Life* (1999), as well as in his novels, *When Nietzsche Wept* (1992) and *The Schopenhauer Cure* (2005), Yalom attempted to detail what an existential psychotherapist actually *does* in the therapeutic session. His book *Staring at the Sun: Overcoming the Terror of Death* (2008) focuses upon the experience and the treatment of high levels of death anxiety.

Other writers who have offered existential approaches to psychotherapy have also furthered its popularity in the United States. Victor Frankl wrote *Man's Search For Meaning* (1956), a widely read and highly influential text that sets out an approach to *logotherapy*, a form of psychotherapy focused on will, freedom, meaning and responsibility. Allen Wheelis (1973), a San Francisco existential psychoanalyst, wrote eloquently about his therapeutic encounters in which the specter of death and the search for meaning play central roles. Of his 14 books, *How People Change* is the best known. He wrote the following of psychotherapy:

> If . . . the determining causes of which we gain awareness lie within, or are brought within, our experience, and if we use this gain in understanding to create present options, freedom will be increased, and with it greater responsibility for what we have been, are, and will become. (1973, p. 117)

Current Status

The spirit of existential psychotherapy has never supported the formation of specific institutes because it deals with the *presuppositions underlying therapy of any kind.* Its concern was with concepts about human beings and not with specific techniques. This leads to the dilemma that existential therapy has been quite influential, but there are very few adequate training courses in this kind of therapy simply because it is not training in a specific technique. Existentially oriented psychotherapists tend to further their knowledge through their own personal therapy and supervision and by reading philosophy and great literature.

Therapists trained in different schools can legitimately call themselves existential if their assumptions are similar to those described in this chapter. Irvin Yalom was trained in a neo-Freudian tradition. Even such an erstwhile behavior therapist as Arnold Lazarus uses some existential presuppositions in his multimodal psychotherapy. Fritz Perls and Gestalt therapy rest on existential grounds. All of this is possible because existential psychotherapy is a way of conceiving the human being.

Existential therapists are centrally concerned with rediscovering the living person amid the dehumanization of modern culture, and in order to do this, they engage in in-depth psychological analysis. Their focus is less on alleviating symptoms and more on greater awareness and freedom in relation to living.

Summing up the existential therapeutic position 25 years after he wrote his classic, influential text, Yalom (2008) describes the need for an inclusive perspective in psychotherapy in these words:

> Psychological distress issues *not only* from our biological genetic substrate (a psycho–pharmacologic model), *not only* from our struggle with suppressed instinctual strivings (a Freudian position), *not only* from our internalized significant adults who may be uncaring, unloving, neurotic (an object relations position), *not only* from disordered forms of thinking (a cognitive–behavioral position), *not only* from shards of forgotten traumatic memories, nor from current life crises involving one's career and relationship with significant others, *but also—but also*—from a confrontation with our existence. (2008, p. 180)

In the contemporary climate of focus on brief, manualized treatments oriented to symptom reduction, driven by market forces rather than human need, all the human-focused approaches to psychotherapy suffer (McWilliams, 2005). In most training programs, across professions, psychotherapy that focuses on the subtleties of human experience is being taught less and less in favor of technological expedience and compliance with the dictates of managed-care companies. Chagrined at seeing the life being squeezed out of psychotherapy as it was becoming more mechanized and less human and intimate, Yalom wrote a highly accessible guide for therapists, both novice and seasoned, titled *The Gift of Therapy* (2002). Judging from its enormous sales, there is a massive wish among psychotherapists to engage the issues of existence and presence with their patients. The tenets of existential psychotherapy will perhaps serve future generations when deeper forms of healing again become more, or more widely, possible.

PERSONALITY

Theory of Personality

In Tolstoy's *The Death of Ivan Illych,* the central character, Ivan Illych, a self-involved, self-satisfied, pompous bureaucrat, is dying in pain and suddenly realizes that he is dying badly because he has lived badly. "'Maybe I did not live as I ought to have done,' it suddenly occurred to him. 'But how could that be, when I did everything properly?'" (p. 145). Ivan Illych's realization of the impoverishment of his life leads him, in the last days of his life, to relate more authentically and empathically to his family, thus redeeming his life at the very end. The existential focus of a theory of personality concerns whether people are living as authentically and meaningfully as possible.

Existential psychotherapy is a *dynamic psychotherapy.* It takes from Freud the model of personality as a system of forces in conflict with one another. The emotions and behavior (both adaptive and pathological) that constitute personality may exist at different levels of consciousness, some entirely out of awareness, and may conflict. Thus, when we speak of the "psychodynamics" of an individual, we refer to that individual's conflicting conscious and unconscious motives and fears. Dynamic psychotherapy is psychotherapy based upon this internal conflict model of personality structure.

Existential Psychodynamics

In contrast to the Freudian model, which posits conflict between instincts and the demands of the environment (or the superego, which is the environment internalized), and in contrast to the interpersonal and object relational models that posit conflict stemming from interactions with significant powerful others in childhood, the existential model of personality postulates that the basic conflict is between the individual and the "givens," the ultimate concerns of existence. Thus, the existential system replaces the Freudian system of

DRIVE → ANXIETY → DEFENSE MECHANISM

with

AWARENESS OF ULTIMATE CONCERN → ANXIETY → DEFENSE MECHANISM

If we "bracket" the outside world, if we put aside the everyday concerns with which we ordinarily fill our lives and reflect deeply upon our situations in the world, then we must confront the dilemmas of the ultimate concerns (detailed above) that are an inescapable part of the human being's existence in the world. The individual's confrontation with each of these constitutes the content of the inner conflict from the existential frame of reference.

As people, we are influenced by the physical environment, the presence or absence of other people, genetics, and social or cultural variables. In other words, we are influenced by our destiny. That is, because we are stimulated in certain ways, we respond in certain ways. As subjects, however, we are aware of the fact that these things are happening to us. We perceive, ponder, and act on this information. We determine which experiences are valuable and which are not and then act according to these personal formulations. What is crucial is "man's capacity to stand outside himself, to know he is the subject as well as the object of experience, to see himself as the entity who is acting in the world of objects" (May, 1967, p. 75). As humans, we view the world, and we can view ourselves viewing it. It is this consciousness of self that allows people to escape determinism and personally influence what they do.

> Consciousness of self gives us the power to stand outside the rigid chain of stimulus and response, to pause, and by this pause to throw some weight on either side, to cast some decision about what the response will be. (May, 1953, p. 161)

A full understanding of a person involves both knowledge of that person's circumstances (the objective part) and how that person subjectively structures and values those circumstances (the subjective part).

Existential psychotherapy does not offer a theory of individual differences, but it attends carefully to how each individual deals with the ultimate concerns. Therefore, the existential understanding of personality is inherently tied to its approach to psychotherapy.

Variety of Concepts

May attributes anxiety to the fundamental clash between being and the threat of nonbeing. A certain amount of anxiety is therefore a normal and inevitable aspect of every personality. Anxiety confronts each of us with a major challenge. This unpleasant emotion intensifies whenever we choose to boldly assert our innate potentials. Emphatically affirming that we exist also brings a reminder that someday we will not. It is all too tempting to repress or intellectualize our understanding of death, deny our being-in-the-world (*Dasein*), and opt for the apparent safety of social conformity and apathy. The healthy course is to accept nonbeing as an inseparable part of being. This will enable us to live what life we have to the fullest:

> To grasp what it means to exist, one needs to grasp the fact that he might not exist, that he treads at every moment on the sharp edge of possible annihilation and can never escape the fact that death will arrive at some unknown moment . . . [Thus] the confronting of death gives the most positive reality to life itself. (May, 1958, p. 47)

Freedom

Ordinarily we do not think of freedom as a source of anxiety or conflict. Quite the contrary—freedom is generally viewed as an unequivocally positive concept. The history of Western civilization is punctuated by a yearning and striving toward freedom. Yet freedom in the existential frame of reference is riveted to dread.

From an existential viewpoint, conflicts over freedom ensue from the reality that the human being enters and ultimately departs an unstructured universe without a coherent, grand design. Freedom refers to the fact that the human being is responsible for and the author of his or her own world, own life design, and own choices and actions. The human being, as Sartre puts it, is "condemned to freedom" (1956, p. 631). Rollo May (1981) holds that freedom, in order to be authentic, requires the individual to confront the limits of his or her destiny. He defined destiny "as the pattern of limits and talents that constitutes the 'givens' in life. . . . Our destiny cannot be cancelled out . . . but we can choose how we shall respond, how we shall live out our talents" (p. 89).

If it is true that we create our self and our world, then it also means that there is no ground beneath us: There is only an abyss, a void, nothingness. This has terrifying implications. Such awareness of freedom and groundlessness conflicts with our deep need and wish for ground and structure, creates anxiety, and invokes a variety of defense mechanisms.

Awareness of freedom implies responsibility for one's life. Individuals differ enormously in the degree of responsibility they are willing to accept for their life situations and in their modes of denying responsibility. For example, some individuals displace responsibility for their situations onto other people, onto life circumstances, onto bosses and spouses, and, when they enter treatment, they transfer responsibility for their therapy to their psychotherapist. Other individuals deny responsibility by experiencing themselves as innocent victims who suffer from external events (and remain unaware that they themselves have set these events into motion). Still others shirk responsibility by temporarily being "out of their minds"—they enter a temporary irrational state in which they are not accountable even to themselves for their behavior.

Another aspect of freedom is *willing*. To be aware of responsibility for one's situation is to enter the vestibule of action or, in a therapy situation, of change. Willing represents the passage from responsibility to action, moving from wishing to deciding (May, 1969). Many individuals have enormous difficulties in experiencing or expressing a wish. Wishing is closely aligned to feeling, and affect-blocked individuals cannot act spontaneously because they cannot feel and thus cannot wish. *Impulsivity* avoids wishing by failing to discriminate among wishes. Instead, individuals act impulsively and promptly on all wishes. *Compulsivity,* another disorder of wishing, is characterized by individuals driven by unconscious inner demands that often run counter to their consciously held desires.

Once an individual fully experiences a wish, he or she is faced with *decision.* Many individuals can be extremely clear about what they wish but still not be able to decide or to choose. Often they experience a decisional panic; they may attempt to delegate the decision to someone else, or they act in such a way that the decision is made for them by circumstances that they, unconsciously, have brought to pass.

Thus, personality is informed by how people deal with the dilemmas of freedom. From the duty-bound to the capricious to the dependent, people have an array of mechanisms to deny or displace their freedom.

Isolation

Coming to terms with existential isolation, our inherent aloneness in the universe, is a second dynamic conflict that structures the personality. Each individual in the dawn of consciousness creates a primary self by permitting consciousness to curl back upon itself and to differentiate a self from the remainder of the world. Only after the individual becomes "self-conscious" can he or she begin to constitute other selves. Yet the individual cannot escape the knowledge that (1) he or she constitutes others and (2) he or she can never fully share his or her consciousness with others. There is no stronger reminder of existential isolation than a confrontation with death. The individual who faces death invariably becomes acutely aware of existential isolation.

Awareness of our fundamental isolation may invoke an unfulfillable wish to be protected, to merge, and to be part of a larger whole. Bugenthal (1976) points out that all relationships are poised on the poles of being *a part of* and *apart from,* the twin perils of merger and isolation. Fear of existential isolation (and the defenses against it) underlies a great deal of interpersonal psychopathology. Often relationships are troubled by the effort of one person to *use* another for some function rather than to *relate* to the other out of caring for that person's being. If one is overcome with dread in the face of isolation, one will not be able to turn toward others but instead will use others as a shield against isolation. In such instances, relationships will be distortions of what might have been authentic relationships.

Some individuals experience panic when they are alone. These individuals begin to doubt their own existence and believe that they exist only in the presence of another, that they exist only so long as they are responded to or are thought about by another individual.

Many attempt to deal with isolation through *fusion:* they soften their ego boundaries and become part of another individual. They avoid personal growth and the sense of isolation that accompanies growth. Fusion underlies the experience of being in love. The wonderful thing about romantic love is that the lonely "I" disappears into the "we." Others may fuse with a group, a cause, a country, or a project. To be like everyone else—to conform in dress, speech, and customs, to have no thoughts or feelings that are different—saves one from the isolation of the lonely self.

Compulsive sexuality is also a common response to terrifying isolation. Promiscuous sexual coupling offers a powerful but temporary respite for the lonely individual. It is temporary because it is only a caricature of a relationship. The sexually compulsive individual does not relate to the whole being of the other but relates only to the part of that individual that meets his or her need. Sexually compulsive individuals do not know their partners; they show and see only those parts that facilitate seduction and the sexual act.

Meaninglessness

The third existential influence on personality is meaninglessness. If each person must die, and if each person constitutes his or her own world, and if each is alone in an indifferent universe, then what possible meaning can life have? Why do we live? How shall we live? If there is no preordained design in life, then we must construct our own meaning in life. The fundamental question then becomes, "Is it possible that a self-created meaning is sturdy enough to bear one's life?" The third internal conflict stems from this dilemma: *How does a being who requires meaning find meaning in a universe that has no meaning?*

The human being appears to require meaning. Our perceptual neuropsychological organization is such that we instantaneously pattern random stimuli. We organize them automatically into figure and ground and may even create a story about them. When confronted with a broken circle, we automatically perceive it as complete. When any situation or set of stimuli defies patterning, we fit the situation into a recognizable pattern.

In the same way that individuals organize random stimuli, so too do they face existential situations: In an unpatterned world, an individual is acutely unsettled and searches for a pattern, an explanation, a meaning for existence.

A sense of meaning of life is necessary for still another reason: From a meaning schema, we generate a hierarchy of values. Values provide us with a blueprint for life conduct; values tell us not only *why* we live but *how* to live.

To grow as a person, one must constantly challenge one's structure of meaning, which is the core of one's existence, and this necessarily causes anxiety. Thus to be human is to have the urge to expand one's awareness, but to do so causes anxiety. Growth, and with it normal anxiety, consists of the giving up of immediate security for the sake of more extensive goals (May, 1967). The authentic person recognizes the hazards of exploring uncharted territory and does so nonetheless. The anxiety associated with moving forward into the unknown is an unfortunate concomitant of exercising one's freedom and realizing a quest for meaning.

As people tell the stories of their lives, their meanings are implicit. Their personal narratives are structured around their purposes and values, and the ways they narrate their lives reflect how they understand themselves as unique individuals and socially located beings. Narrative, then, becomes another dimension or level of personality (McAdams & Pals, 2006) and discloses the sense of personal unity and identity that construct meaning in life.

Death

The fourth and perhaps most central conflict is the confrontation with death. Death is the ultimate existential concern. It is apparent to all that death will come and that there is no escape. It is a terrible truth, and at the deepest levels we respond to it with mortal terror. "Everything," as Spinoza states, "wishes to persist in its own being" (1954, p. 6). From the existential point of view, a core inner conflict is between awareness of inevitable death and the simultaneous wish to continue to live.

Death plays a major role in one's internal experience. It haunts the individual like nothing else does. It rumbles continuously under the membrane of life. The child at an early age is pervasively concerned with death, and one of the child's major developmental tasks is to deal with the terror of obliteration. To cope with this terror, we erect defenses against death awareness. These defenses are denial based; they shape character structure and, if maladaptive, result in clinical maladjustment.

Psychopathology, to a very great extent, is the result of failed death transcendence; that is, symptoms and maladaptive character structure have their origin in the individual terror of death. There are many defense mechanisms that might be employed for dealing with the anxiety emerging from awareness of death, among them an irrational belief in personal "specialness" and an irrational belief in the existence of an "ultimate rescuer" (Yalom, 1980).

Specialness.   Individuals have deep, powerful beliefs in personal inviolability, invulnerability, and immortality. Although at a rational level we recognize the foolishness of these beliefs, nonetheless, at a deeply unconscious level, we believe that the ordinary laws of biology do not apply to us. People can camouflage their fears of death behind a belief that one's specialness will somehow override the dread decree. Again, Tolstoy's Ivan Illych offers an apt example:

In the depth of his heart he knew he was dying, but not only was he not accustomed to the thought, he simply did not and could not grasp it.

> The syllogism he had learnt from Kiezewetter's Logic, "Caius is a man, men are mortal, therefore Caius is moral,' had always seemed to him correct as applied to Caius, but certainly not as applied to himself. That Caius—man in the abstract— was mortal, was perfectly correct, but he was not Caius, not an abstract man, but a creature quite, quite separate from all others. He had been little Vanya, with a mamma and a papa . . . What did Caius know of the smell of that striped leather ball Vanya had been so fond of? Had Caius kissed his mother's hand like that . . . ? Had Caius been in love like that? Could Caius preside at a session as he did? Caius really was mortal, and it was right for him to die, but for me, little Vanya, Ivan Illych, with all my thoughts and emotions, it's altogether a different matter. It cannot be that I ought to die. That would be too terrible. (pp. 131–2)

What psychotherapists might simply label narcissism or entitlement may actually be subterfuge for the belief that specialness is an antidote to death. Similarly, workaholism or preoccupation with getting ahead, with preparing for the future, amassing material goods, or becoming more powerful or more eminent can be compulsive ways of unconsciously trying to ensure immortality.

Where the defense of specialness operates satisfactorily for a time, a crisis in the lives of these individuals occurs when their belief system is shattered and a sense of unprotected ordinariness intrudes. They frequently seek therapy when the defense of specialness is no longer able to ward off anxiety—for example, at times of severe illness or at the interruption of what had always appeared to be an eternal, upward spiral. In cases of trauma, it is sometimes the "Why me?" question that haunts the trauma survivor. To ask, "Why not me?" is to undermine the defensive sense of specialness, a specialness that ultimately (and irrationally) seems to protect against death.

The Belief in the Existence of an Ultimate Rescuer.   A second denial system is belief in an ultimate rescuer. People may imagine their rescuer to be human or divine, but the belief is in someone who is watching over them in an indifferent world. In order to keep the specter of death at bay, people may unconsciously create a belief in a personal omnipotent savior who eternally guards and protects their welfare, who may let them get to the edge of the abyss but who will always bring them back. An excess of this particular defense mechanism results in a character structure displaying passivity, dependency, and obsequiousness. Often such individuals dedicate their lives to locating and appeasing an ultimate rescuer.

One of Yalom's patients, Elva, an elderly woman, came to therapy because she was traumatized by having her purse snatched. Located within and beneath the resulting panic was her inability to let go of her departed husband who, at a very deep level, she believed would continue to protect her. The purse snatching and ensuing sense of vulnerability challenged this belief in her husband as an ultimate rescuer. In this case, we see how such beliefs may be camouflaged by seemingly unrelated experiences.

PSYCHOTHERAPY

Theory of Psychotherapy

A substantial proportion of practicing psychotherapists consider themselves existentially (or humanistically) oriented. Yet few, if any, have received any systematic training in existential therapy. One can be reasonably certain of this because there are few comprehensive training programs in existential therapy. Although many excellent books illuminate some aspect of the existential frame of reference (Becker, 1973; Bugental, 1976; Koestenbaum, 1978; May, 1953, 1967, 1969; May et al., 1958), Yalom's book (1981) is the only one to present a systematic, comprehensive view of the existential therapeutic approach.

Existential therapy is *not* a comprehensive psychotherapeutic system; it is a frame of reference—a paradigm by which one views and understands a patient's suffering in a particular manner. Existential therapists begin with presuppositions about the sources of a patient's anguish and view the patient in human rather than behavioral or mechanistic terms. They may employ any of a large variety of techniques used in other approaches insofar as they are consistent with basic existential presuppositions and a human, authentic therapist–patient encounter.

The vast majority of experienced therapists, regardless of adherence to some particular ideological school, employ many existential insights and approaches. All competent therapists realize, for example, that an apprehension of one's finiteness can often catalyze a major inner shift of perspective, that it is the relationship that heals, that patients are tormented by choice, that a therapist must catalyze a patient's will to act, and that the majority of patients are bedeviled by a lack of meaning in their lives.

It is also true that the therapist's belief system determines the type of clinical data that he or she encounters. Therapists subtly or unconsciously cue patients to provide them with certain material. Jungian patients have Jungian dreams. Freudian patients discover themes of Oedipal competition. Cognitive therapists are attuned to "irrational" beliefs. The therapist's perceptual system is affected by her or his ideological system. Thus, the therapist tunes in to the material that she or he wishes to obtain. So too with the existential approach. If the therapists tune their mental apparatus to the right channel, it is astounding how frequently patients discuss concerns emanating from existential conflicts. Moreover, there are patients who have had a long-term enduring interest in existential issues. These people connect deeply to a therapist who can speak with them about their existential dilemmas and who places importance on the issues that concern them.

An existential therapist is someone with a sensibility to existential issues. No therapist focuses on existential issues all the time. These issues are important to some, not all, patients at some, not all, stages of therapy.

The basic approach in existential therapy is strategically similar to other dynamic therapies. The therapist assumes that the patient experiences anxiety that issues from some existential conflict that is at least partially unconscious and that suffering ensues from "problems in being" (Wheelis, 1973). The patient handles anxiety by a number of ineffective, maladaptive defense mechanisms that may provide temporary respite from anxiety but ultimately so cripple the individual's ability to live fully and creatively that these defenses merely result in still further secondary anxiety. The therapist helps the patient to embark on a course of self-investigation in which the goals are to understand the unconscious conflict, to identify the maladaptive defense mechanisms, to discover their destructive influence, to diminish secondary anxiety by correcting these heretofore restrictive modes of dealing with self and others, and to develop other ways of coping with primary anxiety.

Although the basic strategy in existential therapy is similar to other dynamic therapies, the content is radically different. In many respects, the process differs as well; the existential therapist's different mode of understanding the patient's basic dilemma results in many differences in the strategy of psychotherapy. For example, because the existential view of personality structure emphasizes the depth of experience at any given moment, the existential therapist does not spend a great deal of time helping the patient to recover the past. The existential therapist strives for an understanding of the patient's *current* life situation and *current* enveloping unconscious fears. The existential therapist believes, as do other dynamic therapists, that the nature of the therapist–client relationship is fundamental in good psychotherapeutic work. However, the accent is not upon transference but instead upon the relationship as fundamentally important in itself, especially in regard to engagement and connection. The existential therapist works in the present tense. The individual is to be understood and helped to understand himself or herself from the perspective of a here-and-now *cross-section,* not from the perspective of a historical *longitudinal section.*

Consider the use of the word *deep.* Freud defines *deep* as "early," and so the deepest conflict meant the earliest conflict in the individual's life. Freud's psychodynamics are developmentally based. *Fundamental* and *primary* are to be grasped chronologically: Each is synonymous with "first." Thus, the fundamental sources of anxiety, for example, are considered to be the earliest calamities: separation and castration.

From the existential perspective, *deep* means the most fundamental concerns facing the individual at that moment. The past (i.e., one's memory of the past) is important only insofar as it is part of one's current existence and has contributed to one's current mode of facing ultimate concerns. The immediate, currently existing ground beneath all other ground is important from the existential perspective. Thus, the existential conception of personality is in the awareness of the depths of one's immediate experiences. Existential therapy does not attempt to excavate and understand the past; instead, it is directed toward the future's becoming the present and explores the past only as it throws light on the present. The therapist must continually keep in mind that we create our past and that our present mode of existence dictates what we choose to remember of the past. The therapeutic focus is on the self-experience of the patient and attends to the patient's capacity for self-actualization, even self-transcendence, through engagement in life.

Process of Psychotherapy

In the existential framework, anxiety is so riveted to existence that it has a different connotation from the way anxiety is regarded in other frames of reference. The existential therapist hopes to alleviate crippling levels of anxiety but not to eliminate it. Life cannot be lived (nor can death be faced) without anxiety. The therapist's task, as May reminds us (1977, p. 374), is to reduce anxiety to tolerable levels and then to use the anxiety constructively.

We can best understand the process of psychotherapy in the existential approach by considering the therapeutic leverage inherent in some of the ultimate concerns. Each of the ultimate human concerns (death, freedom, isolation, and meaninglessness) has implications for the process of therapy.

Existential Psychotherapy and Freedom

A major component of freedom is *responsibility*—a concept that deeply influences the existential therapist's therapeutic approach. Sartre equates responsibility with *authorship:* To be responsible means to be the author of one's own life design. The existential therapist continually focuses upon each patient's responsibility for his or her own distress. Bad genes or bad luck do not cause a patient to be lonely or chronically abused or neglected by others. Until patients realize that they are responsible for their own conditions, there is little motivation to change.

The therapist must identify methods and instances of responsibility avoidance and then make these known to the patient. Therapists may use a wide variety of techniques to focus the patient's attention on responsibility. Many therapists interrupt the patient whenever they hear the patient avoiding responsibility. When patients say they "can't" do something, the therapist immediately comments, "You mean you 'won't' do it." As long as one believes in "can't," one remains unaware of one's active contribution to one's situation. Such therapists encourage patients to *own* their feelings, statements, and actions. If a patient comments that he or she did something "unconsciously," the therapist might inquire, "Whose unconscious is it?" The general principle is obvious: Whenever the patient laments about his or her life situation, the therapist inquires how the patient created that situation.

Often it is helpful to keep the patient's initial complaints in mind and then, at appropriate points in therapy, juxtapose these initial complaints with the patient's in-therapy behavior. For example, consider a patient who sought therapy because of feelings of isolation and loneliness. During the course of therapy, the patient expressed at great length his sense of superiority and his scorn and disdain of others. These attitudes were rigidly maintained; the patient manifested great resistance to examining, much less changing, these opinions. The therapist helped this patient to understand his responsibility for his personal predicament by reminding the patient, whenever he discussed his scorn of others, "And you are lonely."

Responsibility is one component of freedom. Earlier we described another, *willing,* which may be further subdivided into *wishing* and *deciding.* Consider the role of *wishing.* How often does the therapist participate with a patient in some such sequence as this:

"What shall I do? What shall I do?"
"What is it that stops you from doing what you want to do?"
"But I don't *know* what I want to do! If I knew that, I wouldn't need to see you!"

These patients know what they should do, ought to do, or must do, but they do not experience what they *want* to do. Many therapists, in working with patients who have a profound incapacity to wish, have shared May's inclination to shout, "Don't you ever *want* anything?" (1969, p. 165). These patients have enormous social difficulties because they have no opinions, no inclinations, and no desires of their own.

Often the inability to wish is imbedded in a more global disorder—the inability to feel. In many cases, the bulk of psychotherapy consists of helping patients to dissolve their affect blocks. This therapy is slow and grinding. Above all, the therapist must persevere and, time after time, must continue to press the patient with, "What do you feel? What do you want?" Repeatedly the therapist will need to explore the source and nature of the block and of the stifled feelings behind it. The inability to feel and to wish is a pervasive characterological trait, and considerable time and therapeutic perseverance are required to effect enduring change.

There are other modes of avoiding wishing in addition to blocking of affect. Some individuals avoid wishing by not discriminating among wishes, by acting impulsively on all wishes. In such instances, the therapist must help the patient to make some internal discrimination among wishes and assign priorities to each. The patient must learn that two wishes that are mutually exclusive demand that one be relinquished. If, for example, a meaningful, loving relationship is a wish, then a host of conflicting interpersonal wishes—such as the wish for conquest or power or seduction or subjugation—must be denied.

Decision is the bridge between wishing and action. Some patients, even though they are able to wish, are still unable to act because they cannot *decide*. One of the more common reasons that deciding is difficult is that every yes involves a no. Renunciation invariably accompanies decision, and a decision requires a relinquishment of other options—often options that may never come again. The patient must come to terms with the unalterable fact that *alternatives exclude.*

The therapist must help patients make choices. Patients must recognize that they themselves, not the therapist, must generate and choose among options. In helping patients to communicate effectively, therapists teach that one must *own* one's feelings. It is equally important that one owns one's decisions. Some patients are panicked by the various implications of each decision. The "what ifs" torment them. *What if I leave my job and can't find another? What if I leave my children alone and they get hurt?* It is often useful to ask the patient to consider the entire scenario of each "what if" in turn, to fantasize it happening with all the possible ramifications, and then to experience and analyze emerging feelings.

Patients may also feel paralyzed by an inability to tolerate uncertainty. A young woman scientist came to therapy because she was unable to decide whether to move back to her hometown to be near her family, which she very much wanted to do, or to stay in her current city and job, neither of which she liked. Most of all, she hoped to meet a man who could be a life partner, something she had been unable to do in any of the cities she had recently lived in while she was studying and pursuing her career goals. In scientific fashion, she had researched all possibilities, exhaustively checking, for example, dating Web sites to see which men were looking for partners in her hometown. None of them seemed suitable. What if she gave up her prestigious job for a lesser one in her hometown and *still* didn't meet anyone? She would then still be lonely and now full of regret and remorse. What she wanted was for someone to tell her what was the right decision. The therapeutic task with her was to help her face the inevitability of uncertainty in life: There are never guarantees, no matter how scientifically one approaches one's decisions.

A general posture toward decision making is to assume that the therapist's task is not to *create* will but instead to *disencumber* it. The therapist cannot flick the decision switch or inspire the patient with resoluteness. It is the therapist's task to help remove the obstacles to decision making. Once that is done, the individual will naturally move into a more autonomous position in just the way, as Karen Horney (1950) put it, an acorn develops into an oak tree.

The therapist must help patients understand that decisions are unavoidable. One makes decisions all the time and often conceals from oneself the fact that one is deciding. It is important to help patients understand the inevitability of decisions and to identify how they make decisions. Many patients decide *passively* by, for example, letting another person decide for them. They may terminate an unsatisfactory relationship by unconsciously acting in such a way that the partner makes the decision to leave. In such instances, the final outcome is achieved, but the patient may be left with many negative repercussions. The patient's sense of powerlessness is merely reinforced, and he or she continues to experience himself or herself as one to whom things happen rather than as the author of his or her own life situation. The *way* one makes a decision is often as important as the content of the decision. An active decision reinforces the individual's active acceptance of his or her own power and resources.

Existential Isolation and Psychotherapy

No relationship can eliminate existential isolation, but aloneness can be shared in such a way that love compensates for its pain. The experience of existential isolation is so anguishing that defenses are fairly quickly and firmly instituted against it. Yet the capacity to acknowledge deeply our isolated situation in existence also makes it possible to move toward authentic relationships with other (similarly isolated) beings. Patients who grow in psychotherapy learn not only the rewards of intimacy but also its limits: They learn what they *cannot* get from others.

An important step in treatment consists of helping patients address existential isolation directly. Those who lack sufficient experiences of closeness and true relatedness in their lives are particularly incapable of tolerating isolation. Adolescents from loving, supportive families are able to grow away from their families with relative ease and to tolerate the separation and loneliness of young adulthood. On the other hand, those who grow up in tormented, highly conflicted families find it extremely difficult to leave the family. The more disturbed the family, the harder it is for children to leave—they are ill equipped to separate and therefore cling to the family for shelter against isolation and anxiety.

Many patients have enormous difficulty spending time alone. Some may feel they exist only in the eyes of others. Consequently, they construct their lives in such a way that they eliminate time alone. Two of the major problems that result from this are the desperation with which they seek certain kinds of relationships and the use of others to assuage the pain accompanying isolation. The therapist must find a way to help the patient confront isolation in a dosage and with a support system suited to that patient. Some therapists, at an advanced stage of therapy, advise periods of self-enforced isolation during which the patient is asked to monitor and record thoughts and feelings.

The anxiety of existential isolation is best assuaged through the creation of meaningful and mutual relationships with others. Many patients who feel unloved actually suffer from difficulties in the capacity to love. Too occupied with what they need from others, they cannot give to others and cannot participate in reciprocity and mutuality. To love means to be actively concerned with the welfare and growth of another. In *The Art of Loving*, Erich Fromm (1956) wrote "the ability to be alone is the condition for the ability to love (p. 94)." Two partners unable to tolerate aloneness create an A-frame that holds them both up but is a poor basis for marriage.

The authentic human encounter must be modeled by the therapist, who is available to meet the patient in the space between "I" and "Thou." It is the therapeutic relationship that heals. Presence, genuineness, and receptiveness on the part of the therapist form the attitude that invites true *meeting* in a real relationship with the patient. The aim of the therapist is to bring something to life in the patient rather than to impose something. The therapist stays with this task selflessly, attempting to enter the patient's world and experience it as the patient experiences it. The existential therapist tries to do this from a position of being a fellow traveler—not as a technique of psychotherapy.

Meaninglessness and Psychotherapy

To deal effectively with meaninglessness, therapists must first increase their sensitivity to the topic, listen differently, and become aware of the importance of meaning in the lives of individuals. For some patients, the issue of meaninglessness is profound and pervasive. Carl Jung once estimated that more than 30% of his patients sought therapy because of a sense of personal meaninglessness (1966, p. 83).

The therapist must be attuned to the overall focus and direction of the patient's life. Is the patient reaching beyond himself or herself? Or is he or she entirely immersed in the daily routine of staying alive? Yalom (1981) reported that his therapy was rarely successful unless he was able to help patients focus on something beyond these pursuits. Simply by increasing their sensitivity to these issues, the therapist can help them focus on values outside themselves. Therapists, for example, can begin to wonder about the patient's belief systems, inquire deeply into the loving of another, ask about long-range hopes and goals, and explore creative interests and pursuits.

Viktor Frankl, who placed great emphasis on the importance of meaninglessness in contemporary psychopathology, stated that "happiness cannot be pursued, it can only ensue" (1963, p. 165). The more we deliberately search for self-satisfaction, the more it eludes us, whereas the more we fulfill some self-transcendent meaning, the more happiness will ensue.

Therapists must find a way to help self-centered patients develop curiosity and concern for others. The therapy group is especially well suited for this endeavor: The pattern in which self-absorbed, narcissistic patients take without giving often becomes highly evident in the therapy group. In such instances, therapists may attempt to increase an individual's ability and inclination to empathize with others by requesting, periodically, that patients guess how others are feeling at various junctures of the group.

But the major solution to the problem of meaninglessness is engagement. Wholehearted engagement in any of the infinite array of life's activities enhances the possibility of one's patterning the events of one's life in some coherent fashion. To fashion a home, to care about other individuals and about ideas or projects, to search, to create, to build—all forms of engagement are twice rewarding: They are intrinsically enriching, and they alleviate the dysphoria that stems from being bombarded with the unassembled brute data of existence.

The therapist must approach engagement with the same attitudinal set used with wishing. The desire to engage life is always there with the patient, and therefore the therapist's activity should be directed toward the removal of obstacles in the patient's way. The therapist begins to explore what prevents the patient from loving another individual. Why is there so little satisfaction from his or her relationships with others? Why is there so little satisfaction from work? What blocks the patient from finding work commensurate with his or her talents and interests or finding some pleasurable aspects of current work? Why has the patient neglected creative or spiritual or self-transcendent strivings?

Death and Psychotherapy

An increased awareness of one's finiteness stemming from a personal confrontation with death may cause a radical shift in life perspective and lead to personal change. A patient named Carlos, dying of cancer, had increased his preoccupation with having sex with as many women as possible. But as Yalom, his therapist, insisted that he reflect on how he had been living his life, Carlos made astonishing change in his last months. As he lay dying, he thanked his therapist for having saved his life.

Death as an Awakening Experience

An *awakening experience* is a type of urgent experience that propels the individual into a confrontation with an existential situation. The most powerful awakening experience is confrontation with one's personal death. Such a confrontation has the power to provide a massive shift in the way one lives in the world. Some patients report that they learn simply that "existence cannot be postponed." They no longer put off living until some time in the future; they realize that one can really live only in the present. The neurotic individual rarely lives in the present but is either continuously obsessed with events from the past or fearful of anticipated events in the future.

A confrontation with an awakening experience persuades individuals to count their blessings, to become aware of their natural surroundings: the elemental facts of life, changing seasons, seeing, listening, touching, and loving. Ordinarily what we *can* experience is diminished by petty concerns, by thoughts of what we cannot do or what we lack, or by threats to our prestige.

Many terminally ill patients, when reporting personal growth emanating from their confrontation with death, have lamented, "What a tragedy that we had to wait till now, till our bodies were riddled with cancer, to learn these truths." This is an exceedingly important message for therapists. The therapist can obtain considerable leverage to help "everyday" patients (i.e., patients who are not physically ill) increase their awareness of death earlier in their life cycle. With this aim in mind, some therapists have employed structured exercises to confront the individual with personal death. Some group leaders begin a brief group experience by asking members to write their own epitaph or obituary, or they provide guided fantasies in which group members imagine their own death and funeral.

Many existential therapists do not believe that artificially introduced death confrontations are necessary or advisable. Instead, they attempt to help the patient recognize the signs of mortality that are part of the fabric of everyday life. If the therapist and the patient are tuned in, there is considerable evidence of death anxiety in every psychotherapy. Every patient suffers losses through death of parents, friends, and associates. Dreams are haunted with death anxiety. Every nightmare is a dream of raw death anxiety. Everywhere around us are reminders of aging: Our bones begin to creak, age spots appear on our skin, we go to reunions and note with dismay how everyone *else* has aged. Our children grow up. The cycle of life envelops us.

An important opportunity for confrontation with death arises when patients experience the death of someone close to them. The traditional literature on grief primarily focuses on two aspects of grief work: loss and the resolution of ambivalence that so strongly accentuates the dysphoria of grief. But a third dimension must be considered: The death of someone close to us confronts us with our own death.

Often grief has a very different tone, depending upon the individual's relationship with the person who has died. The loss of a parent confronts us with our vulnerability: If our parents could not save themselves, who will save us? When parents die, nothing remains between ourselves and the grave. At the moment of our parents' deaths, we ourselves constitute the barrier between our children and their death.

The death of a spouse often evokes the fear of existential isolation. The loss of the significant other increases our awareness that, try as hard as we can to go through the world two by two, there is nonetheless a basic aloneness we must bear. Yalom reports a patient's dream the night after learning that his wife had inoperable cancer.

> I was living in my old house in _____ [a house that had been in the family for three generations]. A Frankenstein monster was chasing me through the house. I was terrified. The house was deteriorating, decaying. The tiles were crumbling and the roof leaking. Water leaked all over my mother. [His mother had died six months earlier.] I fought with him. I had a choice of weapons. One had a curved blade with a handle, like a scythe. I slashed him and tossed him off the roof. He lay stretched out on the pavement below. But he got up and once again started chasing me through the house. (1980, p. 168)

The patient's first association to this dream was "I know I've got a hundred thousand miles on me." Obviously his wife's impending death reminded him that his life and his body (symbolized in the dream by the deteriorating house) were also finite. As a child, this patient was often haunted by the monster who returned in this nightmare.

Children try many methods of dealing with death anxiety. One of the most common is the personification of death—imagining death as some finite creature: a monster, a sandman, a bogeyman, and so on. This is very frightening to children but nonetheless far less frightening than the truth—that they carry the spores of their own death within them. If death is "out there" in some physical form, then possibly it may be eluded, tricked, or pacified.

Milestones provide another opportunity for the therapist to focus the patient on existential facts of life. Even simple milestones, such as birthdays and anniversaries, are useful levers. These signs of passage are often capable of eliciting pain (consequently, we often deal with such milestones by reaction formation, in the form of a joyous celebration).

Major life events, such as a threat to one's career, a severe illness, retirement, commitment to a relationship, and separation from a relationship, can be important awakening experiences that offer opportunities for an increased awareness of death anxiety. Often these experiences are painful, and therapists feel compelled to focus entirely on pain alleviation. In so doing, however, they miss rich opportunities for deep therapeutic work that reveal themselves at those moments.

Birthdays, grief, reunions, dreams, or the empty nest prime the individual for awakening. These become occasions for reflection on how one has lived one's life. In *Thus Spake Zarathustra,* Nietzsche (1954) poses a challenge: what if you are to live the identical life again and again throughout eternity—how would that change you? The idea of living your identical life again and again for all eternity can be jarring, a sort of *petite* existential shock therapy. It often serves as a sobering thought experiment, leading one to consider seriously how one is really living.

Properly used, regret is a tool that can jar patients into taking actions to prevent its further accumulation. One can examine regret both by looking behind and by looking ahead. If regret reflects what has not been fulfilled, one can choose either to amass more regret or to plan one's life to make the changes that will avoid regret. The therapeutic question becomes, "How can you live now without building new regrets? What do you have to do to change your life?"

Death as a Primary Source of Anxiety

The fear of death constitutes a primary fount of anxiety: It is present early in life, it is instrumental in shaping character structure, and it continues throughout life to generate anxiety that results in manifest distress and the erection of psychological defenses. However, it is important to keep in mind that death anxiety exists at the very deepest levels of being, is heavily repressed, and is rarely experienced in its full sense. Often, death anxiety per se is not easily visible in the clinical picture.

Even though death anxiety may not explicitly enter the therapeutic dialogue, a theory of anxiety based on death awareness may provide therapists with a frame of reference that greatly enhances their effectiveness. Death anxiety is directly proportional to the amount of each person's "unlived life." Those individuals who feel they have lived their lives richly, have fulfilled their potential and their destiny, experience less panic in the face of death.

There are patients, however, who are suffused with overt death anxiety at the very onset of therapy. Sometimes, there are life situations in which the patient has such a rush of death anxiety that the therapist cannot evade the issue. In long-term, intensive therapy, explicit death anxiety is always to be found and must be considered in the therapeutic work.

Mechanisms of Psychotherapy

Existential psychotherapy is not limited to and may not even be focused on a discussion of these ultimate concerns, although the alert therapist aims not to shy away from them or change the subject. Still, the mechanisms of existential psychotherapy maximize the possibility of a clear view of these fundamental human experiences by fostering engagement with the anxieties of existence and being. Through authenticity and presence, the therapist strives to counter avoidance and withdrawal. The mechanisms of existential psychotherapy involve a focus on the here and now and a view of the therapist–patient relationship as one of fellow travelers. The therapeutic stance is founded on empathy and may also include the use of dreams. Existential psychotherapy is the synergy of the therapeutic relationship plus ideas.

Empathy

Empathy is the most powerful tool we have in our efforts to connect with other people: It is the glue of human connectedness and permits one to feel, at a deep level, what someone else is feeling. The existential therapist attempts to see the world from the point of view of the patient. *Patients view the therapy hours in very different ways from therapists.* Again and again, therapists, even highly experienced ones, are surprised to rediscover this phenomenon when their patients describe an intense emotional reaction about the previous hour that the therapist cannot recall. It is extraordinarily difficult to really know what the other feels; far too often we, as therapists, project our own feelings onto the other.

Therapists don't have to have had the same experience as patients to be empathetic. They might try to follow the maxim that "I am human and let nothing human be alien to me." This requires that therapists be open to that part of themselves that corresponds to any deed or fantasy offered by patients, no matter how heinous, violent, lustful, or sadistic.

The Here and Now

The nitty-gritty of *doing* therapy involves intense focus on the here and now. What is happening in the interpersonal space between patient and therapist, right here, right now? Therapy is a social microcosm in the sense that sooner or later, if the therapy is not highly structured, the interpersonal and existential problems of the patient will manifest themselves in the here and now of the therapy relationship. If, in life, the patient is demanding or fearful or arrogant or self-effacing or seductive or controlling or judgmental or maladaptive interpersonally in any other way, then these traits will be displayed in living color in the here and now of the therapy hour. The therapist need only be alert to what is happening in the interaction with the patient and to try to find the analogues to what the patient reports to be his or her difficulties in outside relationships. In order to fully access the here and now, therapists have to access their own feelings and use these as a barometer of what is happening in the interaction. If the therapist is bored, there is something the patient is doing to induce that boredom. Perhaps the patient fears intimacy or is silently rageful toward the therapist. Only by acknowledging his or her feelings in the immediacy of the interaction can the therapist access what is being enacted by the patient. To do this well, the therapist must both have deep self-knowledge and the skill to give feedback tactfully and kindly, to avoid accusation of the patient and above all, to be ready when necessary to acknowledge his or her own contribution to the problematic interaction.

Attention to the here and now invites attention to the *immediacy* of the interaction in the moment in which it occurs. Patients may find this unfamiliar or resist the intimacy that here-and-now processing engages. Yet it is here that the greatest vitality in the therapy hour will be manifest as a fully present therapist forges an authentic connection with a fully present patient, both sharing the phenomenology of their experiences.

It is the task of the therapist to maintain focus on what is transpiring in the relationship as it develops. A simple check-in brings this relationship to the center of attention, asking, for example, such questions as: "How are you and I doing today?" "Are there feelings about me you took home from the last session?" "I've noticed a real shift in the session today. At first it seemed we were very distant and in the past 20 minutes, I felt much closer. Was your experience the same? What enabled us to get closer then?" *Therapy is always an alternating sequence of interaction and reflection upon that interaction.*

What occurs in the here and now will always have analogues in the patient's life. As patients take risks with self-experience in the present of the therapy hour, they will become more courageous to take such risks in their outside lives. As patients come to recognize their blocks to full engagement, their constriction, their flights from responsibility, their difficulties in relating to others, they will better understand what impedes their life projects and relationships. Patients develop a new internal standard for the quality of a genuine relationship. Having achieved it with the therapist, they may well have the confidence and willingness to form similarly good relationships in the future.

The therapist never makes decisions for patients and is alert to any internal convictions that s/he knows what is best for the patient. The role of the therapist is "catalytic" (Wheelis, 1973). Therapy is aimed toward removing roadblocks to purposeful living and helping patients assume responsibility for their actions, not providing solutions.

Dreams

Dreams are a very important access road to the inner life of patients. They comment on the therapy relationship, on existential experiences, and on unconscious fantasies and contain metaphors for the deepest aspects of the person. Yalom (2002) recounts the following story in *The Gift of Therapy* to demonstrate how dreams can enliven and direct the therapy. One of his patients had the following dream:

> I was on the porch of my home looking through the window at my father sitting at his desk. I went inside and asked him for gas money for my car. He reached into his pocket and as he handed me a lot of bills he pointed to my purse. I opened my wallet and it already was crammed with money. Then I said that my gas tank was empty and he went outside to my car and pointed to the gas gauge, which said, "full." (p. 232)

In his analysis of this dream, Yalom points out the following:

> The major theme in this dream was emptiness versus fullness. The patient wanted something from her father (and from me since the room in the dream closely resembled the configuration of my office) but she couldn't figure out what she wanted. She asked for money and gasoline but her wallet was already stuffed with money and her gas tank was full. The dream depicted her pervasive sense of emptiness, as well as her belief that I had the power to fill her up if she could only discover the right question to ask. Hence she persisted in craving something from me—compliments, doting, special treatment, birthday presents—all the while knowing she was off the mark. My task in therapy was to redirect her attention—away from gaining supplies from another and towards the richness of her own inner resources. (p. 233)

Fellow Travelers

Sometimes many hours go by without the voicing of any existential content, but the therapist–patient relationship is influenced by the existential perspective in every single session. Existential therapists experience and present themselves as real, self-revealing *fellow travelers.*

We all, whether in the role of patients or therapists or just human beings, must come to terms with our eventual death, with our aloneness in the universe, with finding meaning in life, and with recognizing our freedom and taking responsibility for the lives we lead. The wise therapist recognizes that these are issues with which we must struggle together; the therapist is only privileged in the sense of being able, one hopes, to talk honestly about what these concerns entail.

A stark confrontation with the ultimate concerns of life leads to a recognition of the primacy of connectedness in human life. What is central to existential psychotherapy is the relationship between therapist and patient. But there are no prescribed formulas for this relationship. The therapeutic venture is always spontaneous, creative, and uncertain. Indeed, the therapist creates a new therapy for each patient. The therapist gropes toward the patient with improvisation and intuition. The heart of psychotherapy is a caring, deeply human meeting between two people, one (generally, but not always, the patient) more troubled than the other. Both are exposed to the same existential issues of meaning, isolation, freedom, and death. There is no distinction between "them" (the afflicted) and "us" (the healers).

Genuineness, so crucial to effective therapy, takes on a new dimension when a therapist deals honestly with existential issues. We have to abandon all vestiges of a medical model that posits that a patient suffering from a strange affliction needs a dispassionate, immaculate, expert healer. We all face the same terror, the wound of mortality, the worm at the core of existence. In order to be truly present with patients dealing with death anxiety, the therapist must be open to his or her own death anxiety, not in a glib or superficial way but with a profound awareness. This is no easy task, and no training program prepares therapists for this type of work.

Fellow travelers focusing on the here and now, on the relational space between them, expose together the dilemmas of human interaction that often underlie the blocks to finding the meaning and connection in life that soften the terrors of death. Focus on the dynamics of the therapeutic relationship as it unfolds enables vitality and engagement. The therapist's most valuable instrument is his or her own self and therefore, the personal exploration that can only be conducted in one's own therapy is necessary. Psychotherapy is a psychologically demanding enterprise, and therapists must develop the awareness and inner strength to cope with the many occupational hazards of psychotherapy. Only through personal therapy can therapists become aware of their own blind spots and dark sides and thus become able to empathize with the extensive range of human wishes and impulses. A personal therapy experience also permits the student therapist to experience the therapeutic process from the patient's seat: the tendency to idealize the therapist, the yearning for dependency, the gratitude toward a caring and attentive listener, the power granted to the therapist. Self-knowledge is not achieved once and for all; therapists can only benefit from re-entering therapy at many stages of life.

Therapist Transparency

As a fellow traveler along the same road as the patient, the therapist tries to be as authentic and genuine as possible. The therapist must be willing to disclose his or her feelings in the here and now, fully open to what is being engendered in his or her inner experience by the interaction with the patient. From an existential psychotherapy standpoint, it is the *examined* therapeutic relationship that heals.

Existential therapists are willing to let patients matter to them and also to acknowledge their errors. Disclosure by the therapist always facilitates therapy. Still, the reflective therapist must also be mindful of the boundaries and the meanings of the boundaries on such disclosure and resist temptations to engage in various forms of exploitation of the patient. Therapists reveal themselves when it enhances therapy, not because of their own needs or rules. This is why personal therapy is so important for doing this kind of work.

Therapist disclosure should be primarily about feelings in the here and now, in the relationship with the patient. Such disclosure must be well processed and tactful, never impulsive. For example, the therapist might tell the patient when s/he feels closer to the patient as a result of the patient's sharing, or more distant as a result of the patient's reluctance to confront some more emotionally charged issues. "I find myself afraid of your criticism, probably like others in your life." "I feel that your putting me on a pedestal makes me feel farther away from you." "I feel I have to be very careful about what I say because you seem to scan everything I say for signs of my approval or disapproval." The therapist uses disclosure in the service of the welfare of the patient, not as an end in itself. Therapists must take care not to disclose what might be (or feel) destructive to the patient. They must respect the pace of therapy and what the patient is or is not ready to hear.

APPLICATIONS

Who Can We Help?

The clinical setting often determines the applicability of the existential approach. In each course of therapy, the therapist must consider the goals appropriate to the clinical setting. To take one example, in an acute inpatient setting where the patient will be hospitalized for as brief a time as possible, the goal of therapy is crisis intervention. The therapist hopes to alleviate symptoms and to restore the patient to a precrisis level of functioning. Deeper, more ambitious goals are unrealistic and inappropriate to that situation.

In situations where patients not only desire symptomatic relief but also hope to attain greater personal growth, the existential approach is generally useful. A thorough existential approach with ambitious goals is most appropriate in long-term therapy, but even in briefer approaches, some aspect of the existential mode (e.g., an emphasis on responsibility, deciding, an authentic therapist–patient encounter, grief work, and so on) is often incorporated into the therapy.

An existential approach to therapy is appropriate with patients who confront some boundary situation—that is, a confrontation with death, the facing of some important irreversible decision, a sudden thrust into isolation, or milestones that mark passages from one life era into another. But therapy need not be limited to these explicit existential crises. Existential psychotherapy can be applied to a diverse range of patients in different modalities (Schneider, 2007). In every course of therapy, there is abundant evidence of patients' anguish stemming from existential conflicts. The availability of such data is entirely a function of the therapist's attitudinal set and perceptivity. The decision to work on these levels should be a joint patient–therapist decision.

Treatment

Existential therapy has its primary applications in an individual therapy setting. However, various existential themes and insights may be successfully applied in a variety of other settings, including group therapy, family therapy, couples therapy, and so forth.

The concept of responsibility has particularly widespread applicability. It is a keystone of the group therapeutic process, in which patients learn how their behavior is viewed by others, how their behavior makes others feel, how they create the opinions others have of them, and how others' opinions shapes their views of themselves. Group members begin to understand that they are responsible for how others treat them and for the way in which they regard themselves (Yalom, 2005). Indeed, patients can see how they create in others the very reactions that trouble them in their outside lives (Josselson, 2007).

In group therapy, all members are "born" simultaneously. Each starts out on an equal footing. Each gradually scoops out and shapes a particular life space in the group. Thus, each person is responsible for the interpersonal position he or she creates in the group (and in life). The therapeutic work in the group then not only allows individuals to change their way of relating to one another but also brings home to them in a powerful way the extent to which they have created their own life predicaments—clearly an existential therapeutic mechanism.

Often the therapist uses his or her own feelings to identify the patient's contribution to his or her life predicament. For example, a depressed 48-year-old woman complained bitterly about the way her children treated her: They dismissed her opinions, were impatient with her, and, when some serious issue was at stake, addressed their comments to their father. When the therapist tuned in to his feelings about this patient, he became aware of a whining quality in her voice that tempted *him* not to take her seriously and to regard her somewhat as a child. He shared his feelings with the patient, and it proved enormously useful to her. She became aware of her childlike behavior in many areas and began to realize that her children treated her precisely as she "asked" to be treated.

Not infrequently, therapists must treat patients who are panicked by a decisional crisis. Yalom (1981) describes one therapeutic approach in such a situation. The therapist's basic strategy consisted of helping the patient uncover and appreciate the existential implications of the decision. The patient was a 66-year-old widow who sought therapy because of her anguish about a decision to sell a summer home. The house required constant attention to gardening, maintenance, and protection and seemed a considerable burden to a frail aging woman in poor health. Finances affected the decision as well, and she asked many financial and realty consultants to assist her in making the decision.

The therapist and the patient explored many factors involved in the decision and then gradually began to explore more deeply. Soon a number of painful issues emerged. For example, her husband had died a year ago and she mourned him still. The house was still rich with his presence, and drawers and closets brimmed with his personal effects. A decision to sell the house also required a decision to come to terms with the fact that her husband would never return. She considered her house her "drawing card" and harbored serious doubts whether anyone would visit her without the enticement of her lovely estate. Thus, a decision to sell the house meant testing the loyalty of her friends and risking loneliness and isolation. Yet another reason centered on the great tragedy of her life—her childlessness. She had always envisioned the estate passing on to her children and to her children's children. The decision to sell the house thus was a decision to acknowledge the failure of her major symbolic immortality project. The therapist used the house-selling decision as a springboard to these deeper issues and eventually helped the patient mourn her husband, herself, and her unborn children.

Once the deeper meanings of a decision are worked through, the decision generally glides easily into place, and after approximately a dozen sessions, the patient effortlessly made the decision to sell the house.

Existentially oriented therapists strive toward honest, mutually open relationships with their patients. The patient–therapist relationship helps the patient clarify other relationships. Patients almost invariably distort some aspect of their relationship to the therapist. The therapist, drawing from self-knowledge and experience of how others view him or her, is able to help the patient distinguish distortion from reality.

The experience of an intimate encounter with a therapist has implications that extend beyond relationships with other people. For one thing, the therapist is generally someone whom the patient particularly respects. But even more important, the therapist is someone, often the only one, who *really* knows the patient. To tell someone else all one's darkest secrets and still to be fully accepted by that person is enormously affirmative.

Existential thinkers such as Erich Fromm, Abraham Maslow, and Martin Buber all stress that true caring for another means to care about the other's growth and to want to bring something to life in the other. Buber (1965) uses the term *unfolding,* which he suggests should be the way of the educator and the therapist: One uncovers what was there all along. The term *unfolding* has rich connotations and stands in sharp contrast to the goals of other therapeutic systems. One helps the patient unfold by *meeting,* by existential communication. Perhaps the most important concept of all in describing the patient–therapist relationship is what May et al. term *presence* (1958, p. 80). The therapist must be fully present, striving for an authentic encounter with the patient.

Evidence

Psychotherapy evaluation is always a difficult task. The more focused and specific the approach and the goals, the easier it is to measure outcome. Symptomatic relief or behavioral change may be quantified with reasonable precision. But more ambitious therapies, which seek to affect deeper layers of the individual's mode of being in the world, defy quantification. These problems of evaluation are illustrated by the following vignettes reported by Yalom (1981).

> A 46-year-old mother accompanied the youngest of her four children to the airport, from which he departed for college. She had spent the last 26 years rearing her children and longing for this day. No more impositions, no more incessantly living for others, no more cooking dinners and picking up clothes. Finally she was free.
>
> Yet as she said good-bye she unexpectedly began sobbing loudly, and on the way home from the airport a deep shudder passed through her body. "It is only natural," she thought. It was only the sadness of saying good-bye to someone she loved very much. But it was much more than that, and the shudder soon turned into raw anxiety. The therapist whom she consulted identified it as a common problem: the empty nest syndrome. (p. 336)

Of course she was anxious. How could it be otherwise? For years she had based her self-esteem on her performance as a mother, and suddenly she found no way to validate herself. The whole routine and structure of her life had been altered. Gradually, with the help of Valium, supportive psychotherapy, an assertiveness training group, several adult education courses, a lover or two, and a part-time volunteer job, the shudder shrank to a tremble and then vanished. She returned to her premorbid level of comfort and adaptation.

This patient happened to be part of a psychotherapy research project, and there were outcome measures of her psychotherapy. Her treatment results could be described as excellent on each of the measures used—symptom checklists, target problem evaluation, and self-esteem. Obviously she had made considerable improvement. Yet, despite this, it is entirely possible to consider this case as one of missed therapeutic opportunities.

Consider another patient in almost precisely the same life situation. In the treatment of this second patient, the therapist, who was existentially oriented, attempted to nurse the shudder rather than to anesthetize it. This patient experienced what Kierkegaard called "creative anxiety." The therapist and the patient allowed the anxiety to lead them into important areas for investigation. True, the patient suffered from the empty nest syndrome; she had problems of self-esteem; she loved her child but also envied him for the chances in life she had never had; and, of course, she felt guilty because of these "ignoble" sentiments.

The therapist did not simply allow her to find ways to fill her time but also plunged into an exploration of the *meaning* of the fear of the empty nest. She had always desired freedom but now seemed terrified of it. Why?

A dream illuminated the meaning of the shudder. The dream consisted simply of holding in her hand a 35-mm photographic slide of her son juggling and tumbling. The slide was peculiar, however, in that it showed movement; she saw her son in a multitude of positions all at the same time. In the analysis of the dream, her associations revolved around the theme of time. The slide captured and framed time and movement. It kept everything alive but made everything stand still. It froze life. "Time moves on," she said, "and there's no way I can stop it. I didn't want John to grow up . . . whether I like it or not time moves on. It moves on for John and it moves on for me as well."

This dream brought her own finiteness into clear focus and, rather than rush to fill time with various distractions, she learned to appreciate time in richer ways than previously. She moved into the realm that Heidegger described as *authentic being:* She wondered not so much at the *way* things are but *that* things are. She recognized that life is seriously linear and irreversible, that everything fades, and that she still had time to live purposefully and meaningfully. Although one could argue that therapy helped the second patient more than the first, it would not be possible to demonstrate this conclusion on any standard outcome measures. In fact, the second patient probably continued to experience more anxiety than the first did; but anxiety is a part of existence, and no individual who continues to grow and create will ever be free of it.

These gains continue to elude randomized-control objective forms of research. Yet nearly all psychotherapy research, especially research on common factors, has substantiated a central premise of existential psychotherapy—that it is the relationship that heals (Frank & Frank, 1991; Gelso & Hayes, 1998; Norcross, 2002; Safran & Muran, 1996; Wampold, 2001).

Psychotherapy in a Multicultural World

Existential psychotherapy considers the situation of the whole person located in society and culture. Cultural, racial, or national identities are not add-ons—they are essential aspects of the phenomenology of the client and intrinsic to the treatment. Existential psychotherapy is oriented to all aspects of human uniqueness and difference and takes into account and investigates the meanings of age, sexual orientation, ethnicity, and so on.

All humans, regardless of cultural background, share in the dilemmas of existence and must come to terms with the ultimate concerns of freedom, isolation, meaninglessness, and death. The potential difficulties come when treating people who have adopted wholesale formulas for managing these concerns that were provided by their cultural, often religious, systems.

Yalom had such a struggle with a young orthodox rabbi who requested a consultation with him. The rabbi said he was in training to become an existential therapist but was experiencing some dissonance between his religious background and the psychological formulations of existential psychotherapy. At first deferential during the session, the rabbi's demeanor slowly changed, and he began to voice his beliefs with such zeal as to make Yalom suspect that the real purpose of his visit was to convert him to the religious life.

Yalom acknowledged the fundamental antagonism between their views. The rabbi's belief in an omnipresent, omniscient personal God watching him, protecting him, and providing him a life design was indeed incompatible with the core of the existential stance that we are free, alone, thrown randomly into an uncaring universe, and mortal.

"But you," the rabbi responded with intense concern on his face, "how can you live with only these beliefs? And without meaning? How can you live without belief in something greater than yourself? What meaning would there be if everything is destined to fade? My religion provides me with meaning, wisdom, morality, with divine comfort, with a way to live."

To this, Yalom responded, "I don't consider that a rational response, Rabbi. Those commodities—meaning, wisdom, morality, living well—are *not* dependent on a belief in God. And, yes, *of course,* religious belief makes you feel good, comforted, virtuous— that is exactly what religions are invented to do. You ask how I can live. I believe I live well. I'm guided by human-generated doctrines. I believe in the Hippocratic oath I took as a physician and dedicate myself to helping others heal and grow. I live a moral life. I feel compassion for those about me I live in a loving relationship with my family and friends. I don't need religion to supply a moral compass."

Yalom has never had a desire to undermine anyone's religious faith, but strong religious belief that overshadows personal struggle with the ultimate concerns may preclude exploration of existential issues. Most, perhaps all, cultures create belief systems that defend against the terrors of stark confrontation with existential concerns. The dilemma for the existential therapist is to recognize the way in which these belief systems provide a sense of meaning for the patient, to stay authentic with regard to his or her own beliefs, and still find ways to increase the patient's engagement with purpose and meaning in life.

A depressed patient whose cultural background dictates unquestioning filial obedience found it difficult to pursue her own life goals. Efforts to engage her in addressing her own responsibility for her choices in life were met with her declaring that she must do what her father requires of her. The existential therapist must then help this patient see herself as making a deliberate choice in this regard—to obey her father rather than to follow her own desires. Obedience itself can be an existential choice for which one can take full responsibility.

CASE EXAMPLE

A Simple Case of Divorce

A 50-year-old scientist, whom we will call David, had been married for 27 years and had recently decided to separate from his wife. He sought therapy because of the degree of anxiety he was experiencing in anticipation of confronting his wife with his decision.

The situation was in many ways a typical midlife scenario. The patient had two children; the youngest had just graduated from college. In David's mind, the children had always been the main element binding him and his wife together. Now that the children were self-supporting and fully adult, David felt there was no reasonable point in continuing the marriage. He reported that he had been dissatisfied with his marriage for many years and on three previous occasions had separated from his wife, but, after only a few days, had become anxious and returned, crestfallen, to his home. Bad as the marriage was, David concluded that it was less unsatisfactory than the loneliness of being single.

The reason for his dissatisfaction with his marriage was primarily boredom. He had met his wife when he was 17, a time when he had been extremely insecure, especially in his relationships with women. She was the first woman who had ever expressed interest in him. David (as well as his wife) came from a blue-collar family. He was exceptionally intellectually gifted and was the first member of his family to attend college. He won a scholarship to an Ivy League school, obtained two graduate degrees, and embarked upon an outstanding academic research career. His wife was not gifted intellectually, chose not to go to college, and during the early years of their marriage worked to support David in graduate school.

For most of their married life, his wife immersed herself in the task of caring for the children while David ferociously pursued his professional career. He had always experienced his relationship to his wife as empty and had always felt bored with her company. In his view, she had an extremely mediocre mind and was so restricted characterologically that he found it constraining to be alone with her and embarrassing to share her with friends. He experienced himself as continually changing and growing, whereas his wife, in his opinion, had become increasingly rigid and unreceptive to new ideas. The prototypic scenario of the male in midlife crisis seeking a divorce was made complete by the presence of the "other woman"—an intelligent, vivacious, attractive woman 15 years younger than himself.

David's therapy was long and complex, and several existential themes emerged during the course of therapy. Responsibility was an important issue in his decision to leave his wife. First, there is the moral sense of responsibility. After all, his wife gave birth to and raised his children and had supported him through graduate school. He and his wife were at an age where he was far more "marketable" than she; that is, he had significantly higher earning power and was biologically able to father children. What moral responsibility, then, did he have to his wife?

David had a high moral sense and would, for the rest of his life, torment himself with this question. It had to be explored in therapy, and, consequently, the therapist confronted him explicitly with the issue of moral responsibility during David's decision-making process. The most effective mode of dealing with this anticipatory dysphoria was to leave no stone unturned in his effort to improve the marriage.

The therapist helped David examine the question of his responsibility for the failure of the marriage. To what degree was he responsible for his wife's mode of being with him? For example, the therapist noted that he himself felt somewhat intimidated by David's quick, facile mind: The therapist also was aware of a concern about being criticized or judged by David. How judgmental was David? Was it not possible that he squelched his wife, that had he engaged differently with her, he might have helped her to develop greater flexibility, spontaneity, and self-awareness?

The therapist also helped David consider whether he was displacing onto the marriage dissatisfaction that belonged elsewhere in his life. A dream pointed the way toward some important dynamics:

> I had a problem with liquefaction of earth near my pool. John [a friend who was dying from cancer] sinks into the ground. It was like quicksand. I used a giant power auger to drill down into the quicksand. I expect to find some kind of void under the ground but instead I found a concrete slab five to six feet down. On the slab I found a receipt of money someone had paid me for $501. I was very anxious in the dream about that receipt since it was greater than it should have been.

One of the major themes of this dream had to do with death and aging. First, there was the theme of his friend who had cancer. David attempted to find his friend by using a giant auger. In the dream, David experienced a great sense of mastery and power during the drilling. The symbol of the auger seemed clearly phallic and initiated a profitable exploration of sexuality—David had always been sexually driven, and the dream illuminated how he used sex (and especially sex with a young woman) as a mode of gaining mastery over aging and death. Finally, he is surprised to find a concrete slab (which elicited associations of morgues, tombs, and tombstones).

He was intrigued by the numerical figures in the dream (the slab was "five to six feet" down and the receipt was for precisely $501). In his associations, David made the interesting observation that he was 50 years old and the night of the dream was his 51st birthday. Though he did not consciously dwell on his age, the dream made it clear that at an unconscious level, he had considerable concern about being over 50. Along with the slab that was between five and six feet deep and the receipt that was just over $500, there was his considerable concern in the dream about the amount cited in the receipt being too great. On a conscious level, he denied his aging.

If David's major distress stemmed from his growing awareness of his aging and diminishment, then a precipitous separation from his wife might have represented an attempt to solve the wrong problem. Consequently, the therapist helped David plunge into a thorough exploration of his feelings about his aging and his mortality. The therapist's view was that only by fully dealing with these issues would he be more able to ascertain the true extent of the marital difficulties. The therapist and David explored these issues over several months. He attempted to deal more honestly with his wife than before, and soon he and his wife made arrangements to see a marital therapist for several months.

After these steps were taken, David and his wife ultimately decided that there was nothing salvageable in the marriage and they separated. The months following his separation were exceedingly difficult. The therapist provided support during this time but did not try to help David eliminate his anxiety; instead, he attempted to help David use his anxiety in a constructive fashion. David's inclination was to rush into an immediate second marriage, whereas the therapist persistently urged him to look at the fear of isolation that on each previous separation had sent him back to his wife. It was important now to be certain that fear did not propel him into an immediate second marriage.

David found it difficult to heed this advice because he felt so much in love with the new woman in his life. The state of being in love is one of the great experiences in life.

In therapy, however, being in love raises many problems; the pull of romantic love is so great that it engulfs even the most well directed therapeutic endeavors. David found his new partner to be the ideal woman, no other woman existed for him, and he attempted to spend all his time with her. When with her, he experienced a state of continual bliss: All aspects of the lonely "I" vanished, leaving only a very blissful state of "we-ness."

What finally made it possible for David to work in therapy was that his new friend became somewhat frightened by the power of his embrace. Only then was he willing to look at his extreme fear of being alone and his reflex desire to merge with a woman. Gradually he became desensitized to being alone. He observed his feelings, kept a journal of them, and worked hard on them in therapy. He noted, for example, that Sundays were the worst time. He had an extremely demanding professional schedule and had no difficulties during the week. Sundays were times of extreme anxiety. He became aware that part of that anxiety was that he had to take care of himself on Sunday. If he wanted to do something, he himself had to schedule the activity. He could no longer rely on that being done for him by his wife. He discovered that an important function of ritual in culture and the heavy scheduling in his own life was to conceal the void, the total lack of structure beneath him.

These observations led him, in therapy, to face his need to be cared for and shielded. The fears of isolation and freedom buffeted him for several months, but gradually he learned how to be alone in the world and what it meant to be responsible for his own being. In short, he learned how to be his own mother and father—always a major therapeutic objective of psychotherapy.

SUMMARY

Existential psychotherapy views the patient as a full person, not as a composite of drives, archetypes, conditioning or irrational beliefs or as a "case." People are regarded as struggling, feeling, thinking, and suffering beings who have hopes, fears, and relationships, who wrestle to create meaningful lives. It takes a life-affirming approach to an essentially tragic view of life. Anxiety will always be present but can be channeled into creative, life-enhancing pursuits. Awareness of the inevitability of death can enrich life.

The original criticism of existential therapy as "too philosophical" has lessened as people recognize that all effective psychotherapy has philosophical implications. The genuine human encounter between patient and therapist engenders possibility of new meanings, new forms of relationship and a possibility of self-actualization. The central aim of the founders of existential psychotherapy was that its emphases would influence therapy of all schools. That this has been occurring is quite clear. Existential therapy is not a technique. It is "an encounter with one's own existence in an immediate and quintessential form" (May, 1967, p. 134) in the company of a therapist who is fully present.

Our present age is one of disintegration of cultural and historical mores, of love and marriage, the family, the inherited religions, and so forth. Given these realities, the existential emphasis on meaning, responsibility, and living a finite life fully will become increasingly important.

ANNOTATED BIBLIOGRAPHY

Becker, E. (1973). *Denial of death*. New York: Free Press.
Pulitzer Prize-winning book. Becker's thesis is that human behavior and mental disorder have their deepest roots in our denying our deaths. The book is a useful resource, particularly for therapists, for reflecting on and coming to terms with death anxiety. Among its topics are meditations on the need for illusions and "immortality projects."

Wheelis, A. (1973). *How people change*. New York: Harper & Row.
This is a short, lyrical, highly readable and accessible book that demonstrates the *attitude* of existential psychotherapy. Wheelis dramatizes the difficulty of intentional change and discusses the need for will, courage, and action in the effort to change.

Yalom, I. (1980). *Existential psychotherapy*. New York: Basic Books.
This is the textbook of existential psychotherapy that elucidates in more detail the ideas presented in this chapter. A major task of the book is to build a bridge between theory and clinical application. It includes many case examples as well as the philosophical foundations of this approach.

Yalom, I. D. (2002). *The gift of therapy*. New York: HarperCollins.
This book includes the wisdom of existential psychotherapy in 85 one- to two-page "lessons." Each lesson is illustrated with a brief case example.

CASE READINGS

Lindner, R. (1987). The jet-propelled couch. In *The Fifty-Minute Hour*. New York: Dell.
A great classic in the psychotherapy literature which, while not directly existential in its thinking, demonstrates that we are all more human than otherwise, that we are, quite literally "fellow travelers." No student of psychotherapy should miss this story.

Yalom, I. D. (1989). *Love's executioner and other tales of psychotherapy*. New York: Basic Books. [A case study from this book, "If Rape Were Legal . . . ," is reprinted in D. Wedding & R. J. Corsini (Eds.). (2011). *Case studies in psychotherapy*. Belmont, CA: Brooks/Cole.]
The actual practice of existential psychotherapy is best illustrated in these longer tales of the therapist–patient encounter. Of note are the examples of how therapist genuineness and self-disclosure foster healing.

Yalom, I. D. (1999). *Momma and the meaning of life*. New York: Basic Books.
More tales of psychotherapy. See especially a story entitled "Seven Lessons in the Therapy of Grief," which demonstrates how slow and complex is the process of resolving grief in the face of death anxiety.

Yalom, I. D., & Elkins, G. (1974). *Everyday gets a little closer*. New York: Basic Books.
An illuminating work in which Yalom and his patient, Ginny Elkins, each keep notes and write a record of their therapy sessions. The final product allows an extraordinary look at how differently patient and therapist experience the therapeutic encounter.

REFERENCES

Becker, E. (1973). *Denial of death*. New York: Free Press.

Binswanger, L. (1958). The case of Ellen West. In R. May, E. Angel, & H. Ellenberger (Eds.), *Existence: A new dimension in psychology and psychiatry* (pp. 237–364). New York: Basic Books.

Buber, M. (1965) *The Knowledge of man*. New York: HarperCollins.

Bugental, J. (1976). *The search for existential identity*. San Francisco: Jossey-Bass.

Frank, J. D., & Frank, J. B. (1991). *Persuasion and healing: A comparative study of psychotherapy* (3rd ed.). Baltimore: Johns Hopkins University Press.

Frankl, V. (1963). *Man's search for meaning: An introduction to logotherapy*. New York: Pocket Books.

Fromm, E. (1941). *Escape from freedom*. New York: Holt.

Fromm, E. (1956). *The art of loving*. New York: Holt.

Gelso, C. J., & Hayes, J. A. (1998). *The psychotherapy relationship: Theory, research, and practice*. New York: Wiley.

Horney, K. (1950). *Neurosis and human growth: The struggle toward self-realization*. New York: W.W. Norton.

Josselson, R. (2007). *Playing Pygmalion: How people create one another*. New York: Rowman & Littlefield.

Jung, C. G. (1966). *Collected works: The practice of psychotherapy* (Vol. 16). New York: Pantheon, Bollingen Series.

Koestenbaum, P. (1978). *The new image of man*. Westport, CT: Greenwood Press.

May, R. (1953). *Man's search for himself*. New York: Norton.

May, R. (1958). Contributions of existential psychotherapy. In R. May, E. Angel, & H. F. Ellenberger (Eds.), *Existence: A new dimension in psychiatry and psychology* (pp. 37–91). New York: Basic Books.

May, R. (1967). *Psychology and the human dilemma*. Princeton, NJ: Van Nostrand.

May, R. (1969). *Love and will*. New York: Norton.

May, R. (1977). *The meaning of anxiety* (rev. ed.). New York: Norton.

May, R. (1981). *Freedom and destiny*. New York: Norton.

May, R. (1991). *The cry for myth*. New York: Norton.

May, R., Angel, E., & Ellenberger, H. F. (Eds.). (1958). *Existence: A new dimension in psychiatry and psychology*. New York: Basic Books.

McAdams, D. P., & Pals, J. L. (2006). A new big five: Fundamental principles for an integrative science of personality. *American Psychologist, 61,* 204–217.

McWilliams, N. (2005). Preserving our humanity as therapists. *Psychotherapy: Theory, Research, Practice, Training, 42*(2), 139–151.

Nabokov, V. (1967). *Speak, memory*. New York: Penguin Books.

Nietzsche, F. (1954) *Thus spake Zarathustra.* (Trans. Thomas Common). New York, Modern Library.

Norcross, J. C. (Ed.). (2002). *Psychotherapy relationships that work: Therapist contributions and responsiveness to patients*. New York: Oxford University Press.

Safran, J. D., & Muran, J. C. (1996). The resolution of ruptures in the therapeutic relationship. *Journal of Consulting and Clinical Psychology, 64,* 447–458.

Sartre, J. P (1956) *Being and nothingness*. New York: Philosophical Library.

Schneider, K. (2007). *Existential–integrative psychotherapy: Guideposts to the core of practice*. New York: Routledge.

Spinoza, Baruch de (1954). *L'Éthique,* (trans) Roger Caillois, Paris: Gallimard/Folio essais.

Tolstoy, L. (1981) *The death of Ivan Ilych.* New York : Bantam books,

Wampold, B. E. (2001). *The great psychotherapy debate*. Mahwah, NJ: Erlbaum.

Wheelis, A. (1999) The *Listener: A Psychoanalyst Examines His Life*. New York: W. W. Norton.

Wheelis, A. (1973). *How people change*. New York: Harper & Row.

Yalom, I. D. (1980). *Existential psychotherapy*. New York: Basic Books.

Yalom, I. D. (1989). *Love's executioner and other tales of psychotherapy*. New York: Basic Books.

Yalom, I. D. (1992). *When Nietzsche wept*. New York: Basic Books/Harper.

Yalom, I. D. (1999). *Momma and the meaning of life*. New York: Basic Books.

Yalom, I. D. (2002). *The gift of therapy*. New York: HarperCollins.

Yalom, I. D. (2005). *The Schopenhauer cure*. New York: HarperCollins.

Yalom, I. D. (with M. Lecscz). (2005). *The theory and practice of group psychotherapy* (5th ed.). New York: Basic Books.

Yalom, I. D. (2008). *Staring at the sun: Overcoming the terror of death*. San Francisco: Jossey-Bass.

Yalom, I. D., & Elkins, G. (1974). *Everyday gets a little closer*. New York: Basic Books.

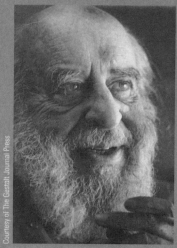

Fritz Perls (1893–1970)

10 | GESTALT THERAPY

Gary Yontef and Lynne Jacobs

OVERVIEW

Gestalt therapy was founded by Frederick "Fritz" Perls and collaborators Laura Perls and Paul Goodman. They synthesized various cultural and intellectual trends of the 1940s and 1950s into a new gestalt, one that provided a sophisticated clinical and theoretical alternative to the two other main theories of their day: behaviorism and classical psychoanalysis.

Gestalt therapy began as a revision of psychoanalysis (F. Perls, 1942/1992) and quickly developed as a wholly independent, integrated system (F. Perls, Hefferline, & Goodman, 1951/1994). Since Gestalt therapy is an experiential and humanistic approach, it works with patients' awareness and awareness skills rather than using the classic psychoanalytic reliance on the analyst's interpretation of the unconscious. Also, in Gestalt therapy, the therapist is actively and personally engaged with the patient rather than fostering transference by remaining in the analytic role of neutrality. In Gestalt therapy theory, a process-based postmodern field theory replaced the mechanistic, simplistic, Newtonian system of classical psychoanalysis.

The Gestalt therapist uses active methods that develop not only patients' awareness but also their repertoires of awareness and behavioral tools. The active methods and active personal engagement of Gestalt therapy are used to increase the awareness, freedom, and self-direction of the patient rather than to direct patients toward preset goals as in behavior therapy and encounter groups.

The Gestalt therapy system is truly integrative and includes affective, sensory, cognitive, interpersonal, and behavioral components (Joyce & Sills, 2009). In Gestalt therapy, therapists and patients are encouraged to be creative in doing the awareness work. There are no prescribed or proscribed techniques in Gestalt therapy.

Basic Concepts

Holism and Field Theory

Most humanistic theories of personality are holistic. Holism asserts that humans are inherently self-regulating, that they are growth oriented, and that persons and their symptoms cannot be understood apart from their environment. Holism and field theory are interrelated in Gestalt theory. Field theory is a way of understanding how one's context influences one's experiencing. Field theory, described elegantly by Einstein's theory of relativity, is a theory about the nature of reality and our relationship to reality. It represents one of the first attempts to articulate a contextualist view of reality (Philippson, 2001). Field theory, born in science, was an early contributor to the current postmodern sensibility that influences nearly all psychological theories today. Schools of thought that emphasize dependence on context build upon the work of Einstein and other field theorists. The combination of field theory, holism, and Gestalt psychology forms the bedrock for the Gestalt theory of personality.

Fields have certain properties that lead to a specific contextual theory. As with all contextual theories, a field is understood to be composed of mutually interdependent elements. But there are other properties as well. For one thing, variables that contribute to shaping a person's behavior and experience are said to be present in one's current field, and therefore, people cannot be understood without understanding the field, or context, in which they live. A patient's life story cannot tell you what actually happened in his or her past, but it can tell you how the patient experiences his or her history in the here and now. That rendition of history is shaped to some degree by the patient's current field conditions.

What happened 3 years ago is not a part of the current field and therefore cannot affect one's experience. What *does* shape one's experience is how one holds a memory of the event, and also the fact that an event 3 years ago has altered how one may organize one's perception in the field. Another property of the field is that the organization of one's experience occurs in the here and now and is ongoing and subject to change based on field conditions. Also, no one can transcend embeddedness in a field; therefore, all attributions about the nature of reality are *relative* to the subject's position in the field. Field theory renounces the belief that anyone, including a therapist, can have an objective perspective on reality.

The *Paradoxical Theory of Change* is the heart of the Gestalt therapy approach (Beisser, 1970). The paradox is that the more one tries to become who one is not, the more one stays the same. Health is largely a matter of being whole, and healing occurs when one is made whole again. The more one tries to force oneself into a mold that does not fit, the more one is fragmented rather than whole.

Organismic self-regulation requires knowing and owning—that is, identifying with—what one senses, feels emotionally, observes, needs or wants, and believes. Growth starts with conscious awareness of what is occurring in one's current existence, including how one is affected and how one affects others. One moves toward wholeness by identifying with ongoing experience, being in contact with what is actually happening, identifying and trusting what one genuinely feels and wants, and being honest with self and others about what one is actually able and willing to do—or not willing to do.

When one knows, senses, and feels one's self here and now, including the possibilities for change, one can be fully present, accepting or changing what is not satisfying.

Living in the past, worrying about the future, and/or clinging to illusions about what one should be or could have been diminishes emotional and conscious awareness and the immediacy of experience that is the key to organismic living and growth.

Gestalt therapy aims for self-knowledge, acceptance, and growth by immersion in current existence, aligning contact, awareness, and experimentation with what is actually happening at the moment. It focuses on the here and now, not on what should be, could be, or was. From this present-centered focus, one can become clear about one's needs, wishes, goals, and values.

The concepts emphasized in Gestalt therapy are contact, conscious awareness, and experimentation. Each concept is described below.

Contact means being in touch with what is emerging here and now, moment to moment. *Conscious awareness* is a focusing of attention on what one is in touch with in situations requiring such attention. Awareness, or focused attention, is needed in situations that require higher contact ability, situations involving complexity or conflict, and situations in which habitual modes of thinking and acting are not working and in which one does not learn from experience. For example, in a situation that produces numbness, one can focus on the experience of numbness and cognitive clarity can emerge.

Experimentation is the act of trying something new in order to increase understanding. The experiment may result in enhanced emotions or in the realization of something that had been kept from awareness. Experimentation, trying something new, is an alternative to the purely verbal methods of psychoanalysis and the behavior control techniques of behavior therapy.

Trying something new, without commitment to either the status quo or the adoption of a new pattern, can facilitate organismic growth. For example, patients often repeat stories of unhappy events without giving any evidence of having achieved increased clarity or relief. In this situation, a Gestalt therapist might suggest that the patient express affect directly to the person involved (either in person or through role playing). The patient often experiences relief and the emergence of other feelings, such as sadness or appreciation.

Contact, awareness, and experimentation have technical meanings, but these terms are also used in a colloquial way. The Gestalt therapist improves his or her practice by knowing the technical definitions. However, for the sake of this introductory chapter, we will try to use the colloquial form of these terms. Gestalt therapy starts with the therapist making contact with the patient by getting in touch with what the patient and therapist are experiencing and doing. The therapist helps the patient focus on and clarify what he or she is in contact with and deepens the exploration by helping focus the patient's awareness.

Awareness Process

Gestalt therapy focuses on the awareness process—in other words, on the continuum of one's flow of awareness. People have patterned processes of awareness that become foci for the work of therapy. This focus enables the patient to become clear about what he or she thinks, feels, and decides in the current moment—and about how he or she does it. This includes a focus on what does not come to awareness. Careful attention to the sequence of the patient's continuum of awareness and observation of nonverbal behavior can help a patient recognize interruptions of contact and become aware of what has been kept out of awareness. For example, whenever Jill starts to look sad, she does not report feeling sad but moves immediately into anger. The anger cannot end as long as it functions to block Jill's sadness and vulnerability. In this situation, Jill can not only gain awareness of her sadness but also gain in skill at self-monitoring by being made aware of her tendency to block her sadness.

That second order of awareness (how she interrupts awareness of her sadness) is referred to as awareness of one's awareness process.

Awareness of awareness can empower by helping the patient gain greater access to himself or herself and clarify processes that had been confusing, improving the accuracy of perception and unblocking previously blocked emotional energy (Joyce & Sills, 2009). Jill had felt stymied by her lover's defensive reaction to her anger. When she realized that she actually felt hurt and sad, and not just angry, she could express her vulnerability, hurt, and sadness. Her lover was much more receptive to this than he was to her anger. In further work, Jill realized that blocking her sadness resulted from being shamed by her family when, as a child, she had expressed hurt feelings.

The Gestalt therapist focuses on the patient's awareness and contact processes with respect, compassion, and commitment to the validity of the patient's subjective reality. The therapist models the process by disclosing his or her own awareness and experience. The therapist is present in as mutual a way as possible in the therapeutic relationship and takes responsibility for his or her own behavior and feelings. In this way, the therapist can be active and make suggestions but also can fully accept the patient in a manner consistent with the paradoxical theory of change.

Other Systems

In the decades up to and including the 1970s, it seemed simple to compare Gestalt therapy with other systems. There were three major systems: classical Freudian psychoanalysis, behavior therapy, and the existential and humanistic therapies. In the 1960s, Gestalt therapy became the most visible of the humanistic existential therapies and a salient alternative to psychoanalysis and behavior modification. However, the theoretical boundaries supporting various schools of therapy have become less distinct over the ensuing decades.

Classical Freudian Psychoanalysis and Gestalt Therapy

At the heart of Freudian psychoanalysis was a belief in the centrality of basic biological drives and in the establishment of relatively permanent structures created by the inevitable conflict between these basic drives and social demands—both legitimate demands and those stemming from parental and societal neurosis. All human development, behavior, thinking, and feeling were believed to be determined by these unconscious biological and social conflicts.

Patients' statements of their feelings, thoughts, beliefs, and wishes were not considered reliable because they were assumed to disguise deeper motivations stemming from the unconscious. The unconscious was a structure to which the patient did not have direct access, at least before completing analysis. However, the unconscious manifested itself in the transference neurosis, and through the analyst's interpretation of the transference, "truth" was discovered and understood.

Psychoanalysis proceeded by a simple paradigm. Through free association (talking without censoring or focusing), the patient provided data for psychoanalytic treatment. These data were interpreted by the analyst according to the particular version of drive theory that he or she espoused. The analyst provided no details about his or her own life or person. He or she was supposed to be completely objective, eschewing all emotional reactions. The analyst had two fundamental rules: the *rule of abstinence* (gratifying no patient wish) and the *rule of neutrality* (having no preferences in the patient's conflict). Any deviation by the analyst was considered countertransference. Any attempt by the patient to know something about the analyst was interpreted as resistance, and any ideas about the analyst were considered a projection from the unconscious of the patient.

Although interpretation of the transference helped bring the focus back to the here and now, unfortunately, the potential of the here-and-now relationship is not realized in classical psychoanalysis because the focus is drawn away from the actual contemporaneous relationship, and the patients' feelings are interpreted as the result of unconscious drives and unresolved conflicts. Discussion in psychoanalysis is usually focused on the past and not on what is actually happening between analyst and patient *in the moment.*

This simple summary of psychoanalysis is not completely accurate, because Adler, Rank, Jung, Reich, Horney, Fromm, Sullivan, and other analysts deviated from core Freudian assumptions in many ways and provided the soil from which the Gestalt therapy system arose. In these derivative systems, as in Gestalt therapy, the pessimistic Freudian view of a patient driven by unconscious forces was replaced by a belief in the potential for human growth and by appreciation for the power of relationships and conscious awareness. These approaches did not limit the data to free association; instead, they valued an explicitly compassionate attitude by the therapist and allowed a wider range of interventions. However, these approaches were still fettered by remaining in the psychoanalytic tradition. Gestalt therapy took a more radical position.

Behavior modification provided a simple alternative: Observe the behavior, disregard the subjective reports of the patient, and control problematic behavior by using either classical or operant conditioning to manipulate stimulus–response relationships. In the behavioral approaches, the emphasis was on what could be measured, counted, and "scientifically" proved.

The behavioral approach was the inverse of the intrapsychic approach of Freudian psychoanalysis. Here-and-now behavior was observed and taken as important data in its own right, but the patient's subjective, conscious experience was not considered reliable data.

A third choice was provided by Gestalt therapy. In Gestalt therapy, the patient's awareness is not assumed to be merely a cover for some other, deeper motivation. Unlike psychoanalysis, Gestalt therapy uses any and all available data. Like behavior modification, Gestalt therapy carefully observes behavior, including observation of the body, and it focuses on the here and now and uses active methods. The patient's self-report is considered real data. And, in a departure from both behavior modification and psychoanalysis, the therapist and the patient codirect the work of therapy.

Client–Centered Therapy, Rational Emotive Behavior Therapy, and Gestalt Therapy

Gestalt therapy and client-centered therapy share common roots and philosophy. Both believe in the potential for human growth, and both believe that growth results from a relationship in which the therapist is experienced as warm and authentic (congruent). Both client-centered and Gestalt therapy are phenomenological therapies that work with the subjective awareness of the patient. However, Gestalt therapy has a more active phenomenological approach. The Gestalt therapy phenomenology is an experimental phenomenology. The patient's subjective experience is made clearer by using awareness experiments. These experiments are often similar to behavioral techniques, but they are designed to clarify the patient's awareness rather than to control her or his behavior.

Another difference is that the Gestalt therapist is more inclined to think in terms of an encounter in which the subjectivity of both patient and therapist is valued. The Gestalt therapist is much more likely than a person-centered therapist to tell the patient about his or her own feelings or experience.

Gestalt therapy provides an alternative to both the confrontational approach of rational emotive behavior therapy (REBT) and the nondirective approach of

Carl Rogers. A person-centered therapist completely trusts the patient's subjective report, whereas a practitioner of REBT confronts the patient, often quite actively, about his or her irrational or dysfunctional ways of thinking. Gestalt therapy uses focused awareness experiments and personal disclosure to help patients enlarge their awareness. (During the 1960s and 1970s, Fritz Perls popularized a very confrontive model for dealing with avoidance, but this model is not representative of Gestalt therapy as it is practiced today.)

Gestalt therapy has become more like the person-centered approach in two important ways. First, Gestalt therapists have become more supportive, compassionate, and kind. In addition, it has become clear that the therapist does not have an "objective" truth that is more accurate than the truth that the patient experiences.

Newer Models of Psychoanalysis and Relational Gestalt Therapy

There have been parallel developments in Gestalt therapy and psychoanalysis. Although the concept of the relationship in Gestalt therapy was modeled on Martin Buber's I–Thou relationship, it was not well explicated until the late 1980s (Hycner, 1985; Jacobs, 1989; Yontef, 1993). In its emerging focus on the relationship, Gestalt therapy has moved away from classical psychoanalysis and drive theory, away from confrontation as a desired therapeutic tool, and away from the belief that the therapist is healthy and the patient is sick.

Psychoanalysis has undergone a similar paradigm shift, and the two systems have somewhat converged. This is possible in part because contemporary psychoanalytic theories (especially relational and intersubjective theories) have rejected the limitations of classical Freudian psychoanalysis. The new theories eschew reductionism and determinism and reject the tendency to minimize the patient's own perspective. This movement brings psychoanalysis closer to the theory and practice of Gestalt therapy. Gestalt therapy was formed in reaction to the same aspects of psychoanalysis that contemporary psychoanalysis is now rejecting.

Basic tenets now shared by contemporary psychoanalysis and Gestalt therapy include the following: an emphasis on the whole person and sense of self; an emphasis on process thinking; an emphasis on subjectivity and affect; an appreciation of the impact of life events (such as childhood sexual abuse) on personality development; a belief that people are motivated toward growth and development rather than regression; a belief that infants are born with a basic motivation and capacity for personal interaction, attachment, and satisfaction; a belief that there is no "self" without an "other"; and a belief that the structure and contents of the mind are shaped by interactions with others rather than by instinctual urges. It is meaningless to speak of a person in isolation from the relationships that shape and define his or her life.

Cognitive Behavior Therapy, REBT, and Gestalt Therapy

The assumption that Gestalt therapy does not engage with patients' thinking processes is inaccurate. Gestalt therapy has always paid attention to what the patient is thinking. Gestalt therapists, like their cognitive therapy colleagues, stress the role of "futurizing" in creating anxiety and, like REBT therapists, discuss the creation of guilt by moralistic thinking and thoughts of unreasonable conditions of worth ("shoulds"). Many of the thoughts that would be labeled irrational in REBT or cognitive behavior therapy have also traditionally been an important focus for Gestalt therapy.

There is one major difference between contemporary Gestalt therapy and REBT or cognitive behavior therapy. In modern Gestalt therapy, the therapist does not pretend to know the truth about what is irrational. The Gestalt therapist observes the process, directs the patient to observe his or her thoughts, and explores alternate ways of thinking in a manner that values and respects what the patient experiences and comes to believe.

HISTORY

Precursors

Gestalt therapy was less a font of substantial original "discoveries" than a groundbreaking integrative system for understanding personality and therapy that developed out of a seedbed of rich and varied sources. Fritz and Laura Perls, and the later American collaborators with whom they wrote, taught, and practiced from the 1940s through the 1960s (Isadore From, Paul Goodman, and others), swam in the turbulent waters of the 20th-century revolutions in science, philosophy, religion, psychology, art, literature, and politics. There was tremendous cross-fertilization between intellectuals in all disciplines during this period.

Frankfurt-am-Main of the 1920s, where Fritz Perls got his M.D. and Laura Perls her D.Sc., was a center of intellectual ferment in psychology. They were directly or indirectly exposed to leading Gestalt psychologists, existential and phenomenological philosophers, liberal theologians, and psychoanalytic thinkers.

Fritz Perls was intimately acquainted with psychoanalysis and in fact was a training analyst. However, Perls chafed under the dogmatism of classical psychoanalysis. For Perls, the revolutionary basic idea that Freud brought to Western culture—the existence of motivations that lay outside of conscious awareness—had to be woven into other streams of thought, particularly holism, Gestalt psychology, field theory, phenomenology, and existentialism.

These intellectual disciplines, each in its own way, were attempting to create a new vision of what it means to be human. Their vision came to be called a "humanistic" vision, and Gestalt therapy introduced that vision into the world of psychotherapy. Freudian analysts asserted the essential truth that human life is biologically determined, conflicted, and in need of constraint; the existentialists asserted the primacy of existence over essence, the belief that people choose the direction of their lives, and the argument that human life is not biologically determined. Within psychoanalysis, Perls was influenced by the more renegade analysts, especially Otto Rank and Wilhelm Reich. Both Rank and Reich emphasized conscious experience, the body as carrier of emotional wisdom and conflicts, and the active process of engagement between the therapist and the patient in the here and now. Reich introduced the important notion of "character armor"—repetitive patterns of experience, behavior, and body posture that keep the individual in fixed, socially determined roles. Reich also thought that how a patient spoke or moved was more important than what the patient said.

Rank emphasized the creative powers and uniqueness of the individual and argued that the client was his or her own best therapist. Like Fritz Perls, Rank stressed the importance of the experience of the here-and-now therapeutic relationship.

Providing a major source of inspiration to Fritz and Laura Perls were European continental philosophers who were breaking away from Cartesian dualism, arguing that the split between subject and object, self and world, was an illusion. These included the existentialists, the phenomenologists, and philosophers such as Ludwig Wittgenstein.

The new approach was influenced by field theory, the Gestalt psychologists, the holism of Jan Smuts, and Zen thought and practice. This thinking was blended by Fritz Perls with the Gestalt psychology of figure/ground perception and with the strongly Gestalt-psychology-influenced work of psychologists Kurt Goldstein and Kurt Lewin (Wulf, 1998).

In his first book, *Ego, Hunger and Aggression* (1942/1992), Perls described people as embedded in a person–environment field; this field was developed by the emergence into consciousness of those needs that organized perception. Perls also wrote about a "creative indifference" that enables a person to differentiate according to what is really needed in a particular situation. With the differentiation emerges the experience of contrast and awareness of the polarities that shape our experience of ourselves as separate. Perls thought of this as a Western equivalent to the Eastern practice of Zen (Wulf, 1998).

Fritz and Laura left Germany during the Nazi era and later fled Nazi-occupied Holland. They went to South Africa, where they started a psychoanalytic training center. During this same period, Jan Smuts, South African prime minister in the 1940s, coined the term *holism* and wrote about it. In time, Fritz and Laura Perls left South Africa because of the beginning of the apartheid policies that Jan Smuts helped to initiate.

The fundamental precept of *holism* is that the organism is a self-regulating entity. For Fritz Perls, Gestalt psychology, organismic theory, field theory, and holism formed a happy union. Gestalt psychology provided Perls with the organizing principles for Gestalt therapy, as well as with a cognitive scheme that would integrate the varied influences in his life.

The word *Gestalt* has no literal English translation. It refers to a perceptual whole or configuration of experience. People do not perceive in bits and pieces, which are then added up to form an organized perception; instead, they perceive in patterned wholes. Patterns reflect an interrelationship among elements such that the whole cannot be gleaned by a study of component parts, but only by a study of the relationship of parts to each other and to the whole. The leading figures in the development of Gestalt psychology were Max Wertheimer, Kurt Koffka, and Wolfgang Kohler.

Kurt Lewin extended this work by applying Gestalt principles to areas other than simple perceptual psychology and by explicating the theoretical implications of Gestalt psychology. He is especially well known for his explication of the field theory philosophy of Gestalt psychology, although this concept did not originate with him. Lewin (1938) discussed the principles by which field theory differed from Newtonian and positivistic thinking. In field theory, the world is studied as a systematic web of relationships, continuous in time, and not as discrete or dichotomous particles. In this view, everything is in the process of becoming, and nothing is static. Reality in this field view is configured by the relationship between the observer and the observed. "Reality," then, is a function of perspective, not a true positivist fact. There may be multiple realities of equal legitimacy. Such a view of the nature of reality opens Gestalt theory to a variety of formerly disenfranchised voices, such as those of women, gays, and non-Europeans.

Lewin carried on the work of the Gestalt psychologists by hypothesizing and researching the idea that a Gestalt is formed by the interaction between environmental possibilities and organismic needs. Needs organize perception and action. Perception is organized by the state of the person-in-relation and the environmental surround. A Gestalt therapy theory of organismic functioning was based on the Gestalt psychology principles of perception and holism. The theory of organismic self-regulation became a cornerstone of the Gestalt therapy theory of personality.

The philosophical tenets of phenomenology and existentialism were popular during the Perlses' years in Germany and in the United States. Gestalt therapy was influenced profoundly by the work of the dialogic existential thinkers, especially Martin Buber, with whom Laura Perls studied directly. Buber's belief in the inextricable existential fact that a self is always a self-with-other was a natural fit with Gestalt thinking, and his theory of the I–Thou relation became, through the teachings of Laura Perls, the basis for the patient–therapist relationship in Gestalt therapy.

Beginnings

Although Fritz Perls's earliest publication was *Ego, Hunger and Aggression* (1942/1992), the first comprehensive integration of Gestalt therapy system is found in *Gestalt Therapy* (F. Perls et al., 1951/1994). This seminal publication represented the synthesis, integration, and new Gestalt formed by the authors' exposure to the intellectual zeitgeist described above. A New York Institute of Gestalt Therapy was soon formed, and the early seminar participants became teachers who spread the word to other cities by running regular training workshops, especially in New York, Cleveland, Miami, and Los Angeles. Intensive study groups formed in each of these cities. Learning was supplemented by the regular workshops of the original study group members, and eventually all of these cities developed their own Gestalt training institutes. The Gestalt Institute of Cleveland has made a special effort to bring in trainees from varied backgrounds and to develop a highly diverse faculty.

Gestalt therapy pioneered many ideas that have influenced humanistic psychotherapy. For instance, Gestalt therapy has a highly developed methodology for attending to experience phenomenologically and for attending to how the therapist and patient experience each other in the therapeutic relationship. *Phenomenology* assumes the reality is formed in the relationship between the observed and the observer. In short, reality is interpreted.

The dialogic relationship in Gestalt therapy derived three important principles from Martin Buber's thought (Jacobs, 1989). First, in a dialogic therapeutic relationship, the therapist practices inclusion, which is similar to empathic engagement. In this, the therapist puts himself or herself into the experience of the patient, imagines the existence of the other, feels it as if it were a sensation within his or her own body, and simultaneously maintains a sense of self. Inclusion is a developed form of contact rather than a merger with the experience of the patient. Through imagining the patient's experience in this way, the dialogic therapist confirms the existence and potential of the patient. Second, the therapist discloses himself or herself as a person who is authentic and congruent and someone who is striving to be transparent and self-disclosing. Third, the therapist in dialogic therapy is committed to the dialogue, surrenders to what happens between the participants, and thus does not control the outcome. In such a relationship, the therapist is changed as well as the patient.

Underlying most existential thought is the existential phenomenological method. Gestalt therapy's phenomenology is a blend of the existential phenomenology of Edmund Husserl and the phenomenology of Gestalt psychology.

Phenomenological understanding is achieved by taking initial perceptions and separating what is actually experienced at the moment from what was expected or merely logically derived. The phenomenological method increases the clarity of awareness by descriptively studying the awareness process. In order to do this, phenomenologists put aside assumptions, especially assumptions about what constitutes valid data. All data are considered valid initially, although they are likely to be refined by continuing phenomenological exploration. This is quite consistent with the Gestalt therapy view that the patient's awareness is valid and should be explored rather than explained away in terms of unconscious motivation.

Although other theories have not fully incorporated the I–Thou relation or systematic phenomenological focusing, they have been influenced by the excitement and vitality of direct contact between therapist and patient; the emphasis on direct experience; the use of experimentation; emphasis on the here and now, emotional process, and awareness; trust in organismic self-regulation; emphasis on choice; and attention to the patient's context as well as his or her inner world.

Current Status

Gestalt Institutes, literature, and journals have proliferated worldwide in the past 55 years. There is at least one Gestalt therapy training center in every major city in the United States, and there are numbers of Gestalt therapy training institutes in most countries of Europe, North and South America, Australia, and Asia. Gestalt therapists practice all over the world.

Various countries and regions have begun to form umbrella organizations that sponsor professional meetings, set standards, and support research and public education. The Association for the Advancement of Gestalt Therapy is an international membership organization. This organization is not limited to professionals. The association was formed with the intention of governing itself through adherence to Gestalt therapy principles enacted at an organizational level. Regional conferences are also sponsored by a European Gestalt therapy association, the European Association for Gestalt Therapy, and by an Australian and New Zealand association, GANZ.

Gestalt therapy is known for a rich oral tradition, and historically, Gestalt writings have not reflected the full depth of its theory and practice. Gestalt therapy has tended to attract therapists inclined to an experiential approach. The Gestalt therapy approach is almost impossible to teach without a strong experiential component.

Since the publication of a seminal book by the Polsters (Polster & Polster, 1973), the gap between the oral and written traditions of Gestalt therapy has closed. There is now an extensive Gestalt therapy literature, and a growing number of books address various aspects of Gestalt therapy theory and practice. There are now five English-language Gestalt journals: the *International Gestalt Journal* (formerly *The Gestalt Journal*), the *British Gestalt Journal,* the *Gestalt Review, Studies in Gestalt Therapy–Dialogical Bridges,* and the *Gestalt Journal of Australia and New Zealand.* The Gestalt Journal Press also lists a comprehensive bibliography of Gestalt books, articles, videotapes, and audiotapes. This listing can be accessed through the Internet at www.gestalt.org. Another Internet site, *Gestalt! (www.g-gej.org),* provides resources for articles and research and is also an online journal. Gestalt therapy literature has also flourished around the world. There is at least one journal in most languages in Europe, North and South America, and Australia. In addition to the books written in English, translated, and widely read in other countries, there have been important original theoretical works published in French, German, Italian, Portuguese Danish, Korean, and Spanish.

The past decade has witnessed a major shift in Gestalt therapy's understanding of personality and therapy. There has been a growing, albeit sometimes controversial, change in understanding the relational conditions for growth, both in general and (especially) in the therapeutic relationship. There is an increased appreciation for interdependence, a better understanding of the shaming effect of the cultural value placed on self-sufficiency, and greater realization of how shame is created in childhood and triggered in interpersonal relationships (Fairfield & O'Shea, 2008; Jacobs, 2005b; Lee, 2004; Lee & Wheeler, 1996; Yontef, 1993). As Gestalt therapists have come to understand shame and its triggers more thoroughly, they have become less confrontive and more accepting and supportive than in earlier years (Jacobs, 1996).

PERSONALITY

Theory of Personality

Gestalt therapy theory has a highly developed, somewhat complicated theory of personality. The notions of healthy functioning and neurotic functioning are actually quite simple and clear, but they are built upon a paradigm shift, not always easy to grasp, from linear cause-and-effect thinking to a process, field theory world view.

Gestalt therapy is a radical ecological theory that maintains there is no meaningful way to consider any living organism apart from its interactions with its environment—that is, apart from the organism–environment field of which it is a part (F. Perls et al., 1951/1994). Psychologically, there is no meaningful way to consider a person apart from interpersonal relations just as there is no meaningful way to perceive the environment except through someone's perspective. According to Gestalt therapy field theory, it is impossible for perception to be totally "objective."

The "field" that human beings inhabit is replete with other human beings. In Gestalt theory, there is no self separate from one's organism/environmental field; more specifically, self does not exist without other. Self implies self-in-relation. Contact is an integral aspect of all experience—in fact, experience does not exist without contact—but it is the contact between humans that dominates the formation and functions of our personalities.

The field is differentiated by *boundaries*. The contact boundary has dual functions: It connects people with each other but also maintains separation. Without emotional connecting with others, one starves; without emotional separation, one does not maintain a separate, autonomous identity. Connecting meets biological, social, and psychological needs; separation creates and maintains autonomy and protects against harmful intrusion or overload.

Needs are met and people grow through contact with and withdrawal from others. By separating and connecting, a person establishes boundary and identity. Effective self-regulation includes contact in which one is aware of what is newly emerging that may be either nourishing or harmful. One identifies with that which is nourishing and rejects that which is harmful. This kind of differentiated contact leads to growth (Polster & Polster, 1973). The crucial processes regulating this discrimination are awareness and contact.

The most important processes for psychological growth are interactions in which two persons each acknowledge the experience of the other with awareness and respect for the needs, feelings, beliefs, and customs of the other. This form of dialogic contact is essential in therapy.

Organismic Self-Regulation

Gestalt therapy theory holds that people are inherently self-regulating, context-sensitive, and motivated to solve their own problems. Needs and desires are organized hierarchically so that one's most urgent need takes precedence and claims one's attention until this need is met. When this need is met, the next need or interest becomes the center of one's attention.

Gestalt (Figure/Ground) Formation

A corollary to the concept of organismic self-regulation is called Gestalt formation. Gestalt psychology has taught us that we perceive in unified wholes and also that we perceive through the phenomenon of contrast. A figure of interest forms in contrast to a relatively dull background. For instance, the words on this page are a visual figure to the reader, whereas other aspects of the room are visually less clear and vivid until this reference to them leads the reader to allow the words on the page to slip into the background, at which time the figure of a table, chair, book, or soda emerges. One can only perceive one clear figure at a time, although figures and grounds may shift very rapidly.

Consciousness and Unconsciousness

A most important consequence of adapting Gestalt psychology to a theory of personality functioning is that ideas about consciousness and unconsciousness are radically different from those of Freud. Freud believed the unconscious was filled with impersonal, biologically based urges that constantly pressed for release. Competent functioning depended on the successful use of repression and sublimation to keep the contents of the unconscious hidden; these urges could be experienced only in symbolic form.

Gestalt therapy's "unconscious" is quite different. In Gestalt therapy theory, the concepts of awareness and unawareness replace the unconscious. Gestalt therapists use the concepts of awareness/unawareness to reflect the belief in the fluidity between what is momentarily in awareness and what is momentarily outside of awareness. When something vital, powerful, and relevant is not allowed to emerge into foreground, one is unaware. What is background is, for the moment, outside of awareness, but it could instantly become the figure in awareness. This is in keeping with the Gestalt psychology understanding of perception, which is the formation of a figure against a background.

In neurotic patients, some aspect of the phenomenal field is purposely and regularly relegated to the background. This concept is roughly similar to the Freudian dynamic unconscious. However, Gestalt therapists do not believe in a "primary process" unconscious that needs to be translated by the therapist before it can be comprehensible to the patient.

Gestalt therapists maintain that what is being relegated to permanent background status reflects the patient's current conflicts as well as the patient's perspective on current field conditions. When a patient perceives the conditions of the therapy relationship to be safe enough, more and more aspects of previously sequestered subjective states can be brought into awareness through the therapeutic dialogue.

Health

The Gestalt therapy notion of health is actually quite simple. In healthy organismic self-regulation, one is aware of shifting need states; that is, what is of most importance becomes the figure of one's awareness. Being whole, then, is simply identifying with one's ongoing, moment-by-moment experiencing and allowing this identification to organize one's behavior.

Healthy organismic awareness includes awareness of the human and nonhuman environment and is not unreflective or inconsiderate of the needs of others. For example, compassion, love, and care for the environment are all part of organismic functioning.

Healthy functioning requires being in contact with what is actually occurring in the person–environment field. Contact is the quality of being in touch with one's experience in relation to the field. By being aware of what is emerging and by allowing action to be organized by what is emerging, people interact in the world and learn from the experience. By trying something new, one learns what works and what does not work in various situations. When a figure is not allowed to emerge, when it is somehow interrupted or misdirected, there is a disturbance in awareness and contact.

Tendency Toward Growth

Gestalt therapists believe that people are inclined toward growth and will develop as fully as conditions allow. Gestalt therapy is holistic and asserts that people are inherently self-regulating and growth-oriented and that people and their behavior, including symptoms, cannot be understood apart from their environment.

Gestalt therapy is interested in the existential themes of existence—connection and separation, life and death, choice and responsibility, authenticity and freedom. Gestalt therapy's theory of awareness is a bedrock phenomenological orientation toward experience derived from an existential and humanistic ethos. Gestalt therapy attempts to understand human beings by the study of experience. Meaning is understood in terms of what is experienced and how it is experienced.

Life Is Relational

Gestalt therapy regards awareness and human relations as inseparable. Awareness develops in early childhood through a matrix of relations that continues throughout life.

Relationships are regulated by how people experience them. People define themselves by how they experience themselves in relation to others. This derives from how people are regarded by others and how they think and behave toward others. In Gestalt therapy theory, derived from Martin Buber, there is no "I," no sense of self, other than self in relation to others. There is only the "I" of the "I–Thou" or the "I" of the "I–[I]t." As Buber said, "All real living is meeting" (1923/1970, p. 11).

Living is a progression of needs, met and unmet. One achieves homeostatic balance and moves on to whatever need emerges next. In health, the boundary is permeable enough to allow exchange with that which promotes health (connecting) and firm enough to preserve autonomy and exclude that which is unhealthful (separation). This requires the identification of those needs that are most pressing at a particular time and in a particular environment.

Variety of Concepts

Disturbances at the Boundary

Under optimal conditions, there is ongoing movement between connecting and withdrawal. When the experience of coming together is blocked repetitively, one is left in a state of *isolation,* which is a boundary disturbance. It is a disturbance because it is fixed, does not respond to a whole range of needs, and fails to allow close contact to emerge. By the same token, if the need to withdraw is blocked, there is a corresponding boundary disturbance, known as *confluence.* Confluence is the loss of the experience of separate identity.

In optimal functioning, when something is taken in—whether it is an idea, food, or love—there is contact and awareness. The person makes discriminations about what to take in and what meaning to attach to that which is taken in. When things (ideas, identity, beliefs, and so on) are taken in without awareness, the boundary disturbance of *introjection* results. Introjects are not fully integrated into organismic functioning.

In order for one to integrate and be whole, what is taken in must be assimilated. *Assimilation* is the process of experiencing what is to be taken in, deconstructing it, keeping what is useful, and discarding what is not. For example, the process of assimilation allows the listener to select and keep only what is useful from a lecture she or he attends.

When a phenomenon that occurs in one's self is falsely attributed to another person in an effort to avoid awareness of one's own experience, the boundary disturbance of *projection* occurs. When an impulse or desire is turned into a one-person event instead of a two-person event (an example is caressing oneself when one wants another person to do the [caressing]), there is the boundary disturbance of *retroflection.* In each of these processes, some part of the person is disowned and not allowed to become figural or to organize and energize action.

Creative Adjustment

When all the pieces are put together, people function according to an overarching principle called creative adjustment. "All contact is creative adjustment of the organism and the environment" (F. Perls et al., 1951/1994, p. 230/6). All organisms live in an environment to which they must adjust. Nevertheless, people also need to shape the environment so that it conforms to human needs and values.

The concept of creative adjustment follows from the notion that people are growth oriented and will try to solve their problems in living in the best way possible. This means solving the problem in a way that makes the fullest use of their own resources and those of the environment. Since awareness can be concentrated on only one figure at a time, those processes that are not the object of creative awareness operate in a habitual mode of adjustment until it is their turn to come into full awareness.

The term *creative adjustment* reflects a creative balance between changing the environment and adjusting to current conditions. Since people live only in relation, they must balance adjusting to the demands of the situation (such as societal demands and the needs of others) and creating something new according to their own, individual interests. This is a continual, mutual, reciprocal negotiation between one's self and one's environment.

The process whereby a need becomes figural, is acted on, and then recedes as a new figure emerges is called a *Gestalt formation cycle.* Every Gestalt formation cycle requires creative adjustment. Both sides of the polarity are necessary for the resolution of a state of need. If one is hungry, one must eat new food taken from the environment. Food that has already been eaten will not solve the problem. New actions must occur, and the environment must be contacted and adapted to meet the individual's needs.

On the other hand, one cannot be so balanced on the side of creating new experience that one does not draw on prior learning and experience, established wisdom, and societal mores. For example, one must use yesterday's learning to be able to recognize aspects of the environment that might be used as a source of food, while at the same time being creative in experimenting with new food possibilities.

Maturity

Good health has the characteristics of a good Gestalt. A *good Gestalt* consists of a perceptual field organized with clarity and good form. A well-formed figure clearly stands out against a broader and less distinct background. The relation between that which stands out (figure) and the context (ground) is meaning. In a good Gestalt, meaning is clear.

Health and maturity result from creative adjustment that occurs in a context of environmental possibility. Both health and maturity require a person whose Gestalt formation process is freely functioning and one whose contact and awareness processes are relatively free of excessive anxiety, inhibition, or habitual selective attention.

In health, the figure changes as needed; that is, it shifts to another focus when a need is met or superseded by a more urgent need. It does not change so rapidly as to prevent satisfaction (as in hysteria) or so slowly that new figures have no room to assume dominance (as in compulsivity). When the figure and ground are dichotomized, one is left with a figure out of context or a context without focus (as in impulsivity) (F. Perls et al., 1951/1994).

The healthy person is in creative adjustment with the environment. The person adjusts to the needs of the environment and adjusts the environment to his or her own needs. Adjustment alone is conformity and breeds stagnation. On the other hand, unbridled creativity in the service of the isolated individual would result in pathological narcissism.

Disrupted Personality Functioning

Mental illness is simply the inability to form clear figures of interest and identify with one's moment-by-moment experience and/or to respond to what one becomes aware of. People whose contact and awareness processes are disrupted often have been shaped by environments that were chronically impoverished. Impoverished environments diminish one's capacity for creative adjustment.

However, even neurotic self-regulation is considered a creative adjustment. Gestalt therapists assume that neurotic regulation is the result of a creative adjustment that was made in a difficult situation in the past and then not readjusted as field conditions changed. For example, one patient's father died when she was 8 years old. The patient was terribly bereft, frightened, and alone. Her grief-stricken mother, the only adult in her life, was unavailable to help her assimilate her painful and frightening reactions to her father's death. The patient escaped her unbearable situation by busying herself to the point of distraction. That was a creative adjustment to her needs in a field with limited resources. But as an adult, she continues to use the same means of adjustment, even though the field conditions have changed. This patient's initial creative adjustment became hardened into a repetitive character pattern. This often happens because the original solution worked well enough in an emergency, and current experiences that mimic the original emergency trigger one's emergency adaptation.

Neurotic self-regulation tends to replace organismic self-regulation. Patients frequently cannot trust their own self-regulation because repeated use of a solution from an earlier time erodes their ability to respond with awareness to the current self-in-field problem. Organismic self-regulation is replaced by "shoulds"—that is, by attempts to control and manage one's experience rather than accepting one's experience. Part of the task of therapy is to create, in the therapy situation, a new "emergency"—but a "safe emergency," one that includes some elements reminiscent of the old situation (such as rising emotional intensity), but also contains health-facilitating elements that can be utilized (for instance, the therapist's affirming and calming presence). The new situation, if safe enough, can promote a new, more flexible and responsive creative adjustment.

Polarities

Experience forms as a Gestalt, a figure against a ground. Figure and ground stand in a polar relation to each other. In healthy functioning, figures and grounds shift according to changing needs and field conditions. What was previously an aspect of the ground can emerge almost instantly as the next figure.

Life is dominated by polarities: life/death, strength/vulnerability, connection/separation, and so on and on. When one's creative adjustments are flowing and responsive to current field conditions, the interaction and continually recalibrating balance of these polarities make up the rich tapestry of existence.

In neurotic regulation, some aspects of one's ground must be kept out of awareness (for instance, the patient's unbearable loneliness), and polarities lose their fluidity and become hardened into dichotomies. In neurotic regulation, a patient may readily identify with his or her strength but may, rather, ignore or disavow the experience of vulnerability. Such selective awareness results in a life filled with insoluble conflicts and plagued by crises or dulled by passivity.

Resistance

The ideas of holism and organismic self-regulation have turned the theory of resistance on its head. Its original meaning in psychoanalysis referred to a reluctance to face a painful truth about one's self. However, the theory of self-regulation posits that all phenomena, even resistance, when taken in context, can be shown to serve an organismic purpose.

In Gestalt theory, resistance is an awkward but crucially important expression of the organism's integrity. Resistance is the process of opposing the formation of a figure (a thought, feeling, impulse, or need) or the imposition of the therapist's figure (or agenda) that threatens to emerge in a context that is judged to be dangerous. For instance, someone may choke back tears, believing the tears would be more for the therapist than for the patient, or that crying would expose him or her to ridicule, or someone who has been ridiculed in the past for showing any vulnerability may assume that the current environmental surround is harsh and unforgiving. The inhibited experience is resisted—usually without awareness. For example, a patient may have pushed all experience of vulnerability out of awareness; however, the experience of vulnerability still lives in the background, quietly shaping and shadowing the figure formation process. Instead of a fluid polar relationship, the patient develops a hardened dichotomy between strength and vulnerability and inevitably experiences anxiety whenever he or she feels vulnerable. The result may be a man who takes risks demonstrating great physical courage but who is terrified by the thought of committing himself to a woman he loves. As the conflict is explored in therapy, he becomes aware that he is terribly frightened of his vulnerable feelings and resists allowing those feelings to be activated and noticed. The resistance protects him by ensuring that his habitual mode of self-regulation remains intact. When the original creative adjustment occurred, the identification with his strength and the banishment of his vulnerability were adaptive. Gestalt theory posits that he has "forgotten" that he made such an adjustment and so remains unaware that he even *has* any vulnerability that might be impeding his ability to make decisions in support of his current figure of interest, the commitment.

Even when the patient becomes vaguely aware, he may not be sure that the current context is sufficiently different that he can dare to change his dichotomized adjustment. Repetitive experiments within the relative safety of the therapeutic relationship may enable him to contact his vulnerable side enough to re-enliven the polarity of strength/vulnerability such that he can resume a more moment-by-moment creative adjustment process.

Emotions are central to healthy functioning because they orient one to one's relationship to the current field, and they help establish the relative urgency of an emergent figure. Emotional process is integral to the Gestalt formation process and functions as a "signal" in a healthy individual. For instance, upon suddenly experiencing shame, the healthy person takes it as a sign that perhaps he or she should not persist in whatever he or she is doing. Unfortunately, the person whose self-regulation has been disrupted cannot experience shame as a signal but instead tends to be overwhelmed by it.

Contact and Support

"*Contact* is possible only to the extent that *support* for it is available. . . . *Support* is everything that facilitates the ongoing assimilation and integration of experience for a person, relationship or society" (L. Perls, 1992). Adequate support is a function of the total field. It requires both self-support and environmental support. One must support oneself by breathing, but the environment must provide the air. In health, one is not out of touch with the present set of self and environmental needs and does not live in the past (unfinished business) or future (catastrophizing). It is only in the present that individuals can support themselves and protect themselves.

Anxiety

Gestalt therapy is concerned with the process of anxiety rather than the content of anxiety (what one is anxious about). Fritz Perls first defined anxiety as excitement minus support (F. Perls, 1942/1992; F. Perls et al., 1951/1994). Anxiety can be created cognitively or through unsupported breathing habits. The cognitive creation of anxiety results from "futurizing" and failing to remain centered in the present. Negative predictions, misinterpretations, and irrational beliefs can all trigger anxiety. When people futurize, they focus their awareness on something that is not yet present. For example, someone about to give a speech may be preoccupied with the potentially negative reaction of the audience. Fears about future failure can have a very negative effect on current performance. Stage fright is a classic example in which physical arousal is mislabeled and misattribution triggers a panic attack.

Anxiety can also be created by unsupported breathing. With arousal there is an organismic need for oxygen. "A healthy, self-regulating individual will automatically breathe more deeply to meet the increased need for oxygen which accompanies mobilization and contact" (Clarkson & Mackewn, 1993, p. 81). When people breathe fully, tolerate increased mobilization of energy, are present centered and cognitively flexible, and put energy into action, they experience excitement rather than anxiety. Breath support requires full inhalation and exhalation, as well as breathing at a rate that is neither too fast nor too slow. When one breathes rapidly without sufficient exhaling, fresh, oxygenated blood cannot reach the alveoli because the old air with its load of carbon dioxide is not fully expelled. Then the person has the familiar sensations of anxiety: increased pulse rate, inability to get enough air, and hyperventilation (Acierno, Hersen, & Van Hasselt, 1993; F. Perls, 1942/1992; F. Perls et al., 1951/1994).

The Gestalt therapy method, with its focus on both body orientation and characterological issues, is ideal for the treatment of anxiety. Patients learn to master anxiety cognitively and physically through cognitive and body-oriented awareness work (Yontef, 1993).

Impasse

An impasse is experienced when a person's customary supports are not available and new supports have not yet been mobilized. The experience is existentially one of terror. The person cannot go back and does not know whether he or she can survive going forward. People in the impasse are paralyzed, with forward and backward energy fighting each other. This experience is often expressed in metaphorical terms: void, hollow, blackness, going off a cliff, drowning, or being sucked into a whirlpool.

The patient who stays with the experience of the impasse may experience authentic existence—that is, existence with minimal illusion, good self-support, vitality, creativity, and good contact with the human and nonhuman environment. In this mode, Gestalt formation is clear and lively, and maximum effort is put into what is important. When support is not mobilized to work through the impasse, the person continues to repeat old and maladaptive behaviors.

Development

Gestalt therapy has not, until recently, had a well-developed theory of childhood development, but current psychoanalytic research and theory support a perspective that Gestalt therapists have held for quite a while. This theory maintains that infants are born with the capacity for self-regulation, that the development and refinement of self-regulatory skills are contingent on mutual regulation between caretaker and infant, that the contact between caretaker and infant must be attuned to the child's emotional states for self-regulation to develop best, and that children seek relatedness through emotionally attuned mutual regulation (Stern, 1985). Gestalt therapist Frank (2001) has used the research of Stern and others to formulate a comprehensive Gestalt theory of development based on embodiment and relatedness. McConville and Wheeler (2003) have used field theory and relatedness in articulating their theories of child and adolescent development.

PSYCHOTHERAPY

Theory of Psychotherapy

People grow and change all through life. Gestalt therapists believe growth is inevitable as long as one is engaged in contact. Ordinarily, people develop increasing emotional, perceptual, cognitive, motoric, and organismic self-regulatory competence. Sometimes, however, the process of development becomes impaired or derailed. To the extent that people learn from mistakes and grow, psychotherapy is not necessary. Psychotherapy is indicated when people routinely fail to learn from experience. People need psychotherapy when their self-regulatory abilities do not lead them beyond the maladaptive repetitive patterns that were developed originally as creative adjustments in difficult circumstances but that now make them or those around them unhappy. Psychotherapy is also indicated with patients who do not deal adequately with crises, feel ill equipped to deal with others in their lives, or need guidance for personal or spiritual growth.

Gestalt therapy concentrates on helping patients become aware of how they avoid learning from experience, how their self-regulatory processes may be closed-ended rather than open-ended, and how inhibitions in the area of contact limit access to the experience necessary to broaden awareness. Of course, awareness is developed through interactions with other people. From the earliest moment of a person's life, both functional and dysfunctional patterns emerge from a matrix of relationships.

Psychotherapy is primarily a relationship between a patient and a therapist, a relationship in which the patient has another chance to learn, to unlearn, and to learn how to keep learning. The patient and the therapist make explicit the patterns of thought and behavior that are manifest in the psychotherapy situation. Gestalt therapists hold that the patterns that emerge in therapy recapitulate the patterns that are manifest in the patient's life.

Goal of Therapy

The only goal of Gestalt therapy is awareness. This includes achieving greater awareness in particular areas and also improving the ability to bring automatic habits into awareness as needed. In the former sense, awareness refers to content; in the latter sense, it refers to process, specifically the kind of self-reflective awareness that is called "awareness of awareness." Awareness of awareness is the patient's ability to use his or her skills with awareness to rectify disturbances in his or her awareness process. Both awareness as content and awareness as process broaden and deepen as the therapy proceeds. Awareness requires self-knowledge, knowledge of the environment, responsibility for choices, self-acceptance, and the ability to contact.

Beginning patients are chiefly concerned with the solution of problems, often thinking that the therapist will "fix" them the way a physician often cures a disease. However, Gestalt therapy does not focus on curing disease, nor is it restricted to talking about problems. Gestalt therapy uses an active relationship and active methods to help patients gain the self-support necessary to solve problems. Gestalt therapists provide support through the therapeutic relationship and show patients how they block their awareness and functioning. As therapy goes on, the patient and the therapist turn more attention to general personality issues. By the end of successful Gestalt therapy, the patient directs much of the work and is able to integrate problem solving, characterological themes, relationship issues with the therapist, and the regulation of his or her own awareness.

How Is the Therapy Done?

Gestalt therapy is an exploration rather than a direct attempt to change behavior. The goal is growth and autonomy through an increase in consciousness. The method is one of direct engagement, whether that engagement is the meeting between therapist and patient or engagement with problematic aspects of the patient's contacting and awareness process. The model of engagement comes directly from the Gestalt concept of contact. Contact is the means whereby living and growth occur, so lived experience nearly always takes precedence over explanation. Rather than maintaining an impersonal professional distance and making interpretations, the Gestalt therapist relates to the patient with an alive, excited, warm, and direct presence.

In this open, engaged relationship, patients not only get honest feedback but also, in the authentic contact, can see, hear, and be told how they are experienced by the therapist, can learn how they affect the therapist, and (if interested) can learn something about the therapist. They have the healing experience of being listened to by someone who profoundly cares about their perspectives, feelings, and thoughts.

What and How; Here and Now

In Gestalt therapy, there is a dual focus: a constant and careful emphasis on *what* the patient does and *how* it is done and also a similar focus on the interactions between therapist and patient. What does the patient do to support himself or herself in the therapy hour in relation to the therapist and in the rest of his or her life?

Direct experience is the primary tool of Gestalt therapy, and the focus is always on the here and now. The present is a transition between past and future. Not being primarily present centered reflects a time disturbance—but so does not being able to contact the relevant past or not planning for the future. Frequently, patients lose their contact with the present and live in the past. In some cases, patients live in the present as though they had no past, with the unfortunate consequence that they cannot learn from the past. The most common time disturbance is living in anticipation of what could happen in the future as though the future were now.

Now starts with the present awareness of the patient. In a Gestalt therapy session, what happens first is not childhood but what is experienced *now*. Awareness takes place *now*. Prior events may be the object of present awareness, but the awareness process is *now*.

Now I can contact the world around me, or *now* I can contact memories or expectations. "Now" refers to *this moment*. When patients refer to their lives outside of the therapy hour, or even earlier in the hour, the content is not considered *now*, but the action of speaking *is* now. We orient more to the now in Gestalt therapy than in any other form of psychotherapy. This "what and how; here and now" method frequently is used to work on characterological and developmental themes. Exploration of past experience is anchored in the present (for example, determining what in the present field triggers this particular old memory). Whenever possible, methods are used that bring the old experience directly into present experience rather than just recounting the past.

There is an emerging awareness in Gestalt therapy that the best therapy requires a binocular viewpoint: Gestalt therapy requires technical work on the patient's awareness process, but at the same time it involves a personal relationship in which careful attention is paid to nuances of what is happening in the contact between therapist and patient.

Awareness

One of the pillars of Gestalt therapy is developing awareness of the awareness process. Does the awareness deepen and develop fully—or is it truncated? Is any particular figure of awareness allowed to recede from the mind to make room for other awarenesses—or does one figure repeatedly capture the mind and shut out the development of other awareness?

Ideally, processes that need to be in awareness come into awareness when and as needed in the ongoing flow of living. When transactions get complex, more conscious self-regulation is needed. If this develops and a person behaves mindfully, the person is likely to learn from experience.

The concept of awareness exists along a continuum. For example, Gestalt therapy distinguishes between merely *knowing* about something and *owning* what one is doing. Merely knowing about something marks the transition between that something's being totally out of awareness and its being in focal awareness. When people report being aware of something and yet claim they are totally helpless to make desired changes, they are usually referring to a situation in which they *know about* something but do not fully feel it, do not know the details of how it works, and do not genuinely integrate it and make it their own. In addition, they frequently have difficulty imagining alternatives and/or believing that the alternatives can be achieved and/or knowing how to support experimenting with alternatives.

Being fully aware means turning one's attention to the processes that are most important for the person and environment; this is a natural occurrence in healthy self-regulating. One must know what is going on and how it is happening. What do I need and what am I doing? What is needed by others? Who is doing what? Who needs what? For full awareness, this more detailed descriptive awareness must be allowed to affect the patient—and he or she has to be able to own it and respond in a relevant way.

Contact

Contact, the relationship between patient and therapist, is another pillar of Gestalt therapy. The relationship is contact over time. What happens in the relationship is crucial. This is more than what the therapist says to the patient, and it is more than the techniques that are used. Of most importance is the nonverbal subtext (posture, tone of voice, syntax, and interest level) that communicates tremendous amounts of information to the patient about how the therapist regards the patient, what is important, and how therapy works.

In a good therapy relationship, the therapist pays close attention to what the patient is doing moment to moment and to what is happening between the therapist and the patient. The therapist not only pays close attention to what the patient experiences but also deeply believes that the patient's subjective experience is just as real and valid as the therapist's "reality."

The therapist is in a powerful position in relation to the patient. If the therapist regards the patient with honesty, affection, compassion, kindness, and respect, an atmosphere can be created in which it is relatively safe for the patient to become more deeply aware of what has been kept from awareness. This enables the patient to experience and express thoughts and emotions that she or he has not habitually felt safe to share. The therapist is in a position to guide the awareness work by entering into the patient's experience deeply and completely. Martin Buber refers to "inclusion" as feeling the experience of the other much as one would feel something within one's own body while simultaneously being aware of one's own self.

There is some tension between the humane urge of the therapist to relieve the patient's pain and the indispensable need of the patient for someone who willingly enters into and understands his or her subjective pain. The therapist's empathic experience of the patient's pain brings the patient into the realm of human contact. However, trying to get the patient to feel better is often experienced by a patient as evidence that the patient is acceptable only to the extent that he or she feels good. The therapist may not intend to convey this message, but this reaction is often triggered when the therapist does not abide by the paradoxical theory of change.

Experiment

In client-centered therapy, the phenomenological work by the therapist is limited to reflecting what the patient subjectively experiences. In modern psychoanalytic work, the therapist is limited to interpretations or reflections. These interventions are both part of the Gestalt therapy repertoire, but Gestalt therapy has an additional experimental phenomenological method. Put simply, the patient and therapist can experiment with different ways of thought and action to achieve genuine understanding rather than mere changes in behavior. As in any research, the experiment is designed to get more data. In Gestalt therapy, the data are the phenomenological experience of the patient.

The greatest risk with experiments is that vulnerable patients may believe that change has been mandated. This danger is magnified if a therapist's self-awareness becomes clouded or if she or he strays from a commitment to the paradoxical theory of change. It is vitally important in Gestalt therapy that the therapist remain clear that the mode of change is the patient's knowledge and acceptance of self, knowing and supporting what emerges in contemporaneous experience. If the therapist makes it clear that the experiments are experiments in awareness and not criticism of what is observed, the risk of adding to the patient's self-rejection is minimized.

Self–Disclosure

One powerful and distinguishing aspect of Gestalt therapy is that therapists are both permitted and encouraged to disclose their personal experience, both in the moment and in their lives. Unlike classical psychoanalysis, in Gestalt therapy data are provided by both the patient and the therapist, and both the patient and the therapist take part in directing therapy through a process of mutual phenomenological exploration.

This kind of therapeutic relationship requires that therapists be at peace with the differences between themselves and their patients. In addition, therapists most truly believe that the patient's sense of subjective reality is as valid as their own. With an appreciation of the relativity of one's subjectivity, it becomes possible for therapists to disclose their reactions to patients without *requiring* that patients change. These conversations, entered into with care and sensitivity, are generally quite interesting and evocative, and they often enhance the patient's sense of efficacy and worthiness.

Dialogue is the basis of the Gestalt therapy relationship. In dialogue, the therapist practices inclusion, empathic engagement, and personal presence (for example, self-disclosure). The therapist imagines the reality of the patient's experience and, in so doing, confirms the existence and potential of the patient. However, this is not enough to make the interaction a real dialogue.

Real dialogue between therapist and patient must also include the therapist surrendering to the interaction and to what emerges from that interaction. The therapist must be open to being changed by the interaction. This sometimes requires the therapist to acknowledge having been wrong, hurtful, arrogant, or mistaken. This kind of acknowledgment puts therapist and patient on a horizontal plane. This sort of open disclosure requires personal therapy for the therapist to reduce defensiveness and the need to pridefully maintain his or her personal self-image.

Process of Psychotherapy

People form their sense of self and their style of awareness and behavior in childhood. These become habitual and often are not refined or revised by new experiences. As a person moves out of the family and into the world, new situations are encountered and the old ways of thinking, feeling, and acting are no longer needed or adaptive in new situations. But the old ways persist because they are not in awareness and hence are not subject to conscious review.

In Gestalt therapy, the patient encounters someone who takes his or her experience seriously, and through this different, respectful relationship, a new sense of self is formed. By combining the Gestalt therapy relationship with phenomenological focusing techniques, the patient becomes aware of processes that previously could not be changed because they were out of awareness. Gestalt therapists believe the contact between therapist and patient sets the stage for development of the capacity to be in contact with one's shifting figures of interest on a moment-by-moment basis.

Gestalt therapy probably has a greater range of styles and modalities than any other system. Therapy can be short term or long term. Specific modalities include individual, couple, family, group, and large systems. Styles vary in degree and type of structure; quantity and quality of techniques used; frequency of sessions; confrontation versus compassionate relating; focus on body, cognition, affect, or interpersonal contact; knowledge of and work with psychodynamic themes; emphasis on dialogue and presence; use of techniques; and so forth.

All styles of Gestalt therapy share a common emphasis on direct experience and experimenting, use of direct contact and personal presence, and a focus on the what and how, here and now. The therapy varies according to context and the personalities of both therapist and patient.

Gestalt therapy starts with the first contact between therapist and patient. The therapist inquires about the desires or needs of the patient and describes how he or she practices therapy. From the beginning, the focus is on what is happening now and what is needed now. The therapist begins immediately to help clarify the patient's awareness of self and environment. In this case, the potential relationship with the therapist is part of the environment.

The therapist and prospective Gestalt therapy patient work together to become clear about what the patient needs and whether this particular therapist is suitable. If there seems to be a match between the two, then the therapy proceeds with getting acquainted. The patient and therapist begin to relate to and understand each other, and the process of sharpening awareness begins. In the beginning, it is often not clear whether the therapy will be short- or long-term or even whether, on further examination, the match between patient and therapist will prove to be satisfactory.

Therapy typically begins with attention to the immediate feelings of the patient, the current needs of the patient, and some sense of the patient's life circumstances and history. A long social history is rarely taken, although there is nothing in Gestalt theory to prevent it. Usually, history is gathered in the process of therapy as it becomes relevant to current therapy work and at a pace comfortable for the patient.

Some patients start with their life story, others with a contemporaneous focus. The therapist helps patients become aware of what is emerging and what they are feeling and needing as they tell their stories. This is done by reflective statements of the therapist's understanding of what the patient is saying and feeling and by suggestions about how to focus awareness (or questions that accomplish that same goal).

For example, a patient might start telling a story of recent events but not say how he was affected by the events. The therapist might ask either what the patient felt when the reported event happened or what the patient is feeling in telling the story. The therapist also might go back over the story, focusing on recognizing and verbalizing the feelings associated with various stages in the story.

The therapist also makes an assessment of the strengths and weaknesses of patients, including personality style. The therapist looks for specific ways in which the patient's self-support is either precarious or robust. Gestalt therapy can be adapted and practiced with virtually any patient for whom psychotherapy is indicated. However, the practice must be adapted to the particular needs of each person. The competent Gestalt therapist, like any other kind of therapist, must have the training and ability to make this determination. A good therapist knows the limits of his or her experience and training and practices within these limits.

Treatment usually starts with either individual or couples therapy—or both. Group therapy is sometimes added to the treatment plan, and the group may become the sole modality for treatment. Fritz Perls claimed that patients could be treated by Gestalt group therapy alone. This belief was never accepted by most Gestalt therapists and is thoroughly rejected today. Gestalt group therapy complements individual and couples work but does not replace it.

Gestalt therapists work with people of all ages, although specialized training is required for work with young children. Gestalt therapy with children is done individually, as part of Gestalt family therapy, and occasionally in groups (Lampert, 2003; Oaklander, 1969/1988).

Mechanisms of Psychotherapy

All techniques in Gestalt therapy are considered experiments, and patients are repeatedly told to "Try this and see what you experience." There are many "Gestalt therapy techniques," but the techniques themselves are of little importance. Any technique consistent with Gestalt therapy principles can and will be used. In fact, Gestalt therapy explicitly encourages therapists to be creative in their interventions.

Focusing

The most common techniques are the simple interventions of focusing. Focusing ranges from simple inclusion or empathy to exercises arising largely from the therapist's experience while being with the patient. Everything in Gestalt therapy is secondary to the actual and direct experience of the participants. The therapist helps clarify what is important by helping the patient focus his or her awareness.

The prototypical experiment is some form of the question "What are you aware of, or experiencing, right here and now?" Awareness occurs continuously, moment to moment, and the Gestalt therapist pays particular attention to the *awareness continuum,* the flow or sequence of awareness from one moment to another.

The Gestalt therapist also draws attention to key moments in therapy. Of course, this requires that the therapist have the sensitivity and experience to recognize these moments when they occur. Some patients feel abandoned if the therapist is quiet for long periods; others feel it is intrusive when the therapist is active. Therefore, the therapist must weigh the possible disruption of the patient's awareness continuum if he or she offers guiding observations or suggestions against the facilitative benefit that can be derived from focusing. This balance is struck via the ongoing communication between the therapist and patient and is not solely directed by the therapist.

One key moment occurs when a patient interrupts ongoing awareness before it is completed. The Gestalt therapist recognizes signs of this interruption, including the non-verbal indications, by paying close attention to shifts in tension states, muscle tone, and/or excitement levels. The therapist's interpretation of the moment is not presumed to be relevant or useful unless the patient can confirm it. One patient may tell a story about events with someone in his life and at a key moment grit his teeth, hold his breath, and not exhale. This may turn out to be either an interruption of awareness or an expression of anger. On another occasion, a therapist might notice that an angry look is beginning to change to a look of sadness—but a sadness that is not reported. The patient might change to another subject or begin to intellectualize. In this case, the sadness may be interrupted either at the level of self-awareness or at the level of expression of the affect.

When the patient reports a feeling, another technique is to "stay with it." This encourages the patient to continue with the feeling being reported and builds the patient's capacity to deepen and work through a feeling. The following vignette illustrates this technique (P = Patient; T = Therapist).

P: [Looks sad.]
T: What are you aware of?
P: I'm sad.
T: Stay with it.
P: [Tears well up. The patient tightens up, looks away, and becomes thoughtful.]
T: I see you are tightening. What are you aware of?
P: I don't want to stay with the sadness.
T: Stay with the not wanting to. Put words to the not wanting to. [This intervention is likely to bring awareness of the patient's resistance to vulnerability. The patient might respond "I won't cry here—it doesn't feel safe," or "I am ashamed," or "I am angry and don't want to admit I'm sad."]

There is an emerging awareness in Gestalt therapy that the moments in which patients change subjects often reflect something happening in the interaction between therapist and patient. Something the therapist says or his or her nonverbal behavior may trigger insecurity or shame in the patient. Most often this is not in the patient's awareness until attention is focused on it by the therapist and explored by dialogue (Jacobs, 1996).

Enactment

The patient is asked to experiment with putting feelings or thoughts into action. This technique might be as simple as encouraging the patient to "say it to the person" (if the person involved is present) or might be enacted using role playing, psychodrama, or Gestalt therapy's well-known empty-chair technique.

Sometimes enactment is combined with the technique of asking the patient to exaggerate. This is not done to achieve catharsis but is, rather, a form of experiment that sometimes results in increased awareness of the feeling.

Creative expression is another form of enactment. For some patients, creative expression can help clarify feelings in a way that talking alone cannot. The techniques of expression include journal writing, poetry, art, and movement. Creative expression is especially important in work with children (Oaklander, 1969/1988).

Mental Experiments, Guided Fantasy, and Imagery

Sometimes visualizing an experience here and now increases awareness more effectively than enacting it, as is illustrated in the following brief vignette (P = Patient; T = Therapist).

P: I was with my girlfriend last night. I don't know how it happened but I was impotent. [Patient gives more details and history.]
T: Close your eyes. Imagine it is last night and you are with your girlfriend. Say out loud what you experience at each moment.
P: I am sitting on the couch. My friend sits next to me and I get excited. Then I go soft.
T: Let's go through that again in slow motion, and in more detail. Be sensitive to every thought or sense impression.
P: I am sitting on the couch. She comes over and sits next to me. She touches my neck. It feels so warm and soft. I get excited—you know, hard. She strokes my arm and I love it. [Pause. Looks startled.] Then I thought, I had such a tense day, maybe I won't be able to get it up.

One can use imagery to explore and express an emotion that does not lend itself to simple linear verbalization. For example, a patient might imagine being alone on a desert, being eaten alive by insects, being sucked in by a whirlpool, and so forth. There are infinite possible images that can be drawn from dreams, waking fantasy, and the creative use of fantasy. The Gestalt therapist might suggest that the patient imagine the experience happening right now rather than simply discussing it. "Imagine you are actually in that desert, right now. What do you experience?" This is often followed by some version of "Stay with it."

An image may arise spontaneously in the patient's awareness as a here-and-now experience, or it may be consciously created by the patient and/or therapist. The patient might suddenly report, "Just now I feel cold, like I'm alone in outer space." This might indicate something about what is happening between the therapist and the patient at that moment; perhaps the patient is experiencing the therapist as not being emotionally present.

Imagery techniques can also be used to expand the patient's self-supportive techniques. For example, in working with patients who have strong shame issues, at times it is helpful for them to imagine a Metaphorical Good Mother, one who is fully present and loving and accepts and loves the patient just as he or she is (Yontef, 1993).

Meditative techniques, many of which are borrowed from Asian psychotherapies, can also be very helpful experiments.

Body Awareness

Awareness of body activity is an important aspect of Gestalt therapy, and there are specific Gestalt therapy methodologies for working with body awareness (Frank, 2001; Kepner, 1987). The Gestalt therapist is especially interested in patterns of breathing. For example, when a person is breathing in a manner that does not support centering and feeling, he or she will often experience anxiety. Usually the breathing of the anxious patient involves rapid inhalation and a failure to fully exhale. One can work with experiments in breathing in the context of an ordinary therapy session. One can also practice a thoroughly body-oriented Gestalt therapy (Frank, 2001; Kepner, 1987).

Loosening and Integrating Techniques

Some patients are so rigid in their thinking—a characteristic derived from either cultural or psychological factors—that they do not even consider alternative possibilities. Loosening techniques such as fantasy, imagination, or mentally experimenting with the opposite of what is believed can help break down this rigidity so that alternatives can at least be considered. Integrating techniques bring together processes that the patient either just doesn't bring together or actively keeps apart (splitting). Asking the patient to join the positive and negative poles of a polarity can be very integrating ("I love him and I abhor his flippant attitude"). Putting words to sensations and finding the sensations that accompany words ("See if you can locate it in your body") are other important integrating techniques.

APPLICATIONS

Who Can We Help?

Because Gestalt therapy is a process theory, it can be used effectively with any patient population the therapist understands and feels comfortable with. Yontef, for instance, has written about its application with borderline and narcissistic patients (1993). If the therapist can relate to the patient and understands the basic principles of Gestalt therapy and how to adjust these principles to fit the unique needs of each new patient, the Gestalt therapy principles of *awareness* (direct experience), *contact* (relationship), and *experimenting* (phenomenological focusing and experimentation) can be applied. Gestalt therapy does not advocate a cookbook of prescribed techniques for specialized groups of individuals. Therapists who wish to work with patients who are culturally different from themselves find support by attending to the field conditions that influence their understanding of the patient's life and culture (for example, see Jacobs, 2000). The Gestalt therapy attitude of dialogue and the phenomenological assumption of multiple valid realities support the therapist in working with a patient from another culture, enabling patient and therapist to mutually understand the differences in background, assumptions, and so forth.

Both Gestalt therapy philosophy and Gestalt therapy methodology dictate that *general principles must always be adapted for each particular clinical situation.* The manner of relating and the choice and execution of techniques must be tailored to each new patient's needs, not to diagnostic categories *en bloc.* Therapy will be ineffective or harmful if the patient is made to conform to the system rather than having the system adjust to the patient.

It has long been accepted that Gestalt therapy in the confrontive and theatrical style of a 1960s Fritz Perls workshop is much more limited in application than the Gestalt therapy described in this chapter. Common sense, professional background, flexibility, and creativity are especially important in diagnosis and treatment planning. Methods, emphases, precautions, limitations, commitments, and auxiliary support (such as medication, day treatment, and nutritional guidance) must be modified with different patients in accordance with their personality organization (for example, the presence of psychosis, sociopathy, or a personality disorder).

The competent practice of Gestalt therapy requires a strong general clinical background and training in more than Gestalt therapy. In addition to training in the theory and practice of Gestalt therapy, Gestalt therapists need to have a firm grounding in personality theory, psychopathology and diagnosis, theories and applications of other systems of psychotherapy, knowledge of psychodynamics, comprehensive personal therapy, and advanced clinical training, supervision, and experience.

This background is especially important in Gestalt therapy because therapists and patients are encouraged to be creative and to experiment with new behavior in and outside of the session. The individual clinician has a great deal of discretion in Gestalt therapy. Modifications are made by the individual therapist and patient according to therapeutic style, personality of therapist and patient, and diagnostic considerations. A good knowledge of research, other systems, and the principles of personality organization are needed to guide and limit the spontaneous creativity of the therapist. The Gestalt therapist is expected to be creative, but he or she cannot abdicate responsibility for professional discrimination, judgment, and proper caution.

Gestalt therapy has been applied in almost every setting imaginable. Applications have varied from intensive individual therapy multiple times per week to crisis intervention. Gestalt therapists have also worked with organizations, schools, and groups; they have worked with patients with psychoses, patients suffering from psychosomatic disorders, and patients with posttraumatic stress disorders. Many of the details about how to modify Gestalt techniques in order to work effectively with these populations have been disseminated in the oral tradition—that is, through supervision, consultation, and training. Written material too abundant to cite has also become available.

Treatment

Patients often present similar issues but need different treatment because of differences in their personality organization and in what unfolds in the therapeutic relationship. In the following two examples, each of the two patients was raised by emotionally abandoning parents.

Tom was a 45-year-old man proud of his intelligence, self-sufficiency, and independence.

He was not aware that he had unmet dependency needs and resentment. This man's belief in his self-sufficiency and denial of dependency required that his therapist proceed with respect and sensitivity. The belief in self-sufficiency met a need, was in part constructive, and was the foundation for the patient's self-esteem. The therapist was able to respond to the patient's underlying need without threatening the patient's pride (P = Patient; T = Therapist).

P: [With pride.] When I was a little kid my mom was so busy I just had to learn to rely on myself.
T: I appreciate your strength, but when I think of you as such a self-reliant kid, I want to stroke you and give you some parenting.
P: [Tearing a little.] No one ever did that for me.
T: You seem sad.
P: I'm remembering when I was a kid . . .

[Tom evoked a sympathetic response in the therapist that was expressed directly to the patient. His denial of needing anything from others was not directly challenged. Exploration led to awareness of a shame reaction to unavailable parents and a compensatory self-reliance.]

Bob was a 45-year-old man who felt shame and isolated himself in reaction to any interaction that was not totally positive. He was consistently reluctant to support himself, conforming to and relying totally on others. Previous empathic or sympathetic responses only served to reinforce the patient's belief in his own inadequacy.

P: [Whiny voice.] I don't know what to do today.
T: [Looks and does not talk. Previous interventions of providing more direction had resulted in the patient following any slight lead by the therapist into talk that was not felt by the patient.]
P: I could talk about my week. [Looks questioningly at therapist.]
T: I feel pulled on by you right now. I imagine you want me to direct you.
P: Yes, what's wrong with that?
T: Nothing. I prefer not to direct you right now.
P: Why not?
T: You can direct yourself. I believe you are directing us now away from your inner self. I don't want to cooperate with that. [Silence.]
P: I feel lost.
T: [Looks alert and available but does not talk.]
P: You are not going to direct me, are you?
T: No.
P: Well, let's work on my believing I can't take care of myself. [The patient had real feelings about this issue, and he initiated a fruitful piece of work that led to awareness of abandonment anxiety and feelings of shame in response to unavailable parents.]

Groups

Group treatment is frequently part of an overall Gestalt therapy treatment program. There are three general models for doing Gestalt group therapy (Frew, 1988; Yontef, 1990). In the first model, participants work one-on-one with the therapist while the other participants remain relatively quiet and work vicariously. The work is then followed by feedback and interaction with other participants, with an emphasis on how people are affected by the work. In the second model, participants talk with each other with emphasis on direct here-and-now communication between the group members. This model is similar to Yalom's model for existential group therapy. A third model mixes these two activities in the same group (Yontef, 1990). The group and therapist creatively regulate movement and balance between interaction and the one-on-one focus.

All the techniques discussed in this chapter can be used in groups. In addition, there are possibilities for experimental focusing that are designed for groups. Gestalt therapy groups usually start with some procedure for bringing participants into the here and now and contacting each other. This is often called "rounds" or "check-in."

A simple and obvious example of Gestalt group work occurs when the therapist has each group member look at the other members of the group and express what he or she is experiencing in the here and now. Some Gestalt therapists also use structured experiments, such as experiments in which participants express a particular emotion ("I resent you for . . . ," "I appreciate you for . . . "). The style of other Gestalt therapists is fluid and organized by what emerges in the group.

Couples and Families

Couples therapy and family therapy are similar to group therapy in that there is a combination of work with each person in the session and work with interaction among the group members. Gestalt therapists vary in where they prefer to strike this balance (see Lee, 2008). There is also variation in how structured the intervention style of the therapist is and in how much the therapist follows, observes, and focuses the spontaneous functioning of the couple or family.

Partners often start couples therapy by complaining and blaming each other. The work at this point involves calling attention to this dynamic and to alternative modes of interaction. The Gestalt therapist also explores what is behind the blaming. Frequently, one party experiences the other as shaming him or her and blames the other, without awareness of the defensive function of the blaming.

Circular causality is a frequent pattern in unhappy couples. In circular causality, A causes B and B causes A. Regardless of how an interaction starts, A triggers a response in B to which A then reacts negatively without being aware of his or her role in triggering the negative response. B likewise triggers a negative response by A without being aware of his or her role in triggering the negative response. Circular causality is illustrated in the following example.

A wife expresses frustration with her husband for coming home late from work every night and not being emotionally available when he comes home. The husband feels unappreciated and attacked, and at an unaware level, he also feels ashamed of being criticized. The husband responds with anger, blaming the wife for not being affectionate. The wife accuses the husband of being defensive, aggressive, insensitive, and emotionally unavailable. The husband responds in kind. Each response in this circle makes it worse. In the worst cases, this circular causality can lead to total disruption in the relationship and may trigger drinking, violence, or sexual acting out.

Underneath the wife's frustration is the fact that she misses her husband, is lonely, worries about him working so hard, really wants to be with him, and assumes that he does not want to be home with her because she is no longer attractive. However, these fears are not expressed clearly. The husband might want to be home with his wife and might resent having to work so hard but might also feel a need to unwind from the stress of work before being emotionally available. The caring and interest of each spouse for the other often get lost in the circular defensive/offensive battle.

Often blaming statements trigger shame, and shame triggers defense. In this kind of toxic atmosphere, no one listens. There is no true contact and no repair or healing. Expressing actual experience, rather than judgments, and allowing oneself to really hear the experience of the spouse are first steps toward healing. Of course, this requires that both of the partners know, or learn, how to recognize their actual experience.

Sometimes structured experiments are helpful. In one experiment, the couple is asked to face each other, pulling their chairs toward each other until they are close enough to touch knees, and then instructed to look at each other and express what they are aware of at each moment. Other experiments include completing sentences such as "I resent you for . . ." or "I appreciate you for . . ." or "I spite you by . . ." or "I feel bad about myself when you . . . "

It is critical in couples therapy for the therapist to model the style of listening he or she thinks will enhance each spouse's ability to verbalize his or her experience, and to encourage each partner to listen as well as to speak. The various experiments help to convey to patients that verbal statements are not something written in stone but are part of an ongoing dialogue. The restoration of dialogue is a sign that therapy is progressing.

As described in the earlier section on psychotherapy, patients may move into various treatment modalities throughout treatment. They may have individual therapy, group therapy, or couples therapy, and they may occasionally participate in workshops. It is not unusual for patients to make occasional use of adjunctive workshops while engaged in ongoing individual therapy.

Gestalt therapists tend to see patients on a weekly basis. As more attention comes to be focused on the therapist–patient relationship, patients are eager to come more often, so some Gestalt therapists see people more often than once a week. Many Gestalt therapists also run groups, and there are therapists who teach and conduct workshops for the general public. Others primarily teach and train therapists. The shape of one's practice is limited only by one's interests and by the exigencies of the work environment.

Evidence

Can Gestalt Therapy Be Evidence Based?

There is research evidence that Gestalt therapy is effective. But what constitutes relevant "evidence"? In 1995, the APA Division of Clinical Psychology published a list of "empirically validated treatments." The task force enshrined only one kind of evidence, randomized controlled trials (RCT). RCT studies the techniques of different types of therapy for removal of the symptoms of particular disorders. This paradigm requires the random assignment of patients to experimental and control groups, blinded raters, manualization of techniques, elimination of the effects of "extraneous" factors (such as the relationship and the personality qualities of the therapist), and orientation to the removal of psychiatric symptoms. This is a paradigm that studies disorders and techniques rather than persons and the whole process of therapy.

RCT is not a suitable research approach for Gestalt therapy, which is a complex system based on the centrality of the dialogue between therapist and patient and on the joint creation of "experiments" useful for that individual person in a specific situation and moment. In the Gestalt framework, therapy evolves or emerges; it is not planned out in advance. It is oriented to the whole person and his or her life rather than to symptom removal alone.

Of course, the APA list endorsed short-term behavioral and cognitive-behavior approaches because the RCT paradigm operates in terms of assumptions derived from the philosophic/epistemological approach of these therapies (Freire, 2006; Westen, Novotny, & Thompson-Brenner, 2004). In response to protests over limiting the evidence to RCT, the concept morphed into "empirically supported treatments" and then into "evidence-based practice." Although 'evidence-based" is a more inclusive term that includes a wider range of types of research, some still consider RCT evidence to be the "gold standard" and give less credence to other types of evidence. When qualitative research—research not governed by the RCT protocol—is included, there is considerable evidence of the efficacy of Gestalt therapy.

Any research that oversimplifies or reduces the Gestalt therapy system in order to get more controlled data may yield important information, but it cannot validate or invalidate the efficacy of the actual practice of Gestalt therapy. Any method that reduces the curative factors of the therapeutic relationship to "extraneous" status is inappropriate for use in validating Gestalt therapy. RCT measures what is easy to measure (Fox, 2006), but it does not well reflect the complexity of actual practice.

Manualizing gives controlled data, but Westen and colleagues (2004) ask what supports these particular data as a valid measure of the effectiveness of therapy. In fact, in a series of meta-analyses, Elliott, Greenberg, and Lietaer (2004) re-analyzed studies comparing humanistic and behavior therapies on the basis of the school of therapy to which the researchers belonged. The factor of the allegiance of a research group proved to be so decisive that there were no further differences between the schools of therapy when it was taken out of the calculations. It appears that the more symptom tests are included in the study, compared to more holistic questions, the more likely the study is to favor behavior therapy (Strümpfel, 2004, 2006). This is consistent with the work of Luborsky et al. (2003), in which the powerful investigator allegiance effect in psychotherapy research predicts 92.5% of the outcome (Westen, Novotny, & Thompson-Brenner, 2004, p. 640).

It has become clear that RCT starts with the bias of the behaviorist philosophy and designs the criteria and method of data collection from within that bias. The positivist, reductionistic philosophic assumptions of this paradigm are contrary to experiential therapies, including Gestalt therapy, psychoanalysis, and humanistic–existential therapies in general (Freire, 2006). Fox goes so far as to assert, "all that has been demonstrated is that EBT, in the form of manualized, brief treatments, are easier to evaluate with RCT methodologies . . . than several other treatments widely used by psychologists—and several of these 'other' treatments have tons of scientific evidence to support them. . . ." (Fox, 2006).

In spite of this bias, Strümpfel claims, on the basis of his meta-analysis and review of the literature, that in no case of clinical comparison between Gestalt therapy and CBT were there significant differences except for one study in which process–experiential/Gestalt therapy led to a greater improvement in mastery of interpersonal problems than cognitive–behavior therapy (Strümpfel, 2006). Given that Gestalt therapy is not a symptom-focused approach to treatment, it is remarkable that it has been shown to be as effective as CBT in removing symptoms (Strümpfel, 2004).

RCT research gains statistical power by controlling "impure" treatments; clinicians gain clinical power by not remaining pure to a "brand-name" protocol (Westen et al., 2004). In actual practice, clinicians use interventions that laboratory research would disallow because they belong to another "brand name." Although they are prevented from using cognitive–behavioral interventions in research, Gestalt therapists and psychodynamic therapists include these techniques in their offices (Ablon, Levy, & Katzenstein, 2006; Westen et al., 2004). By the same token, cognitive–behavior therapists faced with patients with personality dysfunction often explore the dynamic roots of difficulties.

Gestalt therapists are interested in developing research models that are sensitive to the complexities of clinical work and that can obtain evidence, especially of the medium- and long-term effects of various aspects of practice. This has led to a substantial increase in new studies (Strümpfel, 2006). Activity promoting research is also described on

Gestalt therapy listserves and in journals. There is even a new book that instructs readers on conducting research in Gestalt therapy practice (Barber, 2006).

Validation of Therapeutic Relationship and Experiential Techniques

Gathering empirical data on therapeutic relationships is an alternative approach to research on therapy effectiveness (Norcross, 2001, 2002). This approach focuses on enumerating those principles of therapeutic relationship that are empirically supported. This stream of work brings together decades of research on the importance of the quality of the therapeutic contact and alliance, and it documents principles that have been shown to be effective. The evidence from research in this paradigm is more appropriate and useful for Gestalt therapy, and in fact Gestalt therapy can be said to practice within the principles of this line of research.

Ideally, assessments of the effectiveness of psychotherapy practice and theory would have to emphasize both the factors of relationship and the factors of technique (Goldfried & Davila, 2005; Hill, 2005). The effectiveness of combining experiential techniques and a good relationship has been robustly demonstrated by Les Greenberg and associates, who have conducted, over 25 years, a large series of experiments in which process and outcome studies are brought together with attention to context and to the combination of technique and relationship factors. Many of their research reports relate specific interventions with three types of outcome (immediate, intermediate, and final) and three levels of process (speech act, episode, and relationship) (Greenberg, 1991; Greenberg & Paivio, 1997; Greenberg, Rice, & Elliott, 1993).

Greenberg continues to conduct research with increasing sophistication in what he calls process–experiential therapy. This is an active experiential therapy that he describes as an amalgam of a Rogerian client-centered relationship and Gestalt therapy techniques. Greenberg gives evidence of the power of combining a technique with a relational focus, confirming a central tenet in Gestalt therapy. We consider this a form of contemporary, relational Gestalt therapy and include it in our evidence of the effectiveness of Gestalt therapy (Strümpfel, 2006; Strümpfel & Goldman, 2001). For purposes of research, we consider relational Gestalt therapy equivalent to Greenberg's process–experiential therapy, except that Gestalt therapy practice uses a much wider range of techniques than have so far been studied in his program. Although the evidence from a manualized approach (such as Greenberg's use of the empty-chair technique) gives very useful data, it cannot validate or invalidate Gestalt therapy because it is inconsistent with the central tenets of that therapy. On the other hand, his research that combines technique with measures of the efficacy of aspects of the therapy relationship is highly consistent with a Gestalt therapy approach.

Greenberg, Elliott, and Lietaer (1994) reviewed 13 studies comparing experiential therapies with cognitive and behavioral treatments using meta-psychological statistics and found that the cognitive and behavioral interventions were slightly more effective. However, when the seven studies compared directive experiential (process–experiential) therapy with cognitive or behavioral treatment, there was a small, statistically significant difference in favor of the directive experiential approach. This indicates that the directive experiential approach was more effective than either a pure client-centered approach lacking active phenomenological experimentation or the cognitive and behavioral treatments.

Greenberg and various colleagues (see Strümpfel, 2006) have conducted a number of experiments—too numerous to cite individually—in which using the Gestalt therapy two-chair technique resulted in a greater depth of experience than empathic reflection alone and was effective for resolving unfinished emotional issues with significant others. Pre- and posttesting showed that general distress was reduced, and there was a reduction in unfinished business. They have also shown the technique to be effective in healing internal splits because of an increase in the depth of experiencing and from softening the "harsh internal critic" (Greenberg, 1980). Being harsh, critical, or self-rejecting prevents healing and growth. Greenberg also has demonstrated that conflict resolution using the two-chair dialogue occurs via deeper experiencing of previously rejected aspects of self. This confirms Gestalt therapy's paradoxical theory of change. Recent research shows the approach effective in treating depression and maintaining the improvement (Ellison, Greenberg, Goldman, & Angus, 2009) and effective in treating individuals who have been emotionally injured by significant others (Greenberg, Warwar, & Malcom, 2008).

Research that is relevant, realistic, and valid for Gestalt therapy would need to account for the importance of the therapeutic relationship and also for the full range of interventions that are integral to the Gestalt therapy method. Limiting the therapist's interventions in order to achieve scientific precision would achieve uniformity for the research at the expense of misrepresenting the Gestalt therapy methodology. It would also contradict the main tenets of humanistic psychology (Cain & Seeman, 2001).

Specific techniques such as the empty-chair and two-chair techniques can be conveniently studied. However, these tools are not representative of all patients or of the range of techniques used in Gestalt therapy. Some patients are too inhibited to use the empty chair effectively or cannot generate enough affect to do so. A wide range of techniques that accomplish the same function can be used in clinical practice. One advantage of Gestalt therapy is that the therapist has support for using a great variety of techniques within the context of a cohesive theoretical framework.

Neurology, Childhood Development, Affect and Gestalt Therapy

Recent research results in neurology and infant development support the Gestalt therapy viewpoint on the importance of the here and now and the inseparability of emotion and thought (Damasio 1995, 1999; Stern, 2004). In addition, Gestalt therapy's inclusion of work with the body in the methodology of psychotherapy gives it an added power that ideally would be included in the evaluation of psychotherapy efficacy but is not included in most psychotherapy research (Strümpfel, 2006).

Reviews and Meta-Analyses

Cain and Seeman (2001) review issues of validation of humanistic therapies, including Gestalt therapy. They cite relevant research and describe the general results using Carl Rogers's words: "The facts are friendly" (Rogers, 1961/1995, p. 25). The research on Gestalt therapy was reviewed by Yontef (1995).

Strümpfel reviews data from 74 published research studies on therapeutic process and outcome re-analyzed in 10 meta-analyses and adds his own calculations (Strümpfel, 2006). Tests of efficacy were carried out on data for approximately 4,500 patients treated in clinical practice. Of these, approximately 3,000 were treated with Gestalt therapy and 1,500 were control subjects. He also shows 431 sources of evidence that include single case reports. The studies included patients with multiple diagnoses; including such patients is consistent with usual clinical practice, but most laboratory-based studies exclude them in order to get more precise data (Strümpfel, 2006; Westen et al., 2004). Strümpfel discusses comparisons conducted by Elliott (2001) and Elliott et al. (2004) and points out that, relative to the number of measurements undertaken, significant results were found more frequently for the humanistic therapies than for the behavioral and (even more clearly) the psychodynamic approaches. This summary of the data contradicts claims that the behavioral therapies have been demonstrated to be superior.

The variety of different patients, diagnoses, and settings of these studies taken as a whole is evidence for the effectiveness of Gestalt therapy even with highly impaired patients. It confirms the effectiveness of Gestalt therapy adapted to a wide range of clinical disorders (such as schizophrenia, personality disorders, affective and anxiety disorders, substance dependencies, and psychosomatic disorders) and administered in psychosocial preventive health settings. The treatment effects were shown to be stable in the long term. Psychiatric patients with various diagnoses showed significant improvements in their main symptoms, personality dysfunctions, self-concept, and interpersonal relationships after treatment with Gestalt therapy. The patients themselves evaluated the therapy as very helpful. Assessments by nursing staff indicated improvements in the patients' contact and communications functioning (Strümpfel, 2006).

The effects were largest for Gestalt therapy with symptoms of depression, anxiety, and phobias. Studies showed the efficacy of Gestalt and social therapy to drug-dependent patients, with a long-term abstinence rate of 70%. There was also a reduction in symptoms of depression and an improvement in personality development. Studies showed a 55% reduction in pain and in the use of medication with functional disorders.

There was also evidence that Gestalt therapy is effective for schoolchildren with achievement difficulties, for parents who experience their children as having problems, for couples, in preventive health care, and for pregnant women undergoing preparation for delivery (Strümpfel, 2006).

Seventeen studies had follow-up data from 1/2 to 3 years after the end of therapy. The effects of the therapy were stable in all cases except one, in which treatment was administered for only a few hours in a group.

Other studies demonstrated that patients in Gestalt therapy learned strategies to cope successfully with recurrent symptoms (Strümpfel, 2006). Schigl (cited in Strümpfel, 2004, 2006) did follow-up studies with several hundred patients of Gestalt and experiential therapy. Of these, 63% reported attaining their initial goals completely or to a great extent. Use of psychotropic medication was reduced by half and use of tranquillizers by 75%.

In one study cited by Strümpfel (2006), an independent research group evaluated the findings of an evaluation conducted by particular clinics. Based on follow-up data on 117 cases, a comparison was made between patients treated with a combination of psychodynamic and Gestalt therapy, psychodynamic therapy, and/or behavior therapy. The authors reported that Gestalt therapy had improvements with larger-than-average effect sizes on various psychosocial and physical measures. Similarly, Strümpfel (2006) reports on the meta-analysis by Elliott et al. (2004) of 112 studies. Of the various humanistic approaches, process–experiential/Gestalt therapy approaches tended to have the largest effect sizes.

One interesting result found by Strümpfel is that psychiatric patients receiving cognitive–behavior therapy sought social contacts more frequently, but patients were better able to maintain these contacts when treated with a combination of Gestalt therapy and transactional analysis. Strümpfel conducted further exploratory analyses and found indications that the particular effectiveness of Gestalt therapy lies in the domain of social/relational/interpersonal functions. Clinical studies support the finding that Gestalt therapy leads to particularly marked improvement in establishing personal contact, in sustaining relationships, and in managing aggression and conflicts (Strümpfel, 2004, 2006).

The therapeutic method of guiding clients toward their immediate self-experiencing in the process and promoting emotional activation, which was developed in Gestalt therapy, has proved to be an effective mode of therapeutic work. According to a meta-analysis by Orlinsky, Grawe, and Parks (1994), the experiential confrontation process, defined as directing attention to the patient's experience and behavior that are directly activated in the session, is a strong predictor for positive therapeutic outcome.

The active Gestalt therapy interventions have proven to be suitable for intensifying qualities of experience within the therapy session and today can be associated with improved conflict resolution . . . and a reduction in symptoms and problems. In light of these findings and the data on the breadth of its application and efficacy, a number of previous appraisals of Gestalt therapy, e.g., regarding restricted applicability, can be revised. (Strümpfel, 2006)

Psychotherapy comparison studies have provided evidence that the effects of Gestalt therapy are comparable to those of other forms of therapy—or even better (Strümpfel, 2006).

To conclude this section, we suggest a word of caution about using research evidence when endeavoring to understand and evaluate therapeutic efficacy, whether by comparing different approaches or by assessing the value of therapy as a healing enterprise. Any treatment dyad and treatment process has vastly more complex meanings than can possibly be measured. Added to the mix is the fact that each therapist is unique and can practice well only by working within a framework matched to his or her personality. Therefore, even if research suggests most generally that, say, Gestalt therapy is very well suited to support a patient's strivings for enduring relationships, if the therapist is not attracted to working with close attention to moment-by-moment emotional experience, then he or she would probably need to work in another framework in order to be at all helpful to his or her patients. In fact, it is possible that therapists' comfort within their orientations may prove to be a more significant factor for positive outcomes than their specific orientations. Our current research results are limited, as always, by the questions we ask and by the research tools available to us.

Psychotherapy in a Multicultural World

The founders of Gestalt therapy were all cultural/political outsiders. Some were Jews, and some of them were immigrants—including Fritz and Laura Perls—who had fled persecution in Europe. Some were gay. All were interested in developing a process-oriented theory that could provide support and encouragement for people to explore their own life paths, even if those life paths did not fit neatly within extant cultural values. Thus, instead of establishing content goals for successful therapy (e.g., achievement of genital sexuality), they established a process goal: awareness.

Gestalt therapists throughout the world have been involved with, and written about, their involvement in multicultural and intercultural projects, be they the provision of mental health services or community organization or organizational consulting (Bar-Yoseph, 2005). Heiberg (2005) interviewed non-European immigrants and residents of Norway about their experiences and found that shame and a shaming process constantly infused their interactions with members of Norway's dominant culture. Almost all of his respondents had been in therapy with white therapists, and the Gestalt patients spoke most enthusiastically of the chance to explore their experience—especially their shame—on their own terms rather than being analyzed and interpreted. Gaffney (2008) wrote about the subtle and gross difficulties of providing supervision in the divided society of Northern Ireland. Bar-Yoseph (2005) edited a collection of articles by Gestalt therapists engaged in various multicultural endeavors. Articles by American therapists are included.

A common thread in almost all of the literature is that efficacious multicultural interaction requires that the therapist recognize the implications of his or her social/cultural/political situatedness. There are two reasons for this. First, such awareness helps the therapist to relativize his or her own cultural norms so as to help to navigate the inevitable strong emotional reactions that emerge when coming into intimate contact with profoundly different and sometimes disturbing world-views. Second, awareness of the difference between the relative insider status of being a professional and the often marginalized status of the cultural outsider is crucial for opening up meaningful dialogue with one's client. Billies (2005), Jacobs (2005a), and McConville (2005) elaborate this point in exploring what it means to be a white therapist in racially divided America.

All of the authors referred to field theory as a strong support for phenomenological, experiential explorations with their clients. They also emphasized that attention to the contacting and awareness processes and how these processes are shaped by field conditions enhanced the capacity of the therapist and the client to make creative adjustments in their work together.

Another strongly emphasized dimension of Gestalt therapy is the dialogical attitude, a humble attitude that includes a willingness to be affected and changed by the client. In dialogue, the therapist learns from the patient about the patient's culture. This attitude enables the therapist to learn more about his or her own biases, and it also fosters contacting that is often experienced by the client as empowering.

CASE EXAMPLE

Background

Miriam often spoke in a flat voice, seemingly disconnected from her feelings and even from any sense of the meaningfulness of her sentences. She had survived terrifying and degrading childhood abuse, and now, some 35 years after leaving home, she had the haunted, pinched look of someone who expected the abuse to begin again at any moment. She could not even say that she wanted therapy for herself because she claimed not to want or need people in her life. She thought that being in therapy could help her to develop her skills as a consultant more fully. Miriam was quite wary of therapy, but she had attended a lecture given by the therapist and had felt a slight glimmer of hope that this particular therapist might actually be able to understand her.

Miriam's experiential world was characterized by extreme isolation. She was ashamed of her isolation, but it made her feel safe. When she moved about in the world of people, she felt terrified, often enraged, and deeply ashamed. She was unrelentingly self-critical. She believed she was a toxic presence, unwillingly destructive of others. She was unable to acknowledge wants or needs of her own, for such an acknowledgment made her vulnerable and (in her words) a "target" for humiliation and annihilation. Finally, she was plagued by a sense of unreality. She never knew whether what she thought or perceived was "real" or imagined. She knew nothing of what she felt, believed that she had no feelings, and did not even know what a feeling was. At times, these convictions were so strong that she fantasized she was an alien.

Miriam's fundamental conflicts revolved around the polarity of isolation versus confluence. Although she was at most times too ashamed of her desires to even recognize them, when her wish to be connected to others became figural, she was overcome with dread. She recognized that she wanted to just "melt" into the other person, and she could not bear even a hint of distance, for the distance signaled rejection, which she believed would be unbearable to her. She was rigidly entrenched in her isolated world. A consequence of her rigidity was that she was unable to flow back and forth in a rhythm of contact and withdrawal. The only way she could regulate the states of tension and anxiety that emerged as she dared to move toward contact, with the therapist and others, was to suddenly shrink back in shame, retreat into isolation, or become dissociated, which happened quite often. Then she would feel stuck, too ashamed and defeated to dare to venture forward again. She was unable to balance and calibrate the experience of desiring contact while at the same time being afraid of contact.

The following sequence occurred about 4 years into therapy. Miriam was much better at this point in being able to identify with and express feeling, but navigating a contact boundary with another person was still daunting. She had begun this session with a deep sense of pleasure because she finally felt a sense of continuity with the therapist, and she reported that for the first time in her life, she was also connected to some memories. The air of celebration gave way to desperation and panic later as therapist and patient struggled together with her wishes and fears for a closer connection to the therapist.

In a conversation that had been repeated at various times, Miriam's desperation grew as she wanted the therapist to "just reach past" her fear, to touch the tiny, disheveled, and lonely "cave girl" who hid inside. Miriam felt abandoned by the therapist's "patience" (Miriam's word).

P: You're so damn patient!

T: . . . and this is a bad thing? [Said tentatively.]

P: Right now it is.

T: Because you need . . .

P: [Pause.] Something that indicates *something*. [Sounding frightened and exasperated, and confused.]

T: What does my patience indicate to you right now?

P: That I am just going to be left scrambling forever!

T: It sounds like I am watching from too far away—rather than going through this with you—does that sound right?

P: Sounds right . . .

T: So you need something from me that indicates we will get through this together, that I won't just let you drown. [Said softly and seriously.]

[A few minutes later, the exploration of her need for contact and her fear has continued, with Miriam even admitting to a wish to be touched physically, which is a big admission for her to make. Once again Miriam is starting to panic. She is panicked with fear of what may happen now that she has exposed her wish to be touched. She fears the vulnerability of allowing the touch, and she is also panicky about being rejected or cruelly abandoned. The therapist has been emphasizing that Miriam's wish for contact is but one side of the conflict, and that the other side, her fear, needs to be respected as well. The patient was experiencing the therapist's caution as an abandonment, whereas the therapist was concerned that "just reaching past" the patient's fear would reenact a boundary violation and would trigger greater dissociation.]

T: . . . so, we need to honor *both* your fear and your wish. [Miriam looks frightened, on the verge of dissociating.] . . . now you are moving into a panic—speak to me . . .

P: [Agonized whisper.] It's too much.

T: [Softly.] yeah, too much . . . what's that . . . "it's too much"?

P: Somehow if you touch me I will disappear. And I don't want to—I want to—I want to use touch to *connect,* not to disappear!

T: Right, OK, so the fear side of you is saying that the risk in touching is that you'll disappear. Now we have to take that fear into account. And I have a suggestion—that I will move and we sit so that our fingertips can be just an inch or so from each other—and see how that feels to you. Do you want to try? [Therapist moves as patient nods assent. Miriam is still contorted with fear and desperation.] Okay, now, I am going to touch one of your fingers—keep breathing—how is that?

P: [crying] How touch-phobic I am! I shift between "it feels nice" and "it feels horrid!"

T: That is why we have to take this slowly. . . . Do you understand that . . . if we didn't take it slowly you would have to disappear—the horror would make you have to disappear [all spoken slowly and carefully and quietly] . . . do you understand that . . . so it's worth going slowly . . . your fingers feel to me . . . full of feeling?

P: Yes . . . as if all my life is in my fingers . . . not disappeared here, warm . . .

The patient attended a weeklong workshop the next week, after which she reported, with a sense of awe, that she had stayed "in her body" for the whole week, even when being touched. Since this session, this patient has reported that she feels a greater sense of continuity, and as we continue to build on it (even the notion of being able to "build" is new and exciting), she feels less brittle, more open, more "in touch."

As more time has passed, and we continue to work together several times per week, long-standing concerns about feeling alien and about being severely dissociated and fragmented have begun to be resolved. The patient feels increasingly human, able to engage more freely in intimate participation with others.

SUMMARY

Gestalt therapy is a system of psychotherapy that is philosophically and historically linked to Gestalt psychology, field theory, existentialism, and phenomenology. Fritz Perls, his wife Laura Perls, and their collaborator Paul Goodman initially developed and described the basic principles of Gestalt therapy.

Gestalt therapists focus on contact, conscious awareness, and experimentation. There is a consistent emphasis on the present moment and on the validity and reality of the patient's phenomenological awareness. Most of the change that occurs in Gestalt therapy results from an I–Thou dialogue between therapist and patient, and Gestalt therapists are encouraged to be self-disclosing and candid, both about their personal history and about their feelings in therapy.

The techniques of Gestalt therapy include focusing exercises, enactment, creative expression, mental experiments, guided fantasy, imagery, and body awareness. However, these techniques themselves are relatively insignificant and are only the tools traditionally employed by Gestalt therapists. Any mechanism consistent with the theory of Gestalt therapy can and will be used in therapy.

Therapeutic practice is in turmoil in a time when the limitations associated with managed care have encroached on clinical practice. At a time of humanistic growth in theorizing, clinical practice seems to be narrowing, with more focus on particular symptoms and an emphasis on people as products who can be fixed by following the instructions in a procedure manual.

The wonderful array of Gestalt-originated techniques for which Gestalt therapy is famous can be easily misused for just such a purpose. We caution the reader not to confuse the use of technique for symptom removal, however imaginative, with Gestalt therapy. The fundamental precepts of Gestalt therapy, including the paradoxical theory of change, are thoroughly geared toward the development of human freedom, not human conformity, and in that sense, Gestalt therapy rejects the view of persons implied in the managed-care ethos. Gestalt practice, when true to its principles, is a protest against the reductionism of mere symptom removal and adjustment; it is a protest for a client's right to develop fully enough to be able to make conscious and informed choices that shape her or his life.

Since Gestalt therapy is so flexible, creative, and direct, it is very adaptable to short-term as well as long-term therapy. The direct contact, focus, and experimentation can sometimes result in important insight. This adaptability is an asset in dealing with managed care and related issues of funding mental health treatment.

In the 1960s, Fritz Perls prophesied that Gestalt therapy would come into its own during the decade ahead and become a significant force in psychotherapy during the 1970s. His prophecy has been more than fulfilled.

In 1952, there were perhaps a dozen people actively involved in the Gestalt therapy movement. Today there are hundreds of training institutes here and abroad, and there are thousands of well-trained Gestalt therapists practicing worldwide. Unfortunately, there are also large numbers of poorly trained therapists who call themselves Gestalt therapists after attending a few workshops and who do not have adequate academic preparation. It behooves students and patients who are interested in exposure to Gestalt therapy to inquire in depth about the training and experience of anyone who claims to be a Gestalt therapist or who claims to use Gestalt therapy techniques.

Gestalt therapy has pioneered many useful and creative innovations in psychotherapy theory and practice that have been incorporated into the general psychotherapy field. Now Gestalt therapy is moving to further elaborate and refine these innovations. The principles of existential dialogue, the use of direct phenomenological experience for both patient and therapist, the trust of organismic self-regulation, the emphasis on experimentation and awareness, the paradoxical theory of change, and close attention to the contact between the therapist and the patient all form a model of good psychotherapy that will continue to be used by Gestalt therapists and others.

ANNOTATED BIBLIOGRAPHY

Kepner, J. (1993). Body process: *Working with the body in psychotherapy*. San Francisco: Jossey-Bass.
Kepner's book can be read by people who may have no particular interest in Gestalt therapy but want to work effectively with patients while attending to body process as well as verbal communication. It is a beautiful illustration of the holistic approach that Gestalt therapy espouses. Kepner describes how to attend to body process, both observed and experienced, and how to weave work with bodily experience into ongoing psychotherapy. Readers will also get an idea how the therapist's creativity, coupled with the readiness of the patient, can yield fertile Gestalt awareness experiments.

Polster, E., & Polster, M. (1973). *Gestalt therapy integrated*. New York: Vintage Books.
This is one of the most readable and enjoyable therapy books around. There are many illustrative vignettes for people who want to get a sense of what Gestalt therapy is like in practice. The book is written at the level of clinical theory and covers the basics of Gestalt therapy: process, here and now, contact, awareness, and experiments The writing is so lively that the reader is bound to come away with a feel for the Gestalt therapy experience as practiced by some of its finest senior practitioners. A later, equally insightful and rich collection of readings by the Polsters is available in A. Roberts (Ed.). (1999). *From the radical center*, Cleveland, OH: Gestalt Institute of Cleveland Press.

Wheeler, G. (2000). *Beyond individualism: Toward a new understanding of self, relationship and experience*. Hillsdale, NJ: Gestalt Press/Analytic Press.
The author manages to walk the reader, in a simple, lucid, and evocative manner, through the paradigm shift that Gestalt therapy brings to the field of psychotherapy. He offers illustrative experiments along the way. The reader cannot help but have his or her experience of living changed by this book. This book, coupled with the clinical flavor of the Polsters' book *Gestalt Therapy Integrated* (see above), provides a well-rounded beginning for the interested clinician.

Woldt, A., and Toman, S. (2005). *Gestalt therapy: History, theory and practice*. Thousand Oaks, CA: Sage Publications.
Edited collections of articles on various topics are a tradition in Gestalt therapy. For instance, there are collections on Gestalt therapy practice in groups, shame, couples therapy, relationality, cultural issues, etc. Most edited collections in any field are uneven in quality, containing some gems and some lackluster pieces; however, they tend to be worthy reads because they acquaint the reader with multiple viewpoints extant in the area of interest. This particular edited collection of articles with accompanying discussions, thought questions, and experiments can serve as a textbook in that it covers much of the domain of Gestalt therapy. It is useful especially for students and their teachers and is a good foundation before moving on to some of the current controversies and specialized topics of conversation in Gestalt therapy.

Yontef, G. (1993). *Awareness, dialogue and process: Essays on Gestalt therapy*. Highland, NY: Gestalt Journal Press.
A compendium of articles written over a span of 25 years. Some of the articles are for those who are new to Gestalt therapy, but most are for the advanced reader. The essays are sophisticated probes into some of the thornier theoretical and clinical problems that any theory must address. The book comprehensively traces the evolution of Gestalt theory and practice and provides a theoretical scaffolding for its future.

CASE READINGS

Feder, B., & Ronall, R. (1997). *A living legacy of Fritz and Laura Perls: Contemporary case studies.* New York: Feder Publishing.

> This edited collection provides a look at how different clinicians work from a Gestalt perspective. The variety of styles encourages the reader to find his or her own.

Hycner, R., & Jacobs, L. (1995). Simone: Existential mistrust and trust. *The healing relationship in Gestalt therapy: A dialogic, self-psychology approach* (pp. 85–90). Highland, NY: Gestalt Journal Press.

Hycner, R., & Jacobs, L. (1995). Transference meets dialogue. *The healing relationship in Gestalt therapy: A dialogic, self-psychology approach* (pp. 171–195). Highland, NY: Gestalt Journal Press.

> The first case is an example drawn from a workshop conducted in Israel; the second is an interesting case report by a psychoanalytically oriented Gestalt therapist, including verbatim transcripts of three sessions. The second case is analyzed in a panel discussion by two Gestalt therapists and two psychoanalysts in Alexander, Brickman, Jacobs, Trop, & Yontef. (1992). Transference meets dialogue. *Gestalt Journal, 15,* 61–108.

Lampert, R. (2003). *A child's eye view: Gestalt therapy with children, adolescents and their families.* Highland, NY: Gestalt Journal Press.

> Case material is provided throughout this book.

Perls, F. S. (1992). Jane's three dreams. In *Gestalt therapy verbatim* (pp. 284–310). Highland, NY: Gestalt Journal Press.

> Three dreams are presented verbatim. The third dream work is a continuation of unfinished work from the second dream. Portions of this case are also found in D. Wedding & R. J. Corsini (Eds.). (2005). *Case studies in psychotherapy.* Belmont, CA: Brooks/Cole.

Perls, L. P. (1968). Two instances of Gestalt therapy. In P. D. Purlsglove (Ed.), *Recognition in Gestalt therapy* (pp. 42–68). New York: Funk and Wagnalls. [Originally published in 1956.]

> Laura Perls presents the case of Claudia, a 25-year-old woman of color who comes from a lower-middle-class West Indian background, and the case of Walter, a 47-year-old Central European Jewish refugee.

Simkin, J. S. (1967). *Individual Gestalt therapy* [Film]. Orlando, FL: American Academy of Psychotherapists. 50 minutes.

> In this tape of the 11th hour of therapy with a 34-year-old actor, emphasis is on present, nonverbal communications leading to production of genetic material. The use of fantasy dialogue is also illustrated.

Simkin, J. S. (1972). The use of dreams in Gestalt therapy. In C. J. Sager & H. S. Kaplan (Eds.), *Progress in group and family therapy* (pp. 95–104). New York: Brunner/Mazel.

> In a verbatim transcript, a patient works on a dream about his youngest daughter.

Staemmler, F. (Ed.). (2003). The IGJ Transcript Project. *International Gestalt Journal, 26*(1), 9–58.

> In this intriguing project, British Gestalt therapist Sally Denham-Vaughan provides a brief summary of her work with a patient and then an extended transcript of a session. Four therapists from Europe and the United States offer their commentaries on the session, and then Denham-Vaughan replies. The result is not only a good example of a Gestalt therapy process but also a lively discussion of some points of interest and controversy in Gestalt therapy. [Reprinted in D. Wedding & R. J. Corsini. (2011). *Case studies in psychotherapy.* Belmont, CA: Brooks/Cole.]

REFERENCES

Ablon, J., Levy, R., & Katzenstein, T. (2006). Beyond brand names of psychotherapy: Identifying empirically supported change processes. *Psychotherapy: Theory, Research, Practice, Training, 43*(2), 216–231.

Acierno, R., Hersen, M., & Van Hasselt, V. (1993). Interventions for panic disorder: A critical review of the literature. *Clinical Psychology Review, 13,* 561–578.

Bar-Yoseph, T. (Ed.). (2005) *Making a difference: The bridging of cultural diversity.* New Orleans, LA: Gestalt Institute Press.

Barber, P. (2006). *Practitioner researcher: A Gestalt approach to holistic inquiry.* London: Middlesex University Press.

Beisser, A. (1970). The paradoxical theory of change. In J. Fagan & I. Shepherd (Eds.), *Gestalt therapy now* (pp. 77–80). Palo Alto: Science & Behavior Books. Available at gestalttherapy.org.

Billies, M. (2005). Therapist confluence with social systems of oppression and privilege. *International Gestalt Journal, 28*(1), 71–92.

Buber, M. (1923/1970). *I and thou* (W. Kaufmann, Trans.). New York: Scribner's.

Cain, D. J., & Seeman, J. (Eds.). (2001). *Handbook of research and practice.* Washington, DC: American Psychological Association.

Clarkson, P., & Mackewn, J. (1993). *Fritz Perls.* London: Sage.

Damasio, A. (1995). *Descartes' error: Emotion, reason, and the human brain.* New York: Quill.

Damasio, A. (1999). *The feeling of what happens: Body and emotion in the making of consciousness.* New York: Harvest Books.

Elliott, R. (2001). Research on the effectiveness of humanistic therapies: A meta-analysis. In D. Cain & J. Seeman (Eds.), *Humanistic psychotherapies: Handbook on research and practice.* Washington, DC: American Psychological Association.

Elliott, R., Greenberg, L., & Lietaer, G. (2004). Research on experiential psychotherapies. In M. Lambert (Ed.), *Bergin & Garfield's handbook of psychotherapy and behavior change* (5th ed., pp. 493–540). New York: Wiley.

Ellison, J., Greenberg, L, Goldman, R., Angus, L. (2009). Maintenance of gains following experiential therapies for depression. *Journal of Consulting and Clinical Psychology, 77*(1), 103–112.

Fairfield, M., & O'Shea, L. (2008). Getting beyond individualism. *British Gestalt Journal, 17*(2), 24–38

Fox, R. (2006). Psychology's scientific ayatollahs. *Independent Practitioner,* Winter, 11.

Frank, R. (2001). *Body of awareness: A somatic and developmental approach to psychotherapy.* Hillsdale, NJ: GIC/ Analytic Press.

Freire, E. (2006). Randomized controlled clinical trial in psychotherapy research: An epistemological controversy. *Journal of Humanistic Psychology, 46*(3), 323–335.

Frew, J. (1988). The practice of Gestalt therapy in groups. *Gestalt Journal, 11,* 1, 77–96.

Gaffney, S. (2008). Gestalt group supervision in a divided society: Theory, practice, perspective and reflections. *British Gestalt Journal, 17*(1), 27–39.

Goldfried, M., & Davila, J. (2005). The role of relationship and technique in therapeutic change. *Psychotherapy: Theory, Research, Practice, Training, 42*(4), 421–430.

Greenberg, L. (1980). The intensive analysis of recurring events from the practice of Gestalt therapy. *Psychotherapy: Theory, Research and Practice, 17,* 143–152.

Greenberg, L. (1991). Research in the process of change. *Psychotherapy Research, 1,* 14–24.

Greenberg, L., Elliott, R., & Lietaer, G. (1994). Research on experiential psychotherapies. In A. Bergin & S. Garfield (Eds.), *Handbook of psychotherapy and behavior change* (pp. 509–539). New York: Wiley.

Greenberg, L., & Paivio, S. C. (1997). *Working with emotions in psychotherapy.* New York: Guilford Press.

Greenberg, L., Rice, L., & Elliott, R. (1993). *Facilitating emotional change: The moment-by-moment process.* New York: Guilford Press.

Greenberg, L., Warwar, S., & Malcom, W. (2008). Differential effects of emotion-focused therapy and psychoeducation in facilitating forgiveness and letting go of emotional injuries. *Journal of Counseling Psychology, 55*(2), 185–196.

Heiberg, T. (2005). Shame and creative adjustment in a multicultural society. *British Gestalt Journal, 14*(2), 188–127.

Hill, C. (2005). Therapist techniques, client involvement, and the therapeutic relationship: Inextricably intertwined in the therapy process. *Psychotherapy: Theory, Research, Practice, Training, 42*(4), 431–442.

Hycner, R. (1985). Dialogical Gestalt therapy: An initial proposal. *Gestalt Journal, 8*(1), 23–49.

Hycner, R., & Jacobs, L. (1995). *The healing relationship in Gestalt therapy: A dialogic, self-psychology approach.* Highland, NY: Gestalt Journal Press.

Jacobs, L. (1989). Dialogue in Gestalt theory and therapy. *Gestalt Journal, 12*(1), 25–67.

Jacobs, L. (1996). Shame in the therapeutic dialogue. In R. Lee & G. Wheeler (Eds.), *The voice of shame* (pp. 297–314). San Francisco: Jossey-Bass.

Jacobs, L. (2000). Respectful Dialogues. interview in *British Gestalt Journal, 9*(2), 105-116.

Jacobs, L. (2005a). For whites only. In T. Bar-Yoseph (Ed.), *Making a difference: The bridging of cultural diversity* (pp. 225–244). New Orleans, LA: Gestalt Institute Press.

Jacobs, L. (2005b). The inevitable intersubjectivity of selfhood. *International Gestalt Journal, 28*(1), 43–70.

Joyce, P., & Sills, C. (2009). *Skills in Gestalt counseling & psychotherapy* (2nd ed.). Sage: London.

Kepner, J. (1987). *Body process: A Gestalt approach to working with the body in psychotherapy.* New York: Gestalt Institute of Cleveland Press.

Lampert, R. (2003). *A child's eye view: Gestalt therapy with children, adolescents, and their families.* Highland, NY: Gestalt Journal Press.

Lee, R. G. (Ed.). (2004). *The values of connection: A relational approach to ethics.* Cambridge, MA: Gestalt Press/Analytic Press.

Lee, R. G. (2008). *The secret language of intimacy.* New York, Routledge.

Lee, R., & Wheeler, G. (Eds.). (1996). *The voice of shame: Silence and connection in psychotherapy.* San Francisco: Jossey-Bass.

Lewin, K. (1938). The conflict between Aristotelian and Galilean modes of thought in contemporary psychology. In K. Lewin, *A dynamic theory of personality* (pp. 1–42). London: Routledge & Kegan Paul.

Luborsky, L., Rosenthal, R., Diguer, L., Andrusyna, T., Levitt, J., Seligman, D., Berman, J., & Krause, E. (2003). Are some psychotherapies much more effective than others? *Journal of Applied Psychoanalytic Studies, 5*(4), 455–460.

McConville, M., & Wheeler, G. (2003). *Heart of development* (Vols. 1 and 2). Gestalt Press/Analytic Press, Hillsdale, NJ.

McConville, M. (2005). The gift. In T. Bar-Yoseph (Ed.), *Making a difference: The bridging of cultural diversity* (pp. 173–182). New Orleans, LA: Gestalt Institute Press.

Norcross, J., (Ed.). (2001). Empirically supported therapy relationships: Summary report of the Division 29 Task Force. *Psychotherapy, 38*(4), 345–356.

Norcross, J. (Ed.). (2002). *Psychotherapy relationships that work: Therapist contributions and responsibilities to patient needs.* New York: Oxford University Press.

Oaklander, V. (1969/1988). *Windows to our children: A Gestalt therapy approach to children and adolescents.* New York: Gestalt Journal Press.

Orlinsky, D., Grawe, K., & Parks, B. (1994). Process and outcome in psychotherapy. In A. Bergin & S. Garfield (Eds.), *Handbook of psychotherapy and behavior change* (pp. 270–376). New York: Wiley.

Perls, F. (1942/1992). *Ego, hunger and aggression.* New York: Gestalt Journal Press.

Perls, F., Hefferline, R., & Goodman, P. (1951/1994). *Gestalt therapy: Excitement & growth in the human personality.* New York: Gestalt Journal Press.

Perls, L. (1992). *Living at the boundary.* New York: Gestalt Therapy Press.

Philippson, P. (2001). *Self in relation.* New York: Gestalt Journal Press.

Polster, E., & Polster, M. (1973). *Gestalt therapy integrated.* New York: Brunner/Mazel.

Rogers, C. (1961/1995). *On becoming a person.* New York: Houghton Mifflin.

Stern, D. (1985). *The interpersonal world of the infant.* New York: Basic Books.

Stern, D. (2004). *The present moment in psychotherapy and everyday life.* New York: Norton.

Strümpfel, U. (2004). Research on Gestalt therapy. *International Gestalt Journal, 27*(1), 9–54.

Strümpfel, U. (2006). *Therapie Der Gefühle: Forschungsbefunde zur Gestalttherapie.* Cologne, Germany: Edition Humanistiche Psychologie. (Part translation into English: http://www.therapie-der-gefuhle.de/. Translation of the database: http://www.therapie-der-gefuhle.de/database.pdf)

Strümpfel, U., & Goldman, R. (2001). Contacting Gestalt therapy. In D. Cain & J. Seeman (Eds.), *Humanistic psychotherapies: Handbook on research and practice* (pp. 189–219). Washington: American Psychological Association.

Westen, D., Novotny, C., & Thompson-Brenner, H. (2004). The empirical status of empirically supported psychotherapies: Assumptions, findings, and reporting in controlled clinical trials. *Psychological Bulletin, 130*(4), 631–663.

Wheeler, G. (2000). *Beyond individualism.* Hillsdale, NJ: GIC/Analytic Press.

Woldt, A., and Toman, S. (2005). *Gestalt therapy: History, theory and practice.* Thousand Oaks, CA: Sage Publications.

Wulf, R. (1998). The historical roots of Gestalt therapy. *Gestalt Journal, 21*(1), 81–92.

Yontef, G. (1990). Gestalt therapy in groups. In I. Kutash & A. Wolf (Eds.), *Group psychotherapist's handbook* (pp. 191–210). New York: Columbia University Press.

Yontef, G. (1993). *Awareness, dialogue and process: Essays on Gestalt therapy.* New York: Gestalt Journal Press.

Yontef, G. (1995). Gestalt therapy. In A. Gurman & S. Messer (Eds.), *Essential psychotherapies* (pp. 261–303). New York: Guilford Press.

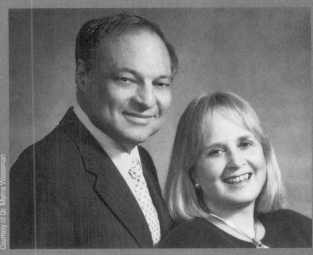

Courtesy of Dr. Myrna Weissman

Gerald Klerman (1929–1992) and Myrna Weissman

11 | INTERPERSONAL PSYCHOTHERAPY

Helen Verdeli and Myrna M. Weissman

OVERVIEW

Basic Concepts

Interpersonal psychotherapy (IPT) is a time-limited, symptom-focused therapy that was originally developed by Gerald Klerman and Myrna Weissman in the 1970s to treat unipolar, nonpsychotic depression in adults (Klerman, Weissman, Rounsaville, & Chevron, 1984; Weissman, Markowitz, & Klerman 2000; Weissman, Markowitz, & Klerman, 2007). The fundamental principle of IPT is that depression occurs in an interpersonal context. Regardless of the *causes* of depression, the *triggers* of depressive episodes involve disruptions of significant attachments and social roles. Four interpersonal problem areas have been defined as depressogenic triggers and become the focus of IPT: grief, interpersonal disputes, role transitions, and interpersonal deficits. While recognizing the genetic, personality, and early childhood factors that contribute to depression, the IPT therapist focuses on the recovery from the current depressive episode by (1) clarifying the relationship between the onset of patient's current depressive symptoms and interpersonal problems and (2) building interpersonal skills to resolve or manage more effectively these interpersonal problems.

The foundation of IPT as an operationalized and manual-based approach has facilitated extensive testing against other psychotherapeutic and pharmacological interventions

(Weissman et al., 2007). In the last 30 years, randomized controlled clinical trials (RCTs) have established IPT as a major evidence-based psychotherapy for a number of mood disorders (major depression, bipolar disorder, postpartum depression, etc.) as well as other conditions (bulimia, binge-eating disorder, PTSD, etc.); populations (adolescents, adults); settings (hospital clinics—inpatient and outpatient, school-based clinics, primary care, prisons); modalities (individual, group, conjoint, via telephone); for various stages of disorder (prevention, acute treatment, maintenance); and cultural contexts (Western countries, sub-Saharan Africa, Asia, and Latin America). Each adaptation adheres to the fundamental elements of the original treatment manual for depression, while emphasizing, adding, and modifying techniques to address the unique needs of the patient population served. The description of the theoretical and empirical basis and principals of IPT can be found in the original manual (Klerman et al., 1984). Current data on efficacy can be found in Weissman and her colleagues (2000), and a simplified clinical manual has been published by Weissman and her co-authors (2007).

Theory of Depression/Psychopathology

In IPT, depression is conceptualized as having three components:

1. Symptom formation
2. Social functioning
3. Personality factors

Historically, IPT has focused on the first two components. Although IPT recognizes the contribution of personality factors in the etiology and maintenance of mental disorders, due to its short-term nature, it has not focused on entrenched aspects of personality that typically take longer to change. Instead, IPT has addressed current symptoms and interpersonal problems that can be improved. Social functioning, symptom formation, and personality factors are all linked, and improvements in interpersonal relations help assuage problems in the other areas of functioning (Weissman et al., 2000). Recently, however, Markowitz and colleagues have adapted IPT to address the more chronic mood disturbances in borderline personality disorder by extending the duration of treatment while preserving its fundamental strategies and techniques (Markowitz, Skodol, & Bleiberg, 2006).

Phases of Treatment

IPT has a "phasic" structure in that it is conducted in three distinct phases (the initial, middle, and termination phases; the specific content of each phase is described in the Process of Psychotherapy section). In that sense, IPT is different from a modular approach to treatment, which characterizes cognitive behavior therapy or dialectical behavior therapy where, for example, cognitive or mindfulness strategies can be conducted before but also after behavioral ones.

Medical Model

Following a medical model of conceptualizing depression, the patient is diagnosed and prescribed the "sick role" in the very beginning of the treatment. The therapist educates the patient about depression, emphasizing that it is a treatable medical problem similar to other illness such as pneumonia, receptive to treatment and not the patient's fault or failure (Klerman et al., 1984). Giving patients' symptoms a name, allowing them to take on the sick role and instilling hope about recovery is in itself a powerful therapeutic strategy that (1) demystifies the patients' symptoms by grouping them as part of a known syndrome; (2) excuses patients from blame for the illness and what it makes them do or renders them incapable of doing; (3) separates patients' disorder from their personality and identifies it as a treatable condition; and (4) gives patients permission to experiment with implementation of new interpersonal strategies.

Interpersonal Problem Areas

IPT identifies four classes of interpersonal problem that may trigger depression: grief, interpersonal disputes, role transitions, and interpersonal deficits. Identifying and addressing these problem areas becomes the central axis of the IPT clinical focus. Right at the outset of the treatment, the therapist and patient review current relationship problems that could be associated with the onset and maintenance of depression symptoms. Together they select and focus on the interpersonal problem area associated with the current episode.

The four interpersonal problem areas of IPT-A are:

- **Grief** (actual death of a significant other or pet)
- **Interpersonal disputes** (overt or covert disagreements with family members, friends and peers, neighbors, etc.)
- **Role transitions** (difficulty making transitions between stages in life and/or changes in life circumstances such as divorce, moving to a new home, promotion, birth of a child, illness in the family, transition to college, etc.)
- **Interpersonal deficits** (social isolation and/or significant communication problems that lead to difficulty in starting or maintaining relationships)

Although many patients present with a variety of problems, in order to organize therapy and maintain focus, one or at most two areas should be identified as initial targets for therapy. It is not necessary to address all the interpersonal problems occurring in a patient's life to reduce depressive symptoms and alleviate the current episode. Developing a sense of mastery in one interpersonal context can transfer over into other areas of a patient's life.

Transcultural adaptations of IPT have shown that the interpersonal problem areas are found across cultures and are universal elements of the human condition. For some disorders (e.g. depression, bulimia nervosa), they are seen as triggers for an episode; in others (e.g. PTSD), they are seen as consequences of the illness that contribute to its maintenance. More generally, the interpersonal context is a paradigm that people universally recognize, unlike intrapsychic or cognitive behavioral perspectives that are much more informed by our Western and Anglophone cultural background, values, and assumptions. Likewise, in parts of the world where there may be a stigma against psychological problems and their treatment, the focus in IPT on resolutions to interpersonal and often group conflict may be more acceptable and less threatening than other approaches.

Time-Limited Duration

The length of treatment is also established in the initial phase and typically ranges between 12 and 16 consecutive weekly sessions. This structure presents a clear, positive expectation of rapid relief from symptoms and improvement in interpersonal functioning and generates mobilization and optimism. It helps establish patient–therapist rapport by promoting confidence in the patient's ability to change. By focusing on the here and now, it also protects against potential risks of long-term treatment such as patient dependency on the therapist, regression, and the reinforcement of avoidance behaviors (Weissman et al., 2000).

Testability

IPT was originally developed as part of a clinical drug trial to be directly comparable to the other treatment arms. This influenced the character and structure of the therapy in two fundamental ways: (1) It is manualized to ensure consistency of treatment delivery and, from a research perspective, to limit threats to internal reliability and validity (although there is considerable flexibility in the therapeutic techniques used, particularly in the middle phase of treatment); (2) regular assessment of the patients' depressive symptoms and functioning is built into the structure of the therapy. These elements are not simply byproducts of the context in which the therapy was developed but may also have important therapeutic effects; for example, tracking patients' illness during treatment (using the Hamilton Rating Scale or some other established measure) gives them and their therapists a clear and objective sense of changes in their clinical picture and so can be used to promote a sense of movement in therapy.

Evidence-Based

The development of IPT was also informed heavily by the scientific ethos of Klerman and colleagues and their conviction that all approaches should be tested empirically and that the strongest source of evidence for a treatment's efficacy derives from RCTs (Klerman et al., 1984). The testability of IPT has facilitated its comparison with other forms of psychotherapeutic and psychopharmacological intervention in a long series of clinical trials. The results of these studies have greatly influenced the evolution of IPT: its adaptation for a range of disorders in different populations, its modification for use in a variety of treatment modalities, and its employment in many different cultures around the world.

Other Systems

Klerman and Weissman's goal in developing IPT was to make explicit and operational a systematic psychotherapeutic approach to depression based on theory, clinical observation, and empirical evidence. Given the genesis of IPT, it is not surprising that its procedures and techniques have much in common with those used in other schools of psychotherapy: Clarification of mood states and linking them to interpersonal events, communication analysis and decision making, interpersonal skill building, and homework are hardly exclusive to IPT. Likewise, IPT shares many common goals with other schools of psychotherapy: helping patients gain a sense of mastery of current social roles, combating social isolation, restoring a sense of group belonging, and assisting patients in finding new meaning in their lives (Klerman et al., 1984).

The focus on reduction of depressive symptoms and interpersonal issues in the here and now distinguishes IPT from more traditional psychoanalytic and dynamic psychotherapies. While psychodynamic psychotherapy focuses heavily on early childhood experiences as determinants of unconscious mental processes and intrapsyhic conflict, IPT does not attempt to explore the patient's behavior as a manifestation of internal conflict but rather in terms of current interpersonal relations. Although the influence of early childhood experiences is recognized as significant, it is not emphasized in IPT. Instead, therapy focuses on patients' current disputes, frustrations, anxieties, and wishes as defined in the interpersonal context. While psychodynamic therapies emphasize unconscious thoughts, IPT works largely at the conscious and preconscious levels. Psychodynamic therapies intervene at the level of personality organization, whereas IPT seeks to improve symptom formation and social adjustment. Psychodynamic therapies are concerned with internalized object relations, whereas IPT looks at interpersonal relations. A psychodynamic therapist listens for a patient's intrapsychic wishes, whereas the IPT therapist listens for the patient's role expectations and interpersonal disputes (Klerman et al., 1984).

These differences between IPT and psychodynamic approaches are not necessarily due to fundamental theoretical differences. In exploring current interpersonal problems with the patient, an IPT therapist may recognize intrapsychic defense mechanisms such as projection, denial, isolation, undoing, or repression but does so without making internal conflict a focus of treatment. Nor do the techniques used in the two forms of therapy necessarily differ greatly: many dynamically trained and psychoanalytically oriented psychotherapists report that they already routinely use many of the concepts and techniques of IPT in their practice.

The interpersonal focus of IPT is quite different from that of another time-limited treatment, cognitive–behavioral therapy (CBT). Aaron Beck's work in defining and describing the procedures of cognitive therapy (CT), from which CBT developed, provided a model for the development of IPT by Klerman and Weissman. In common with CBT, IPT focuses on the here and now, is structured, shares techniques, and addresses patients' limited sense of options available to them. Unlike CBT, IPT does not attempt to uncover distorted thoughts systematically through homework, nor does it attempt to help the patient develop alternative thought patterns through prescribed practice. Instead, the IPT therapist draws attention to patients' exploration and modification of maladaptive communication patterns that trigger and maintain their depressive symptoms. Unlike CBT, negative cognitions and behaviors such as guilt, lack of assertiveness, and negative bias are focused on only through the examination of their impact on the person's relationships and social roles.

Like REBT, IPT views the therapist's role as active and directive. Unlike REBT, IPT does not focus on uncovering irrational thoughts and beliefs through direct confrontation but uses as a point of departure the functional impact of discordant interpersonal and role expectations between the patient and the other parties involved in the interpersonal problem.

Finally, a number of principles of the Rogerian psychotherapy, such as the importance of creating a genuine, accepting, validating, and safe therapeutic environment to promote desire for exploration and growth in the patient, is shared by IPT. However, unlike the Rogerian tradition, IPT therapists believe that making the patient feel safe is a necessary but not sufficient condition for good therapy. Patients need to develop a thorough understanding of how they affect and are affected by their interpersonal problems and then learn and practice concrete skills to manage these problems more effectively.

HISTORY

Precursors

The formative work by Klerman, Weissman, and colleagues was informed by contemporary theories and empirical findings from three different areas.

Interpersonal Context of Depression

The creators of IPT believed that depression was essentially a biological illness but that the onset and recurrence of symptoms were triggered by stress, particularly the loss or threat of an important interpersonal attachment. This idea has its theoretical origins in Adolph Meyer's psychobiological framework of mental illnesses (Meyer, 1957) and the work of Harry Stack Sullivan (Sullivan, 1955).

Meyer was perhaps the most influential figure in American psychiatry during the first decades of the 20th century. Strongly influenced by evolution theory, his concept of psychobiology modified the Darwinian principle of biological adaptation to include the adaptation of the organism to its social environment. Within this model, Meyer viewed mental illness as the result of an individual's *maladaptive* attempt to adjust to the changing environment. Although he considered patients' response to environmental stress and change in adulthood to be determined by early experiences in the family and other important social groups, Meyer put great emphasis on patients' current experience, social relations, and relationship to their environments. He noted that a variety of common life events could be important etiological factors in the development of a disorder and created the "life chart" to track the relationship between life history, illness (physical and psychiatric), and stressful events (Meyer, 1951).

Although the interpersonal approach has its basis in Meyer's ideas, it was Sullivan who developed and fully articulated the interpersonal paradigm. Sullivan went so far as to describe psychiatry as the field of interpersonal relations and defined the discipline as the study of people and the processes between them rather than focusing exclusively on the brain, the individual, or society. Along with his associates, he developed a comprehensive theory of the relationship between psychiatric disorders and interpersonal relations, rooted for the developing child in the family and for the adult in life's many interactions. He maintained that one can only understand and address mental illness by making sense of the person's interpersonal matrix (Sullivan, 1955).

Attachment Theory

If the work of Meyer and then Sullivan established the interpersonal approach to psychiatric practice formalized in IPT, it is John Bowlby's *attachment theory* that provides the theoretical basis for the interpersonal context of depression and the mechanisms underpinning the therapy. Bowlby (1969) proposed that humans have an innate tendency to make strong *affectional bonds* (attachments) and that separation or threat of separation of these bonds causes emotional distress, sadness, and in some cases more severe depression. The underlying premise is that there is a universal human need to develop lasting affectional bonds with primary caregivers. These attachments make it possible for the individual to develop the ability to construct and maintain mental representations of the self and others, namely "internal working models," which organize cognition, affect, and behavior (Bowlby, 1980).

Loss or threat of disruption to these affectional bonds causes emotional distress, sadness, and anxiety. In her famous "Strange Situation" study, Ainsworth (1978) was able to identify three major *attachment styles*: secure attachment, ambivalent–insecure attachment, and avoidant–insecure attachment. A fourth attachment style known as disorganized–insecure attachment was added later (Main & Solomon, 1986). Anxious/ambivalent, avoidant, and disorganized styles are insecure attachment patterns and are considered to be secondary behavioral strategies in response to an insensitive or unavailable caregiver. Although somewhat adaptive, they are considered to be pathogenic because they signify important self-deficits (Peluso, Peluso, White, & Kern, 2004).

Based on these observations, Bowlby proposed that psychotherapy should help patients examine current interpersonal relationships and consider how these relationships developed from experiences with attachment figures earlier in life. In addition, therapeutic strategies should seek to correct the distortions produced by faulty earlier attachments and teach patients how to develop more adaptive and salutary interpersonal relationships. This in turn makes patients less vulnerable to the threats to attachment that might trigger future mental health problems. Contemporary theories and studies of attachment have continued to inform IPT; this research is reviewed in the Theories of Personality section.

Life Events

IPT has also been influenced heavily by the psychosocial and life events literature of depression. Since IPT was first developed, the use of systematic life events interviews within long-term epidemiological studies has begun to clarify the role of life events in the complex matrix of factors that contribute to the development of psychiatric disorders. Eugene Paykel has been an important figure in the development of this research. In an influential 1978 study, he used the measure of relative risk—the ratio of the disease rate among those exposed to a putative causal factor versus the disease rate among people not exposed—to examine the impact of stressful life events on depression. He found the relative risk of developing depression after the most stressful category of events to be a striking 6:1 (Paykel, 1978). Since then, evidence corroborating the role of life stress in the genesis of depression has accumulated from large-scale epidemiological and genetic studies (see Theories of Personality section).

Beginnings

IPT was not originally developed with the intention of creating a new psychotherapy for depression. The motivation was to formulize a psychotherapy for a clinical trial testing the efficacy of antidepressant medication as a maintenance treatment for unipolar depression. Tricyclic antidepressants had shown promise in reducing the acute symptoms of depression, but there were no data on the efficacy of medication in maintaining long-term symptom reduction for depression. Klerman and Weissman felt that as far as possible, clinical trials should mimic clinical practice (Klerman et al., 1984). As the majority of patients at that time received both medication and therapy, they felt a therapy arm should be included, if only to create a milieu effect. Thus an 8-month-long clinical trial was designed for subjects who had shown symptom reduction while on antidepressant medication during their acute phase of depression. Patients were randomly assigned to conditions in which they received amitriptyline, placebo, or no medication with or without weekly psychotherapy sessions.

Prior to conducting the study, the team first needed to define the psychotherapy they would use and the techniques it would incorporate. Psychotherapists could then be trained in this standardized approach and the quality and consistency of the treatment could be tested. A cornerstone of the new therapy was its *time-specific* nature, focus on current problems, and the use of a manual to standardize the procedure. The psychotherapy, initially called "high contact," differed markedly from the open-ended structure of psychodynamic psychotherapy, the predominant treatment method of the time. Another novel feature of the treatment, again reflecting the psychopharmacologic trial of which it was a part, was the use of *standardized assessments* to diagnose patients and follow their clinical course.

The development of the psychotherapy was governed by several guiding principles (Weissman, 2006):

1. It was important to test and establish the efficacy of all treatments, including psychotherapy, in RCTs. (There had been no positive randomized trials of psychotherapy.)

2. Outcomes should be measured across a broad range of standardized measures, including assessments of social functioning and quality of life.

3. Treatment results needed to be replicated before widespread dissemination.

The preliminary step in creating the therapy involved determining its dose, frequency, and diagnostic process. The latter evolved into the first phase of IPT and involved what have become many of IPT's most important and distinctive features: conducting an *interpersonal inventory* of important people currently in the patient's life; giving the patient the "*sick role*"; linking symptoms to *interpersonal situations*; and selecting *problem areas* associated with the onset of the current depressive episode. The four problem areas were chosen to cover the range of problems that lead to disrupted attachment and trigger depression and arose from Klerman and Paykel's ongoing work developing measures to assess the role of life events in depression onset and relapse. The "high contact" treatment manual was developed and revised by reviewing cases and developing scripts based on real practice. In this way, the treatment sequence and procedures were formalized so that therapists could be trained to deliver the therapy in a consistent manner.

The one-year follow-up results from the maintenance study found that medication prevented relapse and the psychotherapy improved social functioning (Klerman, Dimascio, Weissman, Prusoff, & Paykel, 1974). The positive findings for the therapy sparked the team to elaborate the principles of the therapy. It was first termed *interpersonal psychotherapy* at this time. An acute treatment trial involving IPT alone and in combination with medication was also positive, with the combination of IPT and medication proving the most efficacious intervention. This was followed by the NIMH Multisite Collaborative Study testing IPT, cognitive therapy, and drugs as treatments for depression (Elkin et al., 1989). In 1984, the efficacy of IPT was documented by another team, and Klerman, Weissman, and colleagues (1984) published the first IPT manual, *Interpersonal Psychotherapy of Depression*. Since that time, numerous studies and adaptations of IPT for different patient populations have been conducted across a variety of settings and in many different countries.

Current Status

Since it was first developed in the 1970s, clinical and research interest in IPT has grown steadily. IPT has been adapted, tested, and shown to be efficacious as a treatment for a variety of mood and other disorders. Adaptations for mood disorders include IPT as a maintenance treatment of depression, IPT for pregnancy, miscarriage, and postpartum depression, IPT for depression in adolescents and children, IPT for depression in older adults, IPT for depression in medical patients, IPT for dysthymic disorder, and IPT for bipolar disorder. IPT has also been adapted for eating disorders, substance abuse, anxiety disorders, borderline personality disorder (BPD), and posttraumatic stress disorder. The evidence for the efficacy of IPT is strongest for mood disorders (where the most trials have taken place), varies for other adaptations, and remains untested for some of the newest ones.

Although it was developed as an individual psychotherapy, IPT has also been adapted and tested across a variety of treatment modalities: in group, conjoint couple, and telephone formats. These adaptations have been made both for practical reasons (to address barriers to care such as limited funding, poor transportation, and time constraints) and based on a clinical rationale (e.g. to foster a sense of constructive collaboration between patients and destigmatize their problems). Positive evidence has been found for each adaptation, with group therapy in particular supported by a number of RCTs for a variety of disorders, cultures, and patient populations (e.g. Bolton et al., 2003; Wilfley et al., 1993). An abbreviated form of IPT called *interpersonal counseling* (IPC) has also been developed and tested (Weissman & Klerman, 1986) to address the practical restraints of treating patients in certain settings (e.g. patients with depression as a secondary diagnosis being treated for a medical problem in a general hospital setting). A new adaptation, *IPT-EST* (evaluation, support, and triage), developed by Weissman and Verdeli, provides a three-session intervention based on the first phase of the standard IPT (diagnosis, identification of the interpersonal problem area, and management of depression). IPT-EST is designed to be followed by an assessment of the need for ongoing treatment. IPT-EST is currently being refined and tested.

Not only has IPT been tested and used for a range of disorders in a number of different modalities, increasingly it is being used across a variety of cultures, both within and outside the United States. There have been IPT training programs in Australia, Austria, Brazil, the Czech Republic, Ethiopia, Finland, France, Germany, Greece, Hungary, Iceland, India, Italy, Ireland, Japan, Kenya, the Netherlands, New Zealand, Norway, Portugal, Romania, South Korea, Spain, Sweden, Switzerland, Thailand, Turkey, Uganda, and the United Kingdom. In many of these countries, clinical trials have established the efficacy of important new adaptations such as trials of group IPT (IPT-G) with depressed adults in rural southwest Uganda and depressed adolescents in internally displaced persons (IDP) camps in northern Uganda. In the United States, IPT has shown efficacy in clinical trials with black and Hispanic (mainly Puerto Rican and Dominican) minorities. IPT manuals have been translated into French, Spanish, Italian, German, and Japanese, and Portuguese and Danish translations are currently developed.

Ease of training was a priority in the development of IPT, and learning the psychotherapy should be straightforward for anyone with a basic knowledge of clinical psychiatric diagnosis and prior training in standard psychotherapeutic techniques: how to show empathy and warmth, formulate a problem, develop a therapeutic alliance, maintain professional boundaries, and so forth (Weissman, 2006). Within its prescribed, goal-oriented, and three-phased structure, IPT nevertheless affords the therapist considerable autonomy and flexibility to employ a variety of therapeutic techniques common to other forms of therapy.

Despite its widespread dissemination and proven efficacy, few professional training programs for mental heath workers—psychiatrists, psychologists, social workers, or psychiatric nurses—teach IPT as part of a program in evidence-based psychotherapy. Among those that do, typically only a didactic course is offered without the very important training component of hands-on clinical supervision (Weissman et al., 2006).

For students and professionals who are interested in being trained, many of the professional organizational meetings (e.g. the American Psychiatric Associations's annual meetings) offer continuing education courses in IPT. These short half- or full-day courses are primarily didactic. The 2- to 4-day workshops offered by academic centers around the world are much more intensive and include practical, hands-on training. Clinicians interested in becoming trained in IPT should obtain supervision with an experienced IPT therapist. Three supervised IPT cases following didactic training usually suffice for experienced psychotherapists to learn to perform IPT competently (Weissman, 2006). Guidelines for becoming an IPT therapist or trainer can be found at www.interpersonalpsychotherapy.org, the Web site of the International Society for Interpersonal Psychotherapy. Every other year, the organization holds an international meeting at which IPT researchers, students, and clinicians come together to discuss developments in the field and take part in workshops. The 2009 meeting at Columbia University in New York included more than 300 presenters and attendees from Africa, Asia, Australasia, Europe, and North and South America. For clinicians wanting a glimpse of IPT procedures with scripts, the 2007 manual is recommended (Weissman et al., 2007).

PERSONALITY

Theory of Personality

A theory of personality is not relevant to IPT. Within the theoretical framework of IPT, pathology is considered to have three component processes (symptom function, social and interpersonal relations, and personality and character problems). IPT research and practice have historically focused on the first two. IPT investigators were reluctant to focus on personality traits and disorders for a number of reasons. One is the difficulty in reliably diagnosing personality pathology while in a depressive episode: for example, research by Fava and colleagues (2002) has shown that although Axis II diagnoses are common among acutely depressed patients, they drop significantly following successful antidepressant treatment. Therefore, IPT does not make definitive Axis II diagnostic assessment during the acute phase of the depression. Another reason is that a significant number of patients do not want or cannot be in long-term psychotherapy. Even if a personality disorder emerges, brief treatment focuses on acute symptom relief and not on personality restructuring, which has not been shown empirically to be possible to change in a short time. However, there is some evidence that the skills learned in IPT may have an effect on behavior, which is a reflection of personality. IPT aims for specific, measurable changes in how the person feels, relates, and communicates. As Markowitz and colleagues noted:

> . . . although IPT makes no claims to change personality, imparting interpersonal skills such as self-assertion, confrontation, and effective expression of anger is almost as good as effecting personality change. These skills frequently open up new possibilities for interpersonal functioning that patients may never have dared imagine and that can feel enormously empowering. (Markowitz et al., 2006; p. 442)

The terrain of personality traits as determinants and outcomes of the impact of IPT has changed over the last 10 years. One body of evidence comes from attachment research; another comes from a new line of investigation by Markowitz and colleagues on IPT for borderline personality disorder (2006).

Personality Variables and Environment: Contemporary Research on Attachment

As discussed in the Precursors section, Bowlby's attachment theory and its evolution provide an important theoretical basis for IPT. The attachment framework offers a set of organizing principles for the understanding of the various aspects of normal and pathological interpersonal relations and the consequent psychological fitness across the life cycle.

Attachment patterns remain pertinent throughout the human lifespan. Based on Ainsworth's infant–caretaker attachment paradigm, contemporary research has identified similar attachment patterns in adults. According to Bartholomew's four-category model (Bartholomew & Horowitz, 1991), adult attachment is conceptualized as combinations of the internal working models of the self and others. The internal working model of the self constitutes the dimension of *anxiety* and refers to whether the individual has the inner resources for security and self-soothing vis-à-vis an important relationship, whereas the internal working model of others yields the dimension of *avoidance*—that is, whether security is maintained through proximity or, alternatively, self-reliance and emotional distance (Bartholomew & Horowitz, 1991). The combination of these two dimensions results in *four possible attachment styles:* (1) secure anxiety, (2), dismissing, (3) preoccupied, and (4) fearful.

Secure individuals (those with low scores on measures of anxiety and avoidance attachment) are relatively more protected against psychological distress in general (Hammen et al., 1995) and depression in particular (Mickelson, Kessler, & Shaver, 1997). In contrast, insecurely attached individuals tend to have lower self-esteem (Collins & Read, 1990); poorer affect regulation strategies (Brennan & Shaver, 1995); and marked problems with emotional support (Simpson, Rholes, & Nelligan, 1992), and they tend to have a higher number of depressive symptoms (Murphy & Bates, 1997). Moreover, there is evidence that the fearful attachment pattern is correlated with depression. In a maintenance study of 162 female participants with major depression who received IPT, Cyranowski and colleagues (2002) identified 43% as fearfully attached compared to only 22% who were securely attached.

There is evidence that attachment style is associated with treatment response in IPT. Cyranowski and colleagues (2002) found a temporal effect of attachment style on depression remission: Although the proportion of subjects who remitted did not differ by attachment profile, among the patients who did remit, those with secure attachment had significantly more rapid remission compared to subjects with fearful–avoidant attachment. The finding indicates that IPT's brief course may not allow enough time for fearful–avoidant patients to develop a trusting relationship with the therapist.

At the same time, there is emerging evidence that IPT can help improve patients' attachment styles as opposed simply to resolving the interpersonal crises to which insecure attachment may predispose them. In a new line of research, Ravitz (2009) has hypothesized that IPT may ameliorate the anxious and avoidant behaviors of insecurely attached depressed patients. In a recent study of IPT with depressed adults, subjects whose symptoms fully remitted also showed significant decreases in measures of attachment avoidance and anxiety (Ravitz, 2009). Although these results need to be corroborated in future trials, they present an intriguing possibility: IPT may intervene at the level of attachment style as well as influence the current interpersonal environment and in this way reduce vulnerability to future psychopathology.

IPT and Treatment of Borderline Personality Disorder

Although IPT explicitly addresses only Axis I disorders, Markowitz and colleagues (2006) note that there is a strong rationale for treating BPD with IPT. First, BPD is frequently comorbid with mood disorders. Second, BPD is largely about maladaptive social interactions. Markowitz's team at Columbia is currently investigating the effectiveness of IPT in an open trial of an 8-month (34 sessions) adaptation for BPD patients. According to the investigators, BPD is a "mood-inflected chronic illness," interspersed with explosive outbursts of anger, despair, and impulsivity. Due to the chronicity of the disorder, patients find it particularly difficult to link their mood symptoms with current life events and erroneously regard those symptoms as part of their personality.

Markowitz has outlined the therapeutic elements in IPT for BPD: IPT provides the patient *success experiences*, whereby patients learn new skills in order to deal effectively with their life crises. Overcoming the crisis is experienced as an interpersonal victory and results in significant improvement of their self-image and a sense of competence and control. The medical model of IPT allows patients to conceptualize BPD as a chronic yet treatable illness. Also, IPT aims at solving patients' problems in the relationships *outside the office*, which is thought to minimize the possibility of therapeutic rupture (in a clinical population in which rupture poses serious threat to therapeutic relationship). Finally, although IPT does not implement "direct" changes in personality, the patient is given tools to deal with those triggers of mood dysregulation characteristic of BPD (intense episodes of depression and anger) that result in *correction of interpersonal dysfunction*. The latter heralds new possibilities for interpersonal functioning that deeply alter the way patients see the world and themselves (Markowitz et al., 2006).

Variety of Concepts

The development and practice of IPT have been informed by several fields of research that variously place emphasis on the impact of life events, biology, social interaction, and personality in the development of psychopathology. Together they suggest that the etiology of psychiatric disorders is complex and multidetermined, with the various genetic, personality, and environmental factors interacting with one another.

Methodological advances over the years, in particular the use of systematic life events interviews within long-term epidemiological studies, have helped to clarify the role of life events in the complex matrix of factors that coincide in the development of psychiatric disorders. As the isolation of genes related to specific psychiatric disorders becomes a reality, important new advances are being made in our understanding of gene x environment interactions in the development of pathology.

In a landmark study, Caspi and colleagues (2003) examined how genetic differences in the 5-HTT (serotonin transporter) gene moderated the influence of stressful life events on depression. They found that people with one or two copies of the short allele were more likely to become depressed in response to stressful life events than people with a double long allele. In other words, the study showed a *gene x environment interaction* in which the 5-HTT genotype moderated the depressogenic influence of adverse life events. These findings show that psychiatric disorders are genetically complex illnesses in which, like diabetes or hypertension, a genetic predisposition may interact with the environment to produce pathology; the *phenotype* (clinical picture) results from the interaction of the *genotype* and the environment (Weissman et al., 2007). These genetic findings highlight the importance of addressing the pathology of genetically susceptible individuals with treatment that emphasizes current life events.

While the replication of the Caspi findings has recently been called into question, these questions have to do more with the design of the replications than with the original findings of Caspi and colleagues (Risch et al., 2009). Their important findings based on observational epidemiology are being supported by numerous controlled human and animal studies. This work showing the relationship between genes and environmental stress for depression is in its early phase. Most relevant to psychotherapy is the work of Champagne and colleagues showing that attachment stress in mice can be reversed by maternal licking and grooming (Champagne, Francis, Mar, & Meaney, 2003).

There is strong evidence for a relationship between type of life event and the genesis of depression. Kendler, Prescott, Myers and Neale (2003) have found that humiliating events are more strongly associated with depression onset compared to other types of life events. Moreover, personality characteristics influence the impact of life events on the onset of depression (Shahar, Blatt, Zuroff, & Pilkonis, 2003).

While genetic and personality variables that place people at risk for disorders such as depression cannot readily be altered, people's reactions and responses to their social environment can. IPT aims to improve patients' depression by improving interpersonal relations, thus reducing life stress and increasing social support. These improvements in the people's social world are hypothesized to moderate the effects of the genetic, personality, and environmental factors placing the individual at risk for depression.

PSYCHOTHERAPY

Theory of Psychotherapy

IPT aims to improve symptoms and interpersonal functioning by improving the way distressed individuals relate to others. As emphasized earlier, this interpersonal focus is the hallmark of IPT. IPT has not invented new techniques. However, while many of the techniques it uses are common to other time-limited therapies, IPT specifically applies them to interpersonal issues. Much more than collecting a set of techniques, the developers of IPT codified *strategies* organized around active management of depression and the four problem areas into a cohesive therapeutic system.

The language of affect is used more in IPT than in other time-limited therapies such as CBT or REBT. Commenting on how the affect is communicated (verbally and nonverbally) is the bread and butter of IPT: "Your eyes seem so sad as you are talking about her"; "You say you are mad at him, but I noticed you are smiling"; "How did you let your boss know that you were not happy about his decision?"

IPT is also different from simple interpersonal skills training: Although IPT therapists often work with patients on assertiveness, they put the skills within the much bigger context of patients' expectations of other people. This helps patients mourn what was lost or never given and encourages change and mobilization. The goal is to break patients' social isolation, helplessness, and hopelessness by assisting them in generating new options and enabling them to access sources of interpersonal support.

IPT does not maintain that all relationships need to be maintained at all costs. Some ties are destructive for patients in that they do not foster growth and closeness. In other relationships, one of the parties has moved on and does not wish to continue. Helping patients have a balanced view of the strengths and weaknesses of the relationship and a thorough understanding of their own and the other person's desires would determine the outcome of what is frequently asked by the IPT therapist: "Do you think you would like to try one more time?"

A big challenge in IPT, especially for new therapists, is the difficulty in staying focused on the problem area(s) defined as targets for treatment. Dealing with patients' daily crises without putting them into a larger context of a problem area can diffuse and derail the treatment. What often happens is that a general "antidepressant" method of approaching interpersonal situations is learned systematically through work in one problem area. The learning that was generated is frequently transferred to other interpersonal issues that emerge along the way. There are times, of course, when 16 sessions have not been enough and the person, although better, is still not well. In those cases, therapists renew the contract with the patient, setting as new goals the specific interpersonal aims the patient wants to work on in the next set of sessions.

The Therapeutic Relationship

IPT therapists are active, ask questions, and make comments, especially in the first sessions (see Process of Psychotherapy section below). Although therapists are directive, they are not prescriptive; in other words, they try to let patients generate options, ideas, and resources, as opposed to providing them themselves. They do not work through forms (like the dysfunctional thought records or mood monitoring forms used in CBT). They do not interpret dreams or other material that communicates unconscious desires, and they do not encourage regression (like analytic treatment).

Process of Psychotherapy

The usual course of IPT for acute depression is 16 sessions for adults or 12 for adolescents divided into three phases: the initial phase, middle phase, and termination phase. For a detailed account of clinical practice, see Weissman and colleagues (2007). Here we will briefly illustrate the clinical work through a case vignette with segments from the three phases. The patient, Paul, is a 22-year-old college student who presented to his university's student health services with symptoms of depression. It should be noted that prior to initiation of IPT, the therapist had already conducted a thorough clinical interview, evaluated suicidality, and assessed the need for medication (in case of melancholic depression, severe neurovegetative symptoms, etc.).

Initial Phase (first 3–4 sessions)

During the initial phase, therapists administer depression rating scales or symptoms checklists (e.g. the Hamilton Rating Scale for Depression, the Beck Depression Inventory). In addition, therapists evaluate patients' idiosyncratic symptoms of depression: For example, when depressed, some patients become particularly jealous or anxious; some drink or smoke more, while others stop smoking and drinking; some may develop somatic symptoms, such as nausea, headaches, and the like. Following an in-depth clinical interview to determine patients' diagnosis and psychosocial functioning, the initial phase is conducted over three to four sessions.

In this phase, therapists aim to (1) educate patients about depression and give them hope that it is a treatable condition; (2) help patients manage the consequences of depression and create space in their lives to heal from the episode; (3) understand how depression affects and is affected by patients' important social ties and roles; and (4) agree with patients to focus during the rest of the treatment on one or two interpersonal problem areas that are associated with the current depressive episode. Therapists complete the following tasks (Weissman et al., 2007):

- confirm diagnosis of depression and give syndrome a name
- give patients hope
- assign the "sick role": explain to patients that they are suffering from a depression that does not let them function at an optimal level; tell them that they may temporarily need to lower expectations for what they are able to accomplish but need to do the therapeutic work to get out of the current episode
- help patients to rationalize and manage the impact of depression on their lives (e.g. lower expectations, suspend major decisions until depression remission, etc.)

The following is a dialogue between Paul and his therapist from the initial phase:

Therapist: Paul, you described today a number of difficulties you've had in the last 2 months . . . trouble concentrating, which led to a low grade in your stats test and your difficulty in finishing your sociology assignment . . . you also have trouble falling asleep, and you've been waking up at 5:30 every day . . . you told me that you have been feeling sad and empty and that your friends noticed it . . . you get tired easily and need to go to bed . . . and since you don't feel like eating, you've also lost 11 pounds in the last 7 weeks. These are symptoms of depression. Depression is . . .

Paul: I'm screwing everything up (on the verge of tears) . . . I should have . . . I'm just failing in everything . . . now I *am* depressed (covers face with hands).

Therapist: It's not your fault that you have depression. It's not your failure, Paul. Depression is common and the good news is that we have a number of great treatments for it. You will get better. Right now it's important for you to take care of yourself and make sure that the circumstances around you allow you to get better.

Paul: But I don't have the time for that. I'm failing at school, I'm in trouble big time . . . (is tearful and panicked)

Therapist: If you had any other illness right now, say if you had pneumonia . . . have you ever had pneumonia, or a really bad flu? (Paul nods in agreement) Would you expect yourself to do well in your classes, "business as usual"?

Paul: Well, that's different, that's a real illness.

Therapist: Depression is also a real illness. It has symptoms, exactly the types of things you mentioned before: sadness, sleep and appetite problems, low energy and motivation, difficulty concentrating and making decisions . . . This is typical depression. The good news is that we have some very effective ways to treat it. Right now, to get your everyday work done you may need a little extra help from family and friends. For the time being, you may not even be able to do all of the things that you need and want to do. As we make progress in the treatment, you'll start improving, but it's going to take a little time.

Paul: I hope so, this can't go on. I feel terrible that I may fail my stats class . . . maybe I don't have what it takes to be in the program any more, it's crushing me, I may have to just drop out . . .

Therapist: Paul, this is not the right time to make decisions about leaving the program. Depression colors everything in your world and you may not see any options available to you. Why don't we discuss the program some more after you recover from your depression? If you still feel the same, it might be something to consider.

Paul: Ok, I guess . . . (seems somewhat less overwhelmed). But what am I going to do about the stats?

Therapist: Well, given that you are in the midst of a depressive episode, it makes sense that you are struggling a lot with stats. It requires good concentration, maybe more than other classes. What are your options right now for that class?

Paul: It's too late to drop it.

Therapist: I see.

Paul: Maybe I can get an incomplete, I don't know.

Therapist: You came up with a really good idea there. How can you find out what you need to do to get an incomplete?

They then discussed ways in which Paul might go about talking to the professor about getting an incomplete grade due to his depression. Paul said that he wanted to talk to his professor about getting some extra time to complete the outstanding assignments before considering asking for an incomplete. When the therapist asked him about people who could help him through the stats course, Paul thought of asking the class RA to go over some recent difficult material with him. At the end of this part of the discussion, Paul seemed somewhat relieved, "lighter," and less anxious.

The therapist then proceeded to explore the interpersonal context of Paul's depression. She did so through the following strategies:

1.   By finding out what was happening in Paul's life around the onset of his symptoms
2.   By conducting the interpersonal inventory, a detailed exploration of Paul's significant current interpersonal relationships, to understand which contributed to his depression and which were important resources

Therapist: Paul, you said that you started noticing the first depression symptoms at the beginning of the spring semester.

Paul: Yeah, when I came back after I visited home for the holidays.

Therapist: Did anything happen then, during or after the visit?

Here the therapist wanted to explore what problem area had triggered Paul's depression. She asked questions such as: Did anyone important to you die around that time? Or maybe a pet? Did you have a fight with or feel distant from a person who was close to you? Have you felt very lonely or isolated? Were there any big changes in your life around then?

Paul: No big changes, not yet. I have got some big decisions to make about the future, though. I'm not sure what to do after I graduate . . . I have no idea right now . . . I told my parents that during the visit. They asked me, and I told them the truth, I have no idea. I don't know what to do next, I'm not even sure what I want to do.

The therapist started gathering information about an impeding role transition that seemed to be preoccupying Paul. She also wanted to explore the possibility of a dispute (overt or covert) with his parents, since Paul referred emphatically and repeatedly to that interaction.

Therapist: How did they react?
Paul: They didn't say much . . .
Therapist: Do you know how they felt about it?
Paul: I don't know, I don't think they lost sleep over it. We did the usual family stuff. I don't know what happened, it wasn't different from other times, kind of boring . . .
Therapist: Did you expect it to be boring?
Paul: Well, I guess every time I get ready to go home, I have the stupid idea that this time it's going to be different, but nothing ever is.
Therapist: You were disappointed, Paul. You were hoping that this time things would be better, but they were not. (Paul nods) I wonder what you wish was better.
Paul: Well, I know they love me and everything, but . . . I don't know, my sister Sarah was there and . . . Sarah and I are close, she just got engaged and Bill was there as well . . . I guess they didn't have much time for me, so many things to celebrate about Sarah, I guess. She just got accepted into law school, Dad has this ridiculous expression when he looks at her, like she'll continue his practice or something . . . she won't, she's moving to California, where Bill is from, and they're going to school together there. Don't get me wrong, I am really close to Sarah and all, but I don't know, these visits are too much . . .
Therapist: It sounds like this one was especially rough . . .

The therapist had started to form an idea about Paul's problems linked to his depression (a role transition and a covert dispute with his father, who seem to show preference for his successful sister) but felt she needed to get more information. She proceeded to conduct the interpersonal inventory. The therapist elicited examples of interactions and communications to identify strengths and weaknesses in Paul's interpersonal communication patterns.

Therapist: To get a more complete understanding of your life circumstances right now, I think it'd be useful to talk about the important people in your life. Who would you like to start with?

What do you like about ____?

What don't you like about ____?

Have you ever told ____ how you feel?

What stops you? What do you think would happen?

Are there any times that you and ____ enjoy hanging out? What do you guys do?

Are there things that you would like to change in that relationship? What are they?

How would you feel about _____ if those things changed?

Are there things in that relationship that you would like to keep the same? What are they?

Following the inventory, the therapist suspected that Paul's current episode was triggered by two sets of problems: one was his current difficulty in figuring out what to do after he graduated. Paul did not think he would like to pursue graduate studies in sociology (his major). He described being interested in becoming an emergency medical technician (EMT); he had taken and enjoyed an introductory course. However, he was not sure how to investigate this option further. During the inventory, Paul described a strained relationship with his father, a successful attorney, who had always been proud of Paul's older sister's strong personality and academic excellence and who, by contrast, was dismissive and frequently sarcastic toward Paul. Paul reported reacting to his father's comments by leaving the room or "pretending I don't hear him . . . he is full of it . . . I don't care." Paul described being close to his mother and sister, although the latter's success has been hard on him at times ("It's not her fault, but she always gets it right . . . I'm not jealous or anything , that's juvenile, but it's too much, man . . ."). Paul had a few friends, was on "the quiet side," but talked to a couple of friends daily and was particularly close to a female friend, Lisa. He said that he was not dating much this year.

At this point the therapist shared her understanding of Paul's problems, explained the treatment course, and made a treatment contract, also known as the *interpersonal formulation*.

Therapist: From all the information we gathered these 3 weeks, Paul, it seems to me that your depression began shortly after the Christmas vacation. It seems to me like a couple of things were going on for you around that time. Firstly, you started worrying a bit about what you're going to do after you graduate this May, you're not sure what you want to do next. Secondly, the situation isn't helped by the pressure from your father . . . it sounds like he has very high expectations, and can make you feel pretty bad. I think that your anxieties about what to do next, after you finish school, have been made worse by your father's attitude, and that together these two things triggered your depression . . . all the problems you started experiencing about the time you came back to school: your trouble in some of your classes, your difficulty sleeping, the concentration problems, your loss of appetite. Does this sound right to you?

Paul: Sure, I guess.

Therapist: We'll be talking about these important changes that triggered your depression, and we'll try to find ways to help you feel confident to negotiate these problems . . . finishing up with school and thinking about what you want to do next, and how to manage your interactions with your father. I want to remind you that we will be meeting every week for the next 13 weeks. It's important that you come on time and that you reschedule if you need to miss an appointment. Does all that make sense?

Middle Phase

During this phase of treatment, the majority of the interpersonal work takes place: assisting patients in clarifying how they are affected by and affect their interpersonal environments and building antidepressant relational skills to handle interpersonal difficulties better. In Paul's case, the therapist helped clarify his role transition and made him aware of how his father's derogatory remarks affected his depression. Although Paul's difficulties with his father had started a long time previously, the therapist focused on how the dispute manifested itself in the here and now.

The following is an excerpt from session 8:

Therapist: Hi Paul, how have you been since we saw each other last week?

Paul: Kind of mixed.

Therapist: How have your depression symptoms been?

Paul: I don't feel like doing much, I'm sleeping a bit better but still have trouble concentrating

Therapist: How's your appetite? (The therapist asks about whatever depression symptoms the patient has not mentioned.)

Paul: Same.

Therapist: How would you rate your depression on our 1–10 scale (10 being the worst depression you ever felt)?

Paul: I guess a 6.

Therapist: Was it 6 all week?

Paul: No, after I left here on Wednesday it was, I'd say 4, maybe even 3 for a couple of days. Then it kind of went downhill.

Therapist: So you felt really well for a short time. That's wonderful. What happened during those days?

Paul: Lisa called on Wednesday evening, I went over and we watched a couple of movies, Josh and Annie were there too, it was good. Also, I guess what we talked about last time was helpful, how I don't like theoretical stuff and prefer more hands-on work, how happy I felt when I did my EMT work . . . I felt useful, and I was really good at it, Mr. Harris told me so in front of everybody . . . I pulled some info from the Web and made an appointment with the career counselor to see if she can help me find out some more.

Therapist: How did you feel about doing that?

Paul: I felt good, kind of proud, relieved, I guess. I was thinking that things may get better. I also went to speak to the stats professor again. She thinks it makes more sense now to go for the incomplete than trying to finish. She's right, I guess.

Therapist: These were very important steps, Paul. You did a number of things we discussed: you took action and got information to help you decide about your career; you talked with your professor about your stats course; you had a good time with your friends. And look how well you felt after all that. Then things became tough again. When did you start noticing it?

Paul: I'd say on Saturday, I woke up and . . . well, I didn't really feel like getting up.

Therapist: Hmm, that's quite a change. Did something happen on Friday?

Paul: Well, nothing much, I stayed home and watched TV, my parents called, nothing dramatic.

Therapist: Well, as we discussed, subtle things can at times deeply affect people's mood . . . what happened during the call?

Paul: Well, nothing. My mom was telling me about Sarah's new apartment, the furniture they plan to buy and stuff. My father was also on the line, on the other phone. I was yawning, I was tired, they were going on and on about how her in-laws' plan to get them tickets for a trip to Morocco. On and on and on . . . I am failing my stats, I don't know what to do in my life, and I have to hear about Sarah's vacation . . . My dad asked me why I was yawning, and I told him I was tired and wanted to go to bed.

Therapist: What did he say?

Paul: He said, "You're always tired, not quite sure why."

Therapist: How did you feel when he said that?

Paul: I just said, "Oh! Come on, Dad . . . I'm tired, going to bed." Mom said goodnight, he kind of said "alright . . ." or something like that, and we hung up. I went to bed and fell asleep, but woke up at 5 again. I couldn't go back to sleep, so I watched some TV. I was really tired all day, so I cancelled my plans to go out with Annie and Josh.

Therapist: Paul, as you are talking about the event, are you clearer about what affected your mood?

Paul: I guess that discussion with my dad, it didn't sound that bad, but now that I'm talking about it . . .

Therapist: What are you feeling right now?

Paul: I'm pissed . . . he always puts me down, I don't need this shit right now . . .

Therapist: You're right, you sure don't.

Paul: I have so much crap on my plate right now, the least he could do is to leave me alone, just leave me alone . . . (Paul looks tearful but animated).

Therapist: You seem sad and rightfully angry right now, but you don't seem lost. You do have a lot on your plate: you're trying to finish school and decide what your next professional step is, and you are doing this while you're struggling with depression. Have you ever tried to let your father know the effect his remarks have on you?

Paul: I bet he knows.

Therapist: He may know, but I would like now to focus on whether you have tried to make him understand how his comments affect you.

Paul: Not really, we don't get along; I try to stay away from him.

Therapist: From what you said before though, this seems to work only sometimes. Take last week as an example. You were doing a number of things that were making you feel better: you saw your friends, you *were* better, and then after that discussion you felt depressed again, but thankfully not as much as before. As we said in the beginning, you need to make some space for you to heal from your depression and make the changes that will help you move on. Remember what we said about how important it is to have options, not to let yourself be cornered. What are your options right now about contact with your father?

Paul: I can't just stop talking to him, when Mom calls, he says he wants to talk to me, Mom always lets him talk to me. They do the same with Sarah . . . family tradition, I guess.

Therapist: You've said that you feel well after you talk to your mother. Is there any way you can ask her to talk to you without your father present?

Paul: Knowing her, no. She'll be kind of hurt and ask me why, and insist . . . My Mom likes to pretend that everything is fine . . . she won't do that.

Therapist: I wonder if you could have a direct discussion with your father.

Paul: And what would I say?

Therapist: Good question. What would you like to get across?

Paul: (smiles) You asshole, you are ruining my life . . .

Therapist: (laughs) There you go . . .

Paul: (laughing) OK, OK . . . Maybe I don't know, I could tell him that I'm depressed right now, and listening to him saying things like that isn't really helpful.

Therapist: You know, that was a very clear message. How about we role-play that . . .

Termination Phase (last 2 sessions)

During the initial phase of IPT, the duration of treatment is determined. In IPT, every two to three meetings, therapists explicitly make patients aware of the number of remaining sessions. Having a "deadline" facilitates mobilization and a sense of momentum and keeps patients active. During termination, therapists (1) evaluate patients' depressive symptoms with them to determine if they are full or partial responders; (2) address patients' sadness and/or anxiety about ending treatment (differentiating this from depression); (3) increase patients' competence and independence in continuing therapeutic gains; (4) review what skills were useful; and (5) reduce guilt if IPT has not been successful (e.g., "the treatment failed you, you did not fail the treatment, and we have other options available to you").

One of the therapeutic options after termination is maintenance IPT. The maintenance model consists of monthly therapy sessions for a year after termination of the acute treatment. Therapists emphasize the interpersonal skills learned and practiced during acute treatment while addressing any new interpersonal stressors that could potentially trigger further depressive episodes.

The following is an excerpt from Paul's penultimate therapy session:

Therapist: Paul, you have made some significant gains in the last 4 months. First of all, your depression symptoms have improved: you're sleeping better, you're eating better, you're feeling more motivated and energetic, and your concentration has improved. All these improvements have helped you pass all your courses this semester. You also negotiated the problem with your stats professor by arranging to receive an incomplete. On top of all that, you've found the time to think about you want to do next, once you graduate. You've looked into a career as an EMT and signed up to take another course to help decide if it's the right job for you. Also, you've done really well in finding a way to communicate effectively with your father. Now that he understands that you've been depressed, he's interfering less. In addition, you've identified people in your life who you can look to for support and encouragement moving forward. I'd like to hear what you think about what I've just said.

Paul: Yeah, I'm happy about the semester. I didn't think I'd make it. But I'm feeling better than I did. But even though Dad has gotten off my back, I don't think he really gets it. He still wants me to be a success, which in his mind doesn't include becoming an EMT.

Therapist: That's one of the things that remain for you to keep working on going forward from here. But what you've done during the last few months has been enough to improve your mood. The work you'll do in the future should help keep you from getting depressed again. We're almost finished for today. Next week is our last session, and I'd like to hear about your feelings about termination, to look at what situations might arise in your future that you think might trigger another depression, and to look at what skills you've developed during our work that you might use to manage those situations.

During the final session, therapists complete the tasks of termination that were not addressed in the penultimate session.

Mechanisms of Psychotherapy

IPT aims to reduce the helplessness and hopelessness inherent in depression. Its therapeutic power involves:

- demystifying depression (it is an illness and can be treated; it does not happen out of the blue but is triggered by interpersonal problems)
- generating options for interpersonal communication and action
- increasing mastery
- realizing the antidepressant effect of healthy expression of anger
- clarifying expectations from individuals and roles
- reducing social isolation

At the beginning of each session, therapists assess patients' depressive symptoms, noting any changes that occurred over the course of the week and linking symptom changes to interpersonal interactions and events. Following the review of symptoms, together they address the tasks specific to each IPT phase. The following are the strategies associated with each problem area used in the middle phase:

GOALS	STRATEGIES

Grief—death of people (or animals) important to the patient

GOALS	STRATEGIES
• Facilitate mourning of the deceased loved one • Re-engage with the world by breaking social isolation and refocusing on relationships and interests	• Start with the sequence of events before, during, and after the death • Help the patient to reconstruct the relationship with the deceased and to view it in a balanced way • Assist the patient in facing the future without the loved one, in developing new skills, and in deepening social support

Interpersonal Disputes—overt or covert disagreements with a significant other

GOALS	STRATEGIES
• Identify the stage of the dispute* • Identify and modify mismatched expectations and/or maladaptive communication between the two parties • Assist the patient in actively resolving the dispute	• Explore interactions between the parties to identify discordant expectations that led to the dispute • Explore patient's wishes about the relationship • Modify maladaptive communication patterns • Support the patient in trying out new communication skills to resolve the dispute (and as a result either improve a relationship or end a destructive one).

Role Transitions—positive or negative life changes

GOALS	STRATEGIES
• Mourn the loss of the old role • Develop new skills and social support to handle the new role	• Elicit feelings about loss of the old role • Identify positive and negative aspects of the old role • Identify positive and negative aspects of the new role • Assist patient in reducing social isolation and in finding resources and skills to handle the new role better

Interpersonal Deficits—difficulty in starting and/or sustaining relationships

GOALS	STRATEGIES
• Reduce social isolation by improving social skills	• Review past and current relationships to identify recurrent patterns • Rehearse new social skills for the formation of new relationships and the deepening of existing relationships

*Stages of Disputes

Renegotiation:	The two parties are still communicating, and both want to resolve dispute, but have been unsuccessful so far.
Impasse:	The parties have failed in resolving the dispute and have stopped trying. They still want to be together but are "stuck." The therapist helps to move the impasse into either a renegotiation or a dissolution.
Dissolution:	One or both parties want to end the relationship. The therapist explores whether the person wants to try one more time. If this fails, the therapist helps the patient in moving away from the relationship.

APPLICATIONS

Who Can We Help?

IPT was originally developed for the treatment of unipolar, nonpsychotic depression. However, since the development of IPT, the treatment has been adapted to other depressed populations with good results. In all these adaptations, the founding principles of IPT remain the same, with therapy focusing on the interpersonal context. A growing body of literature suggests that no single treatment is appropriate for all patients with the same disorder. Indeed, outcome research has recently begun to focus not on what works in general, but what works for whom and under what circumstances. Thus, through randomized controlled trials, researchers have been trying to identify those characteristics that influence clinical outcome differently, depending on the treatment modality. These characteristics are commonly cited in clinical and epidemiological research as *moderators* or *effect modifiers*.

A moderator suggests for whom or under what conditions a treatment works (Baron & Kenny, 1986). It is a pretreatment or baseline characteristic that is independent of received treatment and has an interactive effect with treatment modalities on therapeutic outcome. Identifying moderators of treatment is central for both researchers and clinicians: Moderators clarify the best choice for exclusion/inclusion criteria and stratification to maximize power in subsequent RCTs, and they help clinicians identify the most appropriate treatment for a patient (Kraemer, Frank, & Kupfer, 2006). Though the literature in the area of moderators of response to IPT is in its infancy, some moderating characteristics have been identified.

Evidence for *baseline depressive severity* as a moderator of treatment outcome is equivocal. Findings from some studies (e.g. Elkin et al., 1989) suggest that the benefits of IPT (particularly in combination with medication) compared to other psychotherapeutic interventions such as CBT may only emerge in relation to more depressed individuals, with patients with less severe baseline depression fairing equally well across different treatments. However, this association has not been found consistently across all trials.

Somatic anxiety (anxiety of a more physiological nature) appears to reduce response to IPT. Feske and colleagues (1998) found that patients whose depression did not remit following IPT experienced significantly higher levels of somatic anxiety and were more likely to meet lifetime criteria for panic disorder compared to those who did remit. Whereas depression with comorbid anxiety disorder is generally responsive to IPT, when that anxiety is more somatic in nature (as in the case of panic disorder), pharmacotherapy may be required as well.

Social functioning has been shown to moderate the relationship between treatment condition and depression outcome, with patients with low baseline social dysfunction responding significantly better to IPT (Sotsky et al., 1991). This led Sotsky and colleagues to hypothesize that for IPT to be effective, a minimum baseline level of social functioning may be required.

Attachment avoidance also seems to moderate treatment outcome in depression, with findings from McBride and colleagues (2006) suggesting that patients with high attachment avoidance do better in CBT than IPT. They proposed that avoidant individuals' tendency to deny the importance of close relationships and to value cognition over emotion as a defense against attachment insecurity may mean they respond better to CBT, which focuses on cognitions and behaviors, than IPT, which focuses on interpersonal relationships (McBride, Atkinson, Quilty, & Bagby, 2006).

Treatment

IPT works in depression by providing understanding of the symptoms and their origin within the current context, changing the context and making the symptoms understandable and manageable, identifying the problem, and providing ways of resolving it to generate mastery. In the sections above, we outlined the strategies through which the interpersonal goals are realized. We will now present the IPT techniques used to carry out those strategies:

1. Linking mood to the interpersonal event:

Example: "Patient: I am sad." "Therapist: What happened?" or "Patient: I had a terrible fight with my boyfriend." "Therapist: how did it make you feel?"

This is a very important technique, since it provides the interpersonal context in patients' communications and behavior. By understanding that context, patients start realizing which interpersonal interactions contribute to their depression and also which contribute to their recovery.

2. Conducting communication analysis (analyzing frame-by-frame an interpersonal situation to understand where communication strayed):

Example: Justin, you told me how the argument with your boss worsened your mood for the rest of the week. It is important to understand what happened during that argument. How did it start? What did you say? How did he respond? How did you feel when he said that? What did you say in turn? What did you wish you had said? Etc.

The aim of communication analysis is to help patients understand the interpersonal message they wish to convey and clarify what stood in the way of conveying that message or whether the message conveyed was not what they wanted or needed to get across.

Many times, the therapist uses the metaphor of the camera ("I would like to get a sense of what happened with the detail of a video camera"). Communication analysis helps patients to increase their awareness and responsibility for the interpersonal message they need to send.

3. Generating options (e.g., conducting decision analysis): In contrast with analytic work, in IPT therapists always ask patients, "What do you plan to do about his?" Teaching patients to generate options counters the hopelessness and helplessness of depression. Therapists help patients come up with alternative ways of dealing with the situation at hand and support them in thinking how to choose one or a combination of them.

4. Role playing: After a specific option is chosen, therapists and patients play it out (like a dress rehearsal for action). They may take turns playing the roles of the different parties involved. Therapists give feedback on how patients' communications came across; they also instruct patients about interpersonal skills needed to carry out the communication effectively. For example: The need to find an appropriate time for an important discussion, when both parties will be receptive; the importance of focusing on the current issue as opposed to talking about similar issues from the past; characterizing the action but not the person; being direct in what one is asking for; etc.

5. Assigning homework (to implement the options that came out of the session guided by the role play): Homework in IPT is less prescriptive than in CBT. Patients are instructed to try to implement a certain interpersonal interaction before the next session, when they review how the interaction went.

Evidence

The rules of evidence should apply equally to studies of psychotherapy and studies of medication. We believe that a controlled clinical trial with randomization of treatment (RCT) is the highest level of evidence. This phase of research, known as *efficacy testing*, typically tests the treatment within a relatively homogenous group, under optimal clinical circumstances, and with the therapy performed by highly trained experts. *Effectiveness studies*, which by contrast include a broad range of participants and are typically conducted in real-life settings by community clinicians, are the next step in the psychotherapy development sequence (Weissman et al., 2007).

This section offers an overview of the evidence for the various adaptations of IPT. For a more complete discussion of the studies that have contributed evidence for the efficacy of IPT, please refer to Weissman et al. (2007).

IPT for Mood Disorders

In the trial of maintenance antidepressant medication for which it was developed, IPT was shown to improve social functioning. This positive clinical trial, the first for any form of psychotherapy, was followed by a series of studies that established IPT as a leading evidence-based treatment for acute adult unipolar depression. These showed the efficacy of IPT both as a monotherapy and in combination with medication (e.g., Elkin et al., 1989).

Since then, IPT has been adapted to a number of depressed populations. In their adaptation of IPT for *depressed adolescents* (IPT-A), Mufson and colleagues (1999) tailored the therapy through several important modifications: (1) reduction of treatment from 16 to 12 sessions, since in general adolescents do not want to be in treatment for a long time; (2) telephone contact, especially during the initial phase, to increase active participation in the treatment; and (3) engaging in a collaborative relationship with the parents and school. The efficacy of IPT-A has been validated through a number of RCTs (e.g. Mufson, Dorta, & Wickramaratne, 2004). In addition, Young and colleagues have used group IPT focused on interpersonal skills training as a preventive intervention for adolescents at risk for depression (Young, Mufson, & Davies, 2006). At the opposite end of the age spectrum, IPT has also shown efficacy as a treatment for *geriatric depression* across a number of studies (see Hinrichsen & Clougherty, 2006).

IPT has been successfully adapted and tested for *pregnancy* and *postpartum depression*, based on the following rationale: (1) given the potentially damaging effects of medication on fetus development, psychotherapeutic alternatives for pregnant, depressed women may be especially important; (2) IPT lends itself to the issues most frequently encountered in pregnancy and childbirth: major role transition, disputes, and grief (e.g., due to miscarriage).

IPT has also been used for *medical patients*, who often suffer from depression comorbid with their primary diagnosis. Serious medical illness frequently results in social and interpersonal distress: role transitions due to the incapacitating effects of the illness, interpersonal disputes with family and medical staff, and in some cases grief in anticipation of one's impending death. IPT has shown efficacy in treating depression in primary care patients, to include patients with medical syndromes such as human immunodeficiency virus (HIV), cancer, and coronary disease.

Although it is widely acknowledged that *bipolar disorder* has a major biological component and that treatment requires pharmacotherapy, there are also aspects of the clinical picture that suggest that psychotherapy—and IPT in particular—may make a useful adjunct to medication. The depressive, manic, and psychotic symptoms of the disorder are often extremely disruptive to interpersonal relationships. IPT treats the depressive phase of the illness much like unipolar depression: focusing on interpersonal disputes, role transitions associated with depressive episodes, and—in a variation on the grief problem area—patients' "grief for the lost healthy self." However, as IPT is not equipped to deal with the manic aspect of the illness, in their adaptation Frank and colleagues integrated a behavioral component, social rhythm therapy (SRT), aimed at helping patients avoid the disruptions to their daily routine that can trigger manic episodes. IPSRT aims not to treat mania once it has arisen, but to prevent its recurrence by regularizing daily social activities and improving interpersonal relationships. In combination with medication, IPSRT has shown efficacy in increasing the length of time between episodes (see Frank, 2005).

Adapting IPT for *dysthymia* has necessitated some important theoretical modifications. The IPT model, which identifies and targets an interpersonal problem as a trigger of the current depressive episode, makes less sense for a disorder characterized by chronically impaired mood and psychosocial functioning. Thus, IPT for dysthymia (IPT-D) has developed the concept of an iatrogenic role transition: Here the doctor makes treatment itself a role transition through which patients start to understand maladaptive interpersonal patterns, explore new options, and realize that dysthymia is a treatable disorder (Markowitz, 1998). The efficacy of IPT as an adjunct to medication has been established as both an individual and group therapy for dysthymia.

IPT for Nonmood Disorders

IPT for *bulimia nervosa* (IPT-BN) focuses on the interpersonal problems that may trigger binge episodes. One significant modification from IPT for depression is the lack of focus on the primary symptoms of the illness. In IPT-BN, the therapist tries to steer discussion away from eating topics and toward their interpersonal context and to explore with the patient the affective and interpersonal problems that may be triggering and maintaining eating symptomatology. In clinical trials comparing IPT-BN to CBT for bulimia nervosa (e.g. Fairburn, Jones, Peveler, Hope, & O'Connor, 1993), IPT patients have taken longer to attain symptom reduction but have caught up over the course of treatment and shown significant and lasting improvement. These findings support IPT-BN's putative mediating mechanism: Rather than addressing eating problems head-on (like CBT), IPT helps patients improve the interpersonal problems driving their illness, which then leads to reduction in disordered eating. IPT has also shown efficacy in trials for *binge eating disorder*. IPT has also been tested as a treatment for *anorexia nervosa*, but failed to demonstrate efficacy.

In the case of *posttraumatic stress disorder* (PTSD), which by definition occurs in response to a traumatic event, it is less appropriate to conceptualize an interpersonal trigger of pathology. Instead, IPT for PTSD focuses on the management of interpersonal relationships that may become difficult as a result of the disorder: Many patients with PTSD become mistrustful, have difficulty expressing their emotions, and retreat from their social environment. Unlike most treatments, IPT for PTSD does not utilize exposure as a means of confronting past trauma. However, as patients improve, often they voluntarily expose themselves to reminders of past traumas. Initial trials (e.g. Bleiberg & Markowitz, 2005) have shown promising results. In addition to improving patients' PTSD symptoms, IPT appears to help alleviate the depression that is commonly comorbid with this disorder. Adaptations of IPT for *social phobia* and *panic disorder* have also shown promise in open trials but require further testing.

Some of the central characteristics of IPT, such as its short time frame and attention to the reduction of acute symptoms, reflect its development as a treatment for Axis I disorders. The adaptation of IPT for borderline personality disorder (BPD) by Markowitz and colleagues (2006) therefore represents a new departure for the treatment and remains under testing. For further discussion of IPT for BPD, see the Theories of Personality section.

The use of IPT to treat *substance abuse* is based on a double rationale: Patients may abuse drugs or alcohol to compensate for poor interpersonal relationships, or substance abuse may damage existing relationships and in turn intensify the disorder in a vicious cycle. The goal of IPT with this population is to help patients resolve current interpersonal problems and interpersonal deficits and in doing so counter the need for further substance use. However, in initial trials IPT has failed to demonstrate efficacy for substance abuse, although Markowitz and colleagues (2008) showed an antidepressant effect for IPT in alcoholics with comorbid depression in a recent open trial.

Other Applications

The adaptation of IPT to a format has a number of potential benefits. In clinical terms, *group IPT* (IPT-G) can help validate the sick role by showing patients that other people suffer from the same illness, reducing patients' social isolation, allowing them to practice interpersonal skills within therapy, and providing gratification for patients who feel they are helping one another. On a practical level, the group format allows therapists to see a larger number of patients, making it a potentially cost-effective alternative to individual treatment. One potential drawback of IPT-G, especially if different members of a group present with different problem areas, is diminished focus on each individual's particular interpersonal difficulty. Wilfley and colleagues (1993) successfully developed IPT-G as an adaptation for nonpurging bulimic women. To counteract some of the potential problems of the group format, their treatment included two individual sessions before starting the group format (during which the interpersonal inventory was conducted and the case formulation presented), the issuing of homework specific to each patient's case throughout therapy, and the assigning of the interpersonal deficits problem area to all group members. Subsequent studies have provided additional support for the efficacy of IPT-G, including an adaptation of IPT-G for depressed adults in Uganda, which will be discussed in detail in the Psychotherapy in a Multicultural World section below.

Interpersonal counseling (IPC) is a form of IPT with fewer, shorter sessions. IPC was developed by for use with medical patients with comorbid depression (Weissman & Klerman, 1986) and is currently being tested as a treatment for use in primary care settings.

Conjoint (couples) IPT has been used to treat couples in which one or both spouses are depressed. Before the conjoint phase of treatment, therapists conduct individual sessions with each spouse during which they make their diagnosis, complete the interpersonal inventory, and propose a case formulation. Interpersonal disputes and role transitions have emerged as common problem areas with this population. A pilot study by Foley and colleagues (1989) found that while conjoint IPT and individual IPT resulted in similar reduction in depressive symptoms, subjects from the conjoint IPT arm reported greater improvements in marital satisfaction.

Telephone IPT has been tested successfully in a number of small pilot studies and open trials for populations to include homebound cancer patients with comorbid depression who were too ill to come to sessions, depressed patients in partial remission, and patients with subsyndromal depression following miscarriage. Following an initial in-person session to determine the patient's diagnosis and level of suicidality, all sessions take place over the phone. However, in other respects the approach is the same as that used in standard IPT.

Psychotherapy in a Multicultural World

IPT has been successfully practiced with patients in many countries and cultures throughout the globe. Often with minimal modifications, IPT has been used effectively with minority populations in the United States and in more than 30 countries on 6 continents. Moreover, even when adapting IPT for use in sub-Saharan Africa, researchers and clinicians have been struck by the similarity in the issues faced by people in rural Uganda and urban America despite the considerable cultural and socioeconomic differences between the two societies.

A number of features illustrated in the work in Sub-Saharan Africa were prerequisites to make IPT *feasible, acceptable, ecologically valid, effective,* and *sustainable* (Verdeli, 2008):

- Understand the mental health issues and needs of the community.
- Validate assessment scales (not just translate and back-translate) to capture local mental health syndromes.

- Intervene when community recognizes the need for assistance and consents to the intervention plans.

- Choose and adapt the therapy for ecological validity by engaging in ongoing dialogue with the trainees and key informants.

- Develop a practical and feasible intervention by choosing as mental health providers educated local laypeople.

- Develop collaborations among domestic and international academic centers, nongovernment organizations (NGOs), and local communities to test and, if found effective, disseminate the treatment.

- Have a strong commitment from the international experts to gradually make themselves redundant by withdrawing and letting the local experts take over.

An Example of IPT Adaptation: Group IPT in Southwest Uganda

The adaptation of IPT for use in Southwest Uganda serves as a model for the psychotherapy adaptation process. Bolton and colleagues tested the efficacy of IPT to treat adults suffering from depression in the Masaka and Rakai districts of southwestern Uganda, with the long-term goal of making IPT sustainable following the end of the project (Bolton et al., 2003).

Qualitative Research to Inform the Adaptation. Epidemiological studies conducted over the last 25 years have indicated an elevated level of depression in Uganda, with prevalence rates as high as 21% (Bolton et al., 2003). Local people cited the HIV epidemic in Uganda, a country with one of the highest rates of HIV infection in the world, as the cause of this depression. In 2000, an ethnographic study was conducted and two local syndromes were found to be particularly prevalent: "*y'okwetchawa*" (self-loathing) and "*okwekubagiza*" (self-pity). The symptoms experienced within these syndromes overlapped considerably with the DSM-IV criteria for depression (e.g. sadness, poor sleep and appetite, low energy, and feelings of worthlessness). However, these local syndromes also included a number of additional symptoms not recognized with the DSM criteria, such as not responding when greeted and not appreciating assistance when it was provided. The lack of physicians and high cost of medication prohibited the use of antidepressants. Psychotherapy was seen as a viable alternative provided that (1) laypeople with no previous experience as therapists could be trained to deliver the intervention (due to the scarcity of mental health professionals); (2) the therapy could be conducted in groups to increase coverage and reduce cost; and (3) its effectiveness could be established.

IPT seemed like a potentially good fit for this population for three principal reasons: the established efficacy of IPT for depression, its compatibility with the importance local Ugandan culture gives to interpersonal relations, and the match between the IPT problem areas and the types of issues the population surveyed seemed to be experiencing (Verdeli et al., 2003). Grief in the local communities was typically associated with the death of a family member or close friend, often due to AIDS or other epidemics. Some sources of interpersonal dispute were disagreements with neighbors about property boundaries, political fights, and wives protesting an HIV-affected husband's demands to have sex without using condoms. Role transitions included becoming sick with AIDS and other illnesses, getting married and moving into the husband's home, and dealing with a husband's decision to marry a second wife. Local workers deemed interpersonal deficits less relevant to the local culture, and as a result this problem area was dropped from the treatment (Verdeli et al., 2003).

Task-shifting. A group of workers from World Vision, the organization sponsoring the project, were selected as group leaders. Despite the fact that the majority had no background in mental health work, a 2-week training with IPT experts followed by supervision by telephone during the trial itself proved an effective means of instruction. This approach is consistent with the World Health Organization's *task-shifting model*: the delegation of tasks to less specialized local health workers in order to make the most efficient use possible of available resources and thereby improve health care coverage (WHO, 2007).

Adaptations Made for the Local Context.   The language used during therapy was informed by the Ugandan cultural context. For example, grief was referred to as "death of a loved one," role disputes were termed "disagreements," and transitions were referred to as "life changes" (Clougherty, Verdeli, & Weissman, 2003). In addition, the strategies employed were adapted to local cultural norms. For instance, in the local context, direct confrontation could be interpreted as inappropriate and disrespectful and, therefore, indirect forms of communication had to be employed. One effective strategy was for women to cook bad meals, which indicated to their husbands that something was amiss. In another cultural modification, group members understandably had difficulty drawing positives from many of the devastating life changes that had brought about role transitions in Uganda—the AIDS epidemic, tyrannical regimes, and civil war. This problem area was therefore adapted such that therapists worked with group members to identify aspects of life that were under their control and worked on identifying options and building skills that would improve their sense of mastery in these areas (Verdeli et al., 2003).

Results of the Clinical Trial in Southwest Uganda.   An RCT found modified IPT-G for depression to be significantly more effective than the control condition (Bolton et al., 2003). The treatment was very well received by the local community, with excellent attendance and a dropout rate of only 7.8%. Moreover, the groups continued to meet on their own following the official termination.

IPT in Northern Uganda

Effectiveness.   One of the deadliest humanitarian emergencies in the world is the 22-year civil war in Northern Uganda. More than 20,000 children have been abducted and forced to serve and fight for the Lord's Resistance Army rebel movement. In 2005, the Columbia IPT team participated in the adaptation of group IPT for adolescents living in internally displaced persons (IDP) camps in Northern Uganda. Ethnographic studies showed elevated levels of both depression and anxiety in this population (Bolton et al., 2007). Two additional treatment conditions to those used in the adult study in southwest Uganda were included: creative play (CP), which is what NGOs routinely administer in these settings, and wait list. CP was included to control for nonspecific group effects and to discern whether any improvements observed were due to specific elements in IPT over and above generic inclusion in a group. The results of the RCT showed significant improvement of depression in the IPT group compared to the other two conditions (Bolton et al., 2007). Since the study, IDP camp officials have been working with World Vision employees to promote the use of IPT-G among the locally depressed youth, and once again the group leaders have been working extraordinarily hard to cope with the high demand for the treatment.

Sustainability.   Since the initial Ugandan study in 2003, the IPT-G project has been expanded to form new groups and provide services in other provinces. To date, more than 2,500 people in southwest Uganda have been treated as well as adolescents in eight IDP camps in northern Uganda. This stands in contrast to many international projects implemented in developing countries that have dissolved after the initial study (Verdeli, 2008).

Dissemination.   To facilitate the continued development of the IPT work in Africa, a training of trainers was held in Nairobi in 2007. Twelve of the most experienced trainers from the Ugandan projects spent 2 weeks working on including quality assurance and delineation of training standards for trainers and supervisors, clarification of theoretical and technical issues, and teaching of training skills. As a result of collaborations between World Vision and other partner organizations, there are now plans to use IPT in many East and West African countries and with depressed and traumatized populations, including female combatants in Liberia, HIV-infected adults in shanty towns in Nairobi, and child soldiers in Uganda.

Finally, IPT is currently being tested with distressed primary care patients in Goa, India, and with depressed Hispanic immigrants in the United States. In their adaptation of IPT to Spanish-speaking patients with Major Depressive Disorder (MDD), Blanco and colleagues (Markowitz et al., 2009) identified several cultural issues that emerged from therapy with Hispanic patients: (1) the centrality of the family (*familismo*); (2) conflicts because of migration and acculturation, since migration is a major role transition; (3) gender issues (*machismo*) aimed at constructing a more desirable but also culturally acceptable gender-based sense of self; and (4) the need for culturally acceptable confrontational approaches.

CASE EXAMPLE

This summary refers to the case of Paul, whose treatment was used to illustrate aspects of IPT in the Process of Psychotherapy section. Paul, a 22-year-old college student, presented to his university's student health services complaining of a number of symptoms he had been experiencing over the past couple of months: feeling sad and empty, difficulty concentrating, poor sleep, loss of appetite, and fatigue.

Paul's clinical interview confirmed a diagnosis of major depression, and his score of 18 on the Hamilton Rating Scale for Depression (HAM-D) confirmed that he was suffering from a severe depressive episode. Based on his low scores on measures of suicidality and neurovegetative symptoms, the therapist decided not to recommend medication at this time.

While taking a psychiatric history, the IPT therapist learned that Paul was the second of two children. His father was a partner in a big law firm, while his mother had stayed at home to raise Paul and his sister, Sarah. Paul had been an anxious child, and although he had always had two or three close friends, he struggled to meet new people. He had always been close to Sarah, who was very protective of her younger brother. While on the one hand his relationship with his sister gave him a sense of security, on occasion it left him feeling deficient. Whereas Paul was shy, an average student, and lacked confidence, by contrast Sarah was outgoing and academically gifted. Paul felt close to his mother but had a difficult relationship with his father, who seemed to identify much more with his sister. While he was quick to praise Sarah and celebrate her academic excellence, he was often dismissive and sarcastic toward Paul, whose lack of direction seemed to puzzle and frustrate him.

Paul had always gotten by at college with mediocre grades, despite having suspected attention deficit hyperactivity disorder (ADHD), although a formal assessment was inconclusive. He was not passionate about any particular subject area and had chosen to major in sociology because it "seemed easy and kind of general." However, now that he was in the spring semester of his final year, this choice of major had left Paul unsure what he wanted after he graduated in the summer. He felt like he might do better with a career that was concrete and action oriented: "less academic and, you know, more practical."

Paul's depressive episode started after the winter break. He was finding it hard to concentrate and struggling with his courses; in particular, his anxiety that he might fail stats had led Paul to think that maybe he should "just drop out." Being given the "sick role" at this point in treatment seemed to reduce somewhat Paul's anxiety and to persuade him to hold off making drastic decisions about his college and professional future. It also helped him to start considering practical solutions to his most pressing current problems, in particular how to handle his failing grade in his stats class.

Having conducted the interpersonal inventory, the IPT therapist hypothesized that Paul's depressive episode had been triggered by his uncertainty about what to do after college (a role transition) and exacerbated by the pressure and high expectations resulting from his tense relationship with his father (an interpersonal dispute). The fact that his sister had recently gotten engaged and been accepted into law school had left Paul feeling even more inadequate and lost. This interpersonal formulation made sense to Paul, and he and the therapist agreed to focus their work together in therapy on his upcoming postcollege role transition and his interpersonal dispute with his father.

In the middle phase of treatment, the therapist worked with Paul to help him clarify his role transition by separating his feelings and views from other people's, coming up with options about his next career step, and identifying individuals who could help him in this transition by providing information or support. The therapist also helped Paul become more aware of how his father's derogatory remarks affected his depression and assisted Paul in learning to set limits with him.

Over the next few weeks, Paul's depressive symptoms began to improve, and increasingly he took an active role in therapy. Paul explained his situation to his stats professor and, based on her advice, decided to take an incomplete grade for the course. He also made an effort to spend more time with his friend Lisa, and in doing so became friends with her roommates. These accomplishments gave Paul a sense of interpersonal mastery and a new sense of confidence. Paul also became more proactive about planning what to do after college. Reflecting on how much he had enjoyed taking an introductory EMT course, he did some Internet research and talked with a career counselor about next steps in exploring this as a potential career. Paul also worked hard at setting limits in his interactions with his father. Although he felt they "weren't any closer," he became better at establishing limits and over the course of therapy their phone conversations began to affect Paul's mood less.

Having declined steadily, four sessions before treatment termination, Paul's HAM-D depression score briefly increased by several points. Reflecting that this was quite normal for a patient nearing the end of treatment, the therapist assuaged Paul's anxiety about ending therapy, reminding him of the considerable progress he had made over the prior few months. In the final phase of treatment, Paul and his therapist took stock of the progress he had made: the improvements in his depression, his increased interpersonal mastery, and the progress he had made in his postcollege role transition and interpersonal dispute with his father. This discussion became a springboard to discuss Paul's ongoing progress after therapy, the problems that might trigger a future depressive episode, and the resources available to Paul to deal with them. Paul reflected that he felt proud of his gains during therapy and pleased about his decision to take a second EMT course after graduating. He was realistic about his relationship with his father, noting that although he was now giving him more space, when it came to his career plans, he still did not really "get it." He felt good about his relationship with his mother, who had been very supportive of his treatment and encouraging with regard to his plans for the future. Now that Paul felt more secure in himself and his future, he was also able to enjoy his sister's success more. When, in the last session, Paul and the therapist discussed treatment termination, Paul reflected that although things "weren't perfect," he felt he would "do all right."

Before the termination of treatment, the therapist made sure to keep the door open by letting Paul know that if ever he needed more help he could recontact her. Eighteen months later, Paul did call. He reported that in general things were going well. He had not had any more depressive episodes, had become a full-time EMT, and was enjoying the work. He had made a few new friends, and although mostly he was focusing on his career, had been dating casually. However, although he was getting on well with his mother and sister, his relationship with his father remained distant. Paul still felt that in his father's eyes he was "just an EMT" and resented feeling "like I somehow disappointed him, or something." Recently, Paul's father had suffered a heart attack, which had left Paul feeling anxious and as though he should try to "patch things up between us." The therapist congratulated Paul on the gains he had made and reminded him of the importance of separating his own feelings and views from those of others. She helped him accept that his current relationship with his father might be "as good as it gets" and gave him an opportunity to mourn the fact that he might not ever get to be as close to his father as he would have liked. This realization, while sad for Paul, made him feel "less bad, less . . . responsible for how things are between Dad and me" and appeared to reduce his anxiety about their relationship.

SUMMARY

Initially designed to represent the psychotherapy arm of a psychopharmacological trial, in IPT Gerald Klerman, Myrna Weissman, and their colleagues sought to create a therapy that brought together a variety of best psychotherapeutic practices and strategies within a cohesive, systematic structure. What they developed was a logical framework within which therapists from different theoretical approaches and backgrounds could place and use their clinical expertise in a coherent and testable fashion. These characteristics also turned out to be the greatest strength of the approach. IPT is neither doctrinaire nor prescriptive; it allows therapists considerable flexibility to incorporate a broad variety of therapeutic tools within a short-term framework that provides shape to therapy and facilitates patient movement and symptom reduction.

This structure has not only made IPT accessible to clinicians from a variety of professional and cultural backgrounds, it has also allowed for ready adaptation of the treatment to a range of disorders and settings. This flexibility and usability within a uniform, overarching structure has allowed IPT to evolve through continuous testing and adaptation.

The interpersonal context of psychopathology upon which IPT focuses and the problem areas of grief, interpersonal deficits, role transitions, and interpersonal deficits that it identifies as triggers of mental illness appear to hold constant across cultures. Research has established IPT as a feasible and efficacious treatment for a variety of disorders spanning political, economic, and cultural contexts. Currently, it is being used to treat patient populations ranging from depressed American adolescents to sub-Saharan trauma survivors.

Weissman has suggested that psychotherapy in the Western world is in crisis. Rendered prohibitively expensive by the exigencies of insurance companies and the pressures of managed care, psychotherapy is being replaced by pharmacotherapy even where there is evidence to support its use either as monotherapy or in combination with medication. Paradoxically, psychotherapy is beginning to flourish in resource-poor parts of the world, where it is frequently much more cost effective than pharmacological approaches. As the first psychotherapeutic treatment to show efficacy in places such as Africa, IPT is at the forefront of this movement.

ANNOTATED BIBLIOGRAPHY AND WEB RESOURCES

Annotated Bibliography

Frank, E. (2005). *Treating bipolar disorder: A clinician's guide to interpersonal and social rhythm therapy.* New York: Guildford Press.
In this manual, Frank describes the framework and process of IPSRT, an evidence-based treatment for bipolar disorder that incorporates the principles and practice of IPT as part of a broader therapy. This book provides practical guidelines for employing this intervention, outlines efficacy data, and provides clinical vignettes.

Hinrichsen, G. A., & Clougherty, K. F. (2006). *Interpersonal psychotherapy for depressed older adults.* Washington: American Psychological Association.

This manual describes the adaptation of IPT for depressed older adults, addresses issues specific to this population, and discusses the empirical and theoretical basis of the approach.

Klerman, G. L., Weissman, M. M., Rounsaville, B. J., & Chevron, E. S. (1984). *Interpersonal psychotherapy of depression.* New York: Basic Books.

This book was the first IPT manual, published by Klerman, Weissman, and colleagues once efficacy for IPT had been shown outside their research group. The nature and prevalence of depression are discussed, the theoretical basis for IPT is described, and detailed treatment strategies are provided for the four IPT problems areas.

Mufson, L., Dorta, K. P., Moreau, D., & Weissman, M. M. (2004). *Interpersonal psychotherapy for depressed adolescents* (2nd ed.). New York: Guildford Press.

Interpersonal Psychotherapy for Depressed Adolescents (IPT-A) presents readers with developmental adaptations for this age group, including the various presentations of depression in teens and the need for parental involvement in treatment. IPT-A is illustrated through case examples.

Weissman, M. M., Markowitz, J. C., & Klerman, G. L. (2000). *Comprehensive guide to interpersonal psychotherapy.* New York: Basic Books.

This second IPT manual builds upon the first by providing an updated description of IPT for depression, discussing the adaptations of IPT for mood and nonmood disorders, and presenting the efficacy research to support these approaches. Case examples and clinical scripts are included.

Weissman, M. M., Markowitz, J. C., & Klerman, G. L. (2007). *Clinician's quick guide to interpersonal psychotherapy.* Oxford: Oxford University Press.

Designed for busy clinicians, this condensed manual describes how to conduct IPT for depression and provides adaptations of the approach for a variety of disorders (e.g., mood and nonmood), populations (e.g., older adults, medical patients), and settings (e.g., developing countries). This text provides clinicians with the outline and course of IPT treatment in a concise and practical format.

Web Resource

www.interpersonalpsychotherapy.org

The Web site of the International Society for Interpersonal Psychotherapy provides students, clinicians, and researchers with information about meetings, training, and developments in IPT research and practice.

CASE READINGS

Crowe, M., & Luty, S. (2005). The process of change in interpersonal psychotherapy (IPT) for depression: A case study for the new IPT therapist. *Psychiatry, 68*(1), 43–54. [Reprinted in D. Wedding & R. J. Corsini (2011). *Case studies in psychotherapy.* Belmont, CA: Brooks/Cole.]

This case provides detailed examples of how IPT was used to treat a 42-year-old divorced woman with a major depressive disorder.

Mufson, L., Verdeli, H., Clougherty, K. F., & Shoum, K. (2009). How to use interpersonal psychotherapy for adolescents (IPT-A). In J. M. Rey & B. Birmaher (Eds.), *Treating child and adolescent depression.* Baltimore: Lippincott Williams & Wilkins.

The chapter provides a session-by-session description of Bill, a depressed adolescent who received IPT-A.

Weissman, M. M., Markowitz, J. C., & Klerman, G. L. (2000). *Comprehensive guide to interpersonal psychotherapy.* New York: Basic Books.

The case of Ellen, a 27-year-old depressed suicidal woman, is described in detail in this book. The case provides a meaningful introduction to key features of IPT.

Weissman, M. M., Markowitz, J. C., & Klerman, G. L. (2007). *Clinician's quick guide to interpersonal psychotherapy.* Oxford: Oxford University Press.

This book includes a number of case examples illustrating the adaptation of IPT to a variety of disorders.

REFERENCES

Ainsworth, M., Blehar, M., Waters, E., & Wall, S. (1978). *Patterns of attachment.* Hillsdale, NJ: Erlbaum.

Baron, R. M., & Kenny, D. A. (1986). The moderator–mediator variable distinction in social psychological research: conceptual, strategic, and statistical considerations. *Journal of Personality and Social Psychology, 51,* 1173–1182.

Bartholomew, K., & Horowitz, L. M. (1991). Attachment styles among young adults: A test of a four-category model. *Journal of Personality and Social Psychology, 61*(2), 226–244.

Bleiberg, K. L., & Markowitz, J. C. (2005). A pilot study of interpersonal psychotherapy for posttraumatic stress disorder. *American Journal of Psychiatry, 162,* 181–183.

Bolton, P., Bass, J., Betancourt, T., Speelman, L., Onyango, G., Clougherty, K. F., et al. (2007). Interventions for depression symptoms among adolescent survivors of war and displacement in northern Uganda: A randomized controlled trial. *Journal of the American Medical Association, 298,* 519–527.

Bolton, P., Bass, J., Neugebauer, R., Clougherty, K., Verdeli, H., Ndogoni, L., et al. (2003). Results of a clinical trial of a group intervention for depression in rural Uganda. *Journal of the American Medical Association, 289,* 3117–3124.

Bowlby, J. (1969) *Attachment and loss: Volume I: Attachment.* New York: Basic Books.

Bowlby, J. (1980). *Loss· Sadness and depression*. New York: Basic Books.

Brennan, K. A., & Shaver, P. R. (1995). Dimensions of adult attachment, affect regulation, and romantic relationship functioning. *Personality and Social Psychology Bulletin, 21*, 267–283.

Caspi, A., Sugden, K., Moffitt, T. E., Taylor, A., Craig, I. W., Harrington, H., et al. (2003). Influence of life stress on depression: Moderation by a polymorphism in the 5-HTT gene. *Science, 301*, 386–389.

Champagne, F. A., Francis, D. D., Mar, A., & Meaney, M. (2003). Variations in maternal care in the rat as a mediating influence for the effects of environment on development. *Physiology and Behavior, 79*, 359–371.

Clougherty, K. F., Verdeli, H., & Weissman, M. M. (2003). *Interpersonal psychotherapy adapted for a group in Uganda (IPT-G-U)*. Unpublished manual available through M. M. Weissman, Ph.D., 1051 Riverside Drive, Unit 24, New York, NY 10032 (mmw3@columbia.edu).

Collins, N. L., & Read, S. J. (1990). Adult attachment, working models, and relationship quality in dating couples. *Journal of Personality and Social Psychology, 58*, 644–663.

Cyranowski, J. M., Shear, M. K., Rucci, P., Fagiolini A., Frank, E., Grochocinski, V. J., et al. (2002). Adult separation anxiety: Psychometric properties of a new structured clinical interview. *Journal of Psychiatric Research, 36*, 77–86.

Elkin, I., Shea, T. M., Watkins, J. T., Imber, S., Sotsky, S. M., Collins, J. F., et al. (1989). National Institute of Mental Health Treatment of Depression Collaborative Research Program: General effectiveness of treatments. *Archives of General Psychiatry, 46*, 971–982.

Fairburn, C. G., Jones, R., Peveler, R. C., Hope, R. A., & O'Connor, M. (1993). Psychotherapy and bulimia nervosa. Longer-term effects of interpersonal psychotherapy, behavioral therapy, and cognitive behavior therapy. *Archives of General Psychiatry, 50*(6), 419–428.

Fava M., Farabaugh A. H., Sickinger A. H., Wright E., Alpert J. E., Sonawalla S., Nierenberg A. A., Worthington J. J. 3rd (2002). Personality disorders and depression. *Psychological Medicine, 32*(6):1049–1057.

Foley, S. H., Rounsaville, B. J., Weissman, M. M., Sholomskas, D., & Chevron, E. (1989). Individual versus conjoint interpersonal psychotherapy for depressed patients with marital disputes. *International Journal of Family Psychiatry, 10*, 29–42.

Frank, E., Kupfer, D. J., & Thase, M. E. (2005). Two-year outcomes for interpersonal and social rhythm therapy in individuals with bipolar I disorder. *Archives of General Psychiatry, 62*, 996–1004.

Feske, U., Frank, E., Kupfer, D. J., Shear, M. K., & Weaver, E. (1998). Anxiety as a predictor of response to interpersonal psychotherapy for recurrent major depression: An exploratory analysis. *Depression and Anxiety, 8*, 135–141.

Hammen, C., Burge, D., Daley, S., Davila, J., Paley, B., & Rudolph, K. D. (1995). Interpersonal attachment cognitions and prediction of symptomatic responses to interpersonal stress. *Journal of Abnormal Psychology, 104*, 436–443.

Hinrichsen, G. A., & Clougherty, K. F. (2006). *Interpersonal psychotherapy for depressed older adults*. Washington, DC: American Psychological Association.

Kendler, K. S., Prescott, C. A., Myers, J., & Neale, M. C. (2003). The structure of genetic and environmental risk factors for common psychiatric and substance use disorders in men and women. *Archives of General Psychiatry, 60*, 929–937.

Klerman, G.L., Dimascio, A., Weissman, M. M., Prussoff, B., & Paykel, E.S. (1974). Treatment of depression by drugs and psychotherapy. *American Journal of Psychiatry, 131*(2): 186–191.

Klerman, G. L., Weissman, M. M., Rounsaville, B. J., & Chevron, E. (1984). *Interpersonal psychotherapy for depression*. New York: Basic Books.

Kraemer, H. C., Frank, E., & Kupfer, D. J. (2006). Moderators of treatment outcomes: Clinical, research, and policy importance. *JAMA, 296*(10), 1286–1289.

Main, M., & Solomon, J. (1986). Discovery of an insecure–disorganized/disoriented attachment pattern: Procedures, findings and implications for the classification of behavior. In T. B. Brazelton & M. Yogman (Eds.), *Affective development in infancy* (pp. 95–124). Norwood, NJ: Ablex.

Markowitz, J. C. (1998). *Interpersonal psychotherapy for dysthymic disorder*. Washington, DC: American Psychiatric Press.

Markowitz, J. C., Skodol, A. E., & Bleiberg, K. (2006). Interpersonal psychotherapy for borderline personality disorder: Possible mechanisms of change. *Journal of Clinical Psychology, 62*(4), 431–444.

Markowitz, J. C., Kocsis, J. H., Christos, P., Bleiberg, K., & Carlin, A. (2008). Pilot study of interpersonal psychotherapy versus supportive psychotherapy for dysthymic patients with secondary alcohol abuse or dependence. *Journal of Nervous and Mental Disease, 196*(6), 468–474.

Markowitz, J. C., Patel, S. R., Balan, I. C., Bell, M. A., Blanco, C., Brave Heart, M. Y. H., Buttacavoli Sosa, S., & Lewis-Fernandez, R. (2009). Toward an adaptation of Interpersonal Psychotherapy for Hispanic patients with DSM-IV Major Depressive Disorder. *Journal of Clinical Psychiatry, 70*(2), 214–222.

McBride, C., Atkinson, L., Quilty, L. C., & Bagby, R. M. (2006). Attachment as a moderator of treatment outcome to major depression: A randomized control trial of interpersonal psychotherapy vs. cognitive behavior therapy. *Journal of Consulting and Clinical Psychology, 74*, 1041–1054.

Meyer, A. (1951). *Collected papers: Volume II*. Baltimore: John Hopkins Press.

Meyer, A. (1957). *Psychobiology: A science of man*. Springfield, IL: Charles C. Thomas.

Mickelson, K. D., Kessler, R. C., & Shaver, P. R. (1997). Adult attachment in a nationally representative sample. *Journal of Personality and Social Psychology, 73*, 1092–1106.

Mufson, L., Dorta, K. P., & Wickramaratne, P. (2004). A randomized effectiveness trial of interpersonal psychotherapy for depressed adolescents. *Archives of General Psychiatry, 61*, 577–584.

Mufson, L., Pollack Dorta, K., Moreau, D., & Weissman, M. M. (2004). *Interpersonal psychotherapy for depressed adolescents* (2nd ed.). New York: Guilford Publications.

Mufson, L., Weissman, M. M., Moreau, D., & Garfinkel, R. (1999). Efficacy of interpersonal psychotherapy for depressed adolescents. *Archives of General Psychiatry, 56,* 573–579.

Murphy, B., & Bates, G. W. (1997). Adult attachment style and vulnerability to depression. *Personality & Individual Differences, 22,* 835–844.

Paykel, E. S. (1978). Contributions of life-events to causation of psychiatric illness. *Psychological Medicine, 8*(2), 245–253.

Peluso, P. R., Peluso, J. P., White, J. F., & Kern, R. M. (2004). A comparison of attachment theory and individual psychology: A review of the literature. *Journal of Counseling and Development, 82,* 139–145.

Ravitz. P. (2009). *Changes in self-reported attachment and interpersonal problems in depressed patients treated with IPT.* Paper presented at the 3rd International Conference on Interpersonal psychotherapy: Global Update, New York.

Risch, N., Herrell, R., Lehner, T., Liang, K. Y., Eaves, L., Hoh, J., et al. (2009). Interaction between the serotonin transporter gene (5-HTTLPR), stressful life events, and risk of depression: a meta-analysis. *JAMA, 301* (23), 2462–2471.

Shahar, G., Blatt, S. J., Zuroff, D. C., & Pilkonis, P. A. (2003). Role of perfectionism and personality disorder features in response to brief treatment for depression. *Journal of Consulting and Clinical Psychology, 71*(3), 629–633.

Simpson, J. A., Rholes, W. S., & Nelligan, J. S. (1992). Support seeking and support giving within couples in an anxiety-provoking situation: The role of attachment styles. *Journal of Personality and Social Psychology, 62,* 434–446.

Sotsky, S. M., Glass, D. R., Shea, M. T., Pilkonis, P. A., Collins, J. F., Elkin, I., et al. (1991). Patient predictors of response to psychotherapy and pharmacotherapy: Findings in the NIMH Treatment of Depression Collaborative Research Program. *The American Journal of Psychiatry, 148,* 997–1008.

Sullivan, H. S. (1955). *The interpersonal theory of psychiatry.* London: Tavistock Publications.

Verdeli, H. (2008). Toward building feasible, efficacious and sustainable treatments for depression. *Depression and Anxiety, 25*(11), 899–902.

Verdeli, H., Clougherty, K., Bolton, P., Speelman, L., Ndogoni, L., Bass, J., et al. (2003). Adapting group interpersonal psychotherapy for a developing country: Experience in rural Uganda. *World Psychiatry, 2,* 114–120.

Weissman, M. M. (2006). A brief history of interpersonal psychotherapy. *Psychiatric Annals, 36*(8), 553–557.

Weissman, M. M., & Klerman, G. L. (1986). Interpersonal Counseling (IPC) for stress and distress in primary care settings. Unpublished manual available through M. M. Weissman, Ph.D., 1051 Riverside Drive, Unit 24, New York, NY 10032 (mmw3@columbia.edu).

Weissman, M. M., Markowitz, J. C., & Klerman, G. L. (2000). *Comprehensive guide to interpersonal psychotherapy.* New York: Basic Books.

Weissman, M. M., Markowitz, J. C., & Klerman, G. L. (2007). *Clinician's quick guide to interpersonal psychotherapy.* New York: Oxford University Press.

Weissman, M. M., Verdeli, H., Gameroff, M. J., Bledsoe, S. E., Betts, K. Mufson, L., et al. (2006). National Survey of Psychotherapy Training in Psychiatry, Psychology, and Social Work. *Archives of General Psychiatry, 63,* 925–934.

Wilfley, D. E., Agras, W. S., Telch, C. F., Rossiter, E. M., Schneider, J. A., Cole, A. G., et al. (1993). Group cognitive–behavioral therapy and group interpersonal psychotherapy for the nonpurging bulimic individual: A controlled comparison. *Journal of Consulting and Clinical Psychology, 61*(2), 296–305.

World Health Organization. (2007). Treat train retain. Task shifting: Global recommendations and guidelines. Retrieved 20 June, 2009, from www.who.int/healthsystems/task_shifting/en/

Young, J. F., Mufson, L., & Davies, M. (2006). Efficacy of interpersonal psychotherapy-adolescent skills training: An indicated preventive intervention for depression. *Journal of Child Psychology and Psychiatry, 47*(12), 1254–1262.

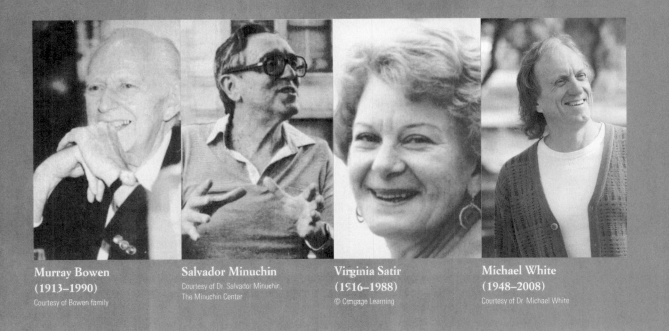

Murray Bowen
(1913–1990)
Courtesy of Bowen family

Salvador Minuchin
Courtesy of Dr. Salvador Minuchin,
The Minuchin Center

Virginia Satir
(1916–1988)
© Cengage Learning

Michael White
(1948–2008)
Courtesy of Dr. Michael White

12 | FAMILY THERAPY

Irene Goldenberg, Herbert Goldenberg, and Erica Goldenberg Pelavin

Family therapy is both a theory and a treatment method. It offers a way to view clinical problems within the context of a family's transactional patterns. Family therapy also represents a form of intervention in which members of a family are assisted in identifying and changing problematic, maladaptive, repetitive relationship patterns, as well as self-defeating or self-limiting belief systems.

Unlike individually focused therapies, in family therapy the *identified patient* (the family member considered to be the problem in the family) is viewed as manifesting troubled or troubling behavior maintained by problematic transactions within the family or perhaps between the family and the outside community. Helping families to change leads to improved functioning of individuals as well as families. In recent years, therapeutic efforts have been directed at broadening the context for understanding family functioning, adopting an ecological focus that takes the individual, the family, and the surrounding cultural community into account (Robbins, Mayorga, & Szapocznik, 2003).

OVERVIEW

Basic Concepts

When a single attitude, philosophy, point of view, procedure, or methodology dominates scientific thinking (and thus assumes the character of a *paradigm*), solutions to problems are sought within the perspectives of that school of thought. If serious problems arise that do not appear to be explained by the prevailing paradigm, however, efforts are made to expand or replace the existing system. Once the old belief system changes, perspectives shift and previous events may take on entirely new meanings. The resulting transition to a new paradigm, according to Kuhn (1970), is a scientific revolution.

In the field of psychotherapy, such a dramatic shift in perspective occurred in the mid-1950s as some clinicians, dissatisfied with slow progress when working with individual patients or frustrated when change in their patients was often undermined by other family members, began to look at the family as the locus of pathology. Breaking away from the traditional concern and investigation of individual personality characteristics and behavior patterns, they adopted a new perspective—a family frame of reference—that provided a new way of conceptualizing human problems, especially the development of symptoms and their alleviation. As is the case with all paradigm shifts, this new viewpoint called for a new set of premises about the nature of psychopathology and stimulated a series of family-focused methods for collecting data and understanding individual functioning.

When the unit of analysis is the individual, clinical theories inevitably look to internal events, psychic organization, and the patient's intrapsychic problems to explain that person's problems. Based on a heritage dating back to Freud, such efforts turn to the reconstruction of the past to seek out root causes of current difficulties, producing hypotheses or explanations for *why* something happened to this person. With the conceptual leap to a family framework, attention is directed to the family context in which individual behavior occurs, to behavioral sequences between individuals, and to *what* is now taking place and *how* each participant influences, and in turn is influenced by, other family members.

This view of *reciprocal causality* provides an opportunity to observe repetitive ways in which family members interact and to use such data to initiate therapeutic interventions. Family therapists therefore direct their attention to the dysfunctional or impaired family unit rather than to a symptomatic person, who is only one part of that family system and, by his or her behavior, is seen as expressing the family's dysfunction.

The Family as a System

By adopting a relationship frame of reference, family therapists pay attention both to the family's *structure* (how it arranges, organizes, and maintains itself at a particular cross section of time) and to its *processes* (the way it evolves, adapts, or changes over time). They view the family as an ongoing, living system, a complex, durable, causal network of related parts that together constitute an entity larger than the simple sum of its individual members. That system, in turn, is part of a larger social context, the outside community.

Several key concepts are central to understanding how systems operate. *Organization* and *wholeness* are especially important. Systems are composed of units that stand in some consistent relationship to one another, and thus we can infer that they are organized around those relationships. In a similar way, units or elements, once combined, produce an entity—a whole—that is greater than the sum of its parts. A change in one part causes a change in the other parts and thus in the entire system. If this is indeed the case, argue systems theorists, then adequate understanding of a system requires study of the whole rather than separate examination of each part. No element within the system can ever be understood in isolation since elements never function separately. The implications for understanding family functioning are clear: A family is a system in which members organize into a group, forming a whole that transcends the sum of its individual parts.

The original interest in viewing a family as a system stems in part from the work of Gregory Bateson, an anthropologist who led an early study in which he and his colleagues hypothesized that schizophrenia might be the result of pathological family interaction (Bateson, Jackson, Haley, & Weakland, 1956). Although not a family thera-pist himself, Bateson (1972) deserves special credit for first seeing how a family might operate as a *cybernetic system*. Current views of the origins of schizophrenia empha-size genetic predispositions exacerbated by environmental stresses, but Bateson's team should be recognized for first focusing attention on the flow of information and the back-and-forth communication patterns that exist within families. Rather than studying the content of what transpires, family therapists were directed to attend to family pro-cesses, the interactive patterns among family members that define a family's functioning as a unit.

A Cybernetic Epistemology

A number of significant shifts in clinical outlook occur with the adoption of a cybernetic epistemology. For example, the locus of pathology changes from the identified patient to the social context, and the interaction between individuals, rather than the troubled person, is analyzed. Instead of assuming that one individual causes another's behavior ("You started it. I just reacted to what you did"), family therapists believe both partici-pants are caught up in a circular interaction, a chain reaction that feeds back on itself, because each family member has defined the situation differently. Each argues that the other person is the cause; both are correct, but it is pointless to search for a starting point in any conflict between people, because a complex, repetitive interaction is occur-ring, not a simple, linear, cause-and-effect situation with a clear beginning and end.

The simple, nonreciprocal view that one event leads to another, in stimulus-response fashion, represents *linear causality*. Family therapists prefer to think in terms of *circular causality:* Reciprocal actions occur within a relationship network by means of a network of interacting loops. From this perspective, any cause is seen as an effect of a previous cause and becomes, in turn, the cause of a later event. Thus, the attitudes and behavior of system members, as in a family, are tied to one another in powerful, durable, recipro-cal ways, and in a never-ending cycle.

The term *cybernetics,* based on a Greek word for "steersman," was coined by math-ematician Norbert Wiener (1948) to describe regulatory systems that operate by means of *feedback loops.* The most familiar example of such a mechanism is the thermostat in a home heating system; set to a desired temperature, the furnace will turn on when the heat drops below that setting, and it will shut off when the desired temperature is reached. The system is balanced around a set point and relies on information fed back into it about the temperature of the room. Thus, it maintains a dynamic equilibrium and undertakes operations to restore that equilibrium whenever the balance is upset or threatened.

So, too, with a family. When a crisis or other disruption occurs, family members try to maintain or regain a stable environment—*family homeostasis*—by activating family-learned mechanisms to decrease the stress and restore internal balance.

Families rely on the exchange of information—a word, a look, a gesture, or a glance that acts as a feedback mechanism, signaling that disequilibrium has been created and that some corrective steps are needed to help the relationship return to its previous bal-anced state. In effect, information about a system's output is fed back into its input, to alter, correct, or govern the system's functioning. *Negative feedback* has an attenuat-ing effect, restoring equilibrium, whereas *positive feedback* leads to further change by accelerating the deviation. In negative feedback, a couple may exchange information during a quarrel that says, in effect, "It is time to pull back or we will regret it later." In positive feedback, the escalation may reach dangerous, runaway proportions; the quarreling couple may escalate an argument to the point when neither one cares about the consequences. In some situations, however, positive feedback, though temporarily destabilizing, may be beneficial if it does not get out of control and if it helps the couple reassess a dysfunctional transactional pattern, reexamine their methods of engagement, and change the system's rules. That is, a system need not revert to its previous level but may instead, as a result of positive feedback, change and function more smoothly at a higher homeostatic level (Goldenberg & Goldenberg, 2008).

Subsystems, Boundaries, and Larger Systems

Following largely from the work of Minuchin, Nichols, & Lee (2006), family therapists view families as comprising a number of coexisting subsystems in which members group together to carry out certain family functions or processes. Subsystems are organized components within the overall system, and they may be determined by generation, sex, or family function. Each family member is likely to belong to several subsystems at the same time. A wife may also be a mother, daughter, younger sister, and so on, thus entering into different complementary relationships with other members at various times and playing different roles in each. In certain dysfunctional situations, families may split into separate long-term coalitions: males opposed to females, parents against children, father and daughter in conflict with mother and son.

Although family members may engage in temporary alliances, three key subsystems will always endure: the spousal, parental, and sibling subsystems (Minuchin, Rosman, & Baker, 1978). The first is especially important to the family: Any dysfunction in the spousal subsystem is bound to reverberate throughout the family, resulting in the scapegoating of children or co-opting them into alliances with one parent against the other. Effective spousal subsystems provide security and teach children about commitment by presenting a positive model of marital interaction. The parental subsystem, when effective, provides child care, nurturance, guidance, limit setting, and discipline; problems here frequently take the form of intergenerational conflicts with adolescents, often reflecting underlying family disharmony and instability. Sibling subsystems help members learn to negotiate, cooperate, compete, and eventually attach to others.

Boundaries are invisible lines that separate a system, a subsystem, or an individual from outside surroundings. In effect, they protect the system's integrity, distinguishing between those considered insiders and those viewed as outsiders. Boundaries within a family vary from being rigid (overly restrictive, permitting little contact among the members of different groups) to being diffuse (overly blurred, so that roles are interchangeable and members are overinvolved in each other's lives). Thus, the clarity of the boundary between subsystems and its permeability are more important than the subsystem's membership. Excessively rigid boundaries characterize *disengaged families* in which members feel isolated from one another, and diffuse boundaries identify *enmeshed families* in which members are intertwined in one another's lives.

Boundaries between the family and the outside world need to be sufficiently clear to allow information to flow to and from the environment. In systems terms, the more flexible the boundaries, the better the information flow; the family is open to new experiences, is able to alter and discard unworkable or obsolete interactive patterns, and is operating as an *open system*. When boundaries are not easily crossed, the family is insular, is not open to what is happening around it, is suspicious of the outside world, and is said to be operating as a *closed system*. In reality, no family system is either completely open or completely closed; rather, all exist along a continuum.

Cybernetics Revisited and the Postmodern Challenge

The early, radical assumptions proposed by systems theory (circular causality, feedback loops, boundaries, subsystems) were groundbreaking in their relationship-focused and holistic character but were limited because they were confined to outside observers attempting to describe what was occurring within a system (Becvar, 2003). A later refinement, sometimes called second-order cybernetics, acknowledged the effect of the observer (the family therapist) on his or her observations; by helping define the problem, the observer influences goals and outcomes. Each family member's perceptions of the presenting problem began to be acknowledged as important and valid, because how each member constructs reality influences and is influenced by a larger social context. Postmodern views, popular today, are especially rejecting of the systems metaphor as based on mechanistic models. Postmodernists argue that our notion of reality is inevitably subjective; there are no universal truths out there ready to be described by "objective observers" (Gergen, 1999).

All family systems thus are influenced by one or more of society's larger systems—the courts, the health care system, schools, welfare, probation, and most currently the psychological challenges inherent in the cybersystem. This frontier presents new challenges to therapists who must be aware and understand the complications of virtual relationships and boundaries. Untangling the web of relationships, both perceived and real, can be difficult for the practitioner and presents both legal and ethical issues. (Pelavin & Moskowitz-Sweet, 2009).

Although such contact with the larger system may be time limited and generally free of long-term conflict, numerous families become entangled with such systems, and this entanglement sometimes impedes the development of family members. Family therapists today pay close attention to such interactions, looking beyond the dysfunctional family itself and integrating the recommendations of the various agencies in order to provide a broad, coordinated set of interventions to achieve maximum effectiveness.

Gender Awareness and Culture Sensitivity

Challenged by postmodern inquiries into the diversity of perspectives for viewing life, as well as by the feminist movement, family therapists have begun to look beyond observable interactive patterns within a family, and today they examine how gender, culture, and ethnicity shape the perspectives and behavior patterns of family members. Indoctrinated early into gender-role behavior in a family, men and women have different socialization experiences and as a result develop distinct behavioral expectations, are granted disparate opportunities, and have differing life experiences. Work and family roles and responsibilities have changed dramatically in the last 30 years, requiring new male–female interactions and family adaptations (Barnett & Hyde, 2001).

Gender, cultural background, ethnicity membership, and social class are interactive; one cannot be considered without the others. As Kliman (1994) notes, the experience of being male or female shapes, and in turn is shaped by, being poor or middle-class or wealthy, or being African American, Chinese, or Armenian. Contemporary views of family therapy emphasize taking a *gender-sensitive outlook* in working with families, being careful not to reinforce (as therapists sometimes did in the past) stereotyped sexist, patriarchal attitudes, or class differences. Today, family therapists pay more attention to differences in power, status, and position within families and in society in general.

Similarly, family therapists today believe a comprehensive picture of family functioning at the minimum requires an understanding of the cultural context (race, ethnic group membership, social class, religion, sexual orientation) and the form of family organization (stepfamily, single parent-led family, gay couples, etc.) of the family seeking help. Adopting a broad, multicultural framework leads to a pluralistic outlook, one that recognizes that attitudes and behavior patterns are often deeply rooted in the family's cultural background. That pluralistic viewpoint also enables therapists to better understand the unique problems inherent in the multitude of families today that do not fit the historical model of the intact family (Sue & Sue, 2007).

Developing a *culturally sensitive therapy* (Prochaska & Norcross, 1999) necessitates moving beyond the white, middle-class outlook from which many therapists operate (prizing self-sufficiency, independence, and individual development) and recognizing that such values are not necessarily embraced by all ethnic groups. For example, many clients from traditional Asian backgrounds are socialized to subordinate their individual needs to those of their families or of society in general. In developing a multicultural framework, the family therapist must recognize that acculturation is an ongoing process that occurs over generations and that ethnic values continue to influence a client family's child-rearing practices, intergenerational relationships, family boundaries, and so forth.

A culturally competent family therapist remains alert to the fact that how he or she accesses or counsels a family is influenced not only by professional knowledge but also by his or her own "cultural filters"—values, attitudes, customs, religious beliefs and practices, and (especially) beliefs regarding what constitutes normal behavior (Madsen, 2007). To ignore such built-in standards is to run the risk of misdiagnosing or mislabeling as abnormal an unfamiliar family pattern that might be perfectly appropriate to that family's cultural heritage (McGoldrick & Hardy, 2008). Similarly, the culturally sensitive therapist must be careful not to overlook or minimize deviant behavior by simply attributing it to cultural differences. According to Falicov (2000), the family therapy encounter is really an engagement between a therapist's and a family's cultural and personal constructions about family life. This includes the role of spirituality on the part of both the clinician and the client, tapping spiritual resources for coping, healing, and resiliency (Walsh, 2009). If religious or previously established family rituals do not satisfy the system's needs, creating collaborative rituals can be healing to the family (Imber-Black, Roberts, & Alva Whiting, 2003).

Therapeutic intervention with a wide variety of families requires the therapist to help family members understand any restrictions imposed on them as a result of such factors as gender, race, religion, social class, or sexual orientation. Cultural narratives (White, 2007) specifying the customary or preferred ways of being in a society are sometimes toxic (racism, sexism, ageism, class bias) and thus inhibiting and subjugating to the individual, family, and group. Here the therapist must provide help in addressing the limitations imposed by the majority culture if the family is to overcome societal restrictions.

Other Systems

Differences between family therapy and other therapeutic approaches are less clear cut than in the past, as systems ideas have permeated other forms of psychotherapy. Although therapists may focus on the individual patient, many have begun to view that person's problems within a broader context, of which the family is inevitably a part, and have adapted family systems methods to individual psychotherapy (Wachtel & Wachtel, 1986). For example, *object relations theory* has emphasized the search for satisfactory "objects" (persons) in our lives, beginning in infancy. Practitioners of psychoanalytically based object relations family therapy, such as Scharff and Scharff (2006), help family members uncover how each has internalized objects from the past, usually as a result of an unresolved relationship with one's parents, and how these imprints from the past—called *introjects*—continue to impose themselves on current relationships, particularly with one's spouse or children. Object relations family therapists search for unconscious relationship-seeking from the past as the primary determinant of adult personality formation, whereas most family therapists deal with current interpersonal issues to improve overall family functioning.

Conceptually, Adlerian psychotherapy is compatible with family therapy formulations. Far less reliant on biological or instinctual constructs than is psychoanalysis,

Adlerian theory emphasizes the social context of behavior, the embeddedness of the individual in his or her interpersonal relationships, and the importance of present circumstances and future goals rather than unresolved issues from childhood. Both Adlerian psychotherapy and family therapy take a holistic view of the person and emphasize intent and conscious choices. Adler's efforts to establish a child guidance movement, as well as his concern with improving parenting practices, reflect his interest beyond the individual to family functioning. However, the individual focus of his therapeutic efforts fails to change the dysfunctional family relationships that underlie individual problems.

The person-centered approach developed by Carl Rogers is concerned with the client's here-and-now issues, is growth oriented, and is applicable to helping families move in the direction of self-actualization. Its humanistic outlook was particularly appealing to experiential family therapists such as Virginia Satir (1972) and Carl Whitaker (Whitaker & Bumberry, 1988), who believed families were stunted in their growth and would find solutions if provided with a growth-facilitating therapeutic experience. Experiential family therapists are usually more directive than Rogerians and, in some cases, act as teachers to help families open up their communication processes (for instance, using methods developed by Virginia Satir).

Existential psychotherapies are phenomenological in nature, emphasizing awareness and the here and now of the client's existence. Considered by most family therapists to be too concerned with the organized wholeness of the single person, this viewpoint nevertheless has found a home among some family therapists, such as Walter Kempler (1991), who argues that people define themselves and their relationships with one another through their current choices and decisions and what they choose to become in the future rather than through their reflections on the past.

Behavior therapists traditionally take a more linear view of causality regarding family interactions than do most systems theory advocates. A child's tantrums, for example, are viewed by behaviorists as maintained and reinforced by parental responses. Systems theorists view the tantrum as an interaction, including an exchange of feedback information, occurring within a family system

Most behaviorists now acknowledge that cognitive factors (attitudes, thoughts, beliefs, expectations) influence behavior, and cognitive–behavior therapy has become a part of mainstream psychotherapy (Dattilio & Epstein, 2005). However, rational emotive behavior therapy's view that problems stem from maladaptive thought processes seems too individually focused for most family therapists (Ellis & Dryden, 2007).

HISTORY

Precursors

Freud, Adler, Sullivan

Family therapy can trace its ancestry to efforts begun early in the last century, led largely by Sigmund Freud, to discover intervention procedures for uncovering and mitigating symptomatic behavior in neurotic individuals. However, although Freud acknowledged in theory the often-powerful impact of individual fantasy and family conflict and alliances (e.g., the Oedipus conflict) on the development of such symptoms, he steered clear of involving the family in treatment, choosing instead to help the symptomatic person resolve personal or intrapsychic conflicts.

Adler went further than Freud in emphasizing the family context for neurotic behavior, stressing the importance of the family constellation (e.g., birth order, sibling rivalry) on individual personality formation. He drew attention to the central role of the family in the formative years, contending that family interactive patterns are the key to understanding a person's current relationships both within and outside the family.

Harry Stack Sullivan, beginning in the 1920s, adopted an interpersonal relations view in working with hospitalized schizophrenics. Sullivan (1953) argued that people were the product of their "relatively enduring patterns of recurrent interpersonal situations" (p. 10). In spite of not working directly with families, Sullivan speculated on the role that family played in the transitional period of adolescence, thought to be the typical time for the onset of schizophrenia. Sullivan's influence on Don Jackson and Murray Bowen, two pioneers in family therapy who trained under Sullivan, as well as on his colleague Frieda Fromm-Reichmann, is apparent both in their adoption of Sullivan's early notion of redundant family interactive patterns and in their active therapeutic interventions with families.

General Systems Theory

Beginning in the 1940s, Ludwig von Bertalanffy (1968) and others began to develop a comprehensive theoretical model embracing all living systems. General systems theory challenged the traditional reductionistic view in science that complex phenomena could be understood by carefully breaking them down into a series of less complex cause-and-effect reactions and then analyzing in linear fashion how A causes B, B causes C, and so forth. Instead, this new theory argued for a systems focus in which the interrelations between parts assume far greater significance: A may cause B, but B affects A, which in turn affects B, and so on in a *circular causality.* General systems theory ideas can be seen in such family systems concepts as circular causality and the belief that symptoms in one family member signal family dysfunction rather than individual psychopathology.

Group Therapy

John Bell (1961) developed a therapeutic approach called *family group therapy,* applying some of the social psychological theories of small-group behavior to the natural group that is the family. Adopting group therapy's holistic outlook, family therapists involve entire families in the therapeutic process, believing that kinship groups are more real situations and provide a greater opportunity for powerful and longer-lasting systems changes as a result of family-level interventions.

Beginnings

Research on Schizophrenia

A number of researchers, working independently, began in the 1950s to zero in on schizophrenia as an area where family influences might be related to the development of psychotic symptoms. Taking a linear viewpoint at first and seeking causes of the schizophrenic condition in early family child-rearing practices, the researchers ultimately branched out into a broader systems point of view. Early efforts by the following are particularly noteworthy: Bateson's group in Palo Alto, Theodore Lidz's project at Yale, and the efforts at the National Institute of Mental Health (NIMH) of Murray Bowen and Lyman Wynne. The idea of seeing family members together for therapeutic purposes came later, as a result of research discoveries and subsequent theorizing.

A landmark paper by Bateson, Jackson, Haley, and Weakland (1956) speculated that *double-bind* communication patterns within a family may account for the onset of schizophrenia in one of its members. Double-bind situations exist when an individual, usually a child, habitually receives simultaneous contradictory messages from the same important person, typically a parent (verbally, "I'm interested in what you are telling me" but nonverbally, by gesture or glance signaling, "Go away, you are bothering me, I don't care about you") who forbids comment on the contradiction. Compelled to respond, but doomed to failure whatever the response, the child becomes confused and ultimately withdraws after repeated exposure to such incongruent messages, unable to understand the true meaning of his or others' communications. Schizophrenia was thus reformulated as an interpersonal phenomenon and as a prototype of the consequences of failure in a family's communication system.

Lidz and his colleagues (Lidz, Cornelison, Fleck, & Terry, 1957) hypothesized that schizophrenics did not receive the necessary nurturance as children and thus failed to achieve autonomy as adults. According to this premise, one or both parents' own arrested development was responsible, especially because the parents were likely to have a conflict-ridden marriage, providing poor role models for children. These researchers distinguished two patterns of chronic marital discord that were common in schizophrenic families. In one, labeled *marital skew,* extreme domination by one emotionally disturbed partner is accepted by the other, who implies to the children that the situation is normal. In the *marital schism* scenario, parents undermine their spouses, threats of divorce are common, and each parent vies for the loyalty and affection of the children.

Bowen was especially interested in the symbiotic mother-child bonds that he hypothesized might lead to schizophrenia. Hospitalizing entire families on the research wards for months at a time in order to observe ongoing family interactions, Bowen (1960) broadened his outlook, observing emotional intensity throughout these families. As a result, he moved from his previous psychoanalytic viewpoint to one that emphasized reciprocal functioning, in what he labeled the *family emotional system.*

Lyman Wynne, who succeeded Bowen at NIMH, turned his attention to the blurred, ambiguous, confused communication patterns he and his associates found in families with schizophrenic members (Wynne, Ryckoff, Day, & Hirsch, 1958). Wynne coined the term *pseudomutuality* to describe a false sense of family closeness in which the family gives the appearance of taking part in a mutual, open, and understanding relationship without really doing so. The members of these families have poorly developed personal identities and doubt their ability to accurately derive meaning from personal experiences outside the family, preferring to remain within the safe and familiar family system with its enclosed boundaries.

Psychodynamics of Family Life

Trained in psychoanalytic work with children, Nathan Ackerman nevertheless saw the value of treating entire families as a unit in assessing and treating dysfunctional families. In his landmark book *The Psychodynamics of Family Life,* often considered the first text to define the new field, Ackerman (1958) argued for family sessions aimed at untangling interlocking pathologies, thus endorsing the systems view that problems of any one family member cannot be understood apart from those of all other members.

By working therapeutically with nonschizophrenic families, Ackerman demonstrated the applicability of family therapy to less disturbed patients. By 1962, he in New York and Don Jackson on the West Coast founded the first journal in the field, *Family Process,* with Jay Haley as editor. This periodical enabled researchers and practitioners to exchange ideas and identify with the growing field of family therapy.

Delinquent Families

One project combining theory and practice was led by Salvador Minuchin (Minuchin, Montalvo, Guerney, Rosman, & Schumer, 1967) at the Wiltwyck School for Boys in upper New York State, a residential setting for delinquent youngsters from urban slums. Recognizing the limitations of traditional methods for reaching these boys, who were generally from poor, underorganized, fatherless homes, Minuchin developed a number of brief, action-oriented therapeutic procedures aimed at helping reorganize unstable family structures.

Current Status

The current trend in family therapy is toward eclecticism and integration of therapeutic approaches (Lebow, 1997) since no single technique fits all clients or situations. Multi-systemic approaches, research-based whenever possible, are being used to treat a variety of behavioral and emotional problems in adolescents and entire families as therapists select and borrow from one another's theories to address a current therapeutic problem. However, according to Goldenberg and Goldenberg (2008), eight theoretical viewpoints and corresponding approaches to family therapy can be identified.

Object Relations Family Therapy

The psychodynamic view is currently best expressed by object relations family therapists (Hughes, 2007 Scharff & Scharff, 2006), who contend that the need for a satisfying relationship with some "object" (i.e., another person) is the fundamental motive of life. From the object relations perspective, we bring *introjects*—memories of loss or unfulfillment from childhood—into current dealings with others, seeking satisfaction but sometimes "contaminating" family relations in the process. Thus, they argue, people unconsciously relate to one another in the present largely on the basis of expectations formed during childhood. Individual intrapsychic issues and family interpersonal difficulties are examined in a therapeutic setting. Helping family members gain insight into how they internalized objects from the past and how these objects continue to intrude on current relationships is the central therapeutic effort, along with providing understanding and instigating change. Treatment is aimed at helping members become aware of those unresolved objects from their families of origin and at increasing their understanding of the interlocking pathologies that have blocked both individual development and fulfillment from family relationships.

Experiential Family Therapy

Experiential family therapists such as Satir and Whitaker believe that troubled families need a "growth experience" derived from an intimate interpersonal experience with an involved therapist. By being real or authentic themselves, and often self-disclosing, experiential therapists contend that they can help families learn to be more honest, more expressive of their feelings and needs, and better able to use their potential for self-awareness to achieve personal and interpersonal growth.

For Virginia Satir, building self-esteem and learning to communicate adequately and openly were essential therapeutic goals. Calling his approach *symbolic—experiential family therapy,* Carl Whitaker gave voice to his own impulses and fantasies and de-pathologized human experiences as he helped family members probe their own covert world of symbolic meanings, freeing them to activate their innate growth processes. Currently, experiential family therapy is best represented by *emotion-focused couple therapy* (Greenberg & Goldman, 2008), an attachment-theory-grounded experiential approach based on humanistic and systemic foundations that attempts to change a couple's negative interactions while helping them cement their emotional connection to each other.

Transgenerational Family Therapy

Murray Bowen argued that family members are tied in thinking, feeling, and behavior to the family system and thus that individual problems arise and are maintained by relationship connections with fellow members. Those persons with the strongest affective connections (or *fusion*) with the family are most vulnerable to personal emotional reactions to family stress. The degree to which an individualized, separate sense of self independent from the family (or *differentiation of self*) occurs is correlated with the ability to resist being overwhelmed by emotional reactivity in the family; the greater the differentiation, the less likely the individual is to experience personal dysfunction.

Bowen (1978) believed that the child most vulnerable to dysfunction is the one most easily drawn into family conflict. He maintained that the most attached child will have the lowest level of differentiation, will be the least mature and thus have the hardest time separating from the family, and is likely to select as a marital partner someone who is also poorly differentiated in his or her family. The least differentiated of their offspring will marry someone equally undifferentiated, and so forth. In this formulation, problems are passed along to succeeding generations by a multigenerational transmission process. Bowen maintained that schizophrenia could result after several generations of increased fusion and vulnerability.

Another transgenerational family therapist, Ivan Boszormenyi-Nagy (1987), emphasizes the ethical dimension (trust, loyalty, entitlements, and indebtedness) in family relationships, extending over generations. He focuses on the relational ethics within a family aimed at preserving fairness and ensuring fulfillment of each member's subjective sense of claims, rights, and obligations in relation to one another. To *contextual therapists* such as Boszormenyi-Nagy, the patterns of relating within a family that are passed down from generation to generation are the keys to understanding both individual and family functioning.

Structural Family Therapy

Minuchin's (1974) structural view focuses on how families are organized and on what rules govern their transactions. He pays particular attention to family rules, roles, alignments, and coalitions, as well as to the boundaries and subsystems that make up the overall family system. Symptoms are viewed as conflict defusers, diverting attention from more basic family conflicts. Therapeutically, structuralists challenge rigid, repetitive transactions within a family, helping to "unfreeze" them to allow family reorganization (Minuchin, Nichols, & Lee, 2006).

Strategic Family Therapy

This approach involves the designing of novel strategies by the therapist for eliminating undesired behavior. Strategists such as Jay Haley (1996) are not particularly interested in providing insight to family members; they are more likely to assign tasks to get families to change those aspects of the system that maintain the problematic behavior. Sometimes indirect tasks, in the form of *paradoxical interventions,* are employed to force clients to abandon symptoms. Therapists at the Mental Research Institute in Palo Alto believe families develop unworkable "solutions" to problems that become problems themselves. Consequently, these therapists have evolved a set of brief therapy procedures employing various forms of paradox aimed at changing undesired family interactive patterns (Watzlawick, Weakland, & Fisch, 1974).

In Milan, Italy, Mara Selvini-Palazzoli and her colleagues (Selvini-Palazzoli, Boscolo, Cecchin, & Prata, 1978) developed *systemic family therapy,* a variation of strategic family therapy that has had its greatest success with psychotic and anorectic patients. Selvini-Palazzoli (1986) believed behavioral symptoms in families represent "dirty games" in which parents and symptomatic children engage in power struggles, the children using their symptoms to try to defeat one parent for the sake of the other. Boscolo and Cecchin (Boscolo, Cecchin, Hoffman, & Penn, 1987) in particular have refined a number of interviewing techniques, such as *circular questioning,* to help family members examine their family belief system in the process of helping empower them to exercise their prerogative of making new choices for their lives. Boscolo and Cecchin offer a systemic epistemology based on second-order cybernetics in which the therapist, rather than attempting to describe the family system as an outside observer, is viewed as part of what is being observed and treated. Like other participants, the therapist is seen as someone with a particular perspective but not a truly objective view of the family or what is best for it. Their approach enhanced the development of the postmodern-influenced social construction therapies.

Cognitive—Behavior Family Therapy

The behavioral perspective—the idea that maladaptive or problematic behavior can be extinguished as the contingencies of reinforcement for that behavior are altered—has been expanded in recent years by including a cognitive viewpoint (Beck & Weishaar, 2005; Berg, Dolan, & Trepper, 2008; Ellis & Dryden, 2007). Working with couples or offering training in parenting skills, cognitive restructuring is designed to help clients overcome dysfunctional beliefs, attitudes, or expectations and to replace their self-defeating thoughts and perceptions with more positive self-statements about themselves and their future. Beyond changing current distorted beliefs, clients are taught how better to evaluate all beliefs. Cognitively based couples therapy is directed at restructuring distorted beliefs (called *schemas*) learned early in life (from the family of origin, the mass media, and/or the family's ethnic and socioeconomic subculture). These negative schemas affect automatic thoughts and emotional responses to others and call for cognitive restructuring to modify or alter faulty perceptions. (Wills, 2009).

Social Constructionist Family Therapy

Influenced primarily by postmodern thinking, social constructionists are at the forefront of challenging systems thinking, especially the simple cybernetic model presented by the early family therapists. They contend that each of our perceptions is not an exact duplication of the world but, rather, a point of view seen through the limiting lens of our assumptions about people. The view of reality each of us constructs is mediated through language and is socially determined through our relationships with others and with the culture's shared set of assumptions. Valuing diversity, these therapists maintain that ethnicity, cultural considerations, gender issues, sexual orientation, and so forth must be addressed in determining a family's functioning level.

Family therapy from a social constructionist outlook requires collaboration between therapist and family members without preconceived notions of what constitutes a functional family or how a particular family should change. Instead, therapist and family members together examine the belief systems that form the basis for the meaning they give to events, and then they jointly construct new options that change past accounts of their lives and allow them to consider new alternatives that offer greater promise. Leading proponents of this view included Steve de Shazer (1991), Berg (Berg, Dolan, & Trepper, 2007) (*solution-focused therapy*) and Harlene Anderson (1997) (*collaborative language systems approach*).

Narrative Therapy

Narrative therapists such as Michael White (1995) argue that our sense of reality is organized and maintained through the stories by which we circulate knowledge about ourselves and the outside world. Families who present negative, dead-end stories about themselves typically feel overwhelmed, inadequate, defeated, and without future choices. Their self-narratives concede being beaten and fail to provide options that would allow change. The dominant cultural narratives also make them feel they cannot live up to what is expected of them. Therapeutic help comes in the form of learning to reduce the power of problem-saturated stories and reclaiming their lives by substituting previously subjugated stories in which they were successful. The therapist's role is not to help clients replace one story with another but to help them view life as multistoried, with numerous options and possibilities.

Narrative therapists are concerned not with how family patterns produced the problem but with how the problem affected the family. The therapist's task, according to narrative therapists, is to help liberate families from such feelings of hopelessness by collaborating with them in exploring alternative stories, making new assumptions about themselves, and opening them up to new possibilities by re-authoring their stories. *Externalization* (viewing the problem as outside themselves rather than as an internal part of their identity) helps them notice alternative choices and paves the way for alternative stories.

White is especially interested in helping clients reexamine the oppressive stories that formed the basis for how they have lived their lives and in working with them to construct new alternatives, whereas de Shazer helps clients view their problems differently, engaging them in dialogue directed at finding new and empowering solutions.

PERSONALITY

Family therapists as a group do not subscribe to a single, unified theory of personality, though all view individual development as embedded in the context of family life. Expanding on Sullivan's (1953) emphasis on the role of interpersonal relationships in personality development, family therapists believe that behavior is the product of one's relationships with others. Symptomatic conduct in any individual family member is a response to that person's current situation, although it may have its roots in past experiences within the family.

Theory of Personality

Clinicians who adopt a family systems outlook have varying theoretical bases. Individual personality is not overlooked but is instead recast as a unit of a larger system, the family, which in turn is seen as part of a larger societal system. Nevertheless, family therapists remain aware that no matter how much individual behavior is related to and dependent on the behavior of others in the family system, individual family members remain flesh-and-blood persons with unique experiences, private hopes, ambitions, outlooks, expectations, and potentials (Nichols, 1987). Most family therapists try to remain focused on family interaction without losing sight of the singularity of the individual. The ultimate goal is to benefit all those who make up the family.

How a therapist views personality development depends largely on her or his initial theoretical framework. In keeping with their psychoanalytic roots, object relations theorists (Hughes, 2007) believe that people's fundamental need is for attachments—seeking closeness and emotional bonding to others, based on how needy or insecure they are as adults as a result of early infant experiences. These therapists investigate individual "object-loss" growing up, believing that if one's relational needs are unmet by parents or other caregivers, the child will internalize both the characteristics of the lost object and the accompanying anger and resentment over the loss. The resulting unresolved unconscious conflict develops into frustration and self-defeating habits in the adult, who continues, unconsciously and unsuccessfully, to choose intimate partners to repair early deprivation.

Behaviorally oriented family therapists believe that all behavior, normal and abnormal, is learned as a result of a process involving the acquisition of knowledge, information, experiences, and habits. Classical conditioning, operant conditioning, and modeling concepts are used to explain how personality is learned. Following the early lead of B. F. Skinner, some strict behaviorists question whether an inner personality exists, maintaining that what we refer to as "personality" is nothing more than the sum of the environmental experiences in one's life. Rejecting explanations that imply the development of internal traits, they search instead for relationships between observable behavior and observable variations in the person's environment. In their view, situations determine behavior.

Those behavior therapists who adopt a more cognitive orientation believe that people do develop personality traits and that their behavior is based at least in part on those traits and does not arise simply in response to situations. These family therapists contend that certain types of cognitions are learned, become ingrained as traits, and mediate a person's behavior. Perceptions of events, attitudes, beliefs, expectations of outcomes, and attributions are examples of such cognitions. Especially when negative or rigid, these cognitions can contribute to negative behavior exchanges within a family. Intervention is an attempt to change maladaptive cognitions.

Many family therapists view personality from a *family life cycle* perspective (Carter & McGoldrick, 2005). This developmental outlook notes that certain predictable marker events or phases (marriage, birth of first child, children leaving home, and so on) occur in all families, regardless of structure or composition or cultural background, compelling each family to deal in some manner with these events. Because there is an ever-changing family context in which individual members grow up, there are many chances for maladaptive responses. Situational family crises (such as the death of a parent during childhood or the birth of a handicapped child) and certain key transition points are periods of special vulnerability.

Both continuity and change characterize family systems as they progress through the life cycle. Ordinarily, such changes are gradual and the family is able to reorganize as a system and adapt successfully. Certain discontinuous changes, however, may be disruptive, transforming a family system so that it will never return to its previous way of functioning. Divorce, becoming part of a stepfamily, serious financial reverses, and chronic illness in a family member are examples of sudden, disruptive changes that cause upheaval and disequilibrium in the family system. Symptoms in family members are especially likely to appear during these critical periods of change as the family struggles to reorganize while negotiating the transition. Family therapists may seize the crisis period as an opportunity to help families develop higher levels of functioning by helping them galvanize their inherent potential for resiliency to better cope with upheaval or loss (Walsh, 2003).

Variety of Concepts

Family Rules

A family is a rule-governed system in which the interactions of its members follow organized, established patterns. Growing up in a family, members all learn what is expected or permitted in family transactions. Parents, children, relatives, males, females, and older and younger siblings all have prescribed rules for the boundaries of permissible behavior—rules that may not be verbalized but are understood by all. Such rules regulate and help stabilize the family system.

Family therapists are especially interested in persistent, repetitive behavioral sequences that characterize much of everyday family life because of what these patterns reveal about the family's typical interactive patterns. The term *redundancy principle* is used to describe a family's usually restricted range of options for dealing with one another. Attending to a family's rules represents an interactive way of understanding behavior rather than attributing that individual behavior to some inferred inner set of motives. Don Jackson (1965), an early observer of family behavioral patterns, believed that family dysfunction was due to a family's lack of rules for accommodating to changing conditions.

Family Narratives and Assumptions

All families develop paradigms about the world (enduring assumptions that are shared by family members). Some families view the world as friendly, trustworthy, orderly, predictable, and masterable and thus are likely to view themselves as competent and to encourage members to share their views, even when disagreement is likely to ensue. Others perceive the world as mostly menacing, unstable, and thus unpredictable and potentially dangerous. This latter group is likely to insist on agreement from all family members on most if not all issues in an effort to present a united front against any intrusion or threat. The narrative the family develops about itself, derived largely from its history and passed from one generation to the next, has a powerful impact on its daily functioning.

Families inevitably create narratives or stories about themselves, linking certain family experiences together in a certain sequence to justify how and why they live as they do. Certain dominant stories (how they were orphaned at an early age, how they lived with alcoholic parents, how their parents' divorce frightened them about commitment to a relationship, how their grandmother's love and devotion made them feel loved and cared for, and so on) explain their current actions and attitudes. Narrative therapists such as White (2007) contend that our sense of reality is organized and maintained through the stories by which we circulate knowledge about ourselves and our view of the world we live in. Beyond personal experiences, the meanings and understandings that families attribute to events and situations they encounter are embedded in their social, cultural, and historical experiences (Anderson & Gehart, 2006).

Pseudomutuality and Pseudohostility

One result of Wynne's NIMH studies of families with schizophrenic members (Wynne, et al., 1958) was his observation of their recurrent fragmented and irrational style of communication. He discovered an unreal quality about how they expressed both positive and negative emotion to one another, a process he labeled *pseudomutuality*. Wynne reported that members in these families were absorbed with fitting together at the expense of developing their separate identities. Rather than encourage a balance between separateness and togetherness, as occurs in well-functioning families, members in Wynne's group seemed concerned with the latter only, apparently dreading expressions of individuality as a threat to the family as a whole. By presenting a facade of togetherness, they learned to maintain a homeostatic balance, but at the expense of not allowing either disagreements or expressions of affection. The tactic kept them from dealing with any underlying conflict, and at the same time, the surface togetherness prevented them from experiencing deeper intimacy with one another.

Wynne's research also identified *pseudohostility,* a similar collusion in which apparent quarreling or bickering between family members is in reality merely a superficial tactic for avoiding deeper and more genuine feelings. Members may appear alienated from one another, and their antagonism may even appear intense, but the turmoil is merely a way of maintaining a connection without becoming either deeply affectionate or deeply hostile to one another. Like pseudomutuality, it represents a distorted way of communicating and fosters irrational thinking about relationships.

Mystification

Another masking effort to obscure the real nature of family conflict and thus maintain the status quo is called *mystification.* First described by R. D. Laing (1965) in analyzing the family's role in a child's development of psychopathology, the concept refers to parental efforts to distort a child's experience by denying what the child believes is occurring. Instead of telling the child, "It's your bedtime," or explaining that they are tired and want to be left alone, parents say, "You must be tired. Go to bed." In effect, they have distorted what the child is experiencing ("I'm not tired"), especially if they add that they know better than the child what he or she is feeling.

Mystification, then, occurs when families deal with conflict by befuddling, obscuring, or masking whatever is going on between members. This device does not deter conflict but rather clouds the meaning of conflict and is called into play when a family member threatens the status quo, perhaps by expressing feelings. A husband who says, in response to his wife's query about why he appears angry, "I'm not angry. Where do you dream up these things?" when he actually is angry is attempting to mystify her. His apparent intent to avoid conflict and return matters to their previous balance only leads to greater conflict within her. If she believes him, then she feels she must be "crazy" to imagine his anger, and if she trusts her own senses, then she must deal with a deteriorating marital relationship. Mystification contradicts one person's perceptions and, in extreme or repeated cases, leads that person to question his or her grip on reality.

Scapegoating

Within some families, a particular individual is held responsible for whatever goes wrong with the family. *Scapegoating* directed at a particular child often has the effect of redirecting parental conflict, making it unnecessary for the family to look at the impaired father–mother relationship, something that would be far more threatening to the family. By conveniently picking out a scapegoat who becomes the identified patient, other family members can avoid dealing with one another or probing more deeply into what is really taking place.

Scapegoated family members are themselves often active participants in the family scapegoating process. Not only do they assume the role assigned them, but they may become so entrenched in that role that they are unable to act otherwise. Particularly in dysfunctional families, individuals may be repeatedly labeled as the "bad child"—incorrigible, destructive, unmanageable, troublesome—and they proceed to act accordingly. Scapegoated children are inducted into specific family roles that over time become fixed and serve as the basis for chronic behavioral disturbance. Because the family retains a vested interest in maintaining the scapegoated person in that role, blaming all their problems on one member, changes in family interactive patterns must occur before scapegoating will cease. Otherwise, the scapegoated person, usually symptomatic, will continue to carry the pathology for the family.

PSYCHOTHERAPY

Theory of Psychotherapy

There is no single theory of psychotherapy for family therapists, although all would probably agree with the following basic premises:

1. People are products of their social connections, and attempts to help them must take family relationships into account.

2. Symptomatic or problematic behavior in an individual arises from a context of relationships, and interventions to help that person are most effective when those faulty interactive patterns are altered.

3. Individual symptoms are maintained externally in current family system transactions.

4. Conjoint sessions, in which the family is the therapeutic unit and the focus is on family interaction, are more effective in producing change than attempts to uncover intrapsychic problems in individuals via individual sessions.

5. Assessing family subsystems and the permeability of boundaries within the family and between the family and the outside world offers important clues regarding family organization and susceptibility to change.

6. Traditional psychiatric diagnostic labels based on individual psychopathology fail to provide an understanding of family dysfunctions and tend to pathologize individuals.

7. The goals of family therapy are to change maladaptive or dysfunctional family interactive patterns and/or to help clients construct alternative views about themselves that offer new options and possibilities for the future.

Systems thinking most often provides the underpinnings for therapeutic interventions with the family. By viewing causality in circular rather than linear terms, it keeps the focus on family transactional patterns, especially redundant maladaptive patterns that help maintain symptomatic behavior. When family interrelationships are emphasized over individual needs and drives, explanations shift from a *monadic* model (based on the characteristics of a single person) to a *dyadic* model (based on a two-person interaction) or *triadic* model (based on interactions among three or more persons).

In a monadic outlook, a husband fails to pay attention to his wife because he is a cold and uncaring person. Adopting a dyadic mode, people are viewed in terms of their interlocking relationships and their impact on one another. Here the therapist looks beyond the separate individuals who make up the couple, focusing instead on how these two individuals organize their lives together and, more specifically, on how each helps define the other. From a dyadic viewpoint, a husband's indifference arouses his wife's emotional pursuit, and she demands attention. Her insistence arouses the fear of intimacy that led to his withdrawal to begin with, and he retreats further. She becomes more insistent and he less available as their conflict escalates. A family therapist helping such a couple will direct attention to their interactive effect, thus making the dyad (and not each participant) the unit of treatment. Seeing the couple conjointly rather than separately underscores the therapist's view that the problem arises from both partners and that both are responsible for finding solutions.

In a triadic model, the family therapist assumes that the presenting problems result from the dyad's inability to resolve the conflict, which causes other family members to be drawn into it. A preteenage son who frustrates his father by refusing to do his homework and thus is performing badly at school may be doing so in alliance with his mother against his father, indirectly expressing her resentment at her husband's authoritarian behavior. The couple's original dyadic conflict has become a triadic one in which multiple interactions occur. Merely to develop a behavioral plan or contract for the boy to receive money or special television or videogame privileges in return for completing school assignments would miss the complex family interaction involved. Family therapists would look at the overall impact of the symptomatic behavior in context; the youngster may or may not be included in the entire treatment, which certainly would deal with the unspoken and unresolved husband–wife conflicts and the recruitment of their child to express or act out their tensions.

In the example just presented, the child's symptom (the school problem) maintains the family homeostasis but obscures the underlying and unexpressed set of family conflicts. Symptoms often function in maintaining family homeostasis; in this case, attention to the school problem keeps the parents from quarreling with each other and upsetting the family balance. If the school problem did not at some level sustain the family organization, it would not be maintained. Thus, the systems-oriented therapist might wonder: (1) Is the family member expressing, through symptoms, feelings that the other members are denying or not permitting themselves to experience? and (2) What would happen to other family members if the identified patient were to become symptom free? (Wachtel, 2007). Symptoms thus serve a protective purpose or are stabilizing devices used in families. As a consequence, although they may not do so consciously, families may be invested in the maintenance of the symptom for homeostatic purposes.

Even though the idea that symptoms may serve a purpose in helping maintain family stability has been a mainstay of family therapy theory, critics argue that it suggests that families need a "sick" member and are willing to sacrifice that person for the sake of family well-being. *Narrative therapists* such as White (2007) reject the notion that a child's problems necessarily reflect more serious underlying family conflict. In White's view, families may be oppressed rather than protected by the symptomatic behavior. White's efforts are directed at getting all family members to unite in wresting control of their lives from the oppressive set of symptoms.

Family therapists usually are active participants with families and concentrate on current family functioning. They attempt to help members achieve lasting changes in the functioning of the family system, not merely superficial changes that will allow the system to return to its former tenuous balance. Watzlawick, Weakland, and Fisch (1974) distinguish between *first-order changes* (changes within the system that do not alter the organization of the system itself) and *second-order changes* (fundamental changes in a system's organization and function). The former term refers to specific differences that take place within the system, and the latter involves rule changes in the system—in effect, changing the system itself.

For example, the following is a first-order change: The Ryan parents were concerned with the repeated school absences of their son Billy, and in an attempt to correct his behavior, they told him that any time they learned he was truant from school, he would be grounded the following Saturday.

The following is a second-order change: The Ryan parents were concerned with the repeated school absences of their son Billy. After consulting with a family therapist for several sessions, they realized that by struggling with Billy, they only encouraged his rebelliousness and thus were involved in sustaining the truant behavior. They also came to recognize that Billy's relationship with the school was truly his own and that they should back off from intruding. Attempting to change the rules and pull themselves out of the struggle, they told Billy that from now on, whether or not he went to school was between him and the school and that henceforth he would be responsible for his education.

As in these examples, a problematic family on their own may try first-order changes by attempting to impose what appear to be logical solutions to their problems. Assuming the problem to be monadic—the result of Billy's rebelliousness—they are employing negative feedback, attempting to do the opposite of what has been occurring. The family actually may make some changes in behavior for a brief period, but they are still governed by the same rules, the cease-fire is not likely to hold, and Billy will probably return to his school absences sooner or later.

Second-order changes, based on positive feedback, call for a change in the way the family organizes itself. Here the rules of the game must change, viewpoints must be altered, and old situations must be seen in a new light, providing a revised context in which new behavior patterns may emerge. Most people try to solve everyday problems by attempting first-order changes and repeating the same solutions in a self-perpetuating cycle, which only makes things worse. Especially with seriously troubled families, fundamental second-order changes in the system are necessary so that the family members can give different meanings to old feelings and old experiences.

Process of Psychotherapy

The Initial Contact

Family therapy begins when the client asks for help. One family member or a coalition of members begins the process by seeking help outside the family, thus acknowledging that a problem exists and that the family has been unsuccessful in its attempts to resolve the problem by themselves. While the caller is assessing whether the right person has been contacted, the therapist is forming tentative hypotheses about the family. How self-aware is the caller? What sort of impression is he or she trying to make? What other members are involved? Are they all willing to attend the initial session?

Initial contact, whether in person or by telephone, provides an opportunity for a mini-evaluation and also represents the therapist's first opportunity to enter into the family system. If the therapist is careful not to get maneuvered into taking sides, be engulfed by family anxiety, or become excessively sympathetic or angry with any member on the basis of what the caller is reporting, then he or she can establish the rules of the game for further family sessions.

The Initial Session

The family therapist usually encourages as many family members as possible to attend the first session. Entering the room, members are encouraged to sit where they wish; their chosen seating arrangement (such as mother and child close together, father sitting apart) offers the therapist an early clue about possible family alliances and coalitions. Welcoming all members separately as equally important participants, the therapist becomes aware that some members may need extra support and encouragement to participate.

Each person's view of the problem must be heard, as well as the first-order solutions the family has attempted. Observing family interactive patterns, particularly repetitive behavioral sequences that occur around a problem, the therapist tentatively begins to redefine the identified patient's symptoms as a family problem in which each member has a stake. Together, therapist and family explore whether they wish to continue working together and who will attend; if they choose to discontinue, outside referrals to other therapists are in order. If they agree to stay, treatment goals are defined.

Engaging the Family

Beginning with the initial session, the therapist tries to build a working alliance with the family, accommodating to their transactional style as well as assimilating their language patterns and manner of affective expression. The therapist tries to create an atmosphere in which each member feels supported and able to voice previously unexpressed or unexplored problems. By "joining" them, the therapist is letting them know they are understood and cared about and that in such a safe climate, they can begin to confront divisive family issues.

Assessing Family Functioning

Like all forms of psychotherapy, family therapy involves some form of assessment, formal or informal, as the clinician attempts, early in the course of therapy, to learn more about the family in order to make more informed treatment decisions. (1) Is treatment for the entire family needed? (2) Who are the appropriate family members with whom to work? (3) What underlying interactive patterns fuel the family disturbance and lead to symptoms in one or more of its members? (4) What specific interventions will most effectively help this family? In later sessions, the therapist continues to revise hypotheses, basing subsequent interventions on assessments of the success of previous attempts to alter dysfunctional repetitive family patterns.

Cognitive–behavior family therapists are apt to make a careful, systematic behavioral analysis of the family's maladaptive behavioral patterns, often using questionnaires, pinpointing precisely which behaviors need to be altered and which events typically precede and follow that behavioral sequence. What exactly does the family mean by their child's "temper tantrums"? How often do these occur, under what circumstances, how long do they last, what specific reactions does each family member have, and what antecedent and subsequent events are associated with the outburst? The therapist tries to gauge the extent of the problem, the environmental cues that trigger the behavior, and the behaviors of various family members that maintain the problem. The assessment, continuously updated, helps the therapist plan interventions to reduce undesired or problematic behaviors.

Experiential family therapists spend less time on a formal family history. They work more in the here and now, helping families examine current interactive patterns with little regard for historical antecedents. Assessment is an informal, ongoing process indistinguishable from the therapeutic process itself. Such therapists attempt to provide families with an experience, using themselves as models to explore their own feelings and give voice to their own impulses. Carl Whitaker, an experiential therapist, insists on controlling the structure of the therapy at the start of treatment, making certain that the family is not successful in imposing its own definition of the upcoming therapeutic relationship and how it should proceed. Later, he believes, the family members must be encouraged to take responsibility for changing the nature of their relationships.

Many family therapists agree with Salvador Minuchin (1974) that they get a better sense of how families function by interacting with them over a period of time than from any formal assessment process. Therapists observe how subsystems carry out family tasks, how alliances and coalitions operate within the family, how flexible are family rules in the face of changing conditions, and how permeable are the boundaries within the family and between the family and the outside world. These observations help family therapists modify and discard hypotheses and adjust intervention strategies on the basis of refined appraisals of family functioning.

History-Taking

As is consistent with their theoretical leanings, object relations family therapists such as Scharff and Scharff (2006) contend that an examination of family history is essential to understanding current family functioning. Because they believe people carry attachments of their parental introjects (memories from childhood) into their current relationships, these therapists are especially interested in such matters as how and why marital partners chose each other. That choice is seen as seeking to rediscover, through the other person, the lost aspects of primary object attachments that had split off earlier in life. Similarly, contextual family therapists (Boszormenyi-Nagy, 1987) examine with their patients those interconnections from the past that bind families together in an effort to help them discover new ways of making fresh inputs into stagnant relationships.

Bowen (1978) began with a set of evaluation interviews aimed at clarifying the history of the presenting problem, especially trying to understand how the symptoms affect family functioning. He tried to assess the family's pattern of emotional functioning as well as the intensity of the emotional process of the symptomatic person. What is this family's relationship system like? How well differentiated are the various members? What are the current sources of stress, and how adaptive is the family?

Because Bowen believed dysfunction may result from family fusion extending back over generations, he probed for signs of poor differentiation from families of origin. To aid in the process, Bowen constructed a family *genogram,* a schematic diagram in the form of a family tree, usually including at least three generations, to trace recurring family behavior patterns. Hypotheses developed from the genogram, such as fusion/ differentiation issues or emotional cutoffs from family, are used to better understand the underlying emotional processes connecting generations. Careful not to become drawn into the family's emotional system, Bowen used this information to coach family members to modify their relationships and especially to differentiate themselves from their families of origin.

Satir (1972) attempted to get families to think about the relevant concepts that formed the basis of their developing relationships by compiling a family life chronology for each family member. More than simply gathering historical facts, this represented an effort to help people understand how family ideology, values, and commitments had emerged in the family and influenced current family functioning. Later, she used the therapeutic technique of family reconstruction, guiding family members back through stages of their lives in an attempt to discover and unlock dysfunctional patterns from the past.

Structural and strategic family therapists pay less attention to family or individual histories, preferring to focus on the current family organization, coalitions, hierarchies, and so on. They are concerned with developing ways to change ongoing dysfunctional family patterns, and they typically show less concern for how these patterns historically emerged.

Social constructionists pay particular attention to how the various family members view their world rather than attempting to act as outside observers evaluating client responses. From their perspective, any preconceived views by the therapist of what constitutes a functional family fail to attend to the diversity inherent in today's pluralistic society. The personal outlook of each family member is privileged, and all such outlooks are valued equally.

Facilitating Change

Family therapists use a number of therapeutic techniques to alter family functioning.

1. *Reframing.* This technique involves relabeling problematic behavior by viewing it in a new, more positive light that emphasizes its good intention. (To an adolescent angry because he believes his mother is invading his privacy: "Your mother is concerned about your welfare and hasn't yet found the best way to help." Labeling her as wishing to do well for her son, rather than agreeing with her son's perception that she does not trust him, alters the context in which he perceives her behavior, thus inviting new responses from him to her behavior.)

Reframing changes the meaning attributed to a behavior without changing the "facts" of the behavior itself. Strategic family therapists are most likely to use this technique because it enables them to help clients change the basis for their perceptions or interpretation of events. This altered perspective leads to a change in the family system as the problematic behavior becomes understood from a new perspective. Reframing, then, is a method for bringing about second-order changes in the family system.

2. *Therapeutic Double-Binds.* Another technique favored by strategic and systemic family therapists is putting the family in a *therapeutic double-bind* by directing families to continue to manifest their presenting symptoms: Obsessive people are asked to think about their problem for a specific period of time each day; quarreling husbands and wives are instructed to indulge in and even exaggerate their fighting. By instructing family members to enact symptomatic behavior, the therapist is demanding that the presentation of the symptom, which they have claimed is "involuntary" and thus out of their control be done voluntarily. Such paradoxical interventions are designed to evoke one of two reactions, either of which is sought by the therapist. If the patient complies, continuing to be symptomatic, there is the admission that the symptomatology is under voluntary control, not involuntary as claimed, and thus can be stopped. On the other hand, if the directive to continue the symptom is resisted, the symptom will be given up.

3. *Enactment.* Most likely to be used by structural family therapists, *enactments* are role-playing efforts to bring the outside family conflict into the session so that family members can demonstrate how they deal with it and the therapist can start to devise an intervention procedure for modifying their interaction and creating structural changes in the family. Encouraged by the therapist, the family members act out their dysfunctional transactions rather than talking about them. This gives the therapist an opportunity to observe the process directly instead of relying on family members' reports of what occurs at home. Also, because of the immediacy of this approach, the therapist can intervene on the spot and witness the results of such interventions as they occur.

Helping "unfreeze" family members from repetitive family interactions that end in conflict, the therapist has a chance to guide them in modifying the interactions. By introducing alternative solutions calling for structural changes in the family, the therapist can help the family create options for new behavior sequences. Treating the family of an anorectic adolescent, Minuchin (Minuchin et al., 1978) might arrange to meet the family for the first session and bring in lunch, thus deliberately provoking an enactment around eating. Observing their struggles over their daughter's refusal to eat, Minuchin can demonstrate that the parental subsystem is not working effectively. If parents begin to cooperate with one another in encouraging their daughter to eat, they form a stronger union. At the same time, the daughter is relieved of the too-powerful and destructive position she has been maintaining. The enactment impels the family to look at the system they have created together and to change the dysfunctional behavior displayed in the session.

4. *Family Sculpting.* Rather than putting their feelings or attitudes toward one another into words, which may be difficult or threatening, family members each take a turn at being a "director"—that is, at placing each of the other members in a physical arrangement in space. The result is often revealing of how the "director" perceives his or her place in the family, as well as that person's perception of what is being done to whom, by whom, and in what manner. Individual perceptions of family boundaries, alliances, roles, and subsystems are typically revealed, even if the "director" cannot, or will not, verbalize such perceptions. The resulting graphic picture of individual views of family life provides active, nonverbal depictions for other members to grasp. Because of its nonintellectualized way of putting feelings into action, family sculpting is especially suited to the experiential approach of Satir.

5. *Circular Questioning.* This technique is often used by systemic family therapists (Boscolo et al., 1987) to focus attention on family connections rather than individual symptomatology. Each question posed to the family by the therapist addresses differences in different members' perceptions about the same events or relationships. By asking several members the same question regarding their attitudes toward those situations, the therapist is able to probe more deeply without being confrontational or interrogating the participants in the relationship. In this nonconfrontational therapeutic situation, the family can examine the origin of the underlying conflict. Advocates of this technique believe questioning is a therapeutic process that allows the family to untangle family problems by changing the ways they view their shared difficulties.

6. *Cognitive Restructuring.* This technique of cognitive–behavior therapists, based on the idea that problematic behavior stems from maladaptive thought processes, tries to modify a client's perceptions of events in order to bring about behavioral change. Thus, a partner may have unrealistic expectations about a relationship and catastrophize a commonplace disagreement ("I am worthless"). As Ellis (2005) suggests, it is the interpretation that causes havoc, not the quarrel itself. Cognitive restructuring can significantly modify perceptions ("It's upsetting that we're arguing, but that doesn't mean I'm a failure or our marriage is doomed").

7. *Miracle Question.* In this solution-focused technique (de Shazer, 1991), clients are asked to consider what would occur if a miracle took place and, upon awakening in the morning, they found the problem they brought to therapy solved. Each family member is encouraged to speculate on how things would be different, how each would change his or her behavior, and what each would notice in the others. In this way, goals are identified and potential solutions revealed.

8. *Externalization.* In an effort to liberate a family from its dominating, problem-saturated story, narrative therapists employ the technique of externalization to help families separate the symptomatic member's identity from the problem for which they sought help. The problem is recast as residing outside the family (rather than implying an internal family deficiency or individual pathological condition) and as having a restraining influence over the life of each member of the family. Instead of focusing on what's wrong with the family or with one of its members, all are called upon to unite to deal with this external and unwelcome story with a will of its own that dominates their lives. Thus, rather than the family concluding that "Mother is depressed" and therefore creating problems for the family, the symptom is personified as a separate, external, burdensome entity ("Depression is trying to control Mother's life"). By viewing the problem as outside themselves, the family is better able to collaborate in altering their way of thinking and developing new options for dealing with the problem rather than merely being mired in it.

Mechanisms of Psychotherapy

Family therapists generally take an active, problem-solving approach with families. Typically, they are more interested in dealing with current dysfunctional interactive issues within the family than in uncovering or helping resolve individual intrapsychic problems from the past. Past family transactional patterns may be explored, but this is done to home in on ongoing behavioral sequences or limiting belief systems that need changing rather than to reconstruct the past.

Depending on their specific emphases, family therapists may try to help clients achieve one or more of the following changes.

1. *Structural Change.* Having assessed the effectiveness of a family's organizational structure and its ongoing transactional patterns, family therapists may actively challenge rigid,

repetitive patterns that handicap optimum functioning of family members. Minuchin, for example, assumes the family is experiencing sufficient stress to overload the system's adaptive mechanisms, a situation that may be temporary due to failure to modify family rules to cope successfully with the demands of transitions. Helping families modify unworkable patterns creates an opportunity to adopt new rules and achieve realignments, clearer boundaries, and more flexible family interactions. Through restructuring, the family is helped to get back on track so that it will function more harmoniously and the growth potential of each member will be maximized.

2. *Behavioral Change.* All family therapists try to help clients achieve desired behavioral changes, although they may go about it in differing ways. Strategic therapists focus treatment on the family's presenting problems: what they came in to have changed. Careful not to allow families to manipulate or subdue the therapist and therefore control the treatment, strategic therapy is highly directive, and practitioners devise strategies for alleviating the presenting problem rather than exploring its roots or hidden meanings. Through directives such as paradoxical interventions, they try to force the symptom bearer to abandon old dysfunctional behavior. Similarly, *systemic therapists* (the Milan approach of Selvini-Palazzoli and her colleagues) may assign tasks or rituals for the family to carry out between sessions. These typically are offered in paradoxical form and call for the performance of a task that challenges an outdated or rigid family rule. Behavioral change follows from the emotional experience gained by the family through enactment of the directive.

3. *Experiential Change.* Therapists such as Satir, Whitaker, and Kempler believe that families need to feel and experience what previously was locked up. Their efforts are directed at growth-producing transactions in which therapists act as models of open communication, willing to explore and disclose their own feelings. Satir was especially intent on helping families learn more effective ways of communicating with one another and on teaching them to express what they are experiencing. Kempler also tries to help family members learn to ask for what they want from one another, thus facilitating self-exploration, risk taking, and spontaneity. Whitaker champions family members giving voice to underlying impulses and symbols. Because he sees all behavior as human experience and not as pathological, clients are challenged to establish new and more honest relationships, simultaneously maintaining healthy separation and personal autonomy. Emotionally focused couples therapists, too, help clients recognize how they have hidden their primary emotions or real feelings (say, fear of rejection) and instead have displayed defensive or coercive secondary emotions (anger or blaming when afraid). Their therapeutic efforts are directed at accessing and reprocessing the emotions underlying the clients' negative interactional sequences.

4. *Cognitive Change.* Psychodynamically oriented family therapists are interested in providing client families with insight and understanding. Boszormenyi-Nagy stresses intergenerational issues, particularly how relationship patterns are passed on from generation to generation, influencing current individual and family functioning. By gaining awareness of one's "family ledger," a multigenerational accounting system of who, psychologically speaking, owes what to whom, clients can examine and correct old unsettled or unredressed accounts. Framo (1992) also helped clients gain insight into introjects reprojected onto current family members to compensate for unsatisfactory early object relations. He had clients meet with members of their families of origin for several sessions to discover what issues from the past they may have projected onto current members and also to have a corrective experience with parents and siblings. Narrative therapists, such as White, open up conversations about clients' values, beliefs, and purposes so that they have an opportunity to consider a wide range of choices and attach new meanings to their experiences.

APPLICATIONS

Who Can We Help?

Individual Problems

Therapists who adopt a family frame of reference attend primarily to client relationships. Even if they work with single individuals, they look for the *context* of problematic behavior in planning and executing their clinical interventions. Thus, for example, they might see a college student, far away from family, for individual sessions but continue to view his or her problems within a larger context in which faulty relations with others have helped create the presenting troublesome behavior and are still maintaining it. Should the parents arrive for a visit, they might join their child for a counseling session or two to provide clues regarding relationship difficulties within the family system and assist in their amelioration.

Intergenerational Problems

Family therapists frequently deal with parent–child issues, such as adolescents in conflict with their parents or with society in general. Minuchin's structural approach might be adopted to help families, particularly at transition points in the family life cycle, adapt to changes and modify outdated rules. Here they are likely to try to strengthen the parental subsystem, more clearly define generational boundaries, and help the family craft new and more flexible rules to account for changing conditions as adolescence is reached. To cite an increasingly common example, families in which the children are raised in this country by foreign-born parents often present intergenerational conflicts that reflect differing values and attitudes. Intervention at the family level is often required if changes in the family system are to be achieved.

Two promising family approaches, aimed at treating delinquency or other behavior problems in adolescents, as well as at reducing recidivism, are functional family therapy (Sexton & Alexander, 1999) and multisystemic therapy (Henggeler, Schoenwald, Borduin, & Rowland, 2009). Both have garnered considerable research support, and both offer systems-based, cost-effective programs that community providers can adopt in working with at-risk adolescents and their families.

Marital Problems

Troubled marriages are common today, and many of the problems involving symptomatic behavior in a family member can be traced to efforts by the family to deal with parents in conflict. In addition to personal problems of one or both spouses that contribute to their unhappiness, certain key interpersonal difficulties are frequently present: ineffective communication patterns; sexual incompatibilities; anxiety over making or maintaining a long-term commitment; conflicts over money, in-laws, or children; physical abuse; and/or conflicts over power and control. These issues, repeated without resolution over a period of time, escalate the marital dissatisfaction of one or both partners, placing the marriage in jeopardy. Couples who enter therapy conjointly, before one or both conclude that the costs of staying together outweigh the benefits, are better able to salvage their relationship than if either or both seek individual psychotherapy.

Treatment

The Family Therapy Perspective

Family therapy represents an outlook regarding the origin and maintenance of symptomatic or problematic behavior as well as a form of clinical intervention directed at changing dysfunctional aspects of the family system. Adopting such an outlook, the therapist may see the entire family together or may see various dyads, triads, or subsystems, depending on what aspects of the overall problem are being confronted by the therapist. Methods of treatment may vary, depending largely on the nature of the presenting problem, the therapist's theoretical outlook, and her or his personal style.

However, family therapy involves more than seeing distressed families as a unit or group. Simply gathering members together and continuing to treat the individuals separately, but in a group setting, fails to make the paradigm shift called for in treating relationships. Nor is it enough to perceive individual psychopathology as the therapist's central concern while acknowledging the importance of the family context in which such psychopathology developed. Rather, family therapy calls for viewing the amelioration of individual intrapsychic conflicts as secondary to improving overall family functioning.

To work in a family systems mode, the therapist must give up the passive, neutral, nonjudgmental stance developed with so much care in conventional individual psychotherapy. To help change family functioning, the therapist must become involved in the family's interpersonal processes (without losing balance or independence); must be supportive and nurturing at some points and challenging and demanding at others; must attend to (but not overidentify with) family members of different ages; and must move swiftly in and out of emotional involvements without losing track of family interactions and transactional patterns (Goldenberg & Goldenberg, 2008).

The *social constructionist family therapies,* which are currently gaining in popularity, place particular emphasis on the egalitarian, collaborative nature of therapist–family relationships. Family members are encouraged to examine the "stories" about themselves that they have lived by as together the therapist–family system searches for new and empowering ways to view and resolve client problems.

Indications and Contraindications

Family therapy is a valuable option in a therapist's repertoire of interventions, not a panacea for all psychological disturbances. However, it is clearly the treatment of choice for certain problems within the family. Wynne (1965) suggests that family therapy is particularly applicable to resolving relationship difficulties (e.g., parent–children; husband–wife), especially those to which all family members contribute, collusively or openly, consciously or unconsciously. Many family therapists go beyond Wynne's position, arguing that all psychological problems of individuals and of groups such as families ultimately are tied to systems issues and thus amenable to intervention at the family level.

Under what circumstances is family therapy contraindicated? In some cases, it may be too late to reverse the forces of fragmentation or too difficult to establish or maintain a therapeutic working relationship with the family because key members are unavailable or refuse to attend. Sometimes one seriously emotionally disturbed member may so dominate the family with malignant and destructive motives and behavior or be so violent or abusive or filled with paranoid ideation that working with the entire family becomes impossible, although some members of the family may continue to benefit from the family therapy perspective.

Length of Treatment

Family therapy may be brief or extended, depending on the nature and complexities of the problem, family resistance to its amelioration, and the goals of treatment. Changes that most benefit the entire family may not in every case be in the best interest of each family member, and some may cling to old and familiar ways of dealing with one another. In general, however, family therapy tends to be relatively short term compared to most individual therapy. In some cases, as few as 10 sessions may eliminate problematic behavior; others may require 20 sessions or more for symptoms to subside. Strategic therapy quickly focuses on what problems require attention, and then the therapist devises a plan of action to change the family's dysfunctional patterns in order to eliminate the presenting problem. Structural approaches tend to be brief as the therapist joins the family, learns of its transactional patterns, and initiates changes in its structure leading to changes in behavior and symptom reduction in the identified patient. The object relations approach, on the other hand, as is consistent with its psychoanalytic foundations, tends to take longer and to deal with material from earlier in clients' lives.

Settings and Practitioners

Outpatient offices, school counselor settings, and inpatient hospital wards all provide places where family therapy may be carried out. No longer out of the mainstream of psychotherapy, where it dwelt in its earlier years, family therapy has been accepted by nearly all psychotherapists. Marital or couples therapy, now considered a part of the family therapy movement, has grown at an astonishing rate since the 1970s, as recently reflected in the American Board of Professional Psychology change of name to American Board of Couples and Family Psychology.

Psychiatrists, psychologists, social workers, marriage and family counselors, and pastoral counselors practice family therapy, although their training and emphases may be different. Three basic kinds of training settings exist today: degree-granting programs in family therapy, freestanding family therapy institutes, and university-affiliated programs.

Stages of Treatment

Most family therapists want to see the entire family for the initial session since overall family transactional patterns are most apparent when all participants are together. (Very young children, although they are encouraged to attend the first session, are not always expected to attend subsequent meetings unless they are an integral part of the problem.) After establishing contact with each member present and assessing the suitability of family sessions for them, therapists who are interested in family history, such as Bowen, may begin to construct a family genogram. Others, such as Haley, may proceed to negotiate with the family about precisely what problem they wish to eliminate. Minuchin's opening move is to "join the family" by adopting an egalitarian role within it, making suggestions rather than issuing orders. He accommodates to the family's style of communicating, analyzes problems, and prepares a treatment plan. Solution-focused therapists, such as de Shazer, discourage clients from the start from speculating on the origin of a particular problem, preferring instead to engage in collaborative "solution talk"—that is, discussing solutions they want to construct together.

The middle phase of family therapy is usually directed at helping the family members redefine the presenting problem or symptomatic behavior in the identified patient as a relationship problem to be viewed within the family context. Here the family becomes the "patient," and together they begin to recognize that all have contributed to the problem and that all must participate in changing ingrained family patterns. If therapy is successful, families, guided by the therapist, typically begin to make relationship changes.

In the final stage of family therapy, families learn more effective coping skills and better ways to ask for what they want from one another. Although they are unlikely to leave problem free, they have learned problem-solving techniques for resolving relationship issues together. Termination is easier in family therapy than in individual therapy because the family has developed an internal support system and has not become over-dependent on an outsider. The presenting complaint or symptom has usually disappeared, and it is time for disengagement.

Evidence

The early family therapy pioneers, eager to create new and exciting techniques for treating families, did so largely without benefit of research support. In the ensuing years, a kind of cultural war developed between researchers and practitioners. The former contended that clinicians too readily adopted trendy techniques without pausing to evaluate their effectiveness beyond anecdotal data, and the latter maintained that the research being published often seemed trivial and unrelated to their daily work with people with real problems. That schism is now being addressed by a set of research investigations that are better integrated with the delivery of clinical services by family therapists (Sprenkle & Piercy, 2005).

In part as a response to the pressure from managed-care companies to provide validated treatment and in part as a result of increased funding for such research from government agencies such as the National Institute of Mental Health, meaningful studies are being undertaken to determine which family therapy procedures offer empirically based intervention techniques for a variety of family-related problems. Some practitioners, accustomed to relying on their individual experiences rather than on research data, are starting to find themselves forced by third-party payers such as HMOs to justify their interventions by supplying evidence-based data, when available, in order to receive reimbursement for their services.

Evidence-based practice refers to an attempt by researchers to assess the strengths and limitations of the current research data on psychotherapy. It has been shown that the treatment method, the therapist, and the treatment relationship are major contributors to the success or failure of therapy. It is less clear from research what the contributions of the system are to the process. There remain many disorders, problems, constellations, and family dysfunctions where data are sparse (Levant, 2005). Therapeutic research efforts typically are directed at *process research* (what actually occurs during a therapy session that leads to a desired outcome) and *outcome research* (what specific therapeutic approaches work best with which specific problems). The former—and more elusive—approach attempts to operationally describe what actually transpires during a successful session. Is it the therapeutic alliance between a caring, competent therapist and a trusting family that builds confidence and offers hope? Is it insight or greater understanding, or perhaps a shared therapeutic experience with a therapist and other family members, that leads to change? Is it the promotion of constructive dialogue encouraged by the therapist or the blocking of negative affect? Are there certain intervention techniques that work best at an early stage of family treatment and others that are more effective during later stages (Christensen, Russell, Miller, & Peterson, 1998; Heatherington, Friedlander, & Greenberg, 2005)?

Linking certain within-session processes with outcome results would lead to developing an empirically validated map to follow, but unfortunately this is not yet available for most models, with some exceptions. *Emotion-focused couple therapy* integrates research with attachment theory and spells out manualized procedures to be followed. *Functional family therapy* successfully combines systems and behavioral theories with carefully designed research backing. In general, evidence-supported studies thus far have been carried out primarily on behavioral and cognitive–behavioral approaches. These brief methods, with specific goals, are not necessarily the most effective, but they are easier to test using traditional research methodology than are other treatment methods.

Outcome research in family therapy must deal with the same problems that hinder such research in individual therapy, with the additional burden of gauging and measuring the various interactions taking place within a large and complex unit (the family) that is in a continuous state of change. Some family members may change more than others, different members may change in different ways, and the researcher must take into account intrapsychic, relationship, communication, and ordinary group variables in measuring therapeutic effectiveness. In addition, attention must be paid to types of families, ethnic and social backgrounds, level of family functioning, and the like. In recent years, qualitative research methods, discovery-oriented and open to multiple perspectives, have become more popular. Unlike more traditional quantitative research methodology, qualitative analyses are apt to rely on narrative reports in which the researcher makes subjective judgments about the meaning of outcome data. Qualitative research (based on case studies, in-depth interviewing, and document analysis) is especially useful for exploratory purposes, whereas quantitative techniques are more likely to be used in evaluating or justifying a set of experimental hypotheses.

Published outcome research today is likely to take one of two forms: *efficacy studies* or *effectiveness studies* (Pinsof & Wynne, 1995). The former, which are more common, attempt to determine whether a particular treatment works under ideal conditions such as those in a university or medical center. Interview methodology is standardized, treatment manuals are followed, clients are randomly assigned to treatment or no-treatment groups, independent evaluators measure outcomes, and so on. Effectiveness studies seek to determine whether the therapy works under normal, real-life conditions, such as in a clinic, social agency, or private practice setting. Most research to date is of the efficacy kind and is encouraging, but it is not always translatable into specific recommendations for therapy under more real-world, consultation room conditions. Overall results from surveys (Shadash, Ragscale, Glaser, & Montgomery, 1995), based mainly on efficacy studies, indicate that clients receiving family therapy did significantly better than untreated control-group clients.

The current thrust of outcome research continues to explore the relative advantages (in terms of costs, length of treatment, and extent of change) of alternative treatment interventions for clients with different specific psychological or behavioral difficulties. Evidence supporting family-level interventions has been especially strong for adolescent high risk, acting out problems, and parent management training, all of which are based on social learning principles. Psychoeducational programs for marital discord have also proved effective, as have programs for reducing relapse and rehospitalization in schizophrenic patients.

The recent rush to develop evidence-based family therapy represents a need for the accountability increasingly expected of professionals in medicine, education, and elsewhere. Within psychotherapy, there is increasing commitment to establishing an empirically validated basis for delivering services that work (Goodheart, Kazdin, & Sternberg, 2006; Nathan & Gorman, 2007). Clinical interventions backed up by research are intended to make the therapeutic effort more efficient, thereby improving the quality of health care and reducing health care costs (Reed & Eisman, 2006), a goal practitioners and researchers share. However laudable, the effort is costly and time consuming, requiring a homogeneous client population, clients randomly assigned to treatment or no-treatment groups, carefully trained and monitored therapists who follow manuals indicating how to proceed, with multiple goals that need to be measured, follow-up studies over extended periods to see whether gains made during therapy are maintained, and so on.

Westen, Novotny, & Thompson-Brenner (2004) argue that researchers might do better by focusing on what works in real-world practice than by devoting their efforts to designing new treatments and manuals from the laboratory. Although everyone would agree that integration of the best available research and clinical expertise represents an ideal solution, the fact remains that practitioners and clinical researchers operate from different perspectives. (The former are client focused and dedicated to improving services; the latter are science focused and dedicated to understanding and testing clinical phenomena.) Experienced practitioners are likely to be integrationists, taking the best from different approaches on the basis of their experience with what works with whom. Now that students are trained in academia on manualized techniques, they are more likely to be able to follow manualized guidelines in treating their clients.

Psychotherapy in a Multicultural World

The 21st century sees an increasing number of challenges for therapists in dealing with the issues stimulated by a multicultural population. As our consulting rooms fill with immigrant populations and the number of mixed-heritage families increases exponentially, we must attend to basic principles in working with "the Other"—people different from ourselves in certain meaningful ways.

It is critical for therapists to understand the movements taking place in the general society and in specific cultural environments. The therapist must be aware of his/her personal strengths and, most importantly, his/her weaknesses, biases, and prejudices (Axelson, 1999).

Understanding when consultation is appropriate or when referral is necessary also is important. Tuning in to the client's internal/external frame of reference allows the therapist to see the world through the client's eyes. Because the family therapist has other members of the family in the room for corroboration, it is easier to differentiate idiosyncratic behavior from culturally determined thinking or action. It is a logical step for the therapist to move from the family to the family of origin to the multicultural family genogram to a global perspective in family therapy (Ng, 2003). That perspective should include information on ethnic, economic, religious and political factors influencing family dynamics.

An important part of the development of the family therapy movement was the corrective action that occurred as a result of the women's movement in the 1980s (McGoldrick, Giordano, & Garcia-Preto, 2005) when the issue of "white male privilege" became a hot topic in family therapy circles. The awareness that gender bias determined the way people were seen and treated in the consulting room was a radical new idea and set the stage for future attention to issues beyond gender, such as race, social class, immigration status, and religion and their influence on the therapy process. Multicultural expertise was recognized as necessary to understand a variety of areas such as boundary lines, communication rules, displays of emotions, gender expectations, rituals, immigrant and refugee status, and the way these variables affect therapy.

The theory of social construction in family therapy has provided an additional philosophical foundation for multicultural counseling. The narrative model of Michael White takes a stand against the imposition of dominant culture imperatives. White recognizes the misuse of power as a central construct in the presentation of dominant culture, giving voice to local alternative knowledges (Epston & White, 1990). Clients are the experts on their own experiences. Working with diverse ethnic and racial groups, including Australian Aborigines, White used a reflecting team approach, which included the participation of traditional and indigenous healers from the community. White believed that therapy does not exist in a vacuum; emerging stories of change must be shared with the client's larger cultural community to be meaningful. This obviates, somewhat, the problem of the personal feelings of the therapist, supplanting them with the reflections of the community. This process can be translated on an international level and can incorporate the voices of other groups within the client's community. It is central to White's philosophy that the therapist collaborates with the client to determine which audience can best witness their stories of change.

CASE EXAMPLE

Background

Although the appearance of troublesome symptoms in a family member is typically what brings the concerned family to seek help, it is becoming increasingly common for couples or entire families to recognize they are having relationship problems that need to be addressed at the family level. Sometimes, too, therapy is seen as a preventive measure. For example, adults with children from previous marriages who are planning to marry may become concerned enough about the potential problems involved in forming a stepfamily that they consult a family therapist before marriage.

Frank, 38, and Michelle, 36, who are to marry within a week, referred themselves because they worried about whether they were prepared or had prepared their children sufficiently for stepfamily life. The therapist saw them for two sessions, which were largely devoted to discussing common problems they had anticipated along with suggestions for their amelioration. Neither Frank's two children, Ann, 13, and Lance, 12, nor Michelle's daughter, Jessica, 16, attended these sessions.

Michelle and Frank had known each other since childhood, although she later moved to a large city and he settled in a small rural community. Their families had been friends in the past, and Frank and Michelle had visited and corresponded with each other over the years. When they were in their early 20s, before Frank went away to graduate school, a romance blossomed between Frank and Michelle and they agreed to meet again as soon as feasible. When her father died unexpectedly, Michelle wrote to Frank, and when he did not respond, she was hurt and angry. On the rebound, she married Alex, who turned out to be a drug user, verbally abusive to Michelle, and chronically unemployed. They divorced after 2 years, and Michelle, now a single mother, began working to support herself and her daughter, Jessica. Mother and daughter became unusually close in the 12 years before Michelle and Frank met again.

Frank also had been married. Several years after his two children were born, his wife developed cancer and lingered for 5 years before dying. The children, although looked after by neighbors, were alone much of the time, with Ann, Frank's older child, assuming the parenting role for her younger brother, Lance. When Frank met Michelle again, their interrupted romance was rekindled, and in a high state of emotional intensity they decided to marry.

Problem

Approximately 3 months after their marriage, Frank and Michelle contacted the therapist again, describing increasing tension between their children. Needing a safe place to be heard (apparently no one was talking to anyone else), the children—Ann and Lance (Frank's) and Jessica (Michelle's)—eagerly agreed to attend family sessions. What emerged was a set of individual problems compounded by the stresses inherent in becoming an "instant family."

Frank, never able to earn much money and burdened by debts accumulated during his wife's long illness, was frustrated and guilty over his feeling that he was not an adequate provider for his family. Michelle was jealous over Frank's frequent business trips, in large part because she felt unattractive (the reason for her not marrying for 12 years). She feared Frank would find someone else and abandon her again, as she felt he had done earlier, at the time of her father's death. Highly stressed, she withdrew from her daughter, Jessica, for the first time. Losing her closeness to her mother, Jessica remained detached from her stepsiblings and became resentful of any attention Michelle paid to Frank. In an attempt to regain a sense of closeness, she turned to a surrogate family—a gang—and became a "tagger" at school (a graffiti writer involved in pregang activities). Ann and Lance, who had not had the time or a place to grieve over the loss of their mother, found Michelle unwilling to take over mothering them. Ann became bossy, quarrelsome, and demanding; Lance, at age 12, began to wet his bed.

In addition to these individual problems, they were having the usual stepfamily problems: stepsibling rivalries, difficulties of stepparents assuming parental roles, and boundary ambiguities.

Treatment

From a systems viewpoint, the family therapist is able to work with the entire family or see different combinations of people as needed. Everyone need not attend every session. However, retaining a consistent conceptual framework of the system is essential.

The therapist had "joined" the couple in the two initial sessions, and they felt comfortable returning after they married and were in trouble. While constructing a genogram, the therapist was careful to establish contact with each of the children, focusing attention whenever she could on their evolving relationships. Recognizing that parent–child attachments preceded the marriage relationship, she tried to help them, as a group, develop loyalties to the new family. Boundary issues were especially important because they lived in a small house with little privacy, and the children often intruded on the parental dyad.

When seeing the couple together without the children present, the therapist tried to strengthen their parental subsystem by helping them to learn how to support one another and share child-rearing tasks. (Each had continued to take primary responsibility for his or her own offspring in the early months of the marriage.) Jealousy issues were discussed, and the therapist suggested they needed a "honeymoon" period that they had never had. With the therapist's encouragement, the children stayed with relatives while their parents spent time alone with each other.

After they returned for counseling, Frank's concerns over not being a better provider were discussed. He and Michelle considered alternative strategies for increasing his income and for his helping more around the house. Michelle, still working, felt less exhausted and thus better able to give more of herself to the children. Frank and Lance agreed to participate in a self-help behavioral program aimed at eliminating bedwetting, thus strengthening their closeness to one another. As Lance's problem subsided, the entire family felt relieved of the mess and smell associated with the bedwetting.

The therapist decided to see Ann by herself for one session, giving her the feeling she was special. Allowed to be a young girl in therapy and temporarily relieved of her job as a parent to Lance, she became more agreeable and reached outside the family to make friends. She and Lance had one additional session (with their father), grieving over the loss of their mother. Michelle and Jessica needed two sessions together to work out their mother–daughter adolescent issues as well as Jessica's school problems.

Follow-Up

Approximately 12 sessions were held. At first the sessions took place weekly, later they were held biweekly, and then they took place at 3-month intervals. By the end of a year, the family had become better integrated and more functional. Frank had been promoted at work and the family had rented a larger house, easing the problems brought about by space limitations. Lance's bedwetting had stopped, and he and Ann felt closer to Michelle and Jessica. Ann, relieved of the burden of acting older than her years, enjoyed being an adolescent and became involved in school plays. Jessica still had some academic problems but had broken away from the gang and was preparing to go to a neighboring city to attend a junior college.

The family contacted the therapist five times over the next 3 years. Each time, they were able to identify the dyad or triad stuck in a dysfunctional sequence for which they needed help. And each time, a single session seemed to get them back on track.

SUMMARY

Family therapy, which originated in the 1950s, turned its attention away from individual intrapsychic problems and placed the locus of pathology on dysfunctional transactional patterns within a family. From this new perspective, families are viewed as systems with members operating within a relationship network and by means of feedback loops aimed at maintaining homeostasis. Growing out of research aimed at understanding communication patterns in the families of schizophrenics, family therapy later broadened its focus to include therapeutic interventions with a variety of family problems. These therapeutic endeavors are directed at changing repetitive maladaptive or problematic sequences within the system. Early cybernetic views of the family as a psychosocial system have been augmented by the postmodern view that rejects the notion of an objectively knowable world, arguing in favor of multiple views of reality.

Symptomatic or problematic behavior in a family member is viewed as signaling family disequilibrium. Symptoms arise from, and are maintained by, current, ongoing family transactions. Viewing causality in circular rather than linear terms, the family therapist focuses on repetitive behavioral sequences between members that are self-perpetuating and self-defeating. Family belief systems also are scrutinized as self-limiting.

Therapeutic intervention may take a number of forms, including approaches assessing the impact of the past on current family functioning (object relations, contextual), those largely concerned with individual family members' growth (experiential), those that focus on family structure and processes (structural) or transgenerational issues, those heavily influenced by cognitive–behavioral perspectives (strategic, behavioral), and those that emphasize dialogue in which clients examine the meaning and organization they bring to their life experiences (social constructionist and narrative therapies). All attend particularly to the context of people's lives in which dysfunction originates and can be ameliorated.

Interest in family systems theory and concomitant interventions will probably continue to grow in the coming years. The stress on families precipitated by the lack of models or strategies for dealing with divorce, remarriage, alternative lifestyles, or acculturation in immigrant families is likely to increase the demand for professional help at a family level.

Consumers and cost-containment managers will utilize family therapy even more often in the future because it is a relatively short-term procedure, solution oriented, dealing with real and immediate problems. Moreover, it feels accessible to families with relationship problems who don't wish to be perceived as pathological. Its preventive quality, helping people learn more effective communication and problem-solving skills to head off future crises, is attractive not only to families but also to practitioners of family medicine, pediatricians, and other primary care physicians to whom troubled people turn. As the field develops in both its research and clinical endeavors, it will better identify specific techniques for treating different types of families at significant points in their life cycles.

ANNOTATED BIBLIOGRAPHY

Goldenberg, H., & Goldenberg, I. (2008). *Family therapy: An overview* (7th ed.). Pacific Grove, CA: Brooks/Cole–Thomson Learning.

This text describes the major theories and the assessment and intervention techniques of family therapy. Systems theory and family life cycle issues are outlined, a historical discussion of the field's development is included, and research, training, and ethical and professional issues are considered.

Goodheart, C. D., Kazdin, A. E., & Sternberg, R. J. (2006). *Evidence-based psychotherapy: Where practice and research meet.* Washington, DC: American Psychological Association.

This timely text outlines the current controversies surrounding the issue of developing an evidence-based body of knowledge to support psychotherapy approaches.

Haley, J., & Richeport-Haley, M. (2007). *Directive family therapy.* New York: Haworth.

This text provides practitioners with directive family techniques to identify client problems, formulate treatment plans, and then carry them out to achieve lasting therapeutic change. Using case examples, this text shows problem-solving directives in action.

McGoldrick, M., & Hardy, K. V. (Eds.). (2008). *Re-visioning family therapy: Race, culture, and gender in clinical practice* (2nd ed.). New York: Guilford Press.

These authors have brought together several dozen experts to provide detailed information about a wide variety of racial and ethnic groupings. Common family patterns are delineated for each group, and suggestions are offered for effective family interventions tied to the unique aspects of each set.

Sue, D. W., & Sue, D. (2007). Counseling the culturally diverse: *Theory and practice* (5th ed.). New York John Wiley.

Authors Derald Wing Sue & David Sue define and analyze the meaning of diversity and multiculturalism, covering racial/ethnic minority groups as well as multiracial individuals, women, gays and lesbians, the elderly, and those with disabilities. This book is up to date and includes new research and a discussion of future direction in the field.

Sexton, T. L., Weeks, G. R., & Robbins, M. S. (Eds.). (2003). *The science and practice of working with families and couples.* New York, Guilford Press.

This useful, up-to-date handbook is filled with discussions of the foundation and theories of family therapy and its application to special populations for whom family therapy is recommended. A large section is devoted to issues surrounding evidence-based couple and family intervention programs.

CASE READINGS

Family therapy trainers commonly make use of videotapes and DVDs of master therapists demonstrating their techniques with real families since these provide a richer sense of the emotional intensity of family sessions than what is available from case readings alone. Tapes are available to rent or purchase from the Ackerman Institute in New York, the Philadelphia Child Guidance Center, the Georgetown University Family Center, the Family Institute of Washington, DC, and many other training establishments.

Three texts deal largely with descriptions and analyses of family therapy from the vantage point of leading practitioners:

Grove, D. R., & Haley, J. (1993). *Conversations on therapy: Popular problems and uncommon solutions.* New York: Norton.

Grove and Haley, apprentice and master therapist, respectively, offer a question-and-answer conversation regarding specific cases seen at the Family Therapy Institute of Washington, DC, and together they devise strategies for intervening effectively in problematic situations.

Napier, A. Y., & Whitaker, C. A. (1978). *The family crucible.* New York: Harper & Row.

This text gives a full account of cotherapy with one family, including both parents; a suicidal, runaway, teenage daughter; an adolescent son; and a 6-year-old daughter.

Satir, V. M., & Baldwin, M. (1983). *Satir step by step: A guide to creative change in families.* Palo Alto, CA: Science and Behavior Books.

Using double columns, Satir presents a transcript of a session accompanied by an explanation for each intervention.

Two recent casebooks contain descriptions offered by family therapists with a variety of viewpoints. Both effectively convey what transpires as family therapists attempt to put theory into practice.

Dattilio, F. (Ed.). (1998). *Case studies in couple and family therapy: Systemic and cognitive perspectives.* New York: Guilford Press.

Leading figures from each school of family therapy briefly summarize their theoretical positions, followed by detailed case studies of actual sessions. The editor offers comments throughout in an attempt to integrate cognitive–behavior therapy with a variety of current family therapy systems.

Golden, L. B. (2003). *Case studies in marriage and family therapy* (2nd ed.). Englewood Cliffs, NJ: Prentice Hall.

This text contains 19 case studies that highlight the major approaches taken to family therapy. Seasoned marriage and family therapists share real-life session data and explore their own decision making and personal experiences.

Other valuable works include the following:

Oxford, L. K., & Wiener, D. J. (2003). Rescripting family dramas using psychodramatic methods. In D. J. Wiener & L. K. Oxford (Eds.), *Action therapy with families and groups: Using creative arts improvisation in clinical practice* (pp. 45–74). Washington, DC: American Psychological Association. [Reprinted in D. Wedding & R. J. Corsini (Eds.). (2008). *Case Studies in Psychotherapy* (5th ed.). Belmont, CA: Brooks/Cole.]

This recent case illustrates how the techniques of psychodrama can be applied in a family therapy context.

Papp, P. (1982). The daughter who said no. In P. Papp, *The process of change* (pp. 67–120). New York: Guilford. [Reprinted in D. Wedding & R. J. Corsini (Eds.). (2011). *Case studies in psychotherapy* (6th ed.). Belmont, CA: Brooks/Cole.]

This classic case illustrates the way a master family therapist treats a young woman with anorexia nervosa.

REFERENCES

Ackerman, N. W. (1958). *The psychodynamics of family life.* New York: Basic Books.

Anderson, H. D. (1997). *Conversation, language, and possibilities: A postmodern approach to therapy.* New York: HarperCollins.

Anderson, H. D., & Gehart, D. R. (2006). *Collaborative therapy: Relationships and conversations that make a difference.* New York: Routledge.

Axelson, J. A. (1999). *Counseling and development in multicultural society* (3rd ed.). Pacific Grove, CA: Brooks/Cole.

Barnett, R. C., & Hyde, J. S. (2001). Women, men, work, family. *American Psychologist, 56,* 781–796.

Bateson, G. (1972). *Steps to an ecology of mind.* New York: Dutton.

Bateson, G., Jackson, D. D., Haley, J., & Weakland, J. (1956). Towards a theory of schizophrenia. *Behavioral Science, 1,* 251–264.

Beck, A. T., & Weishaar, M. (2007). Cognitive therapy. In R. J. Corsini & D. Wedding (Eds.), *Current psychotherapies* (8th ed., pp. 263–294). Belmont, CA: Brooks/Cole.

Becvar, D. S. (2003). Eras of epistemology: A survey of family therapy thinking and theorizing. In T. L. Sexton, G. R. Weeks, & M. S. Robbins (Eds.), *Handbook of family therapy: The science and practice of working with families and couples* (pp. 3–20). New York: Brunner-Routledge.

Bell, J. E. (1961). *Family group therapy.* Public Health Monograph No. 64. Washington, DC: U.S. Government Printing Office.

Berg, I. K., Dolan, Y., & Trepper, T. (Eds.). (2007). *More than miracles: The state of the art of solution-focused brief therapy.* New York: Haworth.

Bertalanffy, L. von (1968). *General systems theory: Foundation, development, applications.* New York: Braziller.

Boscolo, L., Cecchin, G., Hoffman, L., & Penn, P. (1987). *Milan systemic family therapy: Conversations in theory and practice.* New York: Basic Books.

Boszormenyi-Nagy, I. (1987). *Foundations of contextual therapy: Collected papers of Ivan Boszormenyi-Nagy.* New York: Brunner/Mazel.

Bowen, M. (1960). A family concept of schizophrenia. In D. D. Jackson (Ed.), *The etiology of schizophrenia* (pp 346–373). New York: Basic Books.

Bowen, M. (1978). *Family therapy in clinical practice.* New York: Jason Aronson.

Carter, B., & McGoldrick, M. (2005). *The expanded family life cycle: Individual, family, and social perspectives* (3rd ed.). Boston: Allyn & Bacon.

Christensen, L. L., Russell, C. S., Miller, R. B., & Peterson, C. M. (1998). The process of change in couple therapy: A qualitative investigation. *Journal of Marital and Family Therapy, 24,* 177–188.

Dattilio, F. M., & Epstein, N. B. (2005). Introduction to the special section: The role of cognitive–behavioral interventions in couple and family therapy. *Journal of Marital and Family Therapy, 31,* 7–13.

de Shazer, S. (1991). *Putting differences to work.* New York: Norton.

Ellis, A., & Dryden, W. (2007). *The practice of rational emotive behavior therapy* (2nd ed.). Thousand Oaks, CA: Sage.

Epston, D., & White, M. (1990). *Narrative means to therapeutic ends.* Adelaide, Australia: Dulwich Centre.

Falicov, C. J. (2000). *Latino families in therapy: A guide to multicultural practice.* New York: Guilford Press.

Framo, J.L.(1992). *Family-Of-Origin Therapy: An Intergenerational Approach.* New York Brunner Mazel Inc.

Gergen, K. J. (1999). *An invitation to social construction.* Thousand Oaks, CA: Sage.

Goldenberg, I., & Goldenberg, H. (2008). *Family therapy: An overview* (7th ed.). Pacific Grove, CA: Brooks/Cole.

Goodheart, C. D., Kazdin, A. E., & Sternberg, R. J. (2006). *Evidence-based psychotherapy: Where practice and research meet.* Washington, DC: American Psychological Association.

Greenberg, L. S., & Goldman, R. N. (2008). *Emotion-focused couples therapy: The dynamics of emotion, love, and power.* Washington, DC: American Psychological Association.

Haley, J. (1996). *Learning and teaching therapy.* New York: Guilford Press.

Heatherington, L., Friedlander, M. L., & Greenberg, L. (2005). Change process research in couple and family therapy: Methodological challenges and opportunities. *Journal of Family Psychology, 19,* 18–27.

Henggeler, S. W., Schoenwald , S. K., Borduin, C. M., Rowland, M. D., & Cunningham, P. B. (2009). *Multisystemic therapy for antisocial behavior in children and adolescents.* New York: Guillford Press.

Hughes, D. (2007). *Attachment-focused family therapy.* New York: Norton.

Imber-Black, E., Roberts, J., & Alva Whiting, R. (2003). *Rituals in families and family therapy* (rev. ed.). New York: Norton.

Jackson, D. D. (1965). Family rules: Marital quid pro quo. *Archives of General Psychiatry, 12,* 589–594.

Kempler, W. (1991). *Experiential psychotherapy with families.* New York: Brunner/Mazel.

Kliman, J. (1994). The interweaving of gender, class, and race in family therapy. In M. P. Mirkin (Ed.), *Women in context: Toward a feminist reconstruction of psychotherapy* (pp. 25–47). New York: Guilford Press.

Kuhn, T. (1970). *The structure of scientific revolutions.* Chicago: University of Chicago Press.

Laing, R. D. (1965). Mystification, confusion, and conflict. In I. Boszormenyi-Nagy & J. L. Framo (Eds.), *Intensive family therapy: Theoretical and practical aspects* (pp. 343–362). New York: Harper & Row.

Lebow, J. (1997). The integrative revolution in couple and family therapy. *Family Process, 36,* 1–17.

Levant, R. F. (2005, July). *Report of the 2005 Presidential Task Force on Evidence-Based Practice.* Washington, DC: American Psychological Association.

Lidz, T., Cornelison, A., Fleck, S., & Terry, D. (1957). The intrafamilial environment of schizophrenic patients: II. Marital schism and marital skew. *American Journal of Psychiatry, 114,* 241–248.

Madsen, C. W. (2007). *Collaborative therapy with multistressed families* (2nd ed.). New York: Guilford Press.

McGoldrick, M., Giordano, J., & Garcia-Preto, N. (Eds.). (2005). *Ethnicity and family therapy* (3rd ed.). New York: Guilford Press.

McGoldrick, M., & Hardy, K. V. (Eds.). (2008). *Re-visioning family therapy: Race, culture, and gender in clinical practice* (2nd ed.). New York: Guilford Press.

Minuchin, S. (1974). *Families and family therapy.* Cambridge, MA: Harvard University Press.

Minuchin, S., Nichols, M. P., & Lee, W. Y. (2006). *Assessing families and couples: From symptom to system.* Boston: Allyn & Bacon.

Minuchin, S., Montalvo, B., Guerney, B. G., Jr., Rosman, B. L., & Schumer, F. (1967). *Families of the slums: An exploration of their structure and treatment.* New York: Basic Books.

Minuchin, S., Rosman, B. L., & Baker, L. (1978). *Psychosomatic families: Anorexia nervosa in context.* Cambridge, MA: Harvard University Press.

Nathan, P. E., & Gorman, J. M. (2007). *A guide to treatment that works* (3rd ed.). London: Oxford University Press.

Nichols, M. P. (1987). *The self in the system: Expanding the limits of family therapy.* New York: Brunner/Mazel.

Ng, K. S. (2003). *Global perspectives in family therapy: Development, practice, trends* (1st ed.). New York: Brunner-Routledge.

Pelavin, E., & Moskowitz-Sweet, G. (2009). *From common sense to cybersense: A families guide to prevention and response.* Unpublished manuscript, Palo Alto.

Pinsof, W. M., & Wynne, L. C. (1995). The effectiveness and efficacy of marital and family therapy: Introduction to the special issue. *Journal of Marital and Family Therapy, 21,* 341–343.

Prochaska, J. O., & Norcross, J. C. (1999). *Systems of psychotherapy: A transtheoretical analysis* (4th ed.). Pacific Grove, CA: Brooks/Cole.

Reed, G. M., & Eisman, E. J. (2006). Uses and misuses of evidence: Managed care, treatment guidelines, and outcome measurements in professional practice. In C. D. Goodheart, A. E. Kazdin, & R. J. Sternberg (Eds.), *Evidence-based psychotherapy: Where practice and research meet* (pp. 13–36). Washington, DC: American Psychological Association.

Robbins, M. S., Mayorga, C. C., & Szapocznik, J. (2003). The ecosystemic "lens" to understanding family functioning. In T. L. Sexton, G. R. Weeks, & M. S. Robbins (Eds.), *Handbook of family therapy: The science and practice of working with families and couples* (pp. 23–40). New York: Brunner-Routledge.

Satir, V. (1972). *Peoplemaking.* Palo Alto, CA: Science and Behavior Books.

Scharff, J. S., & Scharff, D. E. (2006). *The primer of object relations* (2nd ed.). New York: Jason Aronson.

Selvini-Palazzoli, M. (1986). Towards a general model of psychotic games. *Journal of Marital and Family Therapy, 12,* 339–349.

Selvini-Palazzoli, M., Boscolo, L., Cecchin, G. F., & Prata, G. (1978). *Paradox and counterparadox: A new model in the therapy of the family schizophrenic transaction.* New York: Jason Aronson.

Sexton, T. L., & Alexander, J. F. (1999). *Functional family therapy: Principles of clinical intervention, assessment, and implementation.* Henderson, NV: RCH Enterprises.

Shadash, W. R., Ragsdale, K., Glaser, R. R., & Montgomery, L. M. (1995). The efficacy and effectiveness of marital and family therapy: A perspective from meta-analysis. *Journal of Marital and Family Therapy, 21,* 345–360.

Sprenkle, D. H., & Piercy, F. P. (Eds.). (2005). *Research methods in family therapy* (2nd ed.). New York: Guilford Press.

Sue, D. W., & Sue, D. (2007). *Counseling the culturally diverse: Theory and practice* (5th ed.). New York John Wiley.

Sullivan, H. S. (1953). *The interpersonal theory of psychiatry.* New York: Norton.

Wachtel, P. L. (2007). *Relational theory and the practice of psychotherapy.* New York: Guillford Press.

Wachtel, E. E., & Wachtel, P. L. (1986). *Family dynamics in individual psychotherapy: A guide to clinical strategies.* New York: Guilford Press.

Walsh, F. (2003). Strengths forged through adversity. In F. Walsh (Ed.), *Normal family processes: Growing diversity and complexity* (3rd ed., pp. 356–377). New York: Guilford Press.

Walsh, F. (2009). *Spiritual resources in family therapy* (2nd ed.). New York: Guilford Press.

Watzlawick, P., Weakland, J. H., & Fisch, R. (1974). *Change: Principles of problem formation and problem resolution.* New York: Norton.

Westen, D., Novotny, C. M., & Thompson-Brenner, H. (2004). Empirical status of empirically supported psychotherapies: Assumptions, findings, and reporting in controlled clinical trials. *Psychological Bulletin, 130,* 631–663.

Whitaker, C. A., & Bumberry, W. M. (1988). *Dancing with a family: A symbolic–experiential approach.* New York: Brunner/Mazel.

White, M. (1995). *Re-authoring lives: Interviews and essays.* Adelaide, South Australia: Dulwich Centre Publications.

White, M. (2007). *Maps of narrative practice.* New York: Norton.

Wiener, N. (1948). Cybernetics. *Scientific American, 179*(5), 14–18.

Wills, F. (2009). *Beck's cognitive therapy: Distinctive features.* New York: Routledge.

Wynne, L. C. (1965). Some indications and contraindications for exploratory family therapy. In I. Boszormenyi-Nagy & J. L. Framo (Eds.), *Intensive family therapy: Theoretical and practical aspects* (pp. 289–322). New York: Harper & Row.

Wynne, L. C., Ryckoff, I. M., Day, J., & Hirsch, S. I. (1958). Pseudomutuality in the family relationships of schizophrenics. *Psychiatry, 21,* 205–220.

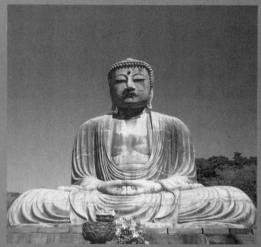

Great Buddha, Kotokuin Temple,
Kamakura, Japan
© Steve Vidler/Superstock

13 | CONTEMPLATIVE PSYCHOTHERAPIES

Roger Walsh

OVERVIEW

Something remarkable is happening. After centuries of separate development, two major disciplines—both designed to explore, heal, and enhance the human mind—are finally meeting. History is being made as contemplative and traditional Western therapies finally meet, mix, challenge, and enrich one another.

Contemplative practices offer benefits to therapists, clients, and the public. Therapeutically, they can offer insight and self-understanding, reduce stress, and ameliorate multiple psychological and psychosomatic disorders. For healthy individuals, they can enhance well-being, unveil latent capacities, and foster psychological development, even beyond conventional levels. On the practical side, they are simple, inexpensive, and often pleasurable.

There are also theoretical benefits. These include new understandings of human nature, as well as of health, pathology, and potentials. For researchers, contemplative practices offer insights into both psychological and neural processes.

Basic Concepts

Varieties of Practices

Contemplative practices—such as contemplation, meditation, and yoga—are found worldwide. They occur in most cultures and are part of every major religion. They include the traditional practices of Taoist and Hindu yogas, Confucian "quiet-sitting," Buddhist meditations, Jewish *Tzeruf,* Islamic Sufi *Zikr,* and Christian contemplation.

In their traditional settings, contemplative practices are usually part of a larger worldview and way of life. For example, they are usually analyzed and explained by a corresponding psychology and philosophy, such as Buddhist philosophy. They are also integrated with other practices intended to facilitate well-being and development such as supportive lifestyles (e.g., ethics) and exercises (e.g., yogic breathing). Originally practiced primarily for attaining religious and spiritual goals, they are now widely used in secular settings for their psychological and psychosomatic benefits. The terms *meditation* and *contemplation* are both used in several ways, but are treated here as synonymous.

There are many kinds of contemplative/meditative practices. The most researched are yogic transcendental meditation (TM) and Buddhist mindfulness, which is also known as *vipassana* (clear seeing), or insight meditation. TM is a mantra (inner sound) practice that begins by directing attention to a repetitive mantra and then allows the mind to settle into a clear, peaceful state. Mindfulness meditation cultivates clear, sensitive awareness by carefully investigating each experience. Indian yoga and Chinese Tai Chi are two other popular but less researched practices. Dozens of other meditations await research. As yet, we have almost no research data comparing different kinds of meditation, so we will usually consider them together.

Definitions

Despite many variations between practices, common themes are evident, and these commonalities suggest the following definitions:

The term *meditation* refers to a family of self-regulation practices that focus on training attention and awareness in order to bring mental processes under greater voluntary control and thereby foster mental well-being and development, as well as specific capacities such as concentration, calm, and clarity.

This definition meets the "demarcation criterion" of a good definition in that it demarcates meditation from other therapeutic and self-regulation strategies such as conventional psychotherapies, visualization, and self-hypnosis. These do not focus primarily on training attention and awareness. Rather, they aim primarily at changing mental contents (objects of attention and awareness) such as emotions, thoughts, and images.

The term *yoga* refers to a family of practices with aims similar to those of meditation. However, yogas are more inclusive disciplines that, in addition to meditation, can encompass ethics, lifestyle, body postures, diet, breath control, study, and intellectual analysis. In the West, the best-known yogic practices are the body postures, which are frequently taken to be the totality of yoga. In fact, they are only one aspect of a far more comprehensive training, a training that was perhaps the first integrative psychotherapy.

Central Assumptions

Contemplative psychologies are based on a "good-news, bad-news" understanding of the mind.

- The *bad news* is that our ordinary state of mind is considerably more uncontrolled, underdeveloped, and dysfunctional than we usually recognize. The result is enormous unnecessary suffering and dysfunction.

- The *good news* is that we can train and develop the mind beyond conventional levels. The results include enhanced well-being, maturity, and psychological capacities.

This good news and bad news can be expanded into eight central assumptions underlying contemplative therapies:

1. Our usual state of mind is significantly underdeveloped, uncontrolled, and dysfunctional.

2. The full extent of this "normal" dysfunction goes unrecognized for two reasons:

   • First, we all share this dysfunction, so it does not stand out. We all live in the biggest cult of all—culture.

   • The second reason is self-masking. Just as psychological defenses distort awareness so that we do not recognize them, so too our usual state of psychological dysfunction (which is partly constituted by defenses) distorts awareness and conceals itself.

3. Psychological suffering is largely a function of this mental dysfunction.

4. It is possible to train and develop mental functions and capacities such as attention, cognition, and emotions.

5. Training the mind in this way is an effective strategy for reducing "normal" dysfunction, enhancing well-being, and developing exceptional capacities such as heightened concentration, compassion, insight, and joy.

6. This mental training allows us to recognize that we underestimate ourselves and suffer from a case of mistaken identity. We recognize that the self-image, self-concept, or "ego" that we usually assume to be our "self" is an image or concept only, and that our real nature is something deeper and far more remarkable.

7. Contemplative disciplines offer effective techniques for training the mind in this way.

8. These claims do not have to be accepted on blind faith; rather, one can, and should, test them for oneself.

A Developmental Perspective

Surveying recent research in developmental psychology will help us to understand contemplative goals and to compare them with other therapies. Developmental psychologists currently recognize three broad levels of development: prepersonal, personal, and transpersonal, which are also called preconventional, conventional, and postconventional (Wilber, 2000a). We are born into the prepersonal, preconventional stage in which we have no coherent sense of self or of social conventions. As we grow, we are gradually acculturated and mature to the personal/conventional stage. Here we establish a more coherent sense of self and largely accept the conventional cultural view of ourselves and the world. Until recently, this conventional stage was widely assumed to be the sum total of our developmental potential.

Yet for centuries, philosophers and sages have lamented the limitations of conventional development and pointed to further possibilities. The conventional stage has been associated with a clouded state of mind that Asian contemplative psychologies describe as "illusion" and some Western psychologists call a "consensus trance" or a "shared hypnosis" (Tart, 1986). Likewise, existentialists describe conventional ways of life as often superficial, defensive, and inauthentic. Too often, they say, we accept cultural beliefs and values unreflectively, follow fads and fashions unquestioningly, and avoid facing the deeper questions and issues about life and ourselves. The result, say existentialists, is a semiconscious submission in "herd mentality" in which we fail to live fully or authentically (Yalom & Josselson, 2010). According to Abraham Maslow (1968), one of the founders of humanistic psychology, the result is that "The normal adjustment of the average, common sense, well-adjusted [person] implies a continued successful rejection of much of the depths of human nature . . ." (p. 142).

This is not a new idea. In fact, Maslow was echoing the words of numerous contemplatives who for centuries have claimed that, as yoga puts it, "You are not fully grown up, there are levels left undeveloped because unattended" (Nisargadatta, 1973, p. 40). Likewise, for Jewish contemplatives, "normality" is regarded as "the 'mentality of childhood' (*mochin de-katnuth*). More advanced modes of thought and states of consciousness, on the other hand, are referred to as the 'mentality of adulthood' (*mochin de-gadluth*). One learns these methods of 'adult thought' through meditation" (Kaplan, 1985, p. 8).

These diverse views—from East and West, from philosophy and religion, and now from psychology—all converge on a startling conclusion of enormous importance: *We are only half grown and half awake.* Development normally proceeds from preconventional to conventional, but then usually grinds to a semiconscious halt.

Fortunately, there is also good news: Further development is possible. Our usual personal, conventional condition may be a form of collective developmental arrest. However, development can proceed beyond what are often assumed to be the upper limits of health and normality. The conventional stage can be a stepping stone rather than a stopping place. Such has long been the claim of contemplative psychologies, and it is now supported by considerable developmental research. Researchers now recognize postconventional stages in motivation, cognition, defenses, moral thinking, and the sense of self (Maslow, 1971; Wilber, 1999, 2000b).

With this developmental background, we can now compare psychotherapeutic systems in two ways. The first is according to the developmental levels they aim to foster. For example, most psychotherapies aim to foster healthy conventional development. Meditative therapies, on the other hand, though capable of facilitating conventional adjustment, traditionally aim for postconventional growth.

A related idea is that psychological systems address three major levels of concerns: pathological, existential, and transpersonal. As this book clearly demonstrates, Western professionals have devised sophisticated techniques for alleviating pathologies, and have begun to focus on the existential issues—such as meaningless, isolation, and death—that all of us inevitably face as part of life (Yalom, 2002; Yalom & Josselson, 2010). However, only recently have Western psychologies begun to explore the transpersonal domains that interest contemplative disciplines.

Other Systems

Principles for Optimal Comparisons of Different Psychotherapies

Each psychotherapy is a rich and complex system, and brief comparisons necessarily do them an injustice. When making comparisons, it is probably wise to assume that:

1. Each system offers a *valuable but only partial* contribution to understanding and treatment.
2. Claims for blanket supremacy of any one approach are suspect.
3. Effective therapies share a variety of methods and mechanisms.
4. Different therapies may be complementary rather than necessarily conflictual.
5. Therapists familiar with only one system are likely to fall into the Procrustean trap of interpreting and treating all clients in the same way. As Abraham Maslow put it, if the only tool you have is a hammer, everything begins to look like a nail. If you know only one therapy, then all clients and conditions begin to look appropriate for it.
6. Good therapists are flexible and familiar with multiple methods. They assess which therapy is likely to work best for each client, and will treat or refer clients appropriately.

These principles are well demonstrated by integrative and integral therapies (Norcross & Beutler, 2010; Wilber, 2000a).

Comparisons with Other Systems

The following comparisons highlight the contributions of contemplative approaches. However, this is in no way to deny the value or many contributions of the following therapies.

Psychoanalysis focuses above all on psychological conflict. It sees humans as necessarily locked and lost in a never-ending inner struggle and assumes that "mental life represents an unrelenting conflict between the conscious and unconscious parts of the mind" (Arlow, 1995, p. 20). Psychoanalysis has made enormous pioneering contributions to our understanding of the unconscious, defenses, the childhood roots of some pathologies, and a variety of therapeutic processes. In fact, it has made major advances over contemplative disciplines in the areas of childhood development, transference, and unconscious dynamics and defenses.

However, from a contemplative perspective, psychoanalysis has tragically underestimated our human nature and potentials. By focusing almost exclusively on conflict, problems, and pathology, it largely overlooks human strengths and possibilities, and what Abraham Maslow (1971) famously called "the farther reaches of human nature." Consequently, psychoanalysis does not recognize possibilities of, for example, exceptional health and well-being, ecstatic experiences, or how to foster transpersonal maturation and exceptional capacities. As several researchers have pointed out, "Freudianism institutionalized the underestimation of human possibility" (Needleman, 1980, p. 60).

Both ancient contemplative claims and recent research call into question psychoanalytic assumptions about the universality of psychological conflict. Contemplative psychologies fully agree that conflict is a given for "normal" people. However, they suggest that these conflicts may largely resolve in the higher reaches of development. This claim is supported by an intriguing Rorschach study of advanced mindfulness meditation teachers.

But first, a word of caution about the Rorschach, which is one of the most famous and controversial of all psychological tests. An American Psychological Association board lauded it as "perhaps the most powerful psychometric instrument ever envisioned," yet *The New York Review of Books* damned it as "a ludicrous but still dangerous relic" (Crews, 2004). Certainly, the Rorschach can still be valuable in exploratory studies such as this examination of mindfulness meditation teachers.

Those teachers at the first of the four classic levels of Buddhist enlightenment showed almost normal amounts of conflict around common issues such as sexuality, dependency, and aggression. However, these conflicts were reported as "encapsulated," meaning that the conflicts had little impact on the teachers' personality or performance. The enlightened practitioners displayed "greater awareness of and openness to conflict but paradoxically less reaction . . ." (Wilber, Engler, & Brown, 1986, p. 210). This is consistent with the behavior of such teachers, who often seem more amused than troubled by their issues.

However, a still more remarkable resolution of conflicts occurred at the third level of enlightenment. An exceptionally advanced female meditation master showed "no evidence of sexual or aggressive drive conflicts" (Wilber et al., 1986, p. 214). Intriguingly, ancient texts not only claim that this type of freedom from conflict and its resultant suffering is possible; they also claim that this freedom occurs at the third level of enlightenment.

One further problem with psychoanalysis is an unfortunate tendency toward grandiosity. Some psychoanalysts make sweeping pronouncements overestimating the scope and supremacy of their own system. Consider, for example, the claims that "Psychoanalysis is the most extensive, inclusive and comprehensive system of psychology" (Arlow, 1995, p. 16), and "When it comes to unraveling the mysteries of the human mind, no body of knowledge approaches that of psychoanalytic theory" (Gabbard, 1995, p. 431). Comparisons with other schools offer little support for such claims. Overestimating the supremacy of one's own school seems directly related to one's ignorance of others. Of course, this trap is widespread among therapeutic schools, including contemplative ones, but is no longer defensible.

In spite of their differences, meditation practices and psychoanalysis (together with other psychodynamic therapies) share certain goals and understandings. Both are based on the recognition that, as Freud (1917/1943, p. 252) put it, "man is not even master in his own house . . . his own mind." Likewise, the two systems emphasize the value of deep introspection, and Freud acknowledged that meditative disciplines "may be able to grasp happenings in the depths of the ego and in the id which were otherwise inaccessible to it. . . . It may be admitted that the therapeutic efforts of psychoanalysis have chosen a similar line of approach" (Freud, 1933/1965, p. 71).

Analytical (Jungian) and contemplative psychologies agree on several major issues. These include the mind's innate drive toward growth, the beneficial effects of transpersonal experiences, and the multilayered nature of the unconscious, including levels below the Freudian.

Meditation traditions tend to agree with Jungian, humanistic, and person-centered Rogerian schools that, in addition to motives such as sex and aggression, the psyche possesses an innate drive toward growth and development. Although the concepts are not perfectly synonymous, there is overlap among Jung's drive for "individuation," Abraham Maslow's "self-actualization" and "self-transcendence," Carl Rogers's "formative tendency," and the contemplative motive for self-transcendence and awakening. All would agree with Abraham Maslow's (1968, p. iv) poignant observation that "Without the transcendent and the transpersonal, we get sick, violent, and nihilistic, or else hopeless and apathetic. We need something 'bigger than we are' to be awed by and to commit ourselves to."

Both Jungian and contemplative perspectives, and now contemporary research, agree that transpersonal experiences can foster psychological healing and growth (Walsh & Vaughan, 1993). Transpersonal experiences are experiences in which the sense of identity or self expands beyond (trans) the individual or personal to encompass wider aspects of humankind and the world. Here one experiences oneself as intimately linked and identified with others, the world, and even the cosmos. As Jung (1973) put it, "the approach to the numinous is the real therapy and inasmuch as you attain to the numinous experience you are released from the curse of pathology" (p. 377).

Jung was one of the first pioneers to recognize adult and postconventional development and transpersonal experiences. Historically, most Western therapies recognized only the first two developmental stages, the prepersonal and personal, and this left them prey to a specific trap. Since transpersonal experiences went unrecognized, they were often confused with prepersonal ones and therefore were mistakenly diagnosed as regressive or pathological. The result was "the pre/post fallacy." For example, Freud interpreted transpersonal experiences as indicative of infantile helplessness, Albert Ellis viewed them as examples of irrational thinking, and the classic text *The History of Psychiatry* referred to "The obvious similarities between schizophrenic regressions and the practices of Yoga and Zen" (Alexander & Selesnich, 1966, p. 372).

However, careful comparisons reveal major differences between prepersonal regression and transpersonal progression, and, as Ken Wilber points out, "pre and trans can be seriously equated only by those whose intellectual inquiry goes no further than superficial impressions" (Wilber, 1999, p. 157). Nevertheless, the pre/trans fallacy was widespread until recently and led to a tragic underestimation of human potentials and of contemplative therapies.

Cognitive, rational emotive, and contemplative therapies share an appreciation of the enormous power of thoughts and beliefs. They agree that we are all prone to numerous erroneous thoughts that all too easily become unrecognized erroneous assumptions. These assumptions are mistaken for reality, and then they bias cognition, distort experience, and produce pathology. These mistaken assumptions are described as "basic mistakes" (Alfred Adler), "cognitive distortions" (cognitive therapy), "irrational beliefs" (Albert Ellis), and "delusion" (Asian therapies). Rumi, one of Sufism's greatest contemplatives and now one of the world's most popular poets, wrote, "Your thinking . . . drives you in every direction under its bitter control (Helminski, 2000, p. 19)," Jewish wisdom holds that "A person's entire destiny—for good or ill—depends on the thoughts in his heart" (Hoffman, 1985, p. 103), and therefore recommends the practice of "elevating strange thoughts." The great Indian leader Mahatma Gandhi, who was a devoted yogic practitioner, summarized it this way: "What you think you become" (Fischer, 1954, p. 146).

Of course, there are also significant differences between schools. Cognitive therapy has made several advances over contemplative approaches. These include recognizing specific cognitive profiles for each psychopathology and experimentally demonstrating the benefits of changing pathogenic beliefs.

On the other hand, because of their refined awareness, meditators can identify and modify layers of thought below those accessible to cognitive and rational emotive therapies. Meditators are able to observe thoughts and their effects with remarkable precision (as will be described), to unearth deep distorted beliefs and cognitive schemas, and to develop remarkable degrees of cognitive control. Advanced meditators may observe each thought that arises, and then reduce harmful thoughts and cultivate beneficial ones. Cognitive therapies recognize the possibility of brief "thought stopping." However, contemplatives can extend thought stopping for prolonged periods, and then rest in the profound calm and clarity that result, a claim now supported by electroencephalogram (EEG) studies (Cahn & Polich, 2006).

Reduction of the usually incessant torrent of thoughts is said to heal, calm, and clarify the mind. This fosters healing and growth and reveals depths of the psyche that are usually obscured, just as the depths of a lake become visible only when surface waves are calmed. Taoism's great philosopher Chuang Tzu wrote, "if water derives lucidity from stillness, how much more the faculties of the mind?" (Giles, 1926/1969, p. 47).

Contemplative therapies can therefore do more than heal the erroneous thoughts and beliefs that underlie clinical psychopathologies. At their best, they can also help us to recognize, transform, and disidentify from deeper thoughts that underlie collective pathology. These are thoughts and beliefs that keep us trapped at conventional levels of development and unaware of our further potentials and deeper identity. So important are thoughts that the Buddha began his teaching with the words:

> We are what we think. All that we are arises with our thoughts. . . .
> It is good to control them, and to master them brings happiness. . . .
> The task is to quieten them, and by ruling them to find happiness. (Byrom, 1976, p. 3, 13)

Existential and contemplative therapies both center on "ultimate concerns," those fundamental challenges of life that all of us inevitably face. These include the inescapable challenges of meaning and purpose, suffering and limitation, isolation and death. Both schools agree that these challenges leave us prey to a deep sense of anxiety (angst). Moreover, this anxiety is not just circumstantial but also existential—that is, it is due not only to our individual circumstances but also to the nature of human existence.

Both schools also emphasize the many ways in which we live superficially and inauthentically, hiding from and deceiving ourselves about these ultimate concerns. Conventional culture often reflects and fosters this inauthenticity, creating what Nietzsche described as a "herd mentality" that functions as a collective defense. This herd mentality encourages us to live conventional lives of what Eric Fromm called "automation conformity": superficial, unreflective lifestyles in which, according to Kierkegaard, we "tranquilize ourselves with trivia."

Contemplative and existential psychologies offer overlapping but distinct solutions. They both urge us to recognize rather than deny our existential condition, and then to face it as fearlessly and defenselessly as we can. Only in this way can we escape the conventional slumber of our herd mentality, go beyond unthinking conformity, and live more fully and authentically. However, for most existentialists, the best we can do is to adopt a heroic attitude, such as courage and authenticity, which involves unflinching openness to the harsh realities of life (Yalom, 2002).

Contemplative therapies agree completely that we need authenticity and courage. However, they also suggest that contemplative practices enable us to deal with life's existential challenges in two additional ways. The first is by cultivating mental qualities such as courage, equanimity, and insight, which help in facing such challenges. The second is by fostering maturation to transpersonal stages. Here the separate "egoic" self that suffers isolation and meaninglessness is transcended in a larger transpersonal identity that recognizes its inherent interconnection with others and with all life, and thereby finds inherent meaning and purpose in this larger identity.

Contemplative disciplines agree with *integrative* and *integral* therapies that the best way to promote healing and growth is by judiciously combining multiple approaches and techniques. In fact, contemplative therapies go further, and suggest that all of life—each experience, activity, and relationship—can become an opportunity for learning. The aim is not just to foster healthy qualities such as calm and clarity during formal practice sessions, but also to both foster and apply these healthy qualities in all activities for the benefit of everyone. The goal is to go into oneself so as to go out into the world more effectively and helpfully, and to go out into the world so as to go into oneself more effectively and deeply.

What Makes Psychotherapy and Psychotherapists Effective? Supershrinks and Pseudoshrinks

One of the most consistent findings in psychotherapy research is that most of the benefits come from so called "nonspecific factors"—such as the quality of the relationship and the clients' and therapists' personal qualities and capacities—rather than from the unique elements of a particular therapy. Moreover, therapists differ enormously in their effectiveness, with "supershrinks" far outperforming "pseudoshrinks." Unfortunately, most research still tries to demonstrate the superiority of one therapy over another in spite of decades of minimal success. Clearly, more (or even most) effort should be going into identifying characteristics of supershrinks and discovering how to emulate them. For example, obtaining feedback is crucial, and using rating scales to obtain feedback from clients in each session on how the session went *dramatically* improves therapy success rates (Duncan, Miller, & Sparks, 2004; Miller, Hubble, & Duncan, 2007).

As yet, we do not know how much of contemplative benefits derive from the specific practices, and how much from the therapist and the relationship. It may be that nonspecific effects are particularly important at the beginning of practice, when teachers or therapists are most active and involved. As practice progresses, the practice and practitioner usually become more independent, and at this stage specific factors unique to meditation or yoga may become increasingly important.

There are probably multiple qualities that characterize contemplative supershrinks. They likely include all the beneficial personal characteristics identified by Carl Rogers, such as accurate empathy, a nonjudgmental positive regard for the client, and personal "congruence" or authenticity. Other beneficial qualities probably include a long-term personal contemplative practice, and development of the psychological qualities and capacities that contemplation has been shown to foster. Therapists of any persuasion can benefit from contemplative practice themselves. Therefore, therapists can learn these practices, and then continue to offer other kinds of therapies to clients while bringing contemplative qualities such as greater calm, clarity, and empathy to their work.

HISTORY

Precursors

The human quest for self-understanding and healing extends back into the dawn of history. The earliest systematic seekers and therapists were ancient healers called shamans, whose 20,000-year-old images decorate cave walls. Shamans were the original general practitioners who functioned as physicians, therapists, and tribal counselors. To fill these multiple roles, they drew on an array of diagnostic and healing techniques that ranged from projective testing to herbal medications, individual counseling, and group therapy (Walsh, 2007). As such, they exemplify Jerome Frank's (1982) famous claim that all psychotherapy methods "are elaborations and variations of age-old procedures of psychological healing" (p. 49).

However, their distinctive practice was the induction and use of altered states of consciousness. Thousands of years ago, they learned how to alter their consciousness through techniques such as fasting, drumming, dancing, and psychedelics. With the heightened sensitivity conferred on them by these altered states, they accessed intuitive knowledge to make diagnoses and recommend treatments. Today, shamanism still plays a vital role in many cultures, making it by far the most enduring of all current psychotherapies (Walsh, 2007).

Beginnings

Meditative and yogic practices emerged when practitioners learned to induce desired states of mind without external aids. Their origins are lost in the mists of history but can be traced back at least 3,000 years.

Beginning some 2,500 years ago, there was a dramatic stirring of human consciousness, a stirring so important that it has been named the Axial Age. In diverse countries, remarkable individuals pioneered new techniques for training the mind, and developed the first systematic meditative, philosophical, and psychological disciplines. In Greece, the first systematic thinkers—and especially the remarkable trio of Socrates, Plato, and Aristotle—established rational inquiry and thereby laid the foundation for Western philosophy and psychology. In India, sages developed yoga and the yoga-based philosophy and psychology that would undergird subsequent centuries of Indian thought. Meanwhile, the Buddha devised new meditations and a corresponding philosophy. In China, Confucius, a veritable one-man university, and Lao Tsu, a semi-legendary sage, laid the foundations of Confucianism and Taoism, respectively. So important was this era to the evolution of human culture and the understanding of human nature that the historian Karen Armstrong (2006) concluded, "All the traditions that were developed during the Axial Age pushed forward the frontiers of human consciousness and discovered a transcendent dimension in the core of their being."

Subsequent Evolution

Each of these traditions evolved over time. Of course, Western contemplative traditions also evolved. However, because these began centuries later and because of space limitations, we will focus on the evolution of the axial traditions that we have already begun to follow.

In China, Taoism split into quite disparate streams. One group degenerated into primitive magic, another developed a systematic philosophy, and a third became yogic and concerned itself with psychological transformation. It is this group whose practices we will examine.

Confucianism started as a social reform movement. Deeply pained by the turmoil and injustice he saw around him, Confucius yearned to improve government and help the downtrodden masses. The philosophy and psychology that he and his followers developed were therefore socially oriented. Only centuries later, when Confucianism incorporated elements of Taoism and Buddhism to create the great synthesis of neo-Confucianism, did the tradition come to include major meditative and yogic components.

In India, yoga developed into several schools emphasizing different but complementary approaches to mind training and self-transformation. Four main approaches, or yogas, emerged that focused on transforming thoughts, emotions, attention, and motivation, respectively.

Buddhism eventually developed a systematic psychology that still stands as one of the world's most remarkable introspective psychologies. It analyzed the contents and processes of mind into some 50 elements of experience. Then it used these elements to describe psychological health and pathology and to guide mental training. Early Western psychology was also largely introspective. However, whereas Western introspectionists failed to create a useful replicable map of experience, the Buddhists succeeded (perhaps because of their far more rigorous training in introspection), and their map has guided meditators for over 2,000 years.

Common Discoveries and Practices

Whenever people search deeply for insight into the great questions and mysteries of life, certain themes emerge. Inevitably, seekers come to recognize the need for developing their own minds and the importance of both wise teachers and periods of silence and introspection. Only in periods of quiet can we disentangle ourselves from the superficial busyness of our lives, reflect on what is truly important, calm our minds, and access our inner wisdom.

Contemplative practices and traditions therefore became part of each of the great religions of both East and West. Christian contemplatives claimed that, for example, "Good speech is silver, but silence is pure gold" (Savin, 1991, p. 127), while Judaism says, "I grew up among the sages. All my life I listened to their words. Yet I have found nothing better than silence" (Shapiro, 1993, p. 18). Likewise, Islamic Sufis recognized that wisdom comes from silence and contemplation. They therefore echoed the words of their founder Mohammad, "Silent is wise; alas, there are not enough who keep silent. . . . Bring your heart to meditation" (Angha, 1995, p. 68, 74). Similar themes echo through Eastern traditions and through the lives of secular contemplatives, too.

Over time, the need for mental training as an essential catalyst for psychological health, wisdom, and spiritual maturity became increasingly apparent. Contemplative practices therefore evolved over the centuries, becoming increasingly refined, systematic, and diverse. Each tradition developed a family of practices aimed at cultivating specific mental capacities—for example, attentional capacities such as concentration and focus, cognitive skills such as insight and wisdom, and valued emotions such as love and compassion. And each tradition came to the crucial, life-changing recognition that within us are untapped potentials, sources of wisdom, and kinds of satisfaction far richer and more profound than we suspect.

"Know yourself" is the key maxim of the contemplative traditions, and it has been stated in numerous ways. The great contemplative Plotinus, who fathered Neoplatonic philosophy, advised, "We must close our eyes and invoke a new manner of seeing . . . a wakefulness that is the birthright of us all, though few put it to use" (O'Brien, 1964, p. 42). Early female Christian contemplatives, who were known as the Christian Desert Mothers because they withdrew from society to practice, quickly learned what so many others before and after them learned:

> Self-awareness is not selfishness but self-connectedness. It is a deep and intense listening to our inner being, learning to be conscious and alert to what our inner world is trying to say to us. With self-awareness and self-knowledge, we understand our reactions toward others, issues that complicate our lives, blind spots we can fall into, as well as our particular strengths and gifts. (Swan, 2001, pp. 36–37)

Current Status

For a long time, Western mental health professionals knew little and misunderstood much about contemplative practices, but recently there has been an explosion of both popular and professional interest. Worldwide, these practices remain among the most widespread and popular of all current psychotherapies. They are now practiced by several thousand therapists and several million laypersons in the United States as well as by hundreds of millions of people around the world (Deurr, 2004). The number of demonstrated psychological and somatic benefits continues to increase, while combination therapies and integrative psychologies that synthesize contemplative and standard Western approaches are proliferating. Several hundred research studies—most on TM and mindfulness—make meditation one of the most extensively researched of all therapies.

Integration of Therapies

Attempts to forge integrations across different Western psychologies and therapies are of three major kinds: (1) the search for underlying common factors, (2) technical eclecticism (combining techniques), and (3) theoretical integration. Similarly, attempts are now being made to integrate meditative and psychological therapies. Therapeutic factors common to both meditations and psychotherapies are discussed below and elsewhere (e.g., Baer, 2005; Kabat-Zinn, 2003; Walsh & Shapiro, 2006).

Contemplative technical eclecticism is proceeding rapidly and most often combines mindfulness with psychotherapeutic techniques. The original inspiration was Jon Kabat-Zinn's (2003) widely used Mindfulness-Based Stress Reduction (MBSR). Recent combinations employing mindfulness include mindfulness-based cognitive, art, and sleep therapies, Mindfulness-Based Eating Awareness Therapy (MB-EAT), relapse prevention for drug abuse, and relationship enhancement. Combinations that employ other or multiple kinds of meditation include dialectical behavior therapy for borderline disorders, acceptance and commitment therapy, and transpersonal and integral therapies. Such approaches have initial research support, and some, such as MBSR, already meet the criteria for "probably efficacious" treatments (Baer, 2005). Nonwestern psychotherapies that incorporate meditative elements include the Japanese *Naikan* and *Morita* therapies.

The success of these combination therapies raises several intriguing questions. An obvious one is "What other combinations will prove efficacious?" A more provocative question, given the many successes so far, may be "Would all mainstream therapies benefit from the addition of mindfulness training?" And perhaps the question that is most important in the long term is "What are the possibilities for using meditation on a widespread social scale, such as in educational systems, to prevent pathologies and problems for which it has already proved therapeutic?"

Theoretical Integrations

There is a growing movement to create integrative theories that synthesize contemplative and Western psychological perspectives. The best-known examples are transpersonal and integral psychologies. *Transpersonal* psychology was founded as the first explicitly integrative school of Western psychology, and as such it sought to honor and synthesize valid insights of all schools, including East and West, psychology and meditation, personal and transpersonal (Walsh & Vaughan, 1993). This synthesis is facilitated by the fact that the meditative and Western psychologies are to some extent complementary, the former focusing on health and the latter on pathology, the former on the transpersonal and the latter on the personal.

The most far-reaching theoretical integration to date is the "integral psychology" of Ken Wilber. His approach traces psychological development, pathologies, and appropriate therapies from infancy to adulthood using primarily Western psychological resources, and then from personal to transpersonal using primarily contemplative resources (Wilber, 1999, 2000b; Wilber et al., 1986).

Therapeutically, the most comprehensive integrative approaches to date are the integral therapies of Ken Wilber and of Michael Murphy, the founder of Esalen Institute. These multimodal therapies address multiple psychological and somatic dimensions, as well as prepersonal, personal, and transpersonal levels. Integral therapies recommend a judicious mix, tailored to the individual, of educational, psychotherapeutic, contemplative, and somatic approaches. Somatic approaches include exercise, mindful movement such as Tai Chi, yogic postures, and diet. Diet has long been a central concern of yoga, which holds that, "As one's food, so is one's mind" (Feuerstein, 1996, p. 63). This ancient wisdom remains vitally important in our modern world, where millions of people consume junk food and die from the complications of obesity, while millions of others die from starvation. Although integral therapies are impressively wide ranging in scope, they lack the research validation that some integrative therapies have amassed (Norcross & Beutler, 2010).

Many therapists now integrate meditative and Western perspectives within their own lives and therapeutic practices. Thousands of Western-trained therapists have now learned contemplative practices, and an increasing number of contemplative teachers are acquiring Western psychological training.

Learning Contemplative Practices

For those who want to learn contemplative practices, there are many popular books (see the Case Readings in this chapter). However, it is extremely helpful to have the guidance of a teacher–therapist. Most teachers are sincere, but there are no licensing procedures or formal regulatory bodies. Good teachers have extensive personal experience, may have been certified to teach by their own instructors, and are likely to be part of an historical contemplative tradition such as TM, Buddhist meditation, or Christian contemplation. Most important, they live and relate in ways consistent with their message, treating everyone with kindness and respect. Therapists who wish to teach these techniques, or to counsel people already using them, need to have done considerable personal practice themselves under expert guidance. Ideally, this would include periods of retreat where, over several days or weeks, one engages in continuous practice that can significantly accelerate learning and growth.

PERSONALITY

Just as there are many types of meditation, there are many contemplative psychologies. Although they vary significantly, there are also recurrent themes. We can therefore outline a contemplative view of mind and human nature, but we need to keep in mind that a specific system may not agree with all the following points.

Theory of Personality

Contemplative practices stem from and lead to views of human nature, health, pathology, and potential that are in some ways very different from traditional Western assumptions. We can discuss these views under the following headings: consciousness, identity, motivation, development, and higher capacities.

Consciousness

A century ago, William James made a famous and provocative claim:

> Our normal waking consciousness . . . is but one special type of consciousness, whilst all about it, parted from it by the filmiest of screens, there lie potential forms of consciousness entirely different. We may go through life without suspecting their existence; but apply the requisite stimulus, and at a touch they are there in all their completeness. . . . No account of the universe in its totality can be final which leaves those other forms of consciousness quite disregarded. (James, 1958, p. 298)

Contemplative psychologies agree fully. They describe a broad spectrum of states of consciousness—many of them as yet unrecognized by mainstream Western psychology—and provide detailed techniques for attaining them. Perceptual sensitivity and clarity, concentration and sense of identity, as well as emotional and cognitive processes all vary with states of consciousness in predictable ways. Some states possess not only the capacities present in our usual condition but also heightened or additional ones, and these are known as "higher states."

If higher states of consciousness exist, then contrary to typical Western assumptions, our usual state must be suboptimal. This is exactly the claim of the contemplative psychologies, which describe our usual state as clouded, hypnotic, and dreamlike. All of us are aware that we sometimes daydream and become lost in thoughts and fantasy. Contemplative psychologies claim that these thoughts and fantasies are significantly more pervasive, distorting, and confusing than we realize.

This claim, like other contemplative claims, is one we can test for ourselves through meditation. Meditative observation quickly reveals that our minds are usually filled with a continual flux of unrecognized thoughts, images, and fantasies that distort and reduce awareness, resulting in unappreciated trance-like states (Kornfield, 1993). As in any hypnotic state, the trance and its attendant constrictions and distortions of awareness easily go unrecognized. The result is said to be a clouding and distortion of daily experience that causes much of our mental suffering, yet remains unrecognized until we subject our perceptual–cognitive processes to direct, rigorous scrutiny, as in meditation.

Thus the "normal" person is considered to be partly "asleep," "dreaming," or in a "consensus trance." When such a "dream" is especially painful or disruptive, it becomes a pathological "nightmare." However, because the vast majority of the population "dreams," the usual more subtle forms remain unrecognized. A central aim of contemplative therapies is to enable people to "awaken" from this waking dream, and this awakening is known by such names as liberation and enlightenment, salvation and *satori, fana,* and nirvana (Walsh, 1999).

To some extent, these concepts simply extend Western psychology. Research shows that we are far less aware of our own cognitive processes than we usually assume, and that we suffer from unrecognized cognitive–perceptual distortions and automaticities. Contemplative psychologies suggest that meditative/yogic training can both enhance awareness and reduce distortions and automaticities. This claim is now supported by studies of advanced meditators who show enhanced perceptual speed, sensitivity, and discrimination (Murphy & Donovan, 1997).

Identity

Contemplative psychologies present a view of our identity or sense of self that differs dramatically from everyday assumptions. Under microscopic meditative examination, what was formerly assumed to be a relatively consistent, permanent self-sense (self, self-construct, self-representation, or ego) is recognized as a continuously changing flux of thoughts, images, and emotions. This discovery is not unique to meditators and can occur whenever people introspect with sufficient care. For example, among Western philosophers, William James spoke of the "stream of consciousness," and David Hume concluded that the self is "nothing but a bundle or collection of different perceptions, which succeed each other with an inconceivable rapidity and are in a perpetual flux and movement" (Jones, 1975, p. 305).

Similarly with psychoanalytic object relations theory. Comparing Buddhist and psychoanalytic systems, the psychologist and meditation teacher Jack Engler (1983) found that in both psychologies:

> What we take to be our "self" and feel to be so present and real is actually an internalized image, a composite representation, constructed by a selective and imaginative "remembering" of past encounters with the object world. In fact, the self is viewed as being constructed anew from moment to moment. But both systems further agree that the self is not ordinarily experienced this way. (p. 33)

Hence both contemplative psychologies and some schools of Western psychology and philosophy conclude that the "self" is very different from our usual unexamined assumptions. The usual sense of the self as being who we "really are" and as being continuous and consistent over time seems to be an illusory construction of imprecise awareness. Closer examination reveals that the self-sense is continuously and selectively constructed from a flux of thoughts, images, and emotions. This is similar to the "flicker fusion phenomenon" by which still photographs projected successively on a movie screen give the illusion of continuity, vitality, and movement.

This bears out a crucial contemplative claim: that we suffer from a case of mistaken identity. We are not who, or even what, we thought we were. What we take to be our real self is merely an illusory construct.

The implications are enormous. We worry over our "self-concept" and obsess about our "self-image" but rarely appreciate the far-reaching significance of this language. If they are merely concepts or images that we have constructed, then they are not who or what we really are. We have mistaken a concept for our self and an image for reality. Then we devote our lives to trying to live up to, defend, or change these concepts and images. In doing so, we become the victims of our own creation. It is as though we painted an ugly picture of ourselves and then cringed in horror. "Pain is caused by false identification," states a classic yoga text (Prabhavananda & Isherwood, 1972, p. 127). The result is delusion and suffering.

When this false identification and its implications are truly recognized, we can become free from the limitations and suffering they produce. Whereas Western therapies teach us that we can modify our self-image, contemplative therapies teach us that we can also do something far more transformative and profound: We can recognize that our self-image is only a fabrication, and can thereby disidentify from it and become free of it.

Contemplative therapies do this by cultivating sensitive, precise awareness. This awareness can penetrate into the depths of the psyche, recognize the false self-image, and thereby loosen its hold. When one is no longer tethered to an illusory, outdated self-image, the mind is free to grow, and this catalyzes development (Walsh & Shapiro, 2006). The self-concept and its boundaries are then increasingly recognized as constructed rather than given, fluid rather than rigid, and capable of considerable expansion. The sense of self can then become transpersonal—extending beyond (trans) the boundaries of the separate person and personality—and identifying with others, and eventually identifying with all humankind and the world. The final culmination is a sense of one's interconnectedness and inherent unity with all, and the result is a natural sense of love and compassion for all.

As meditative–yogic awareness penetrates past arbitrary self-boundaries, it also penetrates into the very depths of the psyche. Below the self-concept, below the thoughts and images that construct this concept, below even the archetypal layers recognized by Jung, awareness uncovers our deep nature and discovers—itself! That is, our deep nature is said to be—not the contents of mind such as thoughts, images and feelings—but rather that which underlies and is aware of them: pure awareness or consciousness. This pure awareness is described in different contemplative traditions as Mind, original Mind, Spirit, Self, Atman, Buddha Nature, and Tao mind. Contemplative traditions agree that the experience of this pure awareness that is our true nature is extremely blissful and far more ecstatic than any other pleasure. After his own discovery of this, Shankara, one of the greatest Indian yogis, exclaimed,

> What is this joy that I feel? Who shall measure it?
> I know nothing but joy, limitless, unbounded! . . .
> I abide in the joy of the Atman. (Prabhavananda & Isherwood, 1978, p. 113)

As a survey of the world's yogas concluded, "This is indeed the great message of all forms of yoga: happiness is our essential nature, and our perpetual quest for happiness is fulfilled only when we realize who we truly are" (Feuerstein, 1996, p.2).

In summary, contemplative training culminates in penetrating insight into the mind and the recognition of one's deep identity. It is recognition of oneself as blissful, pure consciousness, aware of one's connection to all people and all things, and aware of (but no longer identified with, and therefore not controlled by) the thoughts, images, and emotions that parade through the mind. This is the classical unitive experience so widely sought by contemplatives around the world, and it is experienced as the mind's natural, healthy, mature, and ecstatic condition (Wilber, 2000b).

Similar, though transient, ecstatic experiences can emerge under other circumstances. They can be deliberately induced with rituals, fasting, or psychedelics. They may also occur spontaneously in nature, advanced psychotherapy, intensive exercise, during childbirth, and near death (Maslow, 1971). They can also be induced during lovemaking in experiences of "transcendent sex" that advanced tantric yogis use for self-transformation (Feuerstein, 1996; Wade, 2004).

From a contemplative perspective, these are glimpses, or *peak experiences,* of the mind's potentials and our deeper nature, and they can produce significant insights and transformations. However, these experiences are almost always transient. Only mental training can sustain such experiences and thereby transform them into the higher developmental stages and enduring ways of life that are the goals of contemplative disciplines.

Western psychologists periodically rediscover unitive experiences and their benefits. Classic examples include William James's "cosmic consciousness," Carl Jung's "numinous experience," Abraham Maslow's "peak experience," Erich Fromm's "at-onement," and "transpersonal experiences." In fact, some Western researchers have reached conclusions strikingly similar to those of contemplatives; two classic examples are Carl Jung and William James. Jung (1968) argued that "the deeper layers of the psyche . . . become increasingly collective until they are universalized" (p. 291), and William James (1960) suggested that "there is a continuum of cosmic consciousness against which our individuality builds but accidental fences and into which our several minds plunge as into a mother sea" (p. 324). "It is chiefly our ignorance of the psyche if these experiences appear 'mystic,'" claimed Jung (1955, p. 535).

However, Western clinicians usually see ego boundaries dissolve in the ego disintegration of psychoses and borderline disorders. Therefore, it is understandable that healthy ego transcendence was sometimes formerly confused with pathological ego disintegration and therefore dismissed as regressive psychopathology. This unfortunate example of the pre/post fallacy is an outmoded pathologizing interpretation. In fact, unitive experiences occur most often in psychologically healthy individuals and then further enhance health and maturity (Alexander, Rainforth, & Gelderloos, 1991; Maslow, 1971).

Motivation

Contemplative psychologies tend to see motives as organized hierarchically from strong to (initially) weak, from survival to self-transcendence. This ordering is most explicit in Hindu yoga and is similar to the Western theories of Abraham Maslow (1971) and Ken Wilber (1999). Yoga agrees that physiological and survival motives such as hunger and thirst are innately most powerful and predominant. When these needs are fulfilled, drives such as sexual and power strivings may emerge as effective motivators in their turn, and after them, "higher" motives such as love and the pull toward self-transcendence. *Self-transcendence* is the desire to transcend our usual false constricted identity, to awaken to the fullness of our being, and to recognize our true nature and potential. Self-transcendence, lying beyond even self-actualization, was the highest motive recognized by Maslow, but some contemplative psychologies give equal importance to selfless service.

The question of the nature of *the* fundamental human motive (if such there be) has repeatedly split Western psychology. The extremes are represented by Freudian, Marxist, and evolutionary psychologies, on one hand, and by the perspectives of Rogers and Wilber on the other. Freud, Marx, and evolutionary psychology are reductionistic. That is, they view higher motives as expressions of underlying sexual, economic, and survival factors, respectively. By contrast, for Rogers (1959) "the basic actualizing tendency is the only motive which is postulated" (p. 184), while for Wilber (1999), the pull to self-transcendence is fundamental.

This perspective has enormous practical implications for our lives. According to contemplative psychologies, higher motives—what Abraham Maslow called *metamotives,* such as self-actualization, self-transcendence, and selfless service—are part of our very nature. Therefore, ignoring them produces several kinds of pain and pathology.

First, we suffer from a shallow, distorted, and distorting view of ourselves. This has tragic consequences because self-images tend to operate as self-fulfilling prophecies, and as Gordon Allport (1964) pointed out "Debasing assumptions debase human beings" (p. 36).

Second, if metamotives are an essential part of our nature, then overlooking them means that we are starving ourselves of something vital to our well-being. We may need the good, the true, and the beautiful if we are to thrive; we may need to express kindness, care, and compassion if we are to live fully (Walsh & Vaughan, 1993). Therefore, if we do not recognize and express our metamotives, we will live inauthentically and immaturely and remain fundamentally unfulfilled. This is doubly problematic because we will not even recognize the real source of our dissatisfactions, and are likely to blame our malaise on circumstances or other people. These frustrations can mushroom into what Maslow (1971) called *metapathologies,* such as a lack of personal values and guiding principles, a deep sense of meaninglessness and cynicism, distrust of others, and alienation from society.

Maslow worried that many of these metapathologies are rampant in Western society and represent a major threat to our culture. But that is exactly what one would expect given that our culture has denied and starved higher motives. Contemplatives have long emphasized that the recognition and cultivation of metamotives are essential, not only for individuals, but also for cultures and civilization.

The third cost of metamotive blindness is that we then believe that lesser motives—such as gratifying desires for money, sex, prestige, and power—are the only means to happiness. Then we become lost in the seductive illusion that if we can just get enough of them, we will finally be fully and permanently happy.

Unfortunately, there are serious problems with this idea. First, when we believe these lower-order goals are the only means to attain happiness, we become addicted to them. Then whenever we don't have them, we suffer. Worse still, even if we succeed in getting them, we inevitably habituate and need more and more. In order to get the same high, the drug addict needs a bigger hit, the miser more wealth, the consumer yet another shopping binge. This is what contemporary psychologists call the *hedonic treadmill* and what the Buddha was pointing to with his words "The rain could turn to gold, and still your thirst would not be slaked" (Byrom, 1976, p. 70). Finally, obsession with wealth and possessions can tranquilize us with trivia and distract us from what is truly important in our lives. As the Taoist sage Chuang Tsu put it, "you use up all your vital energy on external things and wear out your spirit" (Feng & English, 1974, p. 108).

Recent research supports these claims. For example, considerable evidence shows that once our basic needs are met, further income and possessions add surprisingly little to well-being and that "there is only a slight tendency for people who make lots of money to be more satisfied with what they make" (Myers, 1992, p. 39). In short, money can certainly relieve the suffering of deprivation, but it is curiously ineffective in buying further happiness, which is why so many contemplatives have echoed Mohammad's words: "The richest among you is the one who is not entrapped by greed" (Angha, 1995, p. 21).

None of this is to suggest that pleasures such as money, sex, and prestige are necessarily bad or that seeking them noncompulsively is pathological. But contemplatives do say that when we believe these are the only (or even the most important) pleasures, then we become addicted to them and are doomed to suffer. Contemplative psychologies therefore provide a valuable antidote to the painful misunderstandings about motivation that pervade contemporary culture, and derail so many lives.

Development

A developmental perspective is so crucial to understanding contemplative claims that we will summarize key concepts again and build on them further. Development proceeds through three major stages: prepersonal, personal, and transpersonal (or preconventional, conventional, and postconventional). Whereas Western psychology focuses on the first two stages, contemplatives zero in on the third and recognize several postconventional levels that lie beyond most Western psychological maps. The highest levels merge into experiences that have traditionally been thought of as religious, spiritual, or "mystical" but can now also be understood in psychological terms.

Higher Capacities

Postconventional development can lead to exceptional psychological capacities. These capacities, which are supposedly available to us all if we undertake the necessary contemplative training, are said to include the following (Wilber, 1999).

In the emotional domain, painful emotions such as anger and fear can be greatly reduced (Goleman, 2003). At the same time, positive emotions such as love and joy can mature to become stronger, unconditional, unwavering, and all-encompassing. Cognitive development can proceed beyond Piaget's highest level of linear formal operational thinking to "vision logic" or "network logic," which sees interconnections between groups of ideas simultaneously (Wilber, 1999). Motivation can be redirected up the hierarchy of needs so that motives such as self-transcendence and selfless service grow stronger and eventually predominate. The mind's usual ceaseless agitation can be stilled so that unwavering concentration and profound peace prevail. Wisdom can be developed through sustained reflection on existential issues such as death and the causes of happiness and suffering (Walsh, 1999). A growing body of research, which is reviewed later, now supports several of these claims. More and more, the contemplative view of personality and potentials is coming to seem like a natural extension and enrichment of traditional Western views.

Variety of Concepts

Types of Meditation

There are many kinds of meditation and no fully adequate typology is available. However, one simple division is into two main categories: focused or concentration practices on the one hand, and open or awareness practices on the other.

- *Concentration meditations* hold attention on a single stimulus, such as an image or the sensations of the breath. The aim is to develop the mind's ability to focus and maintain attention.

- *Awareness meditations* allow attention to move from one object to another, exploring the ongoing flux of moment-to-moment experience. The aim is to develop clear sensitive awareness, to explore the nature of mind and experience, and thereby foster mental health and maturation.

Psychopathology

Contemplative views of health and pathology are best understood developmentally. Because they are designed to help with personal and transpersonal levels of development and with existential and transpersonal levels of healing, contemplative approaches by themselves offer little help with major psychopathologies such as psychosis or severe borderline disorder. Rather, their focus is more on "normal pathology," and they agree with Abraham Maslow (1968) that "what we call normal in psychology is really a psychopathology of the average, so undramatic and so widely spread that we don't even notice it ordinarily" (p. 60).

From a contemplative perspective, this "psychopathology of everyday life," as Freud called it, is a reflection of psychological immaturity. Development has proceeded from preconventional to conventional but has then ground to a premature halt far short of our true potentials. The mind is operating suboptimally, multiple beneficial qualities and capacities remain underdeveloped, while unhealthy qualities flourish.

These unhealthy factors are numerous, and each contemplative system describes a long list. They include emotional factors such as hatred and envy, motivational forces such as addiction and selfishness, cognitive distortions such as conceit and mindlessness, and attentional difficulties such as agitation and distractibility. Similar ideas occur in other traditions, but Indian contemplatives emphasize the fundamental role of three specific mental factors in causing psychopathology. These three causes—which Buddhism picturesquely calls "the three poisons"—consist of one cognitive factor (delusion) and two motivation factors (addiction and aversion).

The term *delusion* here refers to an unrecognized mental dullness, mindlessness, or unconsciousness that misperceives and misunderstands the nature of mind and reality. These subtle yet fundamental misunderstandings produce pathogenic motives, beliefs, and behaviors, and the most crucial motives are addiction and aversion. In the words of a famous Zen teacher, "When the deep meaning of things is not understood, the mind's essential peace is disturbed to no avail" (Sengstan, 1975). Contemplatives therefore agree with Albert Ellis (1987) that "virtually all human beings often hold blatant irrational beliefs and therefore are far from being consistently sane and self-helping" (pp. 373–374).

The second root cause of pathology and pain is *craving*. This most closely corresponds to our Western concept of addiction, or what Albert Ellis calls "childish demandingness," and is regarded as a major cause of psychopathology and suffering. Western psychologists emphasize drugs and food. However, contemplatives argue that we can become addicted to almost anything, including people and possessions, our self-image and ideas, and even our ideals. In fact, addictions to material pleasures such as the "physical foursome" of money, sex, power, and prestige are described as "iron chains," while addictions to ideals such as always being good or never getting angry are described as "golden chains" (Walsh, 1999). Being human, we all fall short of our ideals, and if we are addicted to them, then we suffer.

Of course, it is crucial to distinguish craving from simple desire. Desire is mere wanting, craving a compulsive necessity; unfulfilled desires have little impact, unfulfilled addictions yield pain and pathology. Whatever we crave controls us. No wonder yoga claims "Cravings torment the heart" (Prabhavananda & Isherwood, 1972, p. 41).

Along with addiction come painful emotions such as fear, anger, jealousy, and depression. These feelings are intimately tied to craving and reflect the ways it operates in us. We fear that we will not get what we crave, boil with anger toward whoever stands in our way, writhe with jealousy toward people who get what we lust after, and fall into depression when we lose hope. The therapist who recognizes these relationships has an invaluable perspective to offer clients lost in these painful emotions.

Craving is also the basis for many pain-producing life games and lifestyles. These include the "if only game" ("if only I had . . . then I could be happy") and what *transactional analysis* calls the "until game" (I can't be happy until I get . . ."). The amount of suffering in our lives reflects the gap between what we crave and what we have. In fact, for Asian meditative traditions, there is an almost mathematical precision to the relationship between psychological suffering and craving, which we might express in the following formula:

$$\text{Suffering } \alpha \ \Sigma \ \text{Strength of craving} \times (\text{Reality–Craved})$$

What this says is that the amount of psychological suffering in our lives is related to the strength of each craving multiplied by the gap between reality and what is craved. In other words, the greater the number of cravings, the stronger the cravings, and the greater the gap between reality and what we crave, the more we suffer.

Contemplative traditions draw a crucial conclusion. It is possible to reduce psychological conflict and suffering by reducing the number and strength of cravings/addictions, and by accepting reality as it is. In fact, this does more than just reduce suffering. It also allows healthy motives to act more freely and effectively, thereby orienting us towards more healthy and fulfilling goals (Walsh, 1999). No wonder the neo-Confucian sage Wang Yang-ming went so far as to claim that "The learning of the great [person] consists entirely in getting rid of the obscuration of selfish desires [addictions]" (Chan, 1963, p. 660), and the founder of Taoism, Lao Tsu, wrote, "to a land where people cease from coveting, peace comes of course" (Bynner, 1944/1980, p. 48).

Addiction also creates its mirror image, *aversion,* the third of the three root causes of psychopathology. Whereas addiction is a compulsive need to experience and possess desirable stimuli, aversion is a compulsive need to avoid or escape undesirable ones, and it breeds destructive reactions such as anger, fear, and defensiveness. The mind ruled by addiction and aversion is enslaved in a never-ending, pain-fueled quest to get what it wants and avoid what it fears.

From this perspective, psychological pain is no mere nuisance to be ignored, anesthetized, or repressed. Rather, it offers opportunities for learning and growth. For psychological pain is an invaluable feedback signal, a mental alarm pointing to addiction and aversion and the need to relinquish them.

Contemplative traditions of both East and West recognize two possible strategies with regard to addictions. The first is common but tragic, the second rare but beneficial. The first strategy is to devote our lives to satisfying addictions—and thereby mindlessly reinforce and strengthen them. The result is temporary satisfaction and long-term suffering, as drug addicts demonstrate all too well. The second strategy is to reduce and relinquish addictions. This can be difficult at first, but it enhances long-term well-being. This was the basis of Gandhi's recommendation to "renounce and rejoice"—that is, to renounce and relinquish addictions and rejoice in the freedom that follows.

Psychological Health

The contemplative ideal of health extends beyond conventional adjustment and encompasses three shifts:

1. Relinquishment of unhealthy mental qualities such as craving, aversion, and delusion
2. Development of specific healthy mental qualities and capacities
3. Maturation to postconventional, transpersonal levels

Each contemplative tradition has its own list of healthy mental characteristics, but they concur on the crucial importance of seven specific qualities. They agree that psychological health and maturity involve cultivating ethicality, transforming emotions, redirecting motivation, developing concentration, refining awareness, fostering wisdom, and practicing service and contribution to others (Walsh, 1999; Walsh & Vaughan, 1993). These seven central qualities are discussed in detail later.

Compassionate service and contribution are held in particularly high esteem, and in some traditions they represent the culminating expression of health. Obviously, the predominant motives of a person freed of craving and aversion would be very different from those driving most of us. The enlightened individual is said to be minimally driven by the "physical foursome" (money, sensuality, power, and prestige) or indeed by egocentric compulsions in general. According to Zen, "For the unified mind in accord with the Way, all self centered striving ceases" (Sengstan, 1975). For such people, compassion and selfless service are major motives. "Fools think only of their own interest while the sage is concerned with the benefit of others. What a world of difference between them" (Gampopa, 1971, p. 195).

Western theory and research support the idea that altruism is correlated with psychological maturity and well-being. Adler's "social interest," Erikson's "generativity," and the sociologist Sorokin's "creative altruism" are said to be essential expressions of successful adult development, and Maslow (1967, p. 280) claimed that "self-actualizing people, without one single exception, are involved in a cause outside their own skin." Altruism may be central to fostering and expressing psychological health and maturity.

PSYCHOTHERAPY

Theory of Psychotherapy

The central assumption underlying contemplative therapies is that the mind can be trained so that unhealthy qualities diminish, healthy ones flourish, and development ensues. Many techniques can be used, but effective disciplines include seven central kinds of practices to cultivate seven corresponding qualities of mind and behavior.

1. *Ethics.* With rare exceptions, such as integrity groups and ethical therapy, Western therapists have shied away from introducing ethical issues because of understandable concerns about moralizing and advice giving. However, the contemplative understanding of ethics is very different from conventional views and very psychologically astute. "Rare are those who understand virtue," sighed Confucius (Lau, 1979, p. 132).

Contemplative traditions view ethics, not in terms of conventional morality, but rather as an essential discipline for training the mind. Meditative introspection soon makes it painfully apparent that unethical behavior—behavior that aims at inflicting harm—both stems from and strengthens destructive qualities of mind such as greed, anger, and jealousy. In Western terms, unethical behavior reinforces or conditions these destructive qualities; in Asian terms, it deepens their "karmic imprint" on the mind, karma being the psychological residue left by past behavior.

Conversely, ethical behavior—behavior that intends to enhance the well-being of others—does the opposite. It deconditions destructive mental factors while cultivating healthy ones such as kindness, compassion, and calm. From a yogic perspective, ethics is therefore not something imposed from without but rather something sought from within—not a sacrifice but a service to both self and others. The great secret of mature postconventional ethics is recognizing that, as the Buddha pointed out, "Whatever you do, you do to yourself" (Byrom, 1976, p. 118).

At first, ethical behavior involves a struggle to reverse old habits. However, with practice, it becomes increasingly effortless and spontaneous until eventually "whatever is . . . thought to be necessary for sentient beings happens all the time of its own accord" (Gampopa, 1971, p. 271). These heights of contemplative ethics overlap with the highest stages of moral maturity suggested by the Harvard researchers Lawrence Kohlberg and Carol Gilligan.

2. *Emotional Transformation.* There are three components to emotional transformation: reducing problematic emotions such as fear, anger, and jealousy; cultivating positive ones such as love, joy, and compassion; and developing *equanimity*. Although Western therapies have many techniques for reducing negative emotions, they have very few for directly enhancing the positive ones or producing equanimity. In contrast, contemplative therapies contain a wealth of practices for cultivating these beneficial emotions to a remarkable level of intensity. For example, Buddhist and Confucian compassion and the Christian contemplative's *agape* (love) flower fully only when they unconditionally and unwaveringly encompass all creatures, and this is facilitated by the third component of equanimity. Emotional transformation presumably fosters "emotional intelligence," which research suggests is associated with exceptional personal, interpersonal, and professional success (Goleman, 2003).

3. *Redirecting Motivation.* Ethical behavior and emotional transformation work together, along with practices such as meditation, to redirect motivation along healthier paths. Traditionally, it is said that with maturation, motivation becomes less compulsive and addictive, as well as less scattered and more focused, while the things desired become more subtle and internal. There is less concern with material acquisition and more concern with metamotives, especially self-actualization, self-transcendence, and selfless service. Traditionally, this motivational shift was described as "purification"; in contemporary terms it seems analogous to movement up Maslow's (1971) hierarchy of needs.

4. *Training Attention.* Contemplative traditions regard training attention and concentration as essential for psychological well-being. By contrast, Western psychology has long accepted William James's forlorn conclusion that "Attention cannot be continuously sustained" (James, 1899/1962, p51). Yet James went further to suggest that:

The faculty of voluntarily bringing back a wandering attention over and over again is the very root of judgment, character, and will. No one is *compos sui* [master of himself] if he have it not. An education which would improve this faculty would be the education par excellence. . . . It is easier to define this ideal than to give practical direction for bringing it about. (James, 1910/1950, p. 424)

Here, then, we have a stark contrast between traditional Western psychology, which says attention *cannot* be sustained, and meditators who argue that attention can be sustained, indeed *must* be sustained, if we are to mature and realize our potentials.

Developing concentration is valuable for many reasons. First, because controlling attentional wanderlust is crucial for fostering calm and concentration. Second, because the mind tends to take on qualities of the objects to which it attends, and according to yoga, "Whatever we contemplate or place our attention on, that we become" (Feuerstein, 1996, p. 71). For example, thinking of an angry person tends to produce anger, whereas contemplating a loving person elicits feelings of love. People who can control attention can choose what they focus on, and can therefore cultivate desired emotions and motives. The primary tool for developing this capacity is meditation.

5. *Refining Awareness.* The fifth central practice refines awareness by making perception—both external and internal—more sensitive, more accurate, and more appreciative of the freshness and novelty of each moment. This is necessary because, according to Asian psychologies, our awareness is usually insensitive and impaired: fragmented by attentional instability, colored by clouding emotions, and distorted by scattered desires. Similar ideas echo through Western thought, which suggests that we mistake shadows for reality (Plato) because we see through "narrow chinks" (William Blake) or a "reducing valve" (Aldous Huxley).

Meditators report that perception becomes more sensitive and their inner world more available. Both case reports (Walsh, 1984) and research indicate that meditators' perceptual processing becomes more sensitive and rapid, their empathy more accurate, and their introspection more refined (Murphy & Donovan, 1997). Meditators claim that clear awareness can be healing and transformative, and would agree with Fritz Perls (1969), the founder of Gestalt therapy, that "Awareness per se—by and of itself—can be curative" (p. 16).

6. *Wisdom.* Wisdom is deep understanding of, and practical skill in responding to, the central concerns of life, especially existential issues. Existential issues are those crucial, universal concerns that all of us face simply because we are human. They include finding meaning and purpose in a universe vast beyond comprehension, living in inevitable uncertainty and mystery, managing relationships and facing aloneness, and dealing with sickness, suffering, and death (Walsh, 1999). A person who has developed deep insights into these issues and skills for dealing with them is wise indeed.

Wisdom is considerably more than knowledge. Whereas knowledge is gained simply by acquiring information, wisdom requires understanding it. Knowledge is something we have; wisdom is something we must become. Knowledge informs us, whereas wisdom transforms us; knowledge empowers, wisdom enlightens.

Contemplative disciplines regard the cultivation of wisdom as a central goal of life. Among their many strategies, they particularly advise us to seek wisdom from the company of the wise, from the study of their writings, and from reflecting on the nature of life and death. Jewish contemplatives hold that "Wisdom comes from knowing reality" and urge us to "attend to reality with fullness of heart, mind, and action" (Shapiro, 1993, pp. 30, 84). Mature therapists—who have themselves reflected deeply on existential issues—can be of great assistance here, and can offer wise company, recommend readings, encourage introspection, and facilitate reflection.

However, contemplative traditions suggest that social interaction is best balanced with periods of quiet and solitude, especially in nature. These are the conditions that best foster calm, reflection, and introspection. Introspective exploration is crucial, and meditation is the introspective tool par excellence. Neo-Confucian wisdom promises that "If one plumbs, investigates into, sharpens, and refines oneself, a morning will come when one will gain self-enlightenment" (Creel, 1953, p. 213).

7. *Altruism and Service.* Contemplatives regard altruistic service as both a means to and an expression of psychological well-being. "Make it your guiding principle to do your best for others," urged Confucius, and "put service before the reward you get for it" (Lau, 1979, p. 116). Generosity helps transform the mind. Giving inhibits qualities such as craving, jealousy, and fear of loss while strengthening positive emotions such as love and happiness.

In addition, what we want others to experience we tend to experience ourselves. For example, if we plot revenge and pain for others, we tend to experience and reinforce emotions such as anger and hatred. Yet when we desire happiness for others, we feel it ourselves, an experience that Buddhists call "empathic joy." This is why some meditations designed to cultivate benevolent feelings toward others such as love or compassion can produce remarkably ecstatic states in ourselves.

Western psychologists are reaching similar conclusions. Generous people tend to be happier, to be psychologically healthier, and to experience a "helper's high" (Myers, 1992). As people age, they increasingly find it is their legacy—their contribution to the world and to future generations—that gives meaning and satisfaction to their lives. The so-called "paradox of pleasure" is that taking time to make others happy makes us happier than devoting all our efforts to our own pleasure (Myers, 1992). Some therapists have used this principle in their work; for example, Alfred Adler sometimes advised clients to do something for another person each day. Abraham Maslow (1970) summarized the contemplative understanding well when he said, "the best way to become a better helper is to become a better person. But one necessary aspect of becoming a better person is *via* helping other people" (p. xii).

Process of Psychotherapy

Most people who engage in contemplative practices find them slow but cumulative, and it may be several weeks before the benefits of brief daily sessions are clearly evident. Meditation and yoga are skills, and as with any skill, the initial phase can be the least rewarding. However, as with other therapies, perseverance usually brings increasing benefits. Because meditation is central to contemplative approaches, and because it is has been extensively researched and is widely used by psychotherapists, we will focus on it here.

After instruction, practice usually starts with short sessions of perhaps 20 minutes once or twice a day. One of the first discoveries that beginners make is how little control they have over their own attentional and cognitive processes, and just how much their minds and lives run on unconscious, automatic pilot. The following exercises—one a visualization and one focusing on the breath—give a glimpse of this automaticity. Read the following paragraphs. Then put down this book and do the exercises.

Visualization

Seat yourself comfortably and close your eyes. Then visualize an image of a black ring with a black dot in the middle on a white background. Make the image as clear as you can and then try to hold the image clear and stable for one to two minutes. If you become distracted, recreate the image and continue to try to hold it steady. At the end of that period, open your eyes and reflect on your experience. How much of the time were you able to hold the image clear and steady? How often were you distracted? What does this tell you about your mind and its degree of concentration, calm, and clarity? Stop reading and do the visualization now.

Breath Meditation

For this exercise, set an alarm for about 10 minutes. Then take a comfortable seat, close your eyes, and turn your attention to the sensations of breathing in your abdomen. Focus your attention carefully and precisely on the sensations that arise and pass away each instant as the abdominal wall rises and falls. Try not to let your attention wander. If thoughts or feelings arise, just let them be there, and continue to focus your awareness on the sensations.

While you attend to the sensations, start counting the breaths from 1 to 10. After you reach 10, go back to 1 again. However, if you lose count, or if your mind wanders from the sensations of the breath, even for an instant, then go back to 1 and start again. If you get distracted or lost in thoughts or fantasy, just recognize what happened, then gently bring your mind back to the breath and start counting from 1 again. Continue until the alarm tells you to stop.

Open your eyes and estimate how much of the time you were fully aware of the breath. Then take a moment to reflect on what you learned about your mind, its usual state, its concentration and focus, and your amount of control over attentional and cognitive processes. Stop reading and do the exercise now.

Most people are shocked to discover that they could not hold the image of the circle stable or maintain awareness of the breath for more than a few seconds. The mind has a mind of its own. However, with continued practice, concentration gradually improves. As it does, valuable experiences emerge, such as new insights and understandings, greater calm and clarity, and a deepening sense of happiness and well-being.

Stages of Practice

Meditation practice can be divided into six overlapping stages. The first three are stages of recognition or insight: the stages of recognizing mental dyscontrol, habitual patterns, and cognitive insights. The three advanced stages include the development of exceptional capacities, the emergence of transpersonal experiences, and the stabilization of transpersonal development.

The first stage is recognizing the remarkable yet usually unrecognized lack of control we have over our own mental processes. After my own first meditation retreat, I wrote that "Shorn of all my props and distractions, it became clear that I had little more than the faintest inkling of self-control over either thoughts or feelings and that my mind had a mind of its own . . . my former state of mindlessness or ignorance of [this] staggered me" (Walsh, 1984, pp. 265, 266). This recognition of the usual extent of our mindlessness and lack of mental control is an insight of enormous importance, because if our minds are out of control, then our lives are out of control. This recognition can seem overwhelming, but under the guidance of a good therapist, it can also be a powerful incentive to continue practicing and develop mindfulness and control.

The second stage is recognizing habitual patterns. Here, one identifies repetitive mental and behavioral patterns similar to those that insight-oriented psychotherapy unveils. However, as practice deepens, refined awareness unveils the third stage of cognitive insights. Here, one can microscopically investigate parts of the "cognitive unconscious" that are made up of subtle psychological processes such as thought, motivation, and perception. For example, one sees the way a single thought can elicit emotions, color perception, and provoke muscle tension, or how craving evokes tension, grasping at the desired object, fear of loss, and anger toward competitors.

In advanced stages, which we can consider briefly, exceptional capacities and experiences first emerge and eventually stabilize. The fourth stage is marked by the emergence of a variety of exceptional abilities, which are discussed in detail in the research section. In the fifth stage, transpersonal experiences emerge, producing identification with others and compassionate concern for them.

The sixth and final stage is one of stabilization. Here, peak experiences extend into plateau experiences, transient capacities mature into permanent abilities, and temporary transpersonal experiences stabilize into enduring transpersonal stages. For example, a practitioner might initially have brief tastes of calm and joy only during meditation sessions. However, with long-term practice, these may deepen into profound peace and joy and expand to pervade daily life. The remarkable nature of these advanced capacities can be sensed from Jack Kornfield's (2006) interview of a contemporary Buddhist meditation master:

> His mind stays completely steady, silent and free throughout both his waking and sleeping hours. He says, "I haven't experienced a single moment of anger or frustration for over twenty years." He sleeps only one or two hours a night, and describes his inner life, "When I am alone, my mind rests in pure awareness, which has peace and equanimity. Then as I encounter people and experiences, the awareness automatically manifests as loving-kindness or compassion. This is the natural function of pure awareness." (From *The Wise Heart: A Guide to the Universal Teachings of Buddhist Psychotherapies,* 9th Ed., by Jack Kornfield, ©2008 by Jack Kornfield. Used by permission of Bantam Books, a division of Random House, Inc.)

Studies of master meditators from several traditions reveal unique psychometric responses and EEG profiles consistent with some of their claims (Lutz, Dunne, & Davidson, 2007; Walsh & Shapiro, 2006). Needless to say, these advanced experiences and developmental stages are rare and usually require long-term or intensive retreat practice. However, just knowing of them gives a sense of the remarkable potentials that are latent in all of us and that contemplative practices can awaken.

Difficulties

As with any deep uncovering therapy, some experiences can be difficult. The most common are emotional lability, psychosomatic symptoms, unfamiliar perceptual changes, and existential challenges (Walsh & Shapiro, 2006; Wilber et al., 1986).

Emotional lability is probably most frequent. Intense but usually short-lived emotions may surface, such as anger, anxiety, or sadness, sometimes accompanied by psychosomatic symptoms such as muscle spasm. Often, a therapist need only encourage the practitioner to accept and investigate these experiences—and thereby allow them to resolve by themselves in the healing light of awareness.

As perception becomes more sensitive, habitual perceptions and assumptions may be questioned and unfamiliar experiences can emerge. One's sense of self and the world may change, resulting in a sense of unfamiliarity or even unreality that can produce confusion and fear. However, continued practice usually brings greater equanimity and comfort with an ever-widening range of experiences and insights.

Most profound and important are existential and spiritual challenges. Freed from external distractions and trivia, the mind naturally turns to what is most important, and so ponders questions of deep personal and human significance. These include perennial questions about life's meaning and purpose, our inevitable suffering and death, whether one is living honestly and authentically, and the nature of one's mind, identity, and destiny. These are the deepest questions of life, and focusing on them can be unsettling at first. Yet they are the gateway to wisdom, and exploring them is essential to forging a mature, authentic, and well-lived life (Walsh, 1999; Yalom, 2002).

In many cases, meditative difficulties represent the emergence of previously repressed or incompletely experienced memories and conflicts. The initial discomfort of experiencing them may therefore be a necessary price for processing and discharging them. This process is variously described as karmic release (yoga), unstressing (TM), interior purification (Christian contemplation), or catharsis and working through (psychology).

Like other uncovering therapies contemplative practices can sometimes unveil underlying pathology. The most extreme are psychotic reactions, though fortunately these are very rare. They are most likely in individuals with prior psychotic breaks, who are not taking medication, and who do intensive, unsupervised practice (Wilber et al., 1986).

Therapists familiar with both contemplative and traditional Western therapies can be especially helpful with contemplative difficulties. They can recognize and treat common minor difficulties, as well as the less common but more severe underlying pathologies that occasionally surface. Because of their personal familiarity with common difficulties, meditatively experienced therapists can recognize them in their clients, empathize sincerely, and treat them effectively.

There are many useful strategies for treating common difficulties. In many cases they resolve spontaneously with further practice, especially when a therapist provides reassurance and normalization (advice that these are normal and common challenges). *Reframing* and *reattribution* (reinterpreting experiences as potential opportunities for learning and growth) are especially valuable. Common problems can also be treated with standard Western therapeutic techniques such as relaxation or with specific remedies suggested by contemplative disciplines. It can be very valuable to explore the psychological and existential implications of contemplative experiences. Medication is rarely necessary for contemplative difficulties, which are usually transient and better treated with psychological and contemplative strategies. However, medication may be entirely appropriate where contemplatives suffer from severe psychological disorders such as depression (Walsh, Bitner, Victor, & Hillman, 2009).

Mechanisms of Psychotherapy

Explanations of how contemplative therapies work are of three main types: metaphorical, process, and mechanistic. All three are valuable because many factors are involved, and each type illuminates a facet of the rich growth process that meditation catalyzes.

Traditional explanations are usually metaphorical. Common metaphors used to describe the meditative/yogic process include *awakening* from our collective trance, *freeing* us from illusions and conditioning, and *purifying* the mind of toxic qualities. Others include *unfolding* our innate potentials, *uncovering* our true identity, and *enlightening* us about our true identity. These metaphors offer several insights. They suggest that contemplative practices set in motion growth processes that are organic, developmental, therapeutic, and self-actualizing. Some of the ways in which they do this are suggested by the following mechanisms.

Mechanisms Suggested by Contemplative Traditions

Calming the Mind.   The untrained mind is agitated and distracted, continuously leaping from past to future, from thought to fantasy. Contemplative techniques concentrate and calm the mind. As the opening lines of a classic yoga text state,

> Yoga is the settling of the mind into silence. When the mind has settled, we are established in our essential nature, which is unbounded Consciousness. Our essential nature is overshadowed by the activity of the mind. (Shearer, 1989, p. 49)

This process of calming and stilling is the basis for the Western suggestion that meditation works, in part, by producing a "relaxation response."

Enhanced Awareness.   Heightened awareness is emphasized across contemplative practices (Walsh, 1999; Walsh & Shapiro, 2006). It is the primary focus in Buddhist mindfulness and Taoist "internal observation," and is also central to the Sufi practice of "watchfulness of the moment" and the Christian contemplative discipline of "guarding the intellect." Many clinicians also regard it as central to psychotherapy. In fact, "virtually all therapies endorse the expansion of consciousness . . ." (enhanced awareness) (Norcross & Beutler, 2010). Examples include Eugene Gendlin's "experiencing" and the Jungian claim that "therapeutic progress depends on awareness . . ." (Whitmont, 1969, p. 293). Refining awareness may therefore be a central process mediating the benefits of both meditations and psychotherapies. It may also be a necessary precondition for a further important contemplative process: disidentification.

Disidentification.   This is the process by which awareness (mindfulness) precisely observes and therefore ceases to unconsciously identify with mental content such as thoughts, feelings, and fantasies (Walsh & Shapiro, 2006). For example, if the thought "I'm scared" arises but is not carefully observed and recognized as just a thought, then it becomes a belief and is accepted as reality. One identifies with the thought, which is no longer something that is seen; rather, it is that from which and through which one sees. What was an object of awareness has become the subject of awareness; what was "it" has become "me." The self is now identified with or embedded in this thought. One's experiential reality is now "I'm scared," and this identification sets in motion corresponding psychological, neural, and physiological fear responses that appear to validate the reality of the thought. What was actually merely a thought now appears to be reality.

However, if the meditator is sufficiently mindful when the thought "I'm scared" arises, then it is recognized as what it is: merely a thought. It is not mistaken for reality, it has little effect on mind or body, and the neuroendocrine fear response does not occur. Awareness has disidentified from the thought and therefore remains free of its entrapping effects. This can be considered a form of self-dehypnosis. Of course, the meditator can still act on the thought if appropriate, but such action is now a conscious choice rather than an unconscious automaticity.

Western researchers recognize similar processes. For example, the Harvard developmental psychologist Robert Kegan (1982) claims that psychological growth involves "making what was subject into object so that we can 'have' it rather than 'be had' by it—this is the most powerful way I know to conceptualize the growth of the mind . . . [and] is as faithful to the self-psychology of the West as to the 'wisdom literature' of the East" (pp. 33–34).

Similarly, acceptance and commitment therapy describes the process of "defusion," Jean Piaget speaks of "decentration," Ken Wilber speaks of "differentiation," and other therapists speak of "dehypnosis" and "metacognitive awareness" (Wilber, 2000a). All these different terms point to a common principle: When we unconsciously identify with a part of the mind, we are bound by it; when we consciously disidentify from it, we are free. As contemplatives put it "Nonidentification . . . is liberation" (Nisargadatta, 1973, p. 126).

Rebalancing Mental Elements.   Contemplative psychologies commonly divide mental contents into healthy and unhealthy categories. Naturally, a major goal is to increase healthy factors and decrease unhealthy ones, which can be seen as a rebalancing of mental elements and viewed metaphorically as purification.

Buddhist psychology offers a particularly sophisticated map of mental elements and emphasizes the "seven factors of enlightenment." These are seven qualities of mind that, when cultivated and balanced one with another, are said to optimize health and growth.

when cultivated and balanced one with another, are said to optimize health and growth. The first factor is *mindfulness,* a precise conscious awareness of each stimulus that can be regarded as a refinement of the psychoanalytic observing ego. The remaining six mental factors are divided into two groups of three energizing qualities and three calming qualities. The three energizing factors are *effort, investigation* (active exploration of experience), and *rapture* (ecstasy that results from clear, concentrated awareness). The three calming factors are *concentration, calm,* and *equanimity.*

This model of mental health invites interesting comparisons between contemplative and conventional Western therapies (Walsh & Vaughan, 1993). Western therapists recognize that the energizing factors of effort and investigation are essential. However, they are less aware of the potentiating effects of simultaneously developing the calming factors. When the mind is concentrated, calm, and equanimous, then awareness is clearer, insight deeper, and growth quicker. Cultivating and balancing all seven factors is said to be optimal for growth and to lead to the pinnacle of transpersonal maturity: enlightenment.

Mechanisms Suggested by Mental Health Professionals

Western researchers have suggested a range of psychological and physiological mechanisms to account for the effects of meditation. Psychological possibilities include relaxation, desensitization to formerly stressful stimuli, counter-conditioning, and catharsis. Automatic habits may undergo "deautomatization," becoming less automatic and coming under greater voluntary control. Cognitive mechanisms include learning and insight, as well as self-acceptance, self-control, and self-understanding (Baer, 2005). Suggested physiological mechanisms include reduced arousal, stress immunization, hemispheric lateralization (a shift in relative activity of the cerebral hemispheres), and a rebalancing of the autonomic nervous system (Cahn & Polich, 2006).

Probably the most encompassing explanation is developmental. Both contemplatives and psychologists suggest that meditation may work many of its effects by restarting and catalyzing development. In fact, many traditions map progress in developmental terms. Classic examples include the Jewish "stages of ascent," Sufi levels of identity, yogic levels of *samadhi* (concentration), Taoism's "five periods" of increasing calm, and the Buddhist "stages of insight." Research studies of TM are supportive and suggest that it fosters ego, cognitive development, and moral development, as well as coping skills and self-actualization (Alexander et al., 1991). The value of practices that can foster psychological maturity is obvious.

APPLICATIONS

Who Can We Help?

Contemplative practices help with an exceptionally wide range of psychological, somatic, and spiritual issues, and hardly a month goes by without a research study demonstrating yet another effect or application. We can divide the kinds of benefits and areas of application into three groups. First are therapeutic applications for psychological and psychosomatic disorders. Second is the enhancement of well-being, and third are the classic goals that revolve around transpersonal growth and spirituality.

Therapeutic Applications

Psychological Disorders.   Contemplative practices appear helpful with a wide array of psychological and psychosomatic disorders, and stress disorders have been the most extensively researched. For example, mindfulness meditation can ameliorate generalized panic, phobic, and post-traumatic stress disorders, as well as eating disorders (Murphy & Donovan, 1997; Shapiro & Carlson, 2009).

Meditation also reduces anxiety in special populations. Examples include the dying and their caregivers, as well as prisoners who also display reduced aggression and recidivism. Given the large numbers of people languishing in prison, especially in the United States, and their tragically high recidivism rates, these findings are of considerable importance (Alexander, Walton, Orme-Johnson, Goodman, & Pallone, 2003). TM also reduces the use of both legal and illegal drugs (Alexander, Robinson, & Rainforth, 1994). However, TM practitioners are required to stop using drugs for several days before their initial training, so they may be mildly addicted and particularly responsive.

These stress-related benefits are consistent both with classic claims and with physiological studies of meditators. Physiologically, practitioners show lowered readings on stress measures such as muscle tension, galvanic skin response, and stress-related blood chemicals and hormones. Classically, "Relaxation is the alpha and omega of yoga" (Feuerstein, 1996, p. 51), and this claim has been popularized as the idea that meditation involves a "relaxation response." However, the research support for yoga's effectiveness in reducing anxiety and depressive disorders is promising but inconclusive (Kirkwood, Rampes, Tuffrey, Richardson, & Pilkington, 2005; Pilkington, Kirkwood, Rampes, & Richardson, 2005).

We have previously explored some of the many combination therapies that meld mindfulness with conventional Western psychotherapies, and these have proved effective with several additional disorders. The original approach, mindfulness-based stress reduction (MBSR), has been applied to stress, chronic pain, and multiple other conditions. Mindfulness-based approaches targeting specific disorders include mindfulness-based cognitive therapy for recurrent depression (Coelho, Canter, & Ernst, 2007), mindfulness-based eating awareness therapy (MB-EAT) for eating disorders, and mindfulness-based therapy for insomnia. Other interventions that include a meditation component include relapse prevention for alcohol and drug abuse and dialectical behavior therapy for borderline disorders (Baer, 2005). New combinations continue to appear and will doubtless be applied to more and more disorders.

Many therapists have commented on the mutually beneficial interaction that can occur when clients engage in both conventional psychotherapy and a contemplative discipline. Conventional therapies can help clients deal with painful memories and conflicts that emerge during meditation and yoga and with defenses and other blocks inhibiting contemplative progress. Likewise, meditation and yoga can facilitate conventional psychotherapy by cultivating requisite skills, such as calm and introspection, and by allowing clients to work on issues outside the therapeutic hour.

Somatic Disorders.   Contemplative therapies may be useful in helping to treat some diseases and to reduce the anxiety and distress that accompany many diseases. Considerable research has focused on the effects of meditation on psychosomatic disorders, especially those in which stress plays a causal or complicating role, and many disorders are at least partially responsive (Shapiro & Carlson, 2009).

Several benefits occur in the cardiovascular system. High blood pressure and cholesterol are reduced (Anderson, Liu, & Kryscio, 2008), but benefits dissipate if the practice is discontinued. Coronary artery disease, a leading cause of death and disability, was long thought to be irreversible and to require major surgery or cholesterol-lowering drugs. However, research demonstrates that far less dangerous and far more healthy lifestyle changes—especially a combination of low-fat diet, exercise, interpersonal openness, and meditation and yoga—can actually reverse the disorder. These lifestyle changes also seem to slow or perhaps even reverse the progression of prostate cancer (Ornish, 2008).

Hormonal and immune systems are also affected by meditation. Partially responsive hormonal disorders include type II diabetes, primary dysmenorrhea, and premenstrual syndrome, now called premenstrual dysphoric disorder (Murphy & Donovan, 1997). Meditation can also enhance immune function in both healthy people and cancer patients (Kabat-Zinn, 2003), while acceptance and commitment therapy reduced the frequency of epileptic episodes.

Meditation may also enhance conventional treatments. Examples include asthma, psoriasis, prostate cancer, and chronic pain disorders (Kabat-Zinn, 2003). Not surprisingly, meditation and perhaps yoga and Tai Chi can reduce symptoms of distress in a wide array of illnesses, including cancer, fibromyalgia, and rheumatoid arthritis (Klein & Adams, 2004; Ott, 2006; Shapiro & Carlson, 2009). A comprehensive meta-analysis of health-related MBSR interventions concluded that "results suggest that MBSR may help a broad range of individuals to cope with their clinical and nonclinical problems" (Grossman, Niemann, Schmidt, & Walach, 2004, p. 35). Since anxiety and distress are common complicating factors in so many illnesses, contemplative practices will likely prove useful adjuvant therapies for many somatic disorders.

Enhancing Well-Being

Considerable research suggests that contemplative practices can be used by clients, therapists, and the general population to enhance psychological well-being and growth (Murphy & Donovan, 1997; Walsh & Shapiro, 2006). Improvements occur in subjective well-being as well as on multiple measures of personality and performance.

Mental capacities such as perception, cognition, and creativity may be enhanced. Perceptually, measures of sensitivity and empathy improve. So do cognitive skills such as concentration, reaction time, and short- and long-term memory. Not surprisingly, academic performance also improves (Shapiro, Astin, Bishop, & Cordova, 2005).

Personality variables change. As expected, several kinds of meditation appear to reduce trait anxiety. A study of the "big five" personality factors found that conscientiousness remained unaffected, while the other four—extraversion, agreeableness, openness to experience, and especially emotional stability—all increased (Travis, Arenander, & DuBois, 2004). These are striking findings given how little personality usually changes in adulthood.

Since meditation functions as a self-regulation strategy, it is not surprising that practitioners report improved self-control and self-esteem. Likewise, because meditators display greater empathy (Shapiro et al., 2005), it is also not surprising that several studies have demonstrated enhanced interpersonal functioning and marital satisfaction. A mindfulness-based relationship enhancement program was successful in improving multiple measures of both individual and relationship satisfaction in couples. Individuals felt more relaxed and optimistic, and as a couple they felt closer yet also more autonomous, accepting, and satisfied. Benefits persisted through a 3-month follow-up period (Carson, Carson, Gil, & Baucom, 2004).

A classic contemplative goal is to encourage mental maturation, and several studies, most employing TM, are supportive. Meditators tend to score higher on measures of ego, moral, and cognitive development, as well as in self-actualization, coping skills, defenses, and states and stages of consciousness (Alexander et al., 1991; Travis et al., 2004).

Contemplative practices may also be associated with enhanced general psychological and physical health and with reduced signs of aging. TM meditators use approximately half the usual amounts of psychiatric and medical care. Practitioners also score significantly younger on markers of biological age than control subjects, and the extent of improvement correlates with amount of meditation (Alexander, Langer, Newman, Chandler, & Davies, 1989). Meditators also have "younger" chromosomes, greater cortical and hippocampal brain size, and less age-related thinning of the cerebral cortex (Pagnoni & Cekic, 2007). However, it is not clear how much of this superior general health is actually due to meditation, and how much to associated factors such as prior good health and a healthy lifestyle.

One well-designed study demonstrated dramatic effects on elderly retirement home residents whose average age was 81. Those who learned TM performed better on several measures of cognitive function and mental health than residents who were taught relaxation, were given other mental training, or were left untreated. However, the most striking finding was a highly significant (p < 0.001) difference in survival rates. Three years later, all the meditators were still alive, compared to only three-quarters of the untreated study subjects, and only two-thirds of residents who did not participate in the study (Alexander et al., 1989). For thousands of years, yogis have claimed that contemplative practices increase longevity, and this claim now has initial experimental support. Needless to say, studies of this importance deserve careful replication.

Benefits for Health Professionals

Shapiro and Carlson (2009) point out that "Learning to manage stress and enhance self-care should be an essential dimension of clinical training and professional development." In fact, it rarely is. High stress levels are common challenges for health care professions, and both they and their patients pay a price. Clinical observations and research suggest that a personal contemplative practice can ameliorate professionals' stress and offer both personal and professional benefits. For example, meditation reduced symptoms of stress—such as anxiety and depression—while enhancing empathy and life satisfaction, in pre-health care students, medical students, and health care professionals (Shapiro et al., 2005).

Meditation may also enhance essential therapist qualities. Such qualities include Rogers's "accurate empathy," as well as attentional qualities such as Freud's "evenly hovering attention" and Horney's "wholehearted attention." Karen Horney (1952/1998) observed that although "such wholeheartedness is a rare attainment," it is "commonplace in Zen" (p. 36). Other capacities enhanced by meditation—such as self-actualization, self-acceptance, and calm—may also benefit clinicians (Germer, Siegel, & Fulton, 2005).

Therapists report that the deep insights into the workings of their own minds that contemplative practices provide also foster insight into and compassion for their clients. Many therapists feel that their skills are enhanced by these practices and recommend them as part of psychotherapists' training. A study of psychotherapists who were taught mindfulness during their training found that their patients had significantly better treatment outcomes than those of control group therapists (Grepmair, et al., 2007).

Not surprisingly, personal contemplative practice can enhance psychotherapists' ability to work with patients who are themselves contemplatives. Personal practice of meditation deepens clinicians' understanding of contemplative experiences, increases their ability to diagnose and work with meditators' difficulties, and enhances empathy and therapeutic effectiveness (Germer et al., 2005).

Transpersonal Growth

Finally, contemplative disciplines are available for those who wish to practice more intensely in order to foster transpersonal growth. Here, they can be used to explore the mind, to grapple with existential questions, to develop exceptional abilities and well-being, and to seek advanced levels of psychological and spiritual maturity. Coming to voluntary control of one's own mind is a "master aptitude" that fosters multiple capacities.

Although deep insights can occur at any moment, these exceptional capacities and levels often require long-term practice reckoned in years rather than days or weeks. Of course, this is true of any kind of mastery.

Specific Techniques and Skills

The discussion so far has focused on general principles common to most meditation and yoga practices. In addition to these general practices, there are literally hundreds of specific meditative and yogic techniques designed to elicit particular capacities and skills. The following are brief descriptions of two skills—the cultivation of love and lucid dreaming—which until recently Western psychologists considered impossible. Together, they point to the remarkable range of practices and powers of mind that contemplatives have discovered in their 3,000-year-long exploration of our inner universe.

The Cultivation of Love.   There are many specific meditations and techniques for cultivating love. One meditation begins by calming the mind and then focusing attention unwaveringly on an image of someone you love. In a calm, concentrated state, feelings of love arise intensely. After they do, you gradually and successively substitute images of a friend, a stranger, and groups of people, and thereby cultivate and condition the feelings of love to them. Eventually you visualize all people while embracing them in love. Long-term effects include not only deep encompassing feelings of love, but also the reduction of anger, fear, and defensiveness (Kornfield, 1993).

There are also practices for cultivating related emotions such as *empathic joy* (happiness at the happiness of others, which is a superb antidote to jealousy) and *compassion* (the basis for altruism). Western psychologists have recently found evidence for altruism's existence as an independent drive but lament that they know of no way to cultivate it. In contrast, contemplative disciplines contain literally dozens of exercises for fostering altruism.

Lucid Dreaming.   Dream yoga is a 2,000-year-old technique for developing lucid dreaming: the ability to know one is dreaming while still asleep. Adepts are able to observe and modify their dreams so as to continue their explorations and learning during sleep. The most advanced practitioners maintain unbroken awareness throughout the night, during both dream and nondream sleep, thereby combining the benefits of clear awareness and the extreme peace of conscious sleep. The result is continuous lucidity—or "ever-present wakefulness," as the contemplative Plotinus called it—throughout day and night.

Western psychologists dismissed lucid dreaming as impossible for many years until sleep EEGs demonstrated its existence. Since then, further studies have demonstrated even more remarkable abilities. Advanced dream yoga practitioners have long claimed to be able to remain lucid and aware throughout the night, during both dreaming and nondreaming sleep, and recent EEG studies support these claims. Both classic instructions and contemporary induction techniques are now freely available. Consequently, people can now enjoy this ancient yogic skill and can explore and cultivate the mind in the comfort of their own beds (Walsh & Vaughan, 1993). For Freud, dreams were a royal road to the unconscious. For contemplatives, lucid dreams are a royal road to consciousness.

Treatment

As contemplative therapies evolved across centuries, practitioners devised literally thousands of techniques ranging across somatic, psychological, and spiritual domains. These include everything from diet and breathing disciplines through ethical and lifestyle changes to visualizations and meditations (Feuerstein, 1996). In general, novices begin with one or two simple meditative or yogic practices. Over time, they add related exercises and begin more demanding practices so that more and more of their experiences and lives are used for learning and growth. Tailoring the evolving program to the individual practitioner is the mark of a skilled therapist. The following are simple introductory exercises and meditations—from each of the seven practices common to contemplative therapies—that have proved valuable for both clients and therapists.

Ethical Behavior: Say Only What Is True and Helpful

Mark Twain is credited with the line "Truth is so very precious, man is naturally economical in its use," but contemplative disciplines take a different approach. Meditators cannot long escape recognizing the destructive effects—among them anxiety, guilt, and agitation—that unethical behavior such as deceit and aggression has on their own minds. As a result, the desire to live more truthfully and ethically grows stronger.

Truth telling does not imply blurting out everything that comes to mind or being insensitive to people's feelings. Rather, it means bringing careful awareness to each situation to find what we can say that is true to our experience and, wherever possible, helpful to others. When we don't know what is truthful or helpful, it is appropriate either to say we don't know or to remain silent.

Exercise 1: Look for the Lie.   It is intriguing to see how much personal and interpersonal pain is a result of lying, either to oneself or to others. Consequently, a useful exercise during psychotherapy (and life) is to look for the lies that are causing and perpetuating suffering, and then to explore how to end them.

Exercise 2: Say Only What Is True and Helpful for a Day.   An excellent way to begin the practice of truth telling is to commit to doing it for a day. This exercise becomes even more powerful if you carefully record any temptations to lie and identify the motives and emotions underpinning these temptations. On hearing of this exercise, some people obsess over the question of what "the truth" is. However, the point is not to become lost in endless philosophical musings but, rather, to be honest about the only thing we ever know: our experience.

Transforming Emotions: Using Wise Attention to Cultivate Beneficial Emotions

By enhancing concentration, contemplative practices allow us to practice "wise attention." This is the practice of directing attention to people and situations that foster desired qualities (Walsh, 1999). The underlying principle is that we tend to strengthen those qualities to which we give attention. What we focus on, we become. For example, many studies show that watching violence on television can foster aggression. On the other hand, contemplative therapies suggest that when we attend to people who are kind and generous, we cultivate these qualities in ourselves (Kornfield, 1993). What we put into our minds is just as important as what we put into our mouths.

Exercise.   First, relax or meditate and be aware of how you feel. Notice the emotions you are experiencing. Next, visualize or think of someone who tends to be angry and aggressive. Notice any emotions that arise and how you feel. Then take a moment to relax or meditate again. Now visualize or think of someone who is kind and loving and observe the corresponding emotions. Note how differently you feel after visualizing these two people. What we meditate on, we cultivate. Put down the book and do the exercise now.

Transforming Motivation: Exploring the Experience of Craving

Bringing clear awareness to experiences and behavior is crucial to transforming them. Yet when caught by an addiction, we usually focus on what we are trying to get rather than on the actual experience of craving and what it is doing to our mind.

Exercise.   For this exercise, take the opportunity to carefully explore craving. You can do this in two ways: You can wait for an addictive urge to arise spontaneously, or you can choose to think of something you're attached to. For this exercise, it's best to work with a mild craving rather than one that may overwhelm you. When you become aware of a craving, stop whatever you are doing. Then turn attention to your craving and explore it. Try to identify the experiential components that make it up: the underlying emotions, body sensations, thoughts, feelings, and tensions. Bringing careful awareness to the experience of craving rather than mindlessly acting it out gives insight into it and can also decondition and weaken it. In fact, contemplative disciplines suggest that weak addictions "can be removed by introspection and meditation" (Nisargadatta, 1973, p. 112).

Developing Concentration and Calm: Do One Thing at a Time

In our overly busy lives, distractions proliferate, electronic gadgets demand attention, and we often juggle several things simultaneously. New words are emerging to describe our jangled lives and minds, words such as *multitasking, technostress, digital fog, techno-brain burnout, frazzing* (frantic, inefficient multitasking), and *attention-deficit trait,* which is characterized by symptoms similar to those of attention-deficit disorder but is caused by information and work overload.

Multitasking gives an illusion of efficiency. Yet research now shows what contemplative therapies have argued for centuries: Multitasking and attentional fragmentation actually reduce efficiency and creativity while at the same time inflicting anxiety and agitation. Perhaps just as important, they also reduce clarity, thoughtful reflection, and introspection. Distracted, fragmented lives create distracted, fragmented minds.

Contemplative therapies counteract frenzy and fragmentation by fostering concentration and calm. Regular practice of concentration meditation—such as focusing attention on the breath, as described earlier—is an excellent method. The following exercise is a useful addition.

Exercise: Do One Thing at a Time.   To begin, commit a specific time—a day might be good to begin with—to doing only one thing at a time. For this day, give up all multitasking. Give your full attention to each individual activity and each conversation. This very simple exercise can have dramatic effects.

Cultivating Awareness: Mindfulness Meditation and Mindful Eating

After a lifetime of therapeutic work, the Jungian psychiatrist Edward Whitmont (1969) concluded that "Therapeutic progress depends upon awareness; in fact the attempt to become more conscious is the therapy" (p. 293). Contemplative traditions agree and have long emphasized the value of cultivating awareness and introspection. Buddhist meditators are told to observe each experience, while Jewish and Christian contemplatives, respectively, urge us to "Attend to each moment" and "Above all . . . be watchful" (Palmer, Sherrard, & Ware, 1993, p. 97; Shapiro, 1993, p. 17). However, contemplatives recommend that awareness be cultivated not only during therapy sessions but during every waking moment. The goal is to become what Carl Rogers called "fully functioning people [who] are able to experience all their feelings, afraid of none of them, allowing awareness to flow freely in and through their experiences" (Raskin & Rogers, 1995, p. 141). For this, contemplative disciplines recommend mindfulness (awareness) meditation coupled with awareness exercises.

Mindfulness meditation is an art. Like any art, it is best learned via personal instruction, and mastery requires long-term practice. However, even brief experiences can sometimes offer valuable insights, and the following exercise offers a taste of the process. It is best done in quiet surroundings where you will not be disturbed.

Exercise 1: Mindfulness Meditation.   Set an alarm for a period of 10 to 15 minutes, find a comfortable sitting posture, and take a moment to relax. Then, let your attention settle on the sensations of the breath and investigate these physical sensations as sensitively and carefully as you can. Continue to explore those sensations until another stimulus—perhaps a sound, emotion, or sensation—draws attention to it. Then simply explore this stimulus sensitively and carefully until it disappears or is no longer interesting. At this point, return attention to the breath until attracted by another stimulus.

Periodically you will recognize that you have been lost in thoughts and fantasies. At that point, simply return to the breath and start again. Awareness meditation is a gentle dance of awareness in which you begin with the breath, allow attention to move to interesting stimuli, explore them, and then return to the breath.

Simply investigate experiences as carefully as you can, allowing them to come and go without interference, without judging, condemning, or struggling to change them. Not surprisingly, this cessation of struggle can eventually lead to deep peace, but most beginners are initially shocked to discover how agitated their minds are. Take a few minutes now to do the meditation and see for yourself.

Mindfulness meditation is a gentle exercise in cultivating awareness, insight, and acceptance. It is based on the recognition, recently popularized by acceptance and commitment therapy (ACT), that within the mind, whatever we bring awareness to and accept can begin to heal. Conversely, what we resist or attempt to suppress can rebound, producing an "ironic effect" opposite to what we want. Contemplative traditions, and especially mindfulness meditations, therefore emphasize that, to put it poetically,

Be kind to your mind
For what you resist will surely persist,
But what you befriend may come to an end.

Exercise 2: Mindful Eating.   More than 2,000 years ago, Confucius' grandson observed that "Amongst people there are none who do not eat and drink but there are few who really appreciate the taste" (Yu-Lan, 1948, p. 175). Apparently things have not changed much. Often we multitask distractedly, even as we eat. We sit down to a meal and also carry on a conversation, watch television, or read the newspaper. The next thing we notice is that our plate is empty. No wonder that mindful eating is an effective strategy for weight control.

For this exercise, choose a time when you can eat without distraction. Seat yourself comfortably and take a few mindful breaths to relax. Mindfully eating involves attending to and enjoying each sensation and taste, so begin by enjoying the sight and smell of the food. Observe the sensations as you reach for it, the feelings of anticipation, and the touch as it enters the mouth. Then note experiences such as subtle background flavors, the temperature and texture of the food, and feelings of pleasure. Continue to eat each mouthful carefully, consciously, and as enjoyably as you can. Periodically, you will realize that you have been lost in thoughts or fantasies and were quite unaware of the last few mouthfuls. That is how we usually eat and live our lives: in semiconscious distraction. Simply return attention to the experience of eating again and enjoy your meal as fully as you can.

Of course, many meals are social occasions and celebrations, and here mindful eating is more difficult. But the basic issue is the same as with other meditations and therapies. It is the "challenge of generalization," the challenge of generalizing the skills learned in therapy to other areas of life.

Developing Wisdom: Reflecting on Our Mortality

Contemplative therapies offer many techniques for cultivating wisdom, and among them, careful reflections on our life and inevitable death are deemed particularly powerful. Without recognizing our mortality, we tend to squander our lives in inauthentic petty pursuits, to tranquilize ourselves with trivia, and to forget what really matters. Contemplative disciplines emphasize that, as Mohammad stated, "Death is a good advisor" (Angha, 1995, p. 82.) They therefore encourage us to recall that, as Taoists point out, our lives last "but a moment" and that, in Shankara's words, "Youth, wealth and the years of a [person's] life . . . roll quickly away like drops of water from a lotus leaf" (Prabhavananda & Isherwood, 1978, p. 136). When we remember that we don't know how long we and other people will live, we are inspired to live more fully, more lovingly, more boldly, and more impeccably.

Mortality and Wisdom Reflections.   The following questions are common topics for reflection in contemplative disciplines and can be examined in several formats. One approach is to reflect on them in therapy sessions. However, they can also be pondered alone, written about in a journal, or discussed with a trusted friend. Advanced practitioners use the power of concentrated awareness to meditate on them. Consider using one of these formats to explore the following questions:

- Given that we will all die, what is truly important in your life?
- If you were to die tomorrow, what would you regret not having done?
- What relationships remain unhealed in your life, and how could you begin healing them?

These reflections can motivate us to reorder our priorities, to live more fully and authentically, and to heal our relationships (Walsh, 1999).

Generosity and Service: Transforming Pain into Compassion

Research shows that one effective strategy for combating sadness and grief is "downward comparison," in which we compare ourselves with others who are worse off (Myers, 1992). However, contemplative traditions suggest that it can be taken further and used as an effective strategy for cultivating compassion.

Compassion Exercise.   Traditionally, this exercise, like so many contemplative exercises, would be done after a period of meditation. The mind is then calm and concentrated, and this enhances the effects of selected thoughts and images. Therefore, if you already know how to meditate, begin by doing so. Otherwise, simply relax for a moment.

Think of some difficulty you are having, either physical or psychological. Next, think of people who are suffering from related difficulties, perhaps even more than you are. If you know specific individuals suffering in this way, bring them to mind. Think of the pain your difficulty has brought you and of all the pain others must be experiencing. Recognize that, just as you want to be free of pain, so do they. Open yourself to the experience of their suffering and let concern and compassion for them arise. Stop reading and do the exercise now.

Defenseless awareness of the suffering of others arouses compassion and contribution. Contemplative traditions agree that compassionate service to others "clarifies the mind and purifies the heart" (Nisargadatta, 1973, p. 72) and is therefore both a means to and an expression of psychological maturity and well-being.

Contemplative therapies begin by presenting simple introductory meditations and exercises such as these. As skill develops, practitioners are encouraged to practice more deeply and intensely and to move on to more advanced disciplines.

Evidence

The classic approach to evaluating contemplative therapies is via personal experience. For thousands of years, the traditional answer to the question "Do these techniques work?" has been "Try them for yourself." However, several hundred studies now demonstrate these therapies' psychological effects on personality and performance, physiological effects on body and brain, biochemical shifts in chemicals and hormones, and therapeutic benefits for mind and body, patients and therapists.

Exceptional Aspects of the Research

The research on contemplative practices is exceptional in several ways.

- First is the sheer amount, most of it on meditation, making meditation one of the most extensively researched of all psychotherapies.

- Second is the wide array of demonstrated effects. In addition to diverse psychological changes and psychotherapeutic benefits, research has demonstrated developmental, physiological, biochemical, and neural effects—far more than for any other therapy.

- The research demonstrates multiple exceptional abilities.

- Research support is available for most applications (it has been summarized throughout this chapter as specific disorders have been discussed). Consequently, this section focuses on general research principles and on some psychological effects not already covered, especially exceptional abilities. Space precludes detailing the numerous physiological, biochemical, and neural findings.

Several extensive research reviews are available. (For TM studies, see Alexander et al., 1991, 2003. Reviews of mindfulness meditation include Baer, 2005; Didonna, 2009; Germer et al., 2005; and Kabat-Zinn, 2003. Summaries of EEG and brain-imaging studies include Cahn & Polich, 2006 and Lutz et al., 2007. For an overview of the implications of the meeting of meditative disciplines and Western psychology, see Walsh & Shapiro, 2006. For an annotated bibliography of research, see Murphy & Donovan, 1997, and for an overview of clinical applications, see Shapiro & Carlson, 2009.)

Who Benefits?

A crucial question for all therapies is "What type of client is likely to benefit?" TM studies suggest that successful practitioners are likely to be interested in internal experiences, open to unusual ones, and willing to recognize unfavorable personal characteristics. They may also have a sense of self-control, have good concentration, and be less emotionally labile and psychologically disturbed (Alexander et al., 1991; Murphy & Donovan, 1997).

It is still unclear how durable various contemplative effects are. Some simple physiological changes (such as reduced blood pressure) tend to dissipate if practice is discontinued. However, other effects probably persist in the long term, even if practice ceases, depending on factors such as the extent to which they are reinforced and incorporated into lifestyles.

Exceptional Abilities

One thing that sets contemplative approaches apart from traditional Western psychotherapies is their claim to be able to enhance psychological well-being, development, and abilities beyond normal levels (Walsh & Shapiro, 2006). This claim sounds less presumptuous than it once did because of the considerable evidence now available that, under favorable circumstances, development can proceed to postconventional levels. Examples include postconventional morality, Maslow's metamotives, Loevinger's integrated stage of ego development, and post-formal operational cognition. Contemplative disciplines claim to facilitate development to these kinds of stages and beyond, and growing research offers initial support for exceptional abilities such as those described in the following paragraphs.

Attention and Concentration.   William James (1899/1962) famously concluded that "Attention cannot be continuously sustained. . . ." (p. 51). However, contemplative disciplines insist that it can, even to the point of unbroken continuity over hours, as in advanced yogic *samadhi*, Christian *contemplation*, and TM's "cosmic consciousness." For example, in the Buddhist state of "calm abiding," according to the Dalai Lama (2001), "your mind remains placed on its object effortlessly, for as long as you wish" (p. 144). Several studies now offer support for these claims, demonstrating that meditation can enhance concentration and resultant perceptual capacities, even to levels previously though impossible (Carter, Presti, Callistemon, Ungerer, Liu, & Pettigrew, 2009).

Emotional Maturity.   Like Western therapies, contemplative therapies aim to reduce destructive emotions. For Taoists, a goal is "emotions but no ensnarement," and for the Dalai Lama, "the true mark of a meditator is that he has disciplined his mind by freeing it from negative emotions" (Goleman, 2003, p. 26).

Going beyond most Western therapies, contemplative practices also aim to cultivate positive emotions such as joy, love, and compassion. Examples include the intense, unwavering, and all-encompassing love of Buddhist *metta,* yogic *bhakti,* and Christian contemplative *agape,* as well as the compassion of Confucian *jen.* This suggests that negative emotions can be reduced and positive ones strengthened far more than therapists usually assume possible. Experiments demonstrate such shifts. Meditators tend to become happier whether practicing in daily life or more intensely in retreat. They report fewer negative emotions and more positive ones, and their EEG patterns shift accordingly. Advanced practitioners demonstrate EEG shifts associated with exceptionally high levels of well-being (Goleman, 2003; Lutz et al., 2007; Shapiro et al., 2005).

Equanimity.   Equanimity is the capacity for maintaining calm and mental equilibrium in the face of provocative stimuli. Equanimity is the opposite of reactivity, agitation, or emotional lability and is highly valued across contemplative traditions. It is, for example, a basis of the Sufi's "contented self," yogic "evenness," the Christian contemplative's "divine *apatheia,*" and Taoism's "principle of the equality of things." Equanimity extends Western concepts of "stress resistance," "emotional resilience" and "affect tolerance" to include not only tolerance but even serenity in the face of provocative stimuli and has obvious clinical potential. Preliminary experimental support comes from measures of emotional stability and startle response (Goleman, 2003; Travis et al., 2004).

Moral Maturity.   How to foster moral maturity is one of today's most crucial questions, and it is no exaggeration to say that the fate of our species and our planet may depend on how well we answer it. Unfortunately, traditional interventions, such as instruction in moral thinking, produce only modest gains. Contemplative traditions claim to be able to enhance ethical motivation and behavior in several ways. These include reducing problematic motives and emotions (such as greed and anger), strengthening morality-supporting emotions (such as love and compassion), sensitizing awareness to the costs of unethical acts (such as guilt in oneself and pain produced in others), cultivating altruism, and identifying with others via transpersonal experience (Dalai Lama, 2001; Walsh, 1999).

Western research and theory offer partial support. The researcher Lawrence Kohlberg eventually grounded his highest stage of moral maturity in the kinds of transpersonal experiences that meditation induces. Likewise, Carol Gilligan concluded that women develop along a moral trajectory—maturing from *selfish* to *care* to *universal care*—similar to contemplative maturation (Wilber, 2000b). Experimental support comes from TM practitioners whose increased moral development scores correlate with duration of practice and with EEG measures (Travis et al., 2004).

Unique Abilities

In addition to the exceptional capacities described above, advanced meditators have now demonstrated more than a dozen abilities that psychologists once dismissed as impossible (Walsh & Shapiro, 2006). Some of these, such as lucid dream and lucid nondream sleep, have already been described. Mastery of processes that are usually involuntary includes control of both perception and the autonomic nervous system. Other fascinating findings include a unique integrative cognitive style, dramatic reduction of drive conflicts, areas of increased cortical thickness, and the ability to detect fleeting facial expressions of emotion (even more effectively than the previous top scorers, CIA agents).

Initial studies of a single advanced Tibetan Buddhist practitioner found two further unique capacities. The first was almost complete inhibition of the startle response. The second was an ability to respond with compassion and relaxation while observing a video of a severely burned patient that ordinarily elicits intense disgust. The researcher conducting these studies stated that these were "findings that in 35 years of research I'd never seen before" (Goleman, 2003, p. 19).

Coupled with the research on postconventional development, these exceptional and unique abilities hold remarkable implications. They suggest that what we long assumed to be "normality" and the ceiling of psychological development is not fixed. We have greatly underestimated our own potentials, and we are capable of further development. In fact, what we call normality is looking more and more like a kind of unrecognized collective developmental arrest. Both contemplative and conventional research now support Abraham Maslow's startling claim that "what we call 'normal' in psychology is really a psychopathology of the average, so undramatic and so widely spread that we don't even notice it ordinarily" (Maslow, 1968, p. 16). To paraphrase Shakespeare, there are more mysteries within us and more potentials available to us than are dreamed of in our psychology.

Research Limitations

Clearly an enormous amount of exciting, groundbreaking research has been done. Unfortunately, quantity does not always mean quality. In fact, the largest review done to date—a massive analysis of more than 800 reports—found in many cases "the methodological quality of meditation research to be poor" (Ospina, et al., 2007).

The contemplatives studied are usually only beginners, the studies brief, follow-up of long-term effects insufficient, and control groups not ideal. There have also been few comparative analyses, with the result that although it is clear that meditation can be therapeutic, it is less clear how it compares with other psychotherapies, with medications, and with self-regulation strategies such as relaxation, biofeedback, and self-hypnosis. It is also unclear whether specific types of meditation, contemplation, or yoga offer advantages over others.

A further problem is that most research has been "means oriented" rather than "goal oriented" (Maslow, 1971). In other words, researchers have focused on what is easy to measure (the means) rather than on the classic goals of contemplation. Consequently, we know more about effects on heart rate than on heart opening, love, wisdom, or enlightenment.

Of course, this general problem is not unique to contemplative practices. In fact, it is one of the major problems inherent in the quest for empirically supported therapies: What is easiest to measure is not necessarily what is most important. Changes in simple behaviors are relatively easy to study; deeper transformations, existential openings, and postconventional growth are much more difficult. In fact, the more profound the issue, the deeper the question, and the higher the developmental stage, the more challenging assessment may be. Not everything that counts can be easily counted. It will be tragic if the quest for empirical evidence encourages a focus on what can be easily measured rather than on what is truly important.

Psychotherapy in a Multicultural World

Cultural diversity and sensitivity are now topics of considerable discussion. Unfortunately, crucial factors are often overlooked—factors such as the effects of participants' level of psychological maturity and the creative potentials inherent in diversity situations.

A sophisticated approach that integrates such factors is *diversity dynamics*, which aims to study and foster "diversity maturity" (Gregory & Raffanti, in press). Diversity dynamics points out that:

- Diversity occurs in *all* systems, including all (therapeutic) relationships.
- All diversity creates "diversity tension," which has both problematic and beneficial potentials.
- Adults differ on their levels of psychological development, such as levels of ego, cognitive, and moral maturity. For example, research on moral development has identified three major stages—preconventional (egocentric), conventional (ethnocentric), and postconventional (worldcentric). As people mature through these three stages, they tend to identify with and focus their care and concern on first just themselves (egocentric), then on themselves and their community (ethnocentric), and finally on all people (worldcentric). In her studies of women's moral development, Carol Gilligan described this as the maturation from selfishness to care to universal care (Wilber, 2000a).
- People's (and therapists') developmental level influences what they observe and understand in any situation, the range of possible responses they recognize, and therefore how effectively they can respond and help.
- A person's developmental stage will influence attitudes and responses to diversity. For example, consider the markedly different responses of people at three different stages: the conventional ethnocentric, the postconventional "pluralistic," and the postconventional "integral" stages.

At the conventional, ethnocentric stage, people (and therapists) simply assume that their own beliefs and values are basically correct while those of other people and cultures are not. Cultural and diversity sensitivity at this stage therefore means tolerating and accepting other people's (erroneous) beliefs and values.

However, when people mature to the early postconventional "pluralistic" stage, they increasingly question their own assumptions and come to recognize that all beliefs and values are largely personal and cultural constructions. Different beliefs and cultures are therefore considered valid by their own rights, and cultural sensitivity means honoring their validity. The trap at this stage is "cultural relativism," which assumes that all values and beliefs are *equally* valid, and that evaluating or ranking them amounts to cultural imperialism.

At the later postconventional "integral" stage, people are increasingly able to question and evaluate all beliefs and values—their own and other people's—from multiple perspectives. This allows them to remain open to the potential validity of diverse beliefs and values while simultaneously being able to evaluate them according to such criteria as fairness, helpfulness, and maturity.

For people at certain development stages, the idea of development itself can be threatening. However, the recognition of developmental diversity is just one more kind of diversity that needs to be acknowledged, honored, and used to benefit everyone.

- All diversity situations contain creative potentials. As such, they offer participants, including both therapists and patients, opportunities for learning and maturing.

- Once these ideas and findings are recognized, a key concern for diversity training becomes fostering psychological maturity, especially "diversity maturity." Diversity-mature people tend to "always be in discovery mode" (Gregory & Raffanti, in press), constantly seeking ways to transform the challenges of diversity into opportunities for all participants.

The ideas underlying diversity maturity raise a crucial question for psychotherapy: "Does psychotherapy enhance diversity maturity and related qualities such as cultural sensitivity?"

To date, there are few research studies of the effects of psychotherapy on development, and these are largely limited to studies of meditation. Meditation can foster ego, cognitive, moral, and self-actualization development (Alexander et al., 1991). In addition, meditation fosters related capacities such as empathy that presumably underlie diversity sensitivity. Hopefully, this implies that meditation and other therapies do, in fact, enhance diversity sensitivity and maturity.

However, contemplative therapies can and have been taught by people with ethnocentric, sexist views. Any therapy method will be limited by the capacities and maturity of the therapists using it. This is one more reason why all therapists should undergo their own personal psychotherapy in order to recognize and release some of the many limitations, biases, and blind spots to which we are all prone (Yalom, 2002).

CASE EXAMPLE

Clients who have a meditation practice can sometimes make surprisingly rapid progress in psychotherapy, in part because of the psychological work done in meditation sessions, and in part because of greater awareness of their experiences during therapy sessions. Meditators may have an enhanced ability to access their feelings, recognize thoughts and images, plumb deep layers of the psyche, and attend to difficult issues and emotions. Therapists who are themselves meditators can use these clients' abilities to deepen and speed the therapeutic process. The ways in which clients' meditative abilities can speed healing and facilitate insights are evident in the following session with Jan, a thirty-two-year-old female psychiatry trainee who was a long-term yoga practitioner and teacher, and someone who had been meditating for four years before beginning therapy.

Jan requested a consultation to help with intense feelings of dislike toward a fellow female trainee whom she perceived as competent, but also very competitive and duplicitous. Jan literally writhed on the couch as she reported the underhanded actions of the coworker, her own intense feelings of anger and fantasies of revenge, disappointment with herself at having such rage, and anguish over not knowing how to protect herself and others. After listening to her account I asked her where in her body she felt the conflict. "In my stomach" she replied, whereupon I asked her to carefully feel the body sensation and identify its size, shape and texture. This is an excellent way to help someone explore the somatic representation of an emotion or conflict and to keep sustained attention on it.

Jan described the characteristics of the sensation, and identified it as an expression of anger, conflict, and confusion. I asked her to concentrate on the sensation and to notice any changes. Because of her contemplative training, Jan was able to keep her attention focused on the sensation, and over the next few minutes reported that it was becoming smaller, smoother, and fainter. As it did, she noticed she was becoming less angry and agitated, and another sensation was becoming prominent in her chest. This she identified as feelings of sadness at her reactivity and at her inability to protect the other people affected by her coworker. I asked her to simply hold attention on the feeling of sadness and to notice any thoughts or images associated with it. Jan reported a stream of images of herself looking helpless, and of painful anxiety-provoking thoughts such as "I should be able to do something, I should know what to do, what's wrong with me?"

I encouraged her to simply observe the stream of thoughts and images without trying to change them in any way. As she did so, she found that she was becoming less identified with the thoughts and feelings and less reactive to them. She reported that she could feel her mind and body relaxing, and tears came to her eyes as she described feelings of relief welling up inside her along with thoughts such as "I'm only human, It's OK not to know what to do, I don't have to feel responsible for everyone." This spontaneous self-transformation and self-healing of thoughts, images, and emotions as they are observed mindfully—without attempting to change them deliberately—is a frequent finding in meditation, and one of the distinctive differences between many contemplative and traditional psychotherapeutic approaches.

At this stage I simply encouraged Jan to bring a sensitive awareness to the feelings of calm and relief and to see what emerged next. After a pause of perhaps two minutes, she began to describe several insights about how she could handle the situation more effectively. These were accompanied by greater acceptance of her limitations and what she could realistically expect to accomplish, and also by an initial sense of empathy and compassion for her colleague. As we reviewed the session, Jan concluded with, "I can see how she's driven by a need to be in control just like I am, and I want to work on feeling more compassion for her." In subsequent meditation and psychotherapy sessions she did just that.

SUMMARY

Contemplative disciplines include many techniques, of which the best known in the West are meditation, contemplation, Tai Chi, and yoga. Across centuries and cultures, they have been used to plumb the depths of the psyche and the heights of human possibility, and after 3,000 years, they remain the world's most widely used therapies.

The Future of Psychotherapy

Most discussions of the future of psychotherapy focus on local issues, such as novel techniques, empirical validation, and insurance reimbursement. Yet the fact is that the future of psychotherapy will primarily be determined by larger forces at work in the world, forces that will shape not only the future of therapy but also the future of our society and planet.

We have catapulted ourselves into what the Nobel laureate chemist Paul Crutzen calls the "anthropocene epoch," a new phase in Earth's history defined by human effects on the planet, in which the next few decades will determine our collective fate. It is a time of paradox. On the one hand, we possess unprecedented scientific, psychological, and technological resources. On the other hand, millions of people starve, our ecosystem is near collapse, weapons multiply, and our survival is in question.

What is striking is that each of the major threats to humankind is now human-created. For example, overpopulation, pollution, poverty, and conflicts all stem directly from our own behavior. Our global problems are therefore actually global symptoms: symptoms of our individual and collective psychological dysfunctions. The state of the world reflects the state of our minds. This means that to heal our social and global problems, we must also understand and heal the psychological forces within us and between us that spawned them in the first place.

But will our growth in psychological understanding and wisdom be sufficient? This is one of the great questions of our times. The challenge of how to foster widespread psychological and social healing and maturation is no longer an academic question but rather a collective challenge. Clearly, we are in a race between consciousness and catastrophe, the outcome remains uncertain, and mental health professionals are called to contribute. What *is* certain is that if we don't solve these problems, there will be little future for psychotherapy or psychotherapists.

Limits of Psychotherapy Training

Unfortunately, most training of psychotherapists and other mental health professionals is woefully unsuited to deal with many major causes of psychological suffering and pathology, let alone with larger social and global issues. Much psychological suffering has roots in social, educational, and economic factors such as poverty, ignorance, faulty collective beliefs, and inequality. Yet as numerous critiques point out, most psychotherapy training focuses on treating individuals or at most, families. The suffering individual is all too often seen as an isolated monad whose pain and pathology stem primarily from faulty internal forces such as conditioning, psychodynamics, or neurotransmitters.

Likewise, mental health professionals have seriously underestimated the importance of lifestyle factors for mental health. More specifically, mental health professionals have underestimated the importance of lifestyle factors in the causation and treatment of multiple psychopathologies, the enhancement of psychological and social wellbeing, and for optimizing and maintaining cognitive capacities. Yet lifestyle factors—such as diet, exercise, relationships, recreation, time in nature, religion/spirituality, and service to others—can be as therapeutically effective as either psychotherapy or pharmacotherapy, for example, in treating several forms of depression. In the 21st century, therapeutic lifestyles may need to be a central focus of mental, medical, and public health, and psychotherapists have much to contribute.

Compounding this neglect of social and lifestyle factors is an almost exclusive emphasis on tertiary treatment rather than primary prevention. That is, most resources are dedicated to treating illnesses and their complications after they arise, rather than to preventing them arising in the first place. Yet primary prevention is far more effective and efficient than later tertiary treatment. Of course, this bias contaminates not only individual psychotherapists and training institutions, but also the economic and insurance systems that emphasize individual treatment over large-scale prevention, especially in the United States.

Like other professionals, psychotherapists are subject to "professional deformation." This is the harmful distortion of personality, perception, and behavior that results from professional and social forces. Biases and blind spots such as the above are examples of widespread professional deformation.

Granted, psychotherapists are subject to larger social, economic, and cultural forces. But to what extent are we as psychotherapists colluding with and maintaining unhealthy social and economic systems when we merely patch up the worst casualties without also working to question and correct the larger systems and forces that help to create many casualties in the first place? This is a question that has been raised many times—for example, by Adlerian, feminist, social, and postmodern psychologies. Unfortunately, the question and the issues remain unsolved. Yet they provide the "big picture" context within which discussions of psychotherapy must proceed.

Questions for Contemplative Approaches

As contemplative practices become increasingly popular in the West, new opportunities and questions are emerging. These questions include:

- What role should contemplative approaches play in medical and mental health systems?

- How are contemplative methods best combined with conventional psychotherapies?

- To what extent and in what ways should contemplative training become part of psychotherapy training? Much of the effectiveness of psychotherapy is a function of the personal and interpersonal qualities of the therapist. However, meditation is one of the few methods that have been demonstrated to cultivate effective qualities such as empathy, and to specifically enhance therapeutic effectiveness (Grepmair et al., 2007). Accordingly, contemplative practices could be a valuable element of training.

- How can contemplative practices be made more widely available in society, for example in educational, professional, and penal systems?

- Will contemplative therapies prove prophylactic for disorders for which they have already proved therapeutic? If so, how can they be made available for this purpose—for example, within the educational system?

- Can contemplative practices contribute to cultivating the psychological qualities, maturity, and values that our society and times require, and if so, how can we foster these contributions?

- Will our views of human nature, capacities, and potentials expand to encompass the heights long suggested by contemplative therapies and now increasingly supported by research? This is a crucial question because, as Gordon Allport (1964) pointed out, "By their own theories of human nature psychologists have the power of elevating or degrading that same nature. Debasing assumptions debase human beings; generous assumptions exalt them" (p. 36). Contemplative practices offer a generous view of human nature and a means to foster those qualities that exalt it.

ANNOTATED BIBLIOGRAPHY

Baer, R. (Ed.). (2005). *Mindfulness-based treatment approaches: Clinician's guide to evidence base and applications* (Practical resources for the mental health professional). St. Louis, MO: Academic Press.

This comprehensive collection offers a summary of the many mindfulness-based therapies, their applications, and the research on them.

Feuerstein, G. (1996). *The Shambhala guide to yoga.* Boston: Shambhala.

Certain traditional philosophical and metaphysical assumptions are accepted uncritically, but otherwise the book is solid and provides a concise, readable overview.

Shapiro, S., & Carlson, L. (2009). *The art and science of meditation.* Washington, DC: American Psychological Association.

This book lives up to its title. It provides a clearly written introduction to the art of practicing and using meditation and a good survey of the scientific research. The book includes a valuable summary of the benefits that therapists themselves may gain from meditation. This is an excellent introduction to the field.

Walsh, R. (1999). *Essential spirituality: The seven central practices.* New York: Wiley.

This practical book introduces contemplative practices of both Asia and the West. The emphasis is on integrating these practices into one's life in order to foster well-being and growth.

Wilber, K. (1999). *No boundary.* Boston: Shambhala. Ken Wilber is an encyclopedic integrator of multiple schools of psychology and psychotherapy, including both contemplative and conventional Western approaches. *No Boundary* is an easily readable but somewhat dated introduction to his ideas. A more expanded treatment, including related social and philosophical issues, is *A Brief History of Everything. Integral Psychology* summarizes his psychological theory but is rather dense. Extensive reviews of Wilber's writings are available on the Web, and an overview appears at http://cogweb.ucla.edu/CogSci/Walsh_on_Wilber_95.html.

CASE READINGS

Germer, C., Siegel, R., & Fulton, P. (Eds.). (2005). *Mindfulness and psychotherapy.* New York: Guilford Press.

This practical book covers a wide variety of cases demonstrating issues and applications relevant to using contemplative approaches, and especially mindfulness meditation, in psychotherapy. Good case histories are also available in R. Baer's *Mindfulness-based treatment approaches.*

Kabat-Zinn, J. (1990). *Full catastrophe living: Using the wisdom of your body and mind to face stress, pain, and illness.* New York: Delacorte.

Jon Kabat-Zinn was director of the Stress Reduction Clinic at the University of Massachusetts and successfully taught meditation to thousands of people with severe illness and intractable pain. This book summarizes his experience and is both theoretical and practical, clinical and personal, and contains numerous brief clinical vignettes.

Kornfield, J. (1993). *A path with heart.* New York: Bantam.

This book is a wise, practical "how-to" guide for integrating contemplation into daily life in order to deal with the personal, interpersonal, and existential issues that all of us face.

Shapiro, D. (1980). Meditation as a self-regulation strategy: Case study–James Sidney. In *Meditation: Self-regulation strategy and altered states of consciousness* (pp. 55–84). Hawthorne, NY: Aldine. [Also in D. Wedding & R. J. Corsini (Eds.). (2011). *Case studies in psychotherapy* (6th ed.). Belmont, CA: Brooks/Cole.]

This case provides an excellent example of combining contemplative and other approaches. The therapist uses meditation, together with behavior therapy techniques and careful behavioral assessment, to treat insomnia and interpersonal difficulties.

Tart, C. (2001). *Mind science: Meditation training for practical people.* Novato, CA: Wisdom Press.

A clear, simple guide to meditation practice by a psychologist. Other practical introductions to learning meditation include S. Bodian (2006), *Meditation for Dummies,* (New York: IDG Books Worldwide), and, for mindfulness meditation, J. Goldstein (1987), *The Experience of Insight* (Boston: Shambhala Press).

REFERENCES

Alexander, C., Langer, E., Newman, R., Chandler, H., & Davies, J. (1989). Transcendental meditation, mindfulness, and longevity: An experimental study with the elderly. *Journal of Personality and Social Psychology, 57,* 950–964.

Alexander, C. N., Rainforth, M. V., & Gelderloos, P. (1991). Transcendental Meditation, self-actualization, and psychological health. *Journal of Social Behavior and Personality, 6,* 189–247.

Alexander, C. N., Robinson, P., & Rainforth, M. (1994). Treating and preventing alcohol, nicotine, and drug abuse through Transcendental Meditation: A review and statistical meta-analysis. *Alcohol Treatment Quarterly 11,* 13–87.

Alexander, F., & Selesnich, S. (1966). *The history of psychiatry.* New York: New American Library.

Alexander, C., Walton, K., Orme-Johnson, D., Goodman, R., & Pallone, N. (Eds.). (2003). *Transcendental Meditation in criminal rehabilitation and crime prevention.* New York: Haworth Press.

Allport, G. (1964). The fruits of eclecticism: Bitter or sweet? *Acta Psychologica, 23,* 27–44.

Anderson, J. W., Liu, C., & Kryscio, R. J. (2008). Blood pressure response to transcendental meditation: A meta-analysis. *American Journal of Hypertension, 21*(3), 310–316.

Angha, N. (Trans.). (1995). *Deliverance: Words from the Prophet Mohammad.* San Rafael, CA: International Association of Sufism.

Arlow, J. (1995). Psychoanalysis. In R. J. Corsini & D. Wedding (Eds.), *Current psychotherapies* (5th ed., pp. 15–50). Itasca, IL: F. E. Peacock.

Armstrong, K. (2006). *The great transformation: The beginning of our religious traditions.* New York: Knopf.

Baer, R. A. (2005). *Mindfulness-based treatment approaches: Clinician's guide to evidence base and applications.* St. Louis, MO: Academic Press.

Bynner, W. (Trans.). (1944/1980). *The way of life according to Lau Tzu.* New York: Vintage.

Byrom, T. (Trans.). (1976). *The Dhammapada: The sayings of the Buddha.* New York: Vintage.

Cahn, R., & Polich, J. (2006). Meditation states and traits: EEG, ERP, and neuroimaging studies. *Psychological Bulletin, 132,* 180–211.

Carson, J., Carson, K., Gil, K., & Baucom, D. (2004). Mindfulness-based relationship enhancement. *Behavior Therapy, 35,* 471–494.

Carter, O., Presti, D., Callistemon, C., Ungerer, Y., Liu, G., & Pettigrew, J. (2009). Tibetan Buddhist monks. *Current Biology, 15*(11), R412–R413.

Chan, W. (Ed.). (1963). *A sourcebook in Chinese philosophy.* Princeton, NJ: Princeton University Press.

Coelho, H. F., Canter, P. H., & Ernst, E. (2007). Mindfulness-based cognitive therapy: Evaluating current evidence and informing future research. *Journal of Consulting and Clinical Psychology, 75*(6), 1000–1005.

Creel, H. (1953). *Chinese thought from Confucius to Mao Tse-Tung.* Chicago: University of Chicago Press.

Crews, F. (2004, July 15). Out, damned blot! [Review of the book *What's wrong with the Rorschach? Science confronts the controversial inkblot test*]. *New York Review of Books, 51*(12), 22–25.

Dalai Lama. (2001). *An open heart: Practicing compassion in everyday life.* Boston: Little, Brown.

Deurr, M. (2004). *A powerful silence: The role of meditation and other contemplative practices in American life and work.* Northampton, MA: Center for Contemplative Mind in Society.

Didonna, F. (Ed.). (2009). *Clinical handbook of mindfulness.* New York: Springer.

Duncan, B., Miller, S., & Sparks, J. (2004). *The heroic client: A revolutionary way to improve effectiveness through client-directed, outcome-informed therapy* (Rev. ed.). San Francisco: Jossey-Bass.

Ellis, A. (1987). The impossibility of achieving consistently good mental health. *American Psychologist, 42,* 364–575.

Engler, J. H. (1983). Vicissitudes of the self according to psychoanalysis and Buddhism: A spectrum model of objects relations development. *Psychoanalysis and Contemporary Thought, 6,* 29–72.

Feng, G., & English, J. (Trans.). (1974). *Chuang Tsu: Inner chapters.* New York: Vintage Books.

Feuerstein, G. (1996). *The Shambhala guide to yoga.* Boston, MA: Shambhala.

Fischer, L. (1954). *Gandhi.* New York: New American Library.

Frank, J. (1982). *Sanity and survival in the nuclear age: Psychological aspects of war and peace.* New York: Random House.

Freud, S. (1917/1943). *A general introduction to psychoanalysis.* Garden City, NY: Garden City Publishers.

Freud, S. (1933/1965). *New introductory lectures on psychoanalysis* (J. Strachey, Trans.). New York: Norton.

Gabbard, G. (1995). Psychoanalysis. In H. Kaplan & B. Saddock (Eds.), *Comprehensive textbook of psychiatry* (6th ed., Vol. 1, pp. 431–478). Baltimore, MD: Williams & Wilkins.

Gampopa (1971). *The jewel ornament of liberation* (H. Guenther, Trans.). Boston: Shambhala.

Germer, C., Siegel, R., & Fulton, P. (Eds.). (2005). *Mindfulness and psychotherapy.* New York: Guilford Press.

Giles, H. (Trans.). (1926/1969). *Chuang-tzu: Mystic, moralist, and social reformer* (Rev. ed.). Taipei: Ch'eng Wen.

Goleman, D. (Ed.). (2003). *Destructive emotions.* New York: Bantam Books.

Gregory, T. & Raffanti, M. (in press). Integral diversity maturity: Toward a postconventional understanding of diversity dynamics. *Journal of Integral Theory and Practice.*

Grepmair, L., Mittelehner, F., Loew, T., Bachler, E., Rother, W., & Nickel, M. (2007). Promoting mindfulness in psychotherapists in training influences the treatment results of their patients: A randomized, double-blind, controlled study. *Psychotherapy and Psychosomatics, 76*(6), 332–338.

Grossman, P., Niemann, L., Schmidt, S., & Walach, H. (2004). Mindfulness-based stress reduction and health benefits: A meta-analysis. *Journal of Psychosomatic Research, 57,* 35–43.

Helminski, K. (Ed.). (2000). *The Rumi collection.* Boston, MA: Shambhala.

Hoffman, E. (1985). *The heavenly ladder: A Jewish guide to inner growth.* San Francisco: Harper & Row.

Horney, K. (1952/1998). *Neurosis and human growth.* New York: Norton.

James, W. (1899/1962). *Talks to teachers on psychology and to students on some of life's ideals.* New York: Dover.

James, W. (1910/1950). *The principles of psychology.* New York: Dover.

James, W. (1958). *The varieties of religious experience.* New York: New American Library.

James, W. (1960). *William James on psychical research* (ed. G. Murphy and R. Ballou). New York: Viking.

Jones, W. (1975). *A history of western philosophy* (Vols. 1–5, 2nd ed.). New York: Harcourt, Brace, Jovanovich.

Jung, C. (1955). *Mysterium conjunctionis: Collected works of Carl Jung* (Vol. 14). Princeton, NJ: Princeton University.

Jung, C. (1968). *The psychology of the child archetype, in collected works of C. J. Jung* (Vol. 9, Part I), Bollingen Series XX (2nd ed.). Princeton, NJ: Princeton University.

Jung, C. (1973). *Letters* (ed. G. Adler). Princeton, NJ: Princeton University Press.

Kabat-Zinn, J. (2003). Mindfulness-based interventions in context: Past, present, and future. *Clinical Psychology: Science and Practice, 10,* 144–156.

Kaplan, A. (1985). *Jewish meditation.* New York: Schocken Books.

Kegan, R. (1982). *The evolving self.* Cambridge, MA: Harvard University Press.

Kirkwood, G., Rampes, H., Tuffrey, V., Richardson, J., Pilkington, K. (2005). Yoga for anxiety: A systematic review of the research evidence. *British Journal of Sports Medicine, 39*(12), 884–891.

Klein, P. J., & Adams, W. D. A. W. (2004). Comprehensive therapeutic benefits of Taiji: A critical review. *American Journal of Physical Medicine and Rehabilitation, 83*(9), 735–745.

Kornfield, J. (1993). *A path with heart.* New York: Bantam.

Kornfield, J. (2006). Unpublished manuscript.

Kornfield, J. (2009). *The wise heart: A guide to the universal teachings of Buddhist psychology.* New York: Bantam Books.

Lau, D. (Trans.). (1979). *Confucius: The analects.* New York: Penguin.

Lutz, A., Dunne, J., & Davidson, R. (2007). Meditation and neuroscience of consciousness. In P. Zelag, M. Moscoritch, & E. Thompson (Eds.), *Cambridge handbook of consciousness* (pp. 499–554). New York: Cambridge University Press.

Maslow, A. (1967). Self-actualization and beyond. In J. Bugental (Ed.), *Challenges of humanistic psychology* (pp. 279–286). New York: McGraw-Hill.

Maslow, A. (1968). *Toward a psychology of being* (2nd ed.). Princeton, NJ: Van Nostrand.

Maslow, A. (1970). *Religions, values and peak experiences.* New York: Viking.

Maslow, A. (1971). *The farther reaches of human nature.* New York: Viking.

Miller, S., Hubble, M., & Duncan, B. (2007). Supershrinks: What's the secret of their success? *Psychology Networker, Nov/Dec,* 26–35.

Murphy, M., & Donovan, S. (1997). *The physical and psychological effects of meditation* (2nd ed.). Petaluma, CA: Institute of Noetic Sciences.

Myers, D. (1992). *The pursuit of happiness.* New York: Avon.

Needleman, J. (1980). *Lost Christianity.* Garden City, NY: Doubleday.

Nisargadatta, S. (1973). *I am that: Conversations with Sri Nisargadatta Maharaj, part II* (M. Friedman, Trans.). Bombay, India: Cheltana.

Norcross, J., & Beutler, L. (2008). Integrative psychotherapies. In R. J. Corsini & D. Wedding (Eds.), *Current psychotherapies* (8th ed., pp. 481–511). Belmont, CA: Brooks/Cole.

O'Brien, E. (Trans.). (1964). *The essential Plotinus.* Indianapolis, IN: Hackett.

Ornish, D. (2008). *The spectrum.* New York: Ballantine Books.

Ospina, M. B., Bond, T. K., Karkhaneh, M., Tjosvold, L., Vandermeer, B., Liang, Y., et al. (2007). *Meditation practices for health: State of the research.* Rockville, MD: Agency for Healthcare Research and Quality.

Ott, M. (2006). Mindfulness meditation for oncology patients: A discussion and critical review. *Integrative Cancer Theories, 5*(2), 98–108.

Pagnoni, G., & Cekic, M. (2007). Age effects on gray matter volume and attentional performance in Zen meditation. *Neurobiological Aging, 28*(10), 1623–627.

Palmer, G., Sherrard, P., & Ware, K. (Trans.). (1993). *Prayer of the heart: Writings from the Philokalia.* Boston: Shambhala.

Perls, F. (1969). *Gestalt therapy verbatim.* Lafayette, CA: Real People Press.

Pilkington, K., Kirkwood, G., Rampes, H., Richardson, J. (2005). Yoga for depression: The research evidence. *Journal of Affective Disorders, 89*(1–3), 13–24.

Prabhavananda, S., & Isherwood, C. (Trans.). (1972). *The song of God: Bhagavad Gita* (3rd ed.). Hollywood, CA: Vedanta Society.

Prabhavananda, S., & Isherwood, C. (Trans.). (1978). *Shankara's crest-jewel of discrimination.* Hollywood: Vedanta Press.

Raskin, N., & Rogers, C. (1995). Person-centered therapy. In R. Corsini & D. Wedding (Eds.), *Current Psychotherapies* (5th ed., pp. 128–161). Itasca, IL: F. E. Peacock.

Rogers, C. (1959). A theory of therapy, personality and interpersonal relationships as developed in the client centered framework. In S. Koch (Ed.), *Psychology: The study of science* (Vol. 3, pp. 184–256). New York: McGraw-Hill.

Savin, O. (Trans.). (1991). *The way of a pilgrim.* Boston, MA: Shambhala.

Sengstan (1975). *Verses on the faith mind* (R. Clarke, Trans.). Sharon Springs, NY: Zen Center.

Shapiro, R. (Trans.). (1993). *Wisdom of the Jewish sages: A modern reading of Pirke Avot.* New York: Bell Tower.

Shapiro, S., & Carlson, L. (2009). *The art and science of mindfulness.* Washington, DC: American Psychological Association.

Shapiro, S., Astin, J., Bishop, S., & Cordova, M. (2005). Mindfulness-based stress reduction and health care professionals: Results from a randomized controlled trial. *International Journal of Stress Management, 12,* 164–176.

Shearer, P. (Trans.). (1989). *Effortless being: The yoga sutras of Patanjali.* London: Unwin.

Swan, L. (2001). *The forgotten Desert Mothers.* Mahaw, NJ: Paulist Press.

Tart, C. (1986). *Waking up: Overcoming the obstacles to human potential.* Boston: New Science Library/Shambhala.

Travis, F., Arenander, A., & DuBois, D. (2004). Psychological and physiological characteristics of a proposed object-referral/self-referral continuum of self-awareness. *Consciousness and Cognition, 13,* 401–420.

Wade, J. (2004). *Transcendent sex.* New York: Paraview.

Walsh, R. (1984). *Staying alive: The psychology of human survival.* Boston: Shambhala.

Walsh, R. (1999). *Essential spirituality: The seven central practices.* New York: Wiley.

Walsh, R. (2007). *The world of shamanism.* Woodbury, MN: Llewellyn Press.

Walsh, R., Bitner, R., Victor, B., & Hillman, L. (2009). Medicate or meditate. *Buddhadharma, (Spring), 30–35,* 87–77.

Walsh, R., & Shapiro, S. (2006). The meeting of meditative disciplines and Western psychology: A mutually enriching dialogue. *American Psychologist, 61*(3), 227–239.

Walsh, R., & Vaughan, F. (Eds.). (1993). *Paths beyond ego: The transpersonal vision.* New York: Tarcher/Putnam.

Whitmont, E. (1969). *The symbolic quest.* Princeton, NJ: Princeton University Press.

Wilber, K. (1999). *The collected works of Ken Wilber: The atman project.* Boston, MA: Shambhala.

Wilber, K. (2000a). *A brief theory of everything.* Boston: Shambhala.

Wilber, K. (2000b). *Integral psychology.* Boston: Shambhala.

Wilber, K., Engler, J., & Brown, D. (Eds.). (1986). *Transformations of consciousness: Conventional and contemplative perspectives on development* (2nd. ed.). Boston: Shambhala.

Yalom, I. (2002). *The gift of therapy.* New York: Harper Collins.

Yalom, I., & Josselson, R. (2011). Existential psychotherapy. In R. Corsini & D. Wedding (Eds.), *Current Psychotherapies* (9th ed., pp. 310–341). Belmont, CA: Brooks/Cole.

Yu Lan, F. (1948). *A short history of Chinese philosophy* (D. Bodde, Trans.). New York: Free Press/Macmillan.

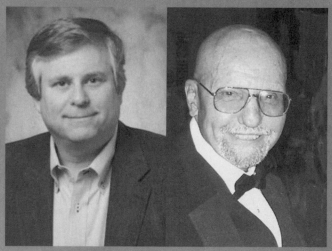

John Norcross
Courtesy of John Norcross

Larry Beutler
Courtesy of Professor Larry Beutler

14 | INTEGRATIVE PSYCHOTHERAPIES[1]

John C. Norcross and Larry E. Beutler

OVERVIEW

Rivalry among theoretical orientations has a long and undistinguished history in psychotherapy, dating back to Freud. In the infancy of the field, therapy systems, like battling siblings, competed for attention, affection, and adherents. Clinicians traditionally operated from within their own theoretical frameworks, often to the point of being blind to alternative conceptualizations and potentially superior interventions. An ideological "cold war" reigned as clinicians were separated into rival schools of psychotherapy.

As the field of psychotherapy has matured, integration has emerged as a mainstay. We have witnessed both a decline in ideological struggle and a movement toward rapprochement. Clinicians now acknowledge that there are inadequacies and potential value in every theoretical system. In fact, many young students of psychotherapy express surprise when they learn about the ideological cold war of the preceding generations.

Psychotherapy integration is characterized by dissatisfaction with single-school approaches and a concomitant desire to look across school boundaries to see how patients can benefit from other ways of conducting psychotherapy. Although various labels are applied to this movement—eclecticism, integration, rapprochement, prescriptive therapy,

[1] Portions of this chapter are adapted from Norcross (2005) and Norcross, Beutler, & Caldwell (2002).

treatment matching—the goals are similar. The ultimate goal is to enhance the efficacy and applicability of psychotherapy.

Applying identical psychosocial treatments to all patients is now recognized as inappropriate and probably impossible. Different folks require different strokes. The efficacy and applicability of psychotherapy will be enhanced by tailoring it to the unique needs of the client, not by imposing Procrustean methods on unwitting consumers of psychological services. The integrative mandate is embodied in Gordon Paul's (1967) famous question: *What* treatment, by *whom,* is most effective for *this* individual with *that* specific problem and under *which* set of circumstances?

Any number of indicators attest to the popularity of psychotherapy integration. *Eclecticism,* or the increasingly favored term *integration,* is the most popular theoretical orientation of English-speaking psychotherapists. Leading psychotherapy textbooks routinely identify their theoretical persuasion as integrative, and an integrative chapter is regularly included in compendia of treatment approaches. The publication of books that synthesize various therapeutic concepts and methods continues unabated; they now number in the hundreds. Handbooks on psychotherapy integration have been published in at least eight countries. This integrative fervor will apparently persist well into the 21st century: A panel of psychotherapy experts predicts the escalating popularity of integrative psychotherapies (Norcross, Hedges, & Prochaska, 2002).

Basic Concepts

There are numerous pathways toward integrative psychotherapies; many roads lead to an integrative Rome. The four most popular routes are technical eclecticism, theoretical integration, common factors, and assimilative integration. Research (Norcross, Karpiak, & Lister, 2005) reveals that each is embraced by a considerable number of self-identified eclectics and integrationists (19% to 28% each). All four routes are characterized by a desire to increase therapeutic efficacy and applicability; all look beyond the confines of single approaches; but all are also distinctive and focus on different levels of patient–therapy process.

Technical eclecticism seeks to improve our ability to select the best treatment techniques or procedures for the person and the problem. This search is guided primarily by research on what specific methods have worked best in the past with similar problems and patient characteristics. Eclecticism focuses on predicting for whom interventions will work; its foundation is actuarial rather than theoretical.

Technical eclectics use procedures drawn from different therapeutic systems without necessarily subscribing to the theories that spawned them, whereas theoretical integrationists draw their concepts and techniques from diverse systems that may be epistemologically or ontologically incompatible. For technical eclectics, no necessary connection exists between conceptual foundations and techniques. "To attempt a theoretical rapprochement is as futile as trying to picture the edge of the universe. But to read through the vast amount of literature on psychotherapy, *in search of techniques,* can be clinically enriching and therapeutically rewarding" (Lazarus, 1967, p. 416).

In *theoretical integration,* two or more therapies are integrated with the hope that the result will be better than the constituent therapies alone. As the name implies, there is an emphasis on integrating the underlying theories of psychotherapy along with the techniques from each. Treatment models that integrate psychoanalytic and interpersonal theories, cognitive and behavioral theories, or systems and humanistic theories illustrate this path.

Theoretical integration involves a commitment to a conceptual or theoretical creation beyond a technical blend of methods. The goal is to create a conceptual framework that synthesizes the best elements of two or more therapies. Integration aspires to more than a simple combination; it seeks an emergent theory that is more than the sum of its parts.

The *common factors* approach seeks to identify core ingredients shared by different therapies, with the eventual goal of creating more parsimonious and efficacious treatments based on those commonalities. This search is predicated on the belief that commonalities are more important in accounting for therapy success than the unique factors that differentiate among them. The common factors most frequently proposed are the development of a therapeutic alliance, opportunity for catharsis, acquisition and practice of new behaviors, and clients' positive expectancies (Grencavage & Norcross, 1990; Tracey, Lichtenberg, Goodyear, Claiborn, & Wampold, 2003).

Assimilative integration entails a firm grounding in one system of psychotherapy, but with a willingness to selectively incorporate (assimilate) practices and views from other systems (Messer, 1992, 2001). In doing so, assimilative integration combines the advantages of a single, coherent theoretical system with the flexibility of a broader range of technical interventions from multiple systems. A cognitive therapist, for example, might use the gestalt two-chair dialogue in an otherwise cognitive course of treatment.

To its proponents, assimilative integration is a realistic way station on the path to a sophisticated integration; to its detractors, it is a waste station of people unwilling to commit themselves to a full evidence-based eclecticism. Both camps agree that assimilation is a tentative step toward full integration: Most therapists gradually incorporate parts and methods of other approaches once they discover the limitations of their original approach. Inevitably, therapists gradually integrate new methods into their home theory.

Of course, these four integrative pathways are not mutually exclusive. No technical eclectic can disregard theory, and no theoretical integrationist can ignore technique. Without some commonalities among different schools of psychotherapy, theoretical integration would be impossible. Assimilative integrationists and technical eclectics both believe that synthesis should occur at the level of practice, rather than theory, by incorporating therapeutic methods from multiple schools. And even the most ardent proponent of common factors cannot practice "nonspecifically" or "commonly" on their own; specific techniques must be applied.

In some circles, the terms *integrative* and *eclectic* have acquired emotionally ambivalent connotations because of their alleged disorganized and indecisive nature. However, much of this opposition should be properly redirected to *syncretism*—uncritical and unsystematic combinations. This haphazard approach is primarily an outgrowth of pet techniques and inadequate training. It is an arbitrary blend of methods without systematic rationale or empirical verification (Eysenck, 1970).

Psychotherapy integration, by contrast, is the product of years of painstaking training, research, and experience. It is integration by design, not default; that is, clinicians competent in several therapeutic systems systematically select interventions and concepts on the basis of comparative outcome research and patient need. The strengths of systematic integration lie in the ability to be taught, replicated, and evaluated.

Our own approach to psychotherapy is broadly characterized as integrative and is specifically labeled *systematic eclectic* or *systematic treatment selection*. We intentionally blend several of the four paths toward integration. Concisely put, we attempt to customize psychological treatments and therapeutic relationships to the specific and varied needs of individual patients as defined by a multitude of diagnostic and particularly nondiagnostic considerations. We do so by drawing on effective methods across theoretical schools (eclecticism), by matching those methods to particular clients on the basis of evidence-based principles (treatment selection), and by adhering to an explicit and orderly (systematic) model.

Although some integrative therapies, particularly those identified with technical eclecticism, provide menus of specific methods, we are committed to defining broader change principles, leaving the selection of specific methods that comply with these principles to the proclivities of the individual therapist. Accordingly, our integrative therapy is expressly designed to transcend the limited applicability of single-theory or "school-bound" psychotherapies. This is accomplished by integrating research-based change principles rather than through a closed theory or a limited set of techniques.

In other words, our integrative therapy ascertains the treatments (and therapeutic relationships) of choice for individual patients rather than restricting itself to a single view of psychopathology and/or change mechanisms. We believe that no theory is uniformly valid and no mechanism of therapeutic action is applicable to all individuals. Thus, we strive to create a new therapy for each patient. We believe that the purpose of integrative psychotherapy is *not* to create a single system or a unitary treatment. Rather, we select different methods according to the patient's response to the treatment goals, following an established set of integrative principles. The result is a more efficient and efficacious therapy—and one that fits both the client and the clinician.

On the face of it, virtually all clinicians endorse matching the therapy to the individual client. After all, who can seriously dispute the notion that psychological treatment should be tailored to the needs of the individual patient in order to improve its success? However, integrative therapy goes beyond this simple acknowledgment in at least four ways.

1. Our treatment selection is derived directly from outcome research rather than from the idiosyncratic theory of the clinician. In our view, empirical knowledge and scientific research are the best arbiters of theoretical differences when it comes to health care.

2. We embrace the potential contributions of multiple systems of psychotherapy rather than working from within a single system. All psychotherapies have a place, but a specific and differential place.

3. Our treatment selection is predicated on multiple diagnostic and nondiagnostic client dimensions, in contrast to the typical reliance on the single, static (and often global) dimension of patient diagnosis. It is frequently more important to know the patient who has the disorder than to know the disorder the patient has.

4. Our aim is to offer treatment methods *and* relationship stances, whereas most theorists focus narrowly on methods alone. Both interventions and relationships, both the instrumental and the interpersonal—intertwined as they are—are required, indeed inevitably involved, in effective psychotherapy.

Other Systems

Integrative psychotherapies gratefully acknowledge the contributions of the traditional, single-school therapy systems, such as psychoanalytic, behavioral, cognitive, experiential, and other unitary systems. Such pure-form therapies are part and parcel of the foundation for integrative approaches. Integration, in fact, could not occur without the constituent elements provided by these respective therapies—their theoretical systems and clinical methods. Integration gathers, in the words of Abraham Lincoln, "strange, discordant, and even, hostile elements from the four winds."

In a narrow sense, pure-form or single-school therapies do not contribute to integration because, by definition, they have no provisions for synthesizing various interventions and conceptualizations. But in a broader and more important sense, they add to the therapeutic armamentarium, enrich our understanding of the clinical process, and produce the process and outcome research from which integration draws. One cannot integrate what one does not know.

The goal of integration, as we have repeatedly emphasized, is to improve the efficacy and applicability of psychotherapy. Toward this end, we must collegially recognize the valuable contributions of pure-form therapies and collaboratively enlist their respective strengths.

Even so, it is important to remember that most single-school therapies also manifest several weaknesses. First, the creation of most psychotherapies is more rational than empirical. Originators developed their therapies without, or with little regard to, the research evidence on their effectiveness. Perhaps as a result, many traditional systems of psychotherapy (classical psychoanalysis, Jungian, and existential, to name a few) have still amassed little controlled outcome research. We highly value empirical evidence, not as an infallible guide to truth, but as the most reliable means to conduct and evaluate psychotherapy, integrative or otherwise.

Second, single-school therapies tend to favor the strong personal opinions, if not pathological conflicts, of their originators. Sigmund Freud found psychosexual conflicts in practically all his patients, Carl Rogers found compromised conditions of worth in practically all his patients, Joseph Wolpe found conditioned anxiety in practically all his patients, and Albert Ellis found maladaptive thinking in practically all his patients. However, patients do not routinely suffer from the favorite problems of famous theorists. It strikes us as far more probable that patients suffer from a multitude of specific problems that should be remedied with a similar multitude of methods.

Third and relatedly, most pure-form systems of psychotherapy recommend their treasured treatment for virtually every patient and problem they encounter. Of course, this simplifies treatment selection—give every patient the same brand of psychotherapy!—but it flies in the face of what we know about individual differences, patient preferences, and disparate cultures. It is akin to seeking the remedy for all ills in a hardware store, simply because it is a "good store." The clinical reality is that no single psychotherapy is effective for all patients and situations, no matter how good it is for some; relational–sensitive, evidence-based practice demands a flexible, if not integrative, perspective. Psychotherapy should be flexibly tailored to the unique needs and contexts of the individual client, not universally applied as one size fits all.

Imposing a parallel situation onto other health care professions drives the point home. To take a medical metaphor, would you entrust your health to a physician who prescribed the identical treatment (say, antibiotics or neurosurgery) for every patient and illness encountered? Or, to take an educational analogy, would you prize instructors who employed the same pedagogical method (say, a lecture) for every educational opportunity? Or would you entrust your child to a child care worker who delivers the identical response (say, a nondirective attitude or a slap on the bottom) to every child and every misbehavior? "No" is probably your resounding answer. Psychotherapy clients deserve no less consideration.

A fourth weakness of pure-form therapies is that they largely consist of descriptions of psychopathology and personality rather than of mechanisms that promote change. They are actually theories of personality rather than theories of psychotherapy; they offer lots of information on the content of therapy but little on the change process. We believe integrative theory should explain how people change. (Specific criticisms of 15 therapy systems from an integrative perspective can be found in Prochaska & Norcross, 2010).

We are convinced of the clinical superiority of a pluralistic or integrative psychotherapy. Among the advantages of integrative psychotherapies are those inferred from the foregoing criticisms of pure-form therapies: Integrative therapies tend to be more empirical in creation and more evidence based in revision; case conceptualization is predicated more on the actual patient than on an abstruse theory; therapy is more likely to be adapted or responsive to the unique patient and the singular situation; and treatment is more focused on the process of change than on the content of personality. In other words, integration promises more evidence, flexibility, responsiveness, and change.

HISTORY

Precursors

Integration as a point of view has probably existed as long as philosophy and psychotherapy. In philosophy, the 3rd-century biographer Diogenes Laertius referred to an eclectic school that flourished in Alexandria in the second century (Lunde, 1974). In psychotherapy, Freud consciously struggled with the selection and integration of diverse methods. As early as 1919, he introduced psychoanalytic psychotherapy as an alternative to classical psychoanalysis in recognition that the more rarified approach lacked universal applicability (Liff, 1992).

More formal ideas on synthesizing the psychotherapies appeared in the literature as early as the 1930s (Goldfried, Pachankis, & Bell, 2005). For example, Thomas French (1933) stood before the 1932 meeting of the American Psychiatric Association and drew parallels between certain concepts of Freud and of Pavlov. In 1936, Sol Rosenzweig published an article that highlighted commonalities among various systems of psychotherapy. These and other early attempts at integration, however, were largely serendipitous, theory driven, and empirically untested.

If not conspiratorially ignored altogether, these precursors to integration appeared only as a latent theme in a field organized around discrete theoretical orientations. Although psychotherapists secretly recognized that their orientations did not adequately assist them in all they encountered in practice, a host of political, social, and economic forces—such as professional organizations, training institutes, and referral networks—kept them penned within their own theoretical school yards and typically led them to avoid clinical contributions from alternative orientations.

Beginnings

Systematic integration was probably inaugurated in the modern era by Frederick Thorne (1957, 1967), who is credited with being the grandfather of eclecticism in psychotherapy. Persuasively arguing that any skilled professional should come prepared with more than one tool, Thorne emphasized the need for clinicians to fill their toolboxes with methods drawn from many different theoretical orientations. He likened contemporary psychotherapy to a plumber who would use only a screwdriver in his work. Like such a plumber, inveterate psychotherapists applied the same treatment to all people, regardless of individual differences, and expected the patient to adapt to the therapist rather than vice versa.

Thorne's admonitions went largely ignored, as did a book published more than a decade later by Goldstein and Stein (1976) that first identified the *Prescriptive Psychotherapies* of its title. This book, far ahead of its time, outlined treatments for different people based on the nature of their problems and on aspects of their living situations.

Since the late 1960s, Arnold Lazarus (1967, 1989) has emerged as the most prominent spokesperson for eclecticism. His influential *multimodal therapy* inspired a generation of mental health professionals to think and behave more broadly. He was joined by the two of us and others soon thereafter (e.g., Beutler, 1983; Frances, Clarkin, & Perry, 1984; Norcross, 1986, 1987).

Simultaneously, efforts were under way to advance common factors. In his classic *Persuasion and Healing,* Jerome Frank (1973) posited that all psychotherapeutic methods are elaborations and variations of age-old procedures of psychological healing. Frank argued that therapeutic change is predominantly a function of four factors common to all therapies: an emotionally charged, confiding relationship; a healing setting; a rationale or conceptual scheme; and a therapeutic ritual. Nonetheless, the features that distinguish psychotherapies from each other receive special emphasis in the pluralistic, competitive American society. Little glory has traditionally been accorded to common factors.

In 1980, Sol Garfield introduced an eclectic psychotherapy predicated on common factors, and Marvin Goldfried published an influential article in the *American Psychologist* calling for the delineation of therapeutic change principles. Goldfried (1980), a leader of the integration movement, argued,

> To the extent that clinicians of varying orientations are able to arrive at a common set of strategies, it is likely that what emerges will consist of robust phenomena, as they have managed to survive the distortions imposed by the therapists' varying theoretical biases. (p. 996)

In specifying what is common across orientations, we may also be selecting what works best among them.

In the late 1970s and the 1980s, several attempts at theoretical integration were introduced. Paul Wachtel authored the classic *Psychoanalysis and Behavior Therapy: Toward an Integration,* which attempted to bridge the chasm between the two systems. His integrative book began, ironically, in an effort to write an article portraying behavior therapy as "foolish, superficial, and possibly even immoral" (Wachtel, 1977, p. xv). But in preparing his article, he was forced for the first time to look closely at what behavior therapy was and to think carefully about the issues. When he observed some of the leading behavior therapists of the day, he was astonished to discover that the particular version of psychodynamic therapy toward which he had been gravitating dovetailed considerably with what a number of behavior therapists were doing. Wachtel's experience should remind us that separate and isolated theoretical schools perpetuate caricatures of other schools, thereby foreclosing basic changes in viewpoint and preventing expansion in practice.

The transtheoretical (across theories) approach of James Prochaska and Carlo DiClemente was also introduced in the late 1970s with the publication of one of the first integrative textbooks, *Systems of Psychotherapy: A Transtheoretical Analysis* (Prochaska, 1979). This book reviewed different theoretical orientations from the standpoint of common change principles and of the stages of change. The transtheoretical approach in general, and the stages of change in particular, are the most extensively researched integrative therapies (Schottenbauer, Glass, & Arnkoff, 2005).

Only within the past 30 years, then, has psychotherapy integration developed into a clearly delineated area of interest. The temporal course of interest in psychotherapy integration, as indexed by both the number of publications and the development of organizations and journals (Goldfried et al., 2005), reveals occasional stirrings before 1970, a growing interest during the 1970s, and rapidly accelerating interest from 1980 to the present. To put it differently, integrative psychotherapy has a long past but a short history as a systematic movement.

Current Status

Between one-quarter and one-half of contemporary clinicians disavow an affiliation with a particular school of psychotherapy, preferring instead the label of *eclectic* or *integrative.* Some variant of integration is routinely the modal orientation of responding psychotherapists. A review of 25 studies performed in the United States between 1953 and 1990 (Jensen, Bergin, & Greaves, 1990) reported a range from 19% to 68%. A more recent review of a dozen studies published during the past decade (Norcross, 2005) found that integration was still the most common orientation in the United States but that cognitive therapy was rapidly challenging it and might soon become the modal theory. That same review also determined that integration receives robust but lower endorsement outside of the United States and Western Europe. Thus, integration is typically the modal orientation in the United States, but not in other countries around the world.

The prevalence of integration can be ascertained directly by assessing endorsement of the integrative orientation (as above) or gleaned indirectly by determining endorsement of multiple orientations. For example, in a study of Great Britain counselors, 87% did *not* take a pure-form approach to psychotherapy (Hollanders & McLeod, 1999). In a study of clinical psychologists in the United States, for another example, fully 90% embraced several orientations (Norcross, Karpiak, & Santoro, 2005). Very few therapists adhere exclusively to a single therapeutic tradition.

The establishment of several international organizations both reflects and reinforces the popularity of integrative psychotherapies. Two interdisciplinary societies, the Society for the Exploration of Psychotherapy Integration (SEPI) and the Society of Psychotherapy Research (SPR), hold annual conferences devoted to the pluralistic practice and ecumenical research of psychotherapy. Both societies also publish international scientific journals: SEPI's *Journal of Psychotherapy Integration* and SPR's *Psychotherapy Research*.

Psychotherapy integration, then, has taken earliest and strongest root in the United States. Nonetheless, it is steadily spreading throughout the world and is becoming an international movement. Both SPR and SEPI now have multiple international chapters and regularly hold their annual meetings outside the United States.

In past years, psychotherapists were typically trained in a single theoretical orientation. The ideological singularity of this training did not always result in clinical competence, but it did reduce clinical complexity and theoretical confusion (Schultz-Ross, 1995). In recent years, psychotherapists have come to recognize that single orientations are theoretically incomplete and clinically inadequate for the variety of patients, contexts, and problems they confront in practice. They are receiving training in several theoretical orientations—or at least are exposed to multiple theories, as evidenced in this book.

The evolution of psychotherapy training has moved the field further toward integration, but this may have been a mixed blessing. On the one hand, integrative training addresses the daily needs of clinical practice, satisfies the intellectual quest for an informed pluralism, and responds to the growing research evidence that different patients prosper under different treatments, formats, and relationships. On the other hand, integrative training increases the pressure for students to obtain clinical competence in multiple methods and formats and, in addition, challenges the faculty to create a coordinated training enterprise (Norcross & Halgin, 2005).

Recent studies indicate that training directors are committed to psychotherapy integration but disagree on the best route toward it. Approximately 80 to 90% of directors of psychology programs and internship programs agree that knowing one therapy system is not sufficient; instead, training in a variety of models is needed. However, their views on the optimal integrative training process differ. About one-third believe that students should be trained first to be proficient in one therapeutic system; about half believe that students should be trained to be at *least* minimally competent in a variety of systems; and the remainder believe that students should be trained in a specific integrative system from the outset (Lampropoulos & Dixon, 2007).

Multimedia procedures may increase the effectiveness of training in integrative psychotherapies. A pilot study using a virtual patient (Beutler & Harwood, 2004) reported case-by-case success in training clinicians to recognize cues suggesting which treatment is likely to be most effective for the patient. A computerized treatment selection procedure has been developed (Harwood & Williams, 2003) to help clinicians plan treatment.

More recently, we launched a user-friendly Web site (www.innerlife.com) that clients can access for free in order to help them select the optimal psychotherapy for them. Taking Systematic Treatment (ST) requires approximately 15 minutes and takes the person through a series of item-branching questions. At completion, ST renders a report addressing six critical treatment issues tailored to the person:

- Potential Areas of Concern
- Treatments to Consider
- Treatments to Avoid
- Compatible Therapist Styles
- Picking a Psychotherapist
- Self-Help Resources

The ensuing treatment recommendations in this system are governed by 30 years of research on identifying evidence-based principles that point to optimal relations among patient characteristics (including diagnosis), treatment methods, and the therapeutic relationship.

Integrative training is both a product and a process. As a product, psychotherapy integration will be increasingly disseminated through books, videotapes, courses, seminars, curricula, workshops, conferences, supervision, postdoctoral programs, and institutional changes. The hope is that educators will develop and deliver integrative products that are less parochial, more pluralistic, and more effective than traditional, single-theory products.

Our more fervent hope is that, as a process, psychotherapy integration will be disseminated in a manner that is consistent with the pluralism and openness of integration itself. The intention of integrative training is not necessarily to produce card-carrying, flag-waving "integrative" psychotherapists. This scenario would simply replace enforced conversion to a single orientation with enforced conversion to an integrative orientation, a change that may be more liberating in content but certainly not in process. Instead, the goal is to educate therapists to think (and, perhaps, to behave) integratively—openly, flexibly, synthetically, but critically—in their clinical pursuits (Norcross & Halgin, 2005).

Integrative therapies respond to the mounting demands for short-term and evidence-based treatments in mental health. With 90% of all patients in the United States covered by some variant of managed care, short-term therapy has become the de facto treatment imperative. Integration, particularly in the form of technical eclecticism, responds to the pragmatic injunction of "whatever therapy works better—and quicker—for this patient with this problem."

The international juggernaut of evidence-based practice (EBP) lends increased urgency to the task of using the best of research and experience to tailor psychological treatment to the client (Norcross, Beutler, & Levant, 2006). Data-based clinical decision making will become the norm. Evidence-based practice has sped the breakdown of traditional schools and the escalation of informed pluralism (Norcross, Hogan, & Koocher, 2008). The particular decision rules for what qualifies as evidence remain controversial, but EBP reflects a pragmatic commitment to "what works for whom." The clear emphasis is on what works, not on what theory applies. Integrative therapies stand ready to meet this challenge.

PERSONALITY

Theory of Personality

Beginning with Freud, most psychotherapy systems have consisted primarily of theories of personality and psychopathology (*what* to change). This is not true of most integrative therapies, which instead emphasize the process of change (*how* to change).

The integration is directly focused on the selection of therapy methods and relationships as opposed to theoretical constructs of how people and psychopathology develop. Although a latent theory necessarily underpins any treatment, integrative therapy is relatively personality-less and immediately change-ful.

Our integrative conceptualization makes no specific assumptions about how personality and psychopathology occur. Such a determination is relatively unimportant if one knows what therapy methods and relationships are likely to evoke a positive response in a specific patient. Effective treatment can be applied from a wide number of theories or from no theoretical framework at all.

To the limited extent that they exist, integrative theories of personality are predictably broad and inclusive. They embrace life-span approaches of developmental psychology. They reflect that humans are, whether functional or dysfunctional, the products of a complex interplay of our genetic endowment, learning history, sociocultural context, and physical environment.

Variety of Concepts

To say that integrative therapies do not rely on a theory of personality is not to say that they pay no heed to personality characteristics. Indeed they do. As detailed in the next section, the patient's personality is a key determinant in integrative therapy, as are the therapist's personality and their mutual match. However, personality characteristics are not separated out into a broader theory of human development and motivation. Like all other patient characteristics in integrative therapy, personality traits are incorporated to the extent that the research evidence has consistently demonstrated that identifying them contributes to effective treatment.

Our data-based therapy eschews the view that one needs to know how a problem developed in order to solve it. Instead, we assert that when one encounters particular behavior patterns or environmental characteristics, it is more important to know what treatment is likely to promote change.

In the next section, we will describe several personality characteristics that the research indicates are useful in helping the clinician improve the efficacy of psychotherapy. To anticipate ourselves, we will present here an example of how personality concepts differ between conventional psychotherapies and integrative therapies.

A patient's coping style is a vital personality characteristic to consider when deciding to conduct insight-oriented or symptom-change methods. Coping style is an enduring quality defined by what one does when confronted with new experience or stress. A person may engage in a cluster of behaviors that disrupt social relationships, such as impulsivity, blaming, and rebellion, on the one hand, or in a cluster of behaviors that increase personal distress, such as self-blame, withdrawal, and emotional constriction, on the other. These clusters are relatively enduring, they cut across situations, and they distinguish among people. Thus, they are personality characteristics. But integrative therapy makes little effort to understand why they occur and makes few efforts to say how they are related to other key qualities of treatment selection, such as the amount of social support and the stage of change. Although there may be correlations among these dimensions, the intercorrelations assume far less importance than knowing how they impact psychotherapy and improve its success.

Our integrative approach is principally concerned with tailoring psychotherapy to the patient's personality, not with developing a theory about that personality. We are committed to the remediation of psychopathology, not preoccupied with its explanation. Let us now move on to the practice of integrative psychotherapy.

PSYCHOTHERAPY

Theory of Psychotherapy

In contrast to the absence of a cohesive theory of personality and psychopathology, integrative psychotherapy strongly values clinical assessment that guides effective treatment. Such assessment is conducted early in psychotherapy to select treatment methods and therapy relationships that are most likely to be effective, throughout therapy to monitor the patient's response and to make mid-course adjustments as needed, and toward the end of psychotherapy to evaluate the outcomes of the entire enterprise. Thus, assessment is continuous, collaborative, and invaluable.

In this section, we begin with an extensive discussion of clinical assessment that fuels and guides treatment selection. This account then segues naturally into the process of psychotherapy, just as it does in actual practice.

Clinical Assessment

Clinical assessment of the patient in integrative therapy is relatively traditional, with one major exception. The assessment interview(s) entail collecting information on presenting problems, relevant histories, and treatment expectations and goals, as well as building a working alliance. As psychologists, we also typically use formal psychological testing as a means of securing additional data and identifying Axis I and Axis II disorders. We recommend both symptomatic rating forms (e.g., Beck Depression Inventory II, Symptom Checklist-90R) and broader measures of pathology and personality (e.g., Minnesota Multiphasic Personality Inventory-II, Millon Clinical Multiaxial Inventory-III).

The one way in which assessment for integrative therapy departs from the usual and traditional is that we collect, from the outset, information on multiple patient dimensions that will guide treatment selection. In fact, the computer-based assessments for both clinicians and clients described earlier enhance the development of treatment plans within the integrative tradition (Beutler & Groth-Marnat, 2003; Harwood & Williams, 2003).

In order to apply treatment-focused assessment, integrative therapy is faced with the central challenge of identifying those patient dimensions and corresponding treatment qualities that will improve our treatment decisions. There are tens of thousands of potential permutations and combinations of patient, therapist, treatment, and setting variables that could contribute. We rely primarily on the available empirical research to identify a limited number of patient dimensions that influence therapy success, and we use focused assessments to target those dimensions that are most predictive of differential treatment response.

This assessment tactic is not without several problems. The main problem has always been the sheer number of potentially valuable patient characteristics that have been researched. Even if all were effective predictors of change, there are far too many of them for clinicians to organize and use consistently. Moreover, researchers may disagree about which characteristics of patients and therapies are the most important. Both of these problems must be overcome before it is possible to balance and weight their contributions in a predictive algorithm.

Fortunately, our programmatic research over the years (see Beutler, Clarkin, & Bongar, 2000) addressed these problems by sequencing three strategies to identify the most potent patient contributors to change and the treatment qualities with which they interact. First, we reviewed an extensive body of research in order to identify what characteristics had been found that contributed to treatment success. Second, these characteristics were reduced in number by a process of iterative discussions and review of research studies. Third, we undertook a cross-validation study on nearly 300 depressed patients. A sophisticated statistical analysis (structural equation modeling) led to further reductions in the numbers of patient and treatment qualities to the most efficient few. Algorithms were developed to predict change, and these were then used to help clinicians plan treatment.

Five Patient Characteristics

In this chapter, we present a sampling of five patient characteristics commonly used by integrative psychotherapists. These patient characteristics guide us in identifying a beneficial fit between patient and treatment. Of course, integrative therapists are not confined to these five considerations in making treatment decisions, but they do illustrate the process of clinical assessment and treatment matching in integrative psychotherapies.

Diagnosis. We organize our treatment planning in part around the disorders as described in DSM-IV. Although diagnosis alone is not sufficient, there are practical reasons why diagnosis is necessary. First, insurance companies demand a diagnosis, and utilization review is done in reference to diagnosis. Second, treatment research is usually organized around the task of determining what is helpful to specific diagnostic groups, and the major symptoms comprising a diagnosis make a suitable way of evaluating the effectiveness of treatment. In order to profit from this research, one must know the patient's diagnosis. Third, specialized and manualized treatments have been developed for many disorders.

At the same time, there are many reasons why diagnosis alone is insufficient for treatment planning. Diagnoses are pathology oriented and neglect a patient's strengths. The criteria established for disorders are multiple, change continually, and select different groups of patients. Axis I patients may also suffer from comorbid Axis I disorders, in addition to one or more Axis II disorders. Few treatments exert effects that are restricted or specific to a particular diagnostic group. It is for these reasons that one must formulate treatment plans for individuals, not for isolated disorders.

We focus on Axis I and Axis II disorders for treatment planning. However, the combination of all five axes—a large array of possibilities—must be considered in treatment planning for the individual. In the multiaxial DSM-IV, the diagnosis is not limited to Axis I (symptoms) and Axis II (personality disorders) considerations but includes environmental stress (Axis IV) and overall functioning (Axis V). This is why it should be no surprise that patients sharing the same Axis I disorder could and should receive quite different treatments. The Axis V or GAF rating may be of particular importance in treatment planning, serving as a simple index of the patient's level of functional impairment.

Stages of Change. The stages represent a person's readiness to change, defined as a period of time as well as a set of tasks needed for movement to the next stage. The stages are behavior and time specific, not enduring personality traits. *Precontemplation* is the stage at which there is no intention to change behavior in the foreseeable future. Most individuals in this stage are unaware or underaware of their problems; however, their families, friends, and employers are often well aware that the precontemplators have problems. When precontemplators present for psychotherapy, they often do so because of pressure or coercion from others. Resistance to recognizing or modifying a problem is the hallmark of precontemplation.

Contemplation is the stage in which people are aware that a problem exists and are seriously thinking about overcoming it but have not yet made a commitment to take action. People can remain stuck in the contemplation stage for years. Contemplators struggle with their positive evaluations of their dysfunctional behavior and the amount of effort, energy, and loss it will cost to overcome it. Serious consideration of problem resolution is the central element of contemplation.

Preparation is a stage that combines intention and behavioral criteria. Individuals in this stage intend to take action in the near future and have unsuccessfully taken action in the past year. Individuals who are prepared for action report small behavioral changes, such as drinking less or contacting health-care professionals. Although they have reduced their problem, they have not yet reached a threshold for effective action, such as abstinence from alcohol abuse. They are intending, however, to take such action in the very near future.

Action is the stage in which individuals modify their behavior, experiences, and/or environment in order to overcome their problems. Action involves the most overt behavioral changes and requires considerable commitment of time and energy. Behavioral changes in the action stage tend to be most visible and externally recognized. Modification of the target behavior to an acceptable level and concerted efforts to change are the hallmarks of action.

Maintenance is the stage in which people work to prevent relapse and consolidate the gains attained during action. For addictive behaviors, this stage extends from 6 months to an indeterminate period past the initial action. For some behaviors, maintenance can be considered to last a lifetime. Being able to remain free of the problem and to consistently engage in a new, incompatible behavior for more than 6 months are the criteria for maintenance.

A patient's stage of change suggests the use of certain treatment methods and relationships. Table 14.1 illustrates where leading systems of therapy are probably most effective in the stages of change. Methods and strategies associated with psychoanalytic and insight-oriented psychotherapies are most useful during the earlier precontemplation and contemplation stages. Existential, cognitive, and interpersonal therapies are particularly well suited to the preparation and action stages. Behavioral methods and exposure therapies are most useful during action and maintenance. Each therapy system has a place, a differential place, in the big picture of behavior change.

The therapist's relational stance is also matched to the patient's stage of change. The research and clinical consensus on the therapist's stance at different stages can be characterized as follows (Prochaska & Norcross, 2002). With precontemplators, often the therapist's stance is like that of a nurturing parent joining with the resistant youngster who is both drawn to and repelled by the prospect of becoming more independent.

TABLE 14.1   Integration of Psychotherapy Systems within the Stages of Change

Stages of Change				
Precontemplation	Contemplation	Preparation	Action	Maintenance
Motivational interviewing				
Strategic family therapy				
Psychoanalytic therapy				
	Analytical therapy			
	Adlerian therapy			
		Existential therapy		
		Rational emotive behavior therapy (REBT)		
		Cognitive therapy		
		Interpersonal therapy (IPT)		
		Gestalt therapy		
			Behavior therapy	
			Structural family therapy	
			EMDR and exposure	

With contemplators, the therapist's role is akin to that of a Socratic teacher who encourages clients to develop their own insights and ideas about their condition. With clients who are preparing for action, the therapist is like an experienced coach who has been through many crucial matches and can provide a fine game plan or can review the person's own action plan. With clients who are progressing into maintenance, the integrative psychotherapist becomes more of a consultant who is available to provide expert advice and support when action is not progressing as smoothly as expected.

Coping Style.   The client's coping style consists of his or her habitual behavior when confronting new or problematic situations. Patients tend to adopt a style of coping that places them somewhere between two extreme but relatively stable types. They are identified by which of the prototypical end points they most resemble when confronted with a problem and the need to make change. Simply, they tend either toward *externalizing* coping (impulsive, stimulation-seeking, extroverted) and *internalizing* coping (self-critical, inhibited, introverted).

Coping style is a marker for whether the psychotherapy should ideally focus on symptomatic reduction or broader thematic objectives. Symptom-focused and skill-building therapies are more effective among externalizing patients. Acting-out children and impulsive adults, for example, are usually best served by reducing their problems via skill development methods. By contrast, a shift from a skill building or symptom focus to the use of insight and awareness-enhancing therapies is typically most effective among internalizing patients. Methods here vary from therapist to therapist but may well include interpretations of the parent–child linkage, analysis of transference and resistance, review of recurrent themes and exercises to enhance awareness of feelings. Nonetheless, research suggests that moving from a symptomatic to an insight focus is most supportive of change among these patients (Beutler, Clarkin, & Bongar, 2000).

Reactance Level.   Patient reactance is a variation of behaviors that are often described as "resistance." A reactant patient is easily provoked by and responds oppositionally to external demands. The propensity to engage in a reactant pattern is a reliable marker for the amount of therapist directiveness to be employed. High reactance indicates the need for nondirective, self-directed, or paradoxical techniques. Conversely, low reactance indicates the patient's accessibility to a wider range of directive techniques, including therapist control. In other words, the use of nondirective and self-directed interventions improves effectiveness with highly resistant patients. By contrast, directive and structured techniques, such as cognitive restructuring, advice, and behavior contracting, improve effectiveness with less resistant patients.

Patient Preferences.   When ethically and clinically appropriate, we accommodate a client's preferences in psychotherapy. These preferences may be heavily influenced by the client's sociodemographics—gender, ethnicity, culture, and sexual orientation, for example—as well as by their attachment styles and previous experiences in psychotherapy. These preferences may be related to the person of the therapist (age, gender, religion, ethnicity/race), to the therapeutic relationship (how warm or tepid, how active or passive, and so on), to therapy methods (preference for or against homework, dream analysis, two-chair dialogues), or to treatment formats (refusing group therapy or medication).

We work diligently in the beginning sessions to identify our patients' strong preferences and subsequently to accommodate these preferences when feasible. Controlled research (Swift & Callahan, 2009) and clinical experience demonstrate that attending to what the patient desires decreases misunderstandings, facilitates the alliance, and establishes collaboration—all relationship qualities connected to therapy success (Norcross,

2002). It would be naïve to assume that patients always know what they want and what is best for them. But if clinicians had more respect for the notion that their clients often sense how they can best be served, fewer relational mismatches might occur (Lazarus, 1993).

Summary.   The five client characteristics listed above serve as reliable markers to systematically tailor treatment to the individual patient, problem, and context. Although this list is likely to change as research progresses, these variables have evolved from extensive reviews and meta-analyses of treatment research. These client characteristics, including but not limited to diagnosis, can be applied independently of a specific theoretical orientation. All of this is to say that psychotherapy has progressed to the point where clinically relevant and readily assessable patient characteristics can suggest specific treatments and thereby enhance the effectiveness of our clinical work.

Process of Psychotherapy

The integrative imperative to match or tailor psychotherapy to the patient can be (and has been) misconstrued as an authority-figure therapist prescribing a specific form of psychotherapy for a passive client. The clinical reality is precisely the opposite. Our goal is for an empathic therapist to work toward an optimal relationship that both enhances collaboration and secures the patient's sense of safety and commitment. The nature of such an optimal relationship is determined both by patient preferences and by therapist's knowledge of how the client's personality determines his or her behavior. If a client frequently resists, for example, then the therapist considers whether she is pushing something that the client finds incompatible (preferences), or the client is not ready to make changes (stage of change), or is uncomfortable with a directive style (reactance). Integrative psychotherapy leads by following the client (Norcross, 2010).

Change takes place through interrelated processes: the nature of the patient–therapist relationship, the treatments that are used, and the way the patient avoids relapse. A comprehensive treatment involves defining the setting in which treatment will be applied, the format of its delivery, its intensity, the role of pharmacotherapy (medications), and the particular therapeutic strategies and techniques.

Therapeutic Relationship

All psychotherapy occurs within the sensitive and curative context of the human relationship. Empirically speaking, therapy success can best be predicted by the properties of the patient and of the therapy relationship (see Norcross, 2002, for reviews); only 10 to 15% of outcome is generally accounted for by any particular treatment technique.

It is a colossal misunderstanding to view treatment selection as a disembodied, technique-oriented process. Integrative psychotherapies attempt to customize not only therapy techniques but also relationship stances to individual clients. One way to conceptualize the matter, paralleling the notion of "treatments of choice" in terms of techniques, is how clinicians determine "therapeutic relationships of choice" in terms of interpersonal stances (Norcross & Beutler, 1997).

In creating and cultivating the therapy relationship, we rely heavily on clinical experience and empirical research on what works. Reviews of hundreds of studies indicate that the therapeutic alliance, empathy, goal consensus, and collaboration are demonstrably effective (Norcross, 2002). Collecting feedback from the client about his/her progress and satisfaction throughout the course of psychotherapy also demonstrably improves success (Lambert, 2005). Therapists' positive regard, congruence, feedback, moderate self-disclosure, and management of their countertransference are probably effective (Norcross, 2002). Conducting the best of evidence-based treatment all comes to naught unless the client feels connected and participates willingly.

Early on, then, we strive to develop a working alliance and to demonstrate empathy for the client's experiences and concerns. We proceed collaboratively in establishing treatment goals, in securing the patient's preferences, in allaying the initially expected distrust and fear, and in presenting ourselves as caring and supportive. Of course, the therapy relationship must also be matched or tailored to the individual patient.

Treatment Planning

Treatment planning invariably involves the interrelated decisions about setting, format, intensity, pharmacotherapy, and strategies and techniques. The important point here is that each client will respond best to a different configuration or mix of components. We cannot and should not assume that the treatment will automatically be outpatient individual therapy on a weekly basis. Below we consider each of these decisions, devoting more time to the strategies and methods.

Treatment Setting.   The setting is where the treatment occurs—a psychotherapist's office, a psychiatric hospital, a halfway house, an outpatient clinic, a secondary school, a medical ward, and so on. The choice of setting depends primarily on the relative need for restricting and supporting the patient, given the severity of psychopathology and the support in the patient's environment.

Each treatment decision is related to the other treatment decisions, as well as to certain patient characteristics (to be considered shortly). The optimal setting, for example, is partially determined by symptomatic impairment and partially reflects reactance level. Those clients who are most impaired and resistant have the greatest need for a restrictive environment. Outpatient treatment is always preferred over a restrictive setting; indeed, preference is nearly always for the least restrictive setting.

Treatment Format.   The format indicates who directly participates in the treatment. It is the interpersonal context within which the therapy is conducted. The typical treatment formats—individual, group, couples, and family—are characterized by a set of treatment parameters, all determined largely by the number and identities of the participants. (See the Treatment section in this chapter for additional remarks on treatment formats.)

Treatment Intensity.   The intensity of psychotherapy is the product of the *duration* of the treatment episode, the *length* of a session, and the *frequency* of contact. It may also involve the use of multiple formats, such as both group and individual therapy or both pharmacotherapy and psychotherapy.

Intensity should be gauged as a function of problem complexity and severity, also taking into account the patient's resources. For example, a patient with a multiplicity of treatment goals, severe functional impairment, few social supports, and a personality disorder is likely to require substantially longer, more intense, and more varied treatment than a patient with a simpler problem. Brief treatments are obviously not for everyone; many patients will need long-term treatment or lifetime care.

Pharmacotherapy.   Decades of clinical research and experience have demonstrated that psychotropic medications are particularly indicated for more severe and chronic disorders. If pharmacotherapy is indicated, the question becomes how it should be prescribed: Which medication in which dosage and for how long?

Unlike some systems of psychotherapy, integrative psychotherapies are well suited to the integration of pharmacotherapy and psychotherapy. This position, of course, is consistent with the pluralism underlying treatment selection.

At the same time, we would offer a cautionary note here. Tightening insurance reimbursements and restrictions on mental health care are unduly favoring pharmacotherapy at the expense of psychotherapy. This situation is clinically and empirically appalling to us because research indicates that, in fact, there is frequently no stronger medicine than psychotherapy (e.g., Antonuccio, 1995; DeRubeis, Hollon, et al., 2005). The preponderance of scientific evidence shows that psychotherapy is generally as effective as medications in treating most nonpsychotic disorders, especially when patient-rated measures and long-term follow-ups are considered. This is not to devalue the salutary impact of pharmacotherapy; rather, it is to underscore the reliable potency of psychotherapy. In addition, we believe that combined treatments should be carefully coordinated and should entail psychoeducation for patients and their support system. Medication alone is not an integrative treatment.

Strategies and Techniques.   When clinicians first meet clients, they are tempted to focus immediately and intensely on particular therapy strategies and techniques. However, as we have noted, treatment selection always involves a cascading series of interrelated decisions. A truly integrated treatment will recursively consider these other decisions before jumping to therapy strategies.

The selection of techniques and strategies is the most controversial component of integrative therapies. Proponents of disparate theoretical orientations endorse decidedly different views of what appear to be the same techniques. Moreover, any given technique can be used in different ways. Thus, rather than focusing on specific techniques per se, we prefer prescribing change principles. These principles can be implemented in a number of ways and with diverse techniques. By mixing and matching procedures from different therapy systems, we tailor the treatment to the particular patient.

Humans, including psychotherapists, cannot process more than four or five matching dimensions at once (Halford, Baker, McCredden, & Bain, 2005). As illustrated above, we principally consider five patient characteristics (diagnosis, stage of change, coping style, reactance level, and patient preferences) that have a proven empirical track record as prescriptive guidelines.

Relapse Prevention.   Tailoring psychotherapy to the individual patient, as we have described, enhances the effectiveness of psychotherapy. But even when psychotherapy is effective, relapse is the rule rather than the exception in many behavioral disorders, particularly the addictive, mood, and psychotic disorders. Thus, teaching relapse prevention to clients toward the end of psychotherapy is strongly advisable in practically all cases.

Relapse prevention helps clients identify "high risks" for regression, makes plans for avoiding such situations, and builds maintenance skills (Marlatt & Donovan, 2007). The patient and therapist examine the environment in which the patient lives, works, and recreates and then pinpoint those locations, people, and situational demands that have characteristically provoked dysfunction This analysis is coupled with teaching the patient to identify cues that signal when he or she is beginning to experience the depression, anxiety, or even euphoria that has typically preceded problem onset. These cues are linked to alternative behaviors that involve help seeking, self-control practice, and avoidance of overwhelming situational stress. Finally, in most circumstances, we try to overcome obstacles that may prevent the patient from seeking help from us or from other mental health professionals once again.

Maintenance sessions are indicated when the problem is complex, when the patient suffers from high functional impairment, and when a personality disorder is present. Maintenance work may also be indicated when the course of treatment is erratic and when symptom resolution is not consistently obtained within a period of 6 months. These features are particularly strong indicators of the tendency to relapse, and maintenance sessions can address emerging problems before they are recognized by the patient.

Mechanisms of Psychotherapy

Integrative psychotherapies do not presume single or universal change mechanisms. The mechanism of action may be very different for different individuals, even though they all may manifest similar symptoms. To an individual who is defensive, the mechanism may be the benevolent, corrective modeling of trust and collaboration offered by an empathic therapist, but for an individual who is trusting and self-reflective, the mechanism of action may be insight and reconceptualization. Similarly, the change mechanism for helping a fearful and anxious patient may be exposure to feared events and supportive reassurance. The point is that there are multiple pathways of change.

Table 14.2 presents nine mechanisms of action or, as we would prefer to call them, change processes. These processes have received the most empirical support to date in our research. The change processes most often used by psychotherapists are consciousness raising and the helping relationship. Virtually all therapies endorse the expansion of consciousness and the therapeutic relationship as potent mechanisms of action or change processes. The least frequently used processes are environmental control and

TABLE 14.2	Nine Change Processes and Representative Therapy Methods
Change Process	**Definition: Representative Methods**
Consciousness raising	Increasing awareness about self and problem: observations; reflections; confrontations; interpretations; bibliotherapy
Self-reevaluation	Assessing how one feels and thinks about oneself with respect to a problem: value clarification; imagery; corrective emotional experience
Emotional arousal	Experiencing and expressing feelings about one's problems: expressive exercises; psychodrama; grieving losses; role playing
Social liberation	Increasing alternatives in society: advocating for rights of oppressed; empowering; policy interventions
Self-liberation	Choosing and committing to act or belief in ability to change: decision-making therapy; logotherapy techniques; commitment-enhancing techniques
Counterconditioning	Substituting incompatible healthy alternatives for problem behaviors: relaxation; desensitization; assertion; cognitive restructuring
Environmental control	Re-engineering environmental stimuli that elicit problem behaviors: adding positive reminders; restructuring the environment; avoiding high-risk cues; fading
Contingency management	Rewarding oneself or being rewarded by others for making changes: contingency contracts; overt and covert reinforcement; self-reward
Helping relationships	Being understood, validated, and supported by a significant other: empathy, collaboration, positive regard, feedback, self-disclosure

Source: Adapted from Prochaska, Norcross, & DiClemente, 1995.

social liberation; the former is seen by some therapists as unduly emphasizing the power of the environment, the latter as improperly bordering on political advocacy.

Integrative therapists experience no hesitation in employing any or all of these change processes; we have no ideological axe to grind. Like therapists from single-school systems, integrative therapists rely heavily on consciousness raising and the therapeutic relationship. But unlike many therapists from single-school approaches, integrative therapists have at their disposal the full range of these change processes, ready to choose among them depending on the specific situation. Some cases call for building skills and implementing environmental control; addicts, in particular, need to learn to avoid people, places, and things that trigger their substance abuse. Other cases call for social liberation; oppressed and minority clients, in particular, profit from a therapist's modeling political advocacy and encouraging liberation strategies.

Moreover, these change processes are differentially effective at different stages of change. In general terms, change processes traditionally associated with the experiential and psychoanalytic persuasions are most useful during the earlier precontemplation and contemplation stages. Change processes traditionally associated with the existential, cognitive, and behavioral traditions, by contrast, are most useful during action and maintenance.

This pattern serves as an important guide. Once a patient's stage of change is evident, the integrative psychotherapist knows which change processes to apply in order to help that patient progress to the next stage of change. Rather than apply the change processes in a haphazard or trial-and-error manner, therapists can begin to use them in a much more systematic and effective way. It is not enough simply to declare that multiple change processes operate in psychotherapy; we must know how they can be selected and sequenced in ways that accelerate psychotherapy and improve its outcome.

We have observed two frequent mismatches in this respect. First, some therapists rely primarily on change processes most indicated for the contemplation stage, such as consciousness raising and self-reevaluation, when clients are moving into the action stage. They try to modify behavior by helping clients become more aware. This is a common criticism of psychoanalysis: Insight alone does not necessarily bring about behavior change. Second, other therapists rely primarily on change processes most indicated for the action stage, such as contingency management, environmental control, and counterconditioning, when clients are still in the precontemplation or contemplation stage. They try to modify behavior by pushing clients into action without the requisite awareness and commitment. This is a common criticism of radical behaviorism: Overt action without insight is likely to lead only to temporary change.

APPLICATIONS

Who Can We Help?

By virtue of its flexibility, integrative psychotherapy is applicable to practically all patient populations and clinical disorders. Children, adolescents, adults, and older adults; diagnosable disorders and growth experiences; private pay or managed care. Avoiding one-size-fits-all treatment and tailoring therapy to the unique individual make it adaptable to a wide range of problems. In fact, we cannot envision a client or a disorder for whom integrative psychotherapy would be contraindicated.

Integrative psychotherapy is particularly indicated for (1) complex patients and presentations, such as clients with multiple diagnoses and comorbid disorders; (2) disorders that have not historically responded favorably to conventional, pure-form psychotherapies, such as personality disorders, eating disorders, PTSD, and chronic mental illness; (3) disorders in which the controlled treatment outcome research is scant; and (4) clients for whom pure-form therapies have failed or have been only partially successful.

The research indicates that patients who are functionally impaired respond best to a comprehensive and integrated treatment. Specifically, more impaired or disabled patients call for more treatment, lengthier treatment, psychoactive medication, multiple therapy formats (individual, couples, group), and explicit efforts to strengthen their social support networks (Beutler, Harwood, Alimohamed, & Malik, 2002). Schizophrenia, borderline personality disorder, and multiple addictions are cases in point; to put it simply, complex problems require complex treatments.

No therapy or therapist is immune to failure. It is at such times that experienced clinicians often wonder whether therapy methods from orientations other than their own might more appropriately have been included in the treatment or whether another orientation's strength in dealing with the particular problems might complement the therapist's own orientational weakness. Integrative therapies assume that each orientation has its particular domain of expertise and that these domains can be linked to maximize their effectiveness (Pinsof, 1995).

When integrative therapy fails, it may be a result of a failure to follow the guiding integrative principles, a lack of skill in implementing a particular treatment, or a poor fit between the particular patient and the particular therapist. Each of these alternatives should be considered when a patient is not accomplishing his or her goals at a rate expected among similar patients.

One clear strength of mixing and matching therapy methods is the ability to address clients' multiple goals. Most clients desire both insight and action; they seek awareness into themselves and their problems, as well as reduction of their distressing symptoms. The integrative therapist can focus on one or both broad goals, depending on the client's preferences. Similarly, integrative psychotherapists can simultaneously tackle improvement in several domains of a client's life: symptoms, cognitions, emotions, relationships, and intrapsychic conflicts. Change in one domain or on a single level nearly always generates synergistic change in another.

Treatment

The term *integration* refers typically to the synthesis of diverse systems of psychotherapy, but it also has a host of other meanings. One is the combination of therapy formats—individual, couples, family, and group. Another is the combination of medication and psychotherapy, also known as combined treatment. In both cases, a strong majority of clinicians (more than 80%) consider these to be part of the meaning of integration (Norcross & Napolitano, 1986).

In practice, integrative psychotherapies are committed to the synthesis of practically all effective, ethical change methods. These include integrating self-help and psychotherapy, integrating Western and Eastern perspectives, integrating social advocacy with psychotherapy, integrating spirituality into psychotherapy, and so on. All are compatible with a comprehensive treatment, but we have restricted ourselves in this chapter to the traditional meaning of integration as the blending of diverse theoretical orientations.

We are impressed by the effectiveness of group, couples, and family therapy. Therapy conducted in these formats is generally as effective as individual therapy, but patients and therapists usually prefer the individual format. Even so, a multiperson format is indicated if social support systems are low and if one or more of the major problems involves a specific other person.

Integrative psychotherapy embraces both long-term and short-term treatments. The length of therapy should be determined not by the therapist's preference or theoretical orientation but by the patient's needs. Virtually every form of brief therapy advertises itself, in comparison to its original long version, as active in nature, collaborative in relationship, and integrative in orientation (Hoyt, 1995). Brief therapy and integrative therapy share a pragmatic and flexible outlook that is contrary to the ideological one that characterized the earlier school domination in the field.

Evidence

The empirical evidence on integrative treatments has grown considerably in recent years, and controlled research has been undertaken on several specific integrative therapies, including our own.

The outcome research supporting integrative psychotherapies comes in several guises. First and most generally, the entire body of psychotherapy research has provided the foundation for the key principles on which integrative treatment rests. This is the basis from which we have systematized the process of treatment selection. A genuine advantage of being integrative is the vast amount of research attesting to the efficacy of psychotherapy and pointing to its differential effectiveness with certain types of disorders and patients. Integration tries to incorporate state-of-the-art research findings into its open framework, in contrast to becoming yet another "system" of psychotherapy.

A second source of research evidence is that conducted on specific integrative treatments. A review of integrative therapies (Schottenbauer, Glass, & Arnkoff, 2005) determined substantial empirical support (defined as four or more randomized controlled studies) for

- Acceptance and commitment therapy
- Cognitive analytic therapy
- Dialectical behavior therapy
- Emotionally focused couple therapy
- Eye movement desensitization and reprocessing (EMDR)
- Mindfulness-based cognitive therapy
- Systematic treatment selection (STS)
- Transtheoretical psychotherapy (stages of change)

Integrative therapists can use these treatments for a particular patient—say, dialectical behavior therapy for a patient suffering from borderline personality disorder. Or integrative therapists can use parts of these treatments for many patients—say, teaching mindfulness or employing EMDR whenever indicated. These treatments and their elements are optimally employed with patients and in situations for which research has found evidence of effectiveness. We hasten to add that the incorporation of these treatments and their parts should occur within a systematic process and an integrative perspective. That is, be integrative, not syncretic.

Another dozen self-identified integrative therapies have garnered some empirical support, defined as between one and four randomized controlled studies. These include behavioral family systems therapy; integrative cognitive therapy; process–experiential therapy; and Lazarus's multimodal therapy.

A third source of research evidence for integrative psychotherapies is the identification of guiding principles on which a clinician of any theoretical orientation can map treatment. Systematic treatment selection (STS), as listed above, does not advocate for specific methods but, instead, proposes the use of research-informed principles. A joint task force of the Society of Clinical Psychology (APA Division 12) and the North American Society for Psychotherapy Research (Castonguay & Beutler, 2006) undertook comprehensive reviews of treatment research on mood, anxiety, personality, and substance abuse disorders. Their mission was to extract, from the more than 5,000 studies reviewed, a set of principles that could be used to guide clinicians in treatment planning.

Research on participant, relationship and treatment variables was undertaken and separately analyzed. The principles ultimately extracted from that literature included the patient characteristics considered in this chapter.

A fourth and specific source of research evidence supporting our particular integrative psychotherapy is the ongoing programmatic research on treatment selection according to client characteristics, including the stages of change. Below we summarize the reviews of research evidence underpinning our approach presented in this chapter in terms of patient characteristics.

Stages of Change

The amount of progress clients make following treatment tends to be a function of their pretreatment stage of change. This has been found to be true for patients suffering from depression, panic, eating disorders, cigarette smoking, brain injury, and cardiac conditions, to name just a few. The strong stage effect applies immediately following intervention, as well as 12 and 18 months afterward (Prochaska, DiClemente, Velicer, & Rossi, 1993). In one representative study of 570 smokers, the amount of success was directly related to the stage they were in before treatment (Prochaska & DiClemente, 1983). Of the precontemplators, only 3% took action by 6 months; of the contemplators, 20% took action; and of those in preparation, 41% attempted to quit by 6 months. These data demonstrate that treatment designed to help people progress just one stage in a month can double the chances of their taking action in the near future.

One of the most powerful findings to emerge from our research is that particular processes of change are more effective during particular stages of change. Twenty-five years of research in behavioral medicine and psychotherapy converge in showing that different processes of change are differentially effective in certain stages of change. A meta-analysis (Rosen, 2000) of 47 cross-sectional studies examining the relationships among the stages and the processes of change showed large effect sizes ($d = .70$ and $.80$) across the stages.

Controlled research on the transtheoretical model indicates that tailoring treatments to the client's stage of change significantly improves outcome across disorders. This stage matching has been demonstrated in large trials for stress management, smoking cessation, bullying violence, and health behaviors (see Prochaska & Norcross, 2010, for review).

In sum, hundreds of studies have demonstrated the effectiveness of tailoring treatment to the client's stage of change. Longitudinal studies affirm the relevance of these constructs for predicting premature termination and treatment outcome. Comparative outcome studies attest to the value of stage-matched treatments and relationships. Population-based studies support the importance of developing interventions that match the needs of individuals at all stages of change (see Prochaska, Norcross, & DiClemente, 1995).

Coping Style

In the research, attention has been devoted primarily to the externalizing (impulsive, stimulation-seeking, extroverted) and internalizing coping styles (self-critical, inhibited, introverted). Approximately 80% of the more than 20 studies investigating this dimension have demonstrated differential effects of the type of treatment as a function of patient coping style. Effect sizes associated with a "good fit" between patient coping style and the therapist's methods has been found to range from .61 to 1.40 (Beutler, in press). Specifically, interpersonal and insight-oriented therapies are more effective among internalizing patients, whereas symptom-focused and skill-building therapies are more effective among externalizing patients (Beutler, in press; Beutler, Harwood, Alimohamed, & Malik, 2002).

Reactance Level

Research confirms what one would expect: that high patient reactance is consistently associated with poorer therapy outcomes (in 82% of more than 25 studies). But matching therapist directiveness to client reactance improves therapy outcome (80% of studies; Beutler et al., 2002). Specifically, clients presenting with high resistance benefited more from self-control methods, minimal therapist directiveness, and paradoxical interventions. By contrast, clients with low resistance benefited more from therapist directiveness and explicit guidance. The strength of this finding has been expressed as an effect size (d) averaging .83 (Beutler, in press).

These client markers provide prescriptive as well as proscriptive guidance on the treatments of choice. In reactance, the prescriptive implication is to match the therapist's amount of directiveness to the patient's reactance, and the proscriptive implication is to avoid meeting high client reactance with high therapist direction. In stages of change, action-oriented therapies are quite effective with individuals who are in the preparation or action stage. However, these same therapies tend to be less effective and even detrimental with individuals in the precontemplation and contemplation stages.

Preferences

Client preferences and goals are frequently direct indicators of the best therapeutic method and relationship for that person. Decades of empirical evidence attest to the benefit of seriously considering, and at least beginning with, the relational preferences and treatment goals of the client (Arnkoff, Glass, & Shapiro, 2002). A meta-analysis of 26 studies, involving 2,300 clients, compared the treatment outcomes of clients matched to their preferred treatment to those clients not matched to a preferred treatment. The findings indicated a small, positive effect ($d = .15$) in favor of clients matched to preferences. But, more importantly, clients who were matched to their preference were only about half as likely to drop out of psychotherapy—a powerful effect indeed (Swift & Callahan, 2009).

Diagnosis

Of the patient characteristics considered here, diagnosis is the one with the least evidence of differential treatment effects. Although we cannot match with certainty, some marriages of disorder and treatment are probably better than others. For example, moderate depressions seem to be most responsive to cognitive therapy, interpersonal therapy, and pharmacotherapy. Behavior therapy and parent training seem to be the treatments of choice for most externalizing child conduct disorders. Some form of exposure seems best for obsessive–compulsive disorders and posttraumatic stress disorder. Conjoint treatments seem best suited for sibling rivalry and couples distress. At the same time, we would reiterate that excessive reliance on diagnosis alone to select a treatment is empirically questionable and clinically suspect.

Psychotherapy in a Multicultural World

The integrative maxim of "different strokes for different folks" converges naturally with multiculturalism. And by culture, we do not refer solely to race, but more broadly to the wonderful diversity of humanity: age and generational influences, disability status, religion, ethnicity, social status, sexual orientation, indigenous heritage, national origin, gender, and so on (Hays, 1996).

Single-school therapies, particularly those born of a dominant "father" and rooted in a culture-bound theory of personality, tend to subtly maintain White, androcentric (male-centered), Western-European, heterosexual norms. Many of the single-school "universal" principles are now rightfully perceived as examples of clinical myopia or cultural imperialism. Integrative therapies, by contrast, rely on neither a particular founder nor a theory of personality. Our sole "universal" principle is that people and cultures differ and should be treated as such. Evidence-based pluralism reigns as integration infuses diversity and flexibility into psychotherapy. No wonder that virtually every feminist, multicultural, and cultural–responsive theory describes itself as eclectic or integrative in practice.

Integrative psychotherapies have been applied cross-culturally and internationally with equal success. As offered to clients, integrative psychotherapies manifest as culturally sensitive or culturally adapted—modified to improve utilization, retention, and outcome. Psychotherapy can be adapted in many ways, such as incorporating the cultural values of the client into therapy, collaborating with indigenous healers, and matching clients with therapists of the same culture who speak, literally, the same language.

As in all practical matters in integrative psychotherapy, incorporating culture should be informed by the cumulative research. A meta-analysis of 76 studies (Griner & Smith, 2006) tells us, inter alia, that adapting therapy to the client's culture exerts a medium, positive effect ($d = .45$), that therapy targeted to a specific cultural group is more effective than that provided to clients from a variety of cultural backgrounds, and that therapy conducted in clients' native language (if other than English) is twice as effective as when it is conducted in English. Moreover, avoid translators in sessions whenever possible as their use is associated with weak alliances, more misdiagnoses (usually more severe than necessary), and higher dropout rates (Paniagua, 2005).

The upshot is for psychotherapists of all persuasions to mutually explore the singular needs and unique cultures of clients from the inception of psychotherapy. One effective practice, especially for historically marginalized populations, is to acquaint beginning clients with the respective roles of patient and therapist. Many patients hold divergent expectations about the process of psychotherapy and may be uncomfortable with mental health treatment. Pretherapy orientation is designed to clarify these expectations and to collaboratively define a more comfortable role for the client.

Another effective practice entails augmenting an individualistic position with a collectivistic orientation to clinical work. The optimal treatment format and therapist team, for example, may well depend on the culture of the particular client. In some cultures, clients will automatically enlist the support of friends, family members, neighbors, clergy, and perhaps traditional healers as part of their treatment and perhaps in their sessions. The culture-sensitive relationship, for another example, may well demand more than ordinary therapist empathy; it may require cultural empathy (Pederson, Crethar, & Carlson, 2008). As defined in the Western culture, empathy takes on an individualistic interpretation of human desire and distress. "I understand your personal feelings." Cultural empathy takes on a more inclusive orientation by placing cultural responsiveness at the center. It is a learned ability to accurately understand the client's self-experience from another culture and then to express that understanding back to the client. "I understand your personal feelings *and* your cultural context."

We enthusiastically embrace multiculturalism in psychotherapy. It's called integration, diversity within unity. Integrative therapy posits that the context for every individual—African, Asian, Latino, or Anglo; straight, gay, bisexual, or trans; Muslim, Christian, Jew, or atheist—is unique. And each psychotherapy needs to be individually constructed to match the needs of a particular person. In some cases, this involves helping individuals become free from social oppression. In other cases, it means helping them become free from mental obsessions. In yet other cases, it involves treatment of biological depression (Prochaska & Norcross, 2010).

CASE EXAMPLE

Ms. A is a 72-year-old European-American widow who was referred for psychotherapy by her son, a practicing psychiatrist in her neighborhood. She sought treatment for anxiety and agoraphobia.

History and Background

Ms. A was raised in Boston as the daughter of a modestly wealthy family. She was the only child of middle-aged and quite rigid parents. She related a poor relationship with her family and especially experienced difficulties with her mother, whom she described as "bossy and unreasonable."

Ms. A related that her first experience of panic when going out of the house occurred when she was 12. At the time, she was staying with a girlfriend while her mother shopped. As they were playing with dolls, Ms. A suddenly experienced a full-blown panic attack. She was overcome with a fear of dying, experienced heart palpitations, and felt short of breath to the point of fearing suffocation. Ms. A ran into the street and tried to yell for help, but she couldn't communicate, and no one heard her or offered assistance. She gradually calmed herself through self-control and forced breath control. She experienced periodic but relatively mild and spontaneous panic attacks through the next 2 years.

At about the age of 16, Ms. A began suffering from panic attacks more frequently and more severely. This resulted in her sleeping with her parents for several months and in her increasingly confining herself to known places and locations. She denied knowing what precipitated the increase in her panic attacks, but they occurred with the development of a relationship with a young man. He pursued her, but she found him unattractive and had no interest in a long-term relationship. He was insistent, and as a result, Ms. A began to see him socially; however, they had a tumultuous relationship punctuated by many separations and reunions. She finally succumbed to his insistence on marriage when she was 17, partially in response to the persuasion of her mother. The couple subsequently moved to Rhode Island to live close to his family.

Throughout the courtship and early years of marriage, the patient endured periodic panic attacks and periods of agoraphobia. Ms. A's symptoms increased and necessitated their moving back to Boston to be close to her family, where she could get the care that she felt she needed. She contemplated divorce and, indeed, separated and moved back with her parents, only to discover that she was pregnant. Ms. A reunited with her husband briefly after the baby's birth, but the panic symptoms became so extreme that she called and begged her mother to allow her to return home, claiming the situation to be a matter of life or death. She subsequently filed for divorce, but her husband fought the marital dissolution and successfully prevailed on the court to disallow the divorce.

Ms. A blamed her parents for her marital difficulties, and when she was unable to obtain a divorce, she left home, leaving the baby in the care of her mother, whom she despised. The patient successfully escaped the pursuit of her husband and her parents for several years. During that time, she experimented with lesbian relationships and came to think of herself as a lesbian. Concomitantly, her symptoms of panic and agoraphobia abated, and she recalled having no panic attacks for a period of about 3 years. The attacks began again, however, shortly after her parents, who had hired a private investigator to find her, reinitiated contact with her through an attorney. She was forced to negotiate an arrangement for the care of her daughter because her parents were getting too old to take care of the girl.

As plans for the future progressed, Ms. A was forced to meet with her estranged husband. For some time before and following these visits, the patient's panic episodes escalated. Through some counseling with the attorney, the patient acceded to her husband's demand that they reconcile and take the child and move away from her parents to "start over." They moved to Oregon.

The patient's effort to reestablish her marriage was successful for only a short period of time. In Oregon, she first sought medical treatment for panic and was briefly hospitalized. She was discharged with medication but stopped taking it after a couple of months. She reported no long-term benefit from the hospitalization. After discharge from the hospital, Ms. A initiated several lesbian affairs, which finally provoked her husband to leave. He subsequently returned to his family on the East Coast and left her to raise the child on her own. He successfully filed for divorce. She struggled to find work and to support her daughter, yet despite this turmoil, the intensity of her panic and agoraphobia abated once again. Nonetheless, she worried about the effect of her lesbian relationships on her daughter.

Soon, Ms. A met a wealthy man who fell in love with her in spite of her "secret" lesbian lifestyle. He proposed marriage to her and vowed to support her and her daughter, to adopt the daughter, and even to tolerate her lovers, on the condition that she would attempt to have children with him. Her daughter and any children that they produced would then be his heirs. After much thought, Ms. A agreed. The marriage lasted 25 years and produced two more children, a boy and a girl. Her husband died of cancer shortly after her youngest daughter graduated from high school. Following her husband's death, she began to live openly as a lesbian, and she has remained unmarried for the past 16 years.

About 10 years ago, Ms. A met a woman with whom she fell in love. They have maintained an ongoing, supportive relationship. It is notable that during this time, even dating back to the end of her second marriage, Ms. experienced only occasional mild anxiety and no panic. She continues to fear the prospect of panic—"the fear of fear"—and describes a general "distaste" for travel, as well as what she calls a "tendency to put off" going out for fear of becoming anxious. She also describes "being uncomfortable" when she is away from home, but she has not had any clinical symptoms of panic or phobia for more than a decade and a half. Even the most dominant and disturbing feeling that has plagued her through most of her life, the sense of being smothered and unable to breathe, disappeared. However, Ms. A does feel despondent and lethargic, has difficulty staying asleep, and has suffered other troubling symptoms of dysphoria and avoidance.

One event was particularly troubling. Approximately 5 years ago, while Ms. A and her lover were on vacation in another country, she awoke disoriented after having sex. She characterized this state as "disassociation" and "amnesia." She was unable to recall where she was, why she was there, and who her lover or her parents were. These symptoms passed within hours, but they recurred several more times, all immediately after having an intense sexual encounter. It was at this time that Ms. A sought psychotherapy for the first time. She saw a psychiatrist who found no medical reason for her dissociative experience and diagnosed it as a "transitory histrionic conversion." The psychiatrist followed Ms. A for about a year and prescribed antidepressants. This work was somewhat helpful, and as a result, Ms. A and her lover decided to cease further sexual contact for fear of triggering another "dissociation" attack. She terminated psychotherapy shortly after that time but has continued to get a variety of tranquilizers from her family physician because she has felt the need for them since that time. Ms. A and her female partner continue to maintain a loving platonic relationship.

Clinical Assessment and Formulation

The integrative therapist took the preceding history, developed a positive alliance with Ms. A, and secured consensus on her treatment goals in the first session. The patient was asked to complete several self-report instruments to evaluate her mental status and to identify those characteristics important in treatment planning. These instruments included the Stages of Change Questionnaire, the MMPI-2, the STS Self-Report Form, the Symptom Checklist 90R (SCL 90-R), and the Beck Depression Inventory-2 (BDI-2).

The results revealed Ms. A to be at the contemplation stage—aware of her problems but uncertain, conflicted, and anxious about how to solve them. She was worried and ruminative, with fears about her continuing ability to take care of herself and with guilt over her past mistakes. Ms. A was especially concerned that she might have harmed her children through ambivalence and neglect. She was, in addition, remorseful over not being able to provide the sexual gratification that her partner desired. These results suggested that the patient would be receptive to exploring her motivations and plans and to seeking understanding about the options that faced her in resolving her concerns.

Diagnostically, Ms. A had suffered from relatively severe panic in the past, but at the time she sought treatment it was considered to be largely in remission. Her agoraphobia, also severe in the past, was only mild to moderate. Like many anxious and agoraphobic patients, Ms. A was suffering from moderate concurrent depression.

Her STS-SR and the MMPI-2 results both suggested relatively mild impairment of daily activities, cognitive focus, and emotional control. Ms. A was able to carry on basic life tasks, to maintain intimate and social relationships, and to provide for her care and comfort. She denied any suicidal ideation and intention. Although driving and traveling caused her some discomfort, she did both on a regular basis. The fear of fear seemed to be more disabling than her actual symptoms. The patient did not warrant an Axis II diagnosis.

The chronicity of Ms. A's problem suggested a guarded prognosis, but she possessed many intellectual strengths and insights that would improve her prognosis. With a mild level of current impairment, a nonintensive treatment was considered sufficient. We agreed on weekly sessions of individual psychotherapy, entailing neither medication nor more frequent sessions.

After some discussion of her "dissociative" experiences, the clinician talked to the patient's family physician, who could not explain the symptoms. The clinician contacted a neurologist and found that a similar, relatively obscure condition had been observed, primarily among older males, to occur following strong exertion, including sexual activity. This condition, known as sudden transient amnesia, had rarely been noted among women, and even among men it was typically experienced only once or twice. It was not thought to be a continuing condition and was probably occasioned by exertion, hyperventilation, and the pattern of entering deep or delta sleep very shortly after the exertion.

Ms. A favored a predominantly internalizing style of coping (versus an externalizing style). Although she had some externalizing qualities, her test scores and interpersonal patterns indicated that her contemplative and ruminative style of functioning were dominant. These results were consistent with her contemplation stage of change and generally favored the use of insight-oriented and awareness-increasing methods.

At the same time, insight-based work should be preceded by efforts to reduce symptoms. This was especially a valued determination, given the patient's concerns with panic and her history of angry, panic-driven behaviors. Thus, we combined both action and insight with Ms. A. We began by using desensitization and exposure to address her fear of panic and her fear of fear. This was followed by stress management methods derived from cognitive analyses of stress. It was necessary to ensure that her panic and fear behaviors were under control before proceeding to insight-based themes.

We examined Ms. A's theme of wishes and avoidance in our insight work. We inspected her persistent phobic response when she was pushed into heterosexual relationships and hypothesized that such relationships may have induced guilt and fear that exacerbated and maintained panic. We hypothesized that the first panic attack may have occurred during sexual play with her playmate at age 12. Based on the strength of this interplay of heterosexual pressure and panic, we explored ways in which Ms. A had been smothered and pressured into these relationships by her parents. Both Ms. A and the therapist believed that the key to insight was understanding her marriages and feelings of being pressured sexually.

The patient's reactance level was assessed by her interpersonal history and her test results on the MMPI-2 and STS-SR. Ms. A's family history was characterized by conflict, mistrust, and forced control. It was associated with her response of moderate to severe rebelliousness. This pattern continued through at least her first marriage but dropped significantly in later relationships. The test results, on the other hand, suggested that at present, Ms. A was reasonably responsive and nonresistant to therapist directiveness. She was willing to take direction and exhibited compliance with structure, as well as the ability to work collaboratively with the therapist. Accordingly, we opted to employ moderate levels of therapist guidance and direction to accomplish both her behavioral action goals and her insight goals.

In the early stages of treatment, therefore, the integrative therapist guided Ms. A into exposure situations and suggested direct contact with feared and avoided activities (e.g., driving, leaving home). Later in treatment, the therapist used interpretations and suggestions about areas of emotional avoidance and thematic patterns in childhood related to the development of panic and agoraphobia. In particular, we focused on the patient's symptoms of "suffocating" within a restricted environment and her subsequent symptom reduction during times when she was less restricted and scrutinized.

In terms of treatment goals, Ms. A expressed a preference for both symptom relief and psychological insight. After a life of fear and avoidance, she sought and was prepared for a therapy that exposed her to her anxiety symptoms associated with driving and traveling and then gradually confronted her thematic conflicts of relationship demands.

In terms of the therapeutic relationship, Ms. A was comfortable with the prospect of a male, heterosexual therapist, declining when asked whether she might be more comfortable with a female therapist. She sought an active collaborator in her growth who would provide direction for her, would be a sounding board, and who would help her discover the origins of her anxiety. Ms. A was eager to engage in homework assignments to facilitate her progress, and although she balked when these assignments required her to drive, she always complied with the therapist's recommendations. On one occasion, she drove 50 miles in a heavy rainstorm to come to psychotherapy, surpassing any accomplishment she thought she would ever achieve.

Treatment Course

The first goal of any psychotherapy is the creation of an empathic, trusting relationship between patient and therapist. Two sessions were spent exploring the patient's feelings and trying to uncover her ambivalence and fear associated with self-expression. We explored feelings of guilt about her children and fears of aging.

The next four sessions were devoted to in vivo work on Ms. A's avoidance patterns. Since her symptoms of panic and agoraphobia were not obvious in the initial evaluation, we tried to produce some of these symptoms through rapid breathing, exposure training, and homework assignments. As we contacted areas of anxiety and fear, we introduced breathing control and cognitive restructuring to help her cope and to provide reassurance. For example, we walked around the neighborhood, spent time doing imagery to evoke arousal, and discussed matters about which she thought she might have anxiety. Interestingly, only momentary and mild anxiety was provoked. Relatively soon (within the first eight sessions), we began exploring her relationships with parents and children that were associated with her guilt and fear.

Ms. A identified her fears of having become like her mother, an authoritarian tyrant. She explained that she blamed herself for having injured her oldest daughter by her demands and abandonment, and she expressed guilt for having "made" her oldest son gay by not being a good role model. With encouragement and supportive advice, Ms. A spoke to these children and was surprised to discover that they were accepting and acknowledging of her difficulties. They also reassured her that they did not feel pressured or smothered by her—the metaphorical symptoms that she loathed as an agoraphobic.

Ms. A's guilt led to discussions of her belief in God. She had been raised in a reformed Jewish family, but her first husband was an orthodox Jew. She found religion troubling and had, she said, largely left her belief in God behind, except in her sense of being punished for neglecting her children. In that domain, try as she might, she still found herself praying to God for forgiveness whenever she thought about her children. To address these concerns, the patient kept a log of her religious thoughts and then used bibliotherapy materials to help her evaluate these thoughts. Specifically, she selected a cognitive therapy self-help book to work on her anxiety and depression. She kept track of thoughts and tried ways of changing those that were most hurtful to her. She kept notes about her progress, and we discussed these at each session.

In these sessions we also discussed Ms. A's negative reaction to having sex with her partner. One session was held with the two of them together, largely because Ms. A's difficulty had never been experienced outside this relationship. We explored their relationship and discussed their sexual desires. Discovering that Ms. A's symptoms of acute amnesia had been described in the medical literature as sudden transient amnesia gave her some relief, but she was still reluctant to go through the experience again. The patient's partner remained devoted and supportive of her decisions, whether or not they could ever restore sexual contact. On one occasion they initiated a sexual encounter, but it was suspended when the patient began having anticipatory fears. They agreed not to try sexual relations again. Although this was not an entirely satisfactory conclusion, the therapist chose to honor the couple's informed decision to seek their own resolution over time.

Outcome and Follow-up

Over the course of 12 sessions, Ms. A impressively reduced her anxiety, minimized her avoidance of driving and traveling, and decreased her concurrent depression. The SCL-90R and BDI-2 were repeated at the end of treatment. Both her anxiety and her depression had dropped substantially (the BDI from 24 to 14 and the SCL-90R from 75T to 54T). Symptomatically, she was better than ever. Ms. A courageously approached and apologized to her grown children for her potentially neglectful actions and negotiated a more satisfying relationship with her partner. Interpersonally, she mourned her losses and was moving forward. Despite all of these positive outcomes, as with most cases in psychotherapy, not all of her goals were realized. Her anticipatory fear of sexual relations led her not to attempt sex again.

Ms. A called the psychotherapist approximately one year after she had ended treatment "just to check in." She indicated that she had made several trips to the East Coast during the year and had experienced only one mild episode of panic. Nonetheless, she was thinking of returning to therapy for a few sessions to work on some "family issues." An appointment was made, but Ms. A called and cancelled, indicating that she would call again if she couldn't resolve the problem herself. An inadvertent contact with the patient's family some months later suggested that she was doing very well and had experienced no further difficulties.

Case Commentary

We have deliberately chosen to illustrate our integrative treatment with a patient that psychotherapy has historically neglected: elderly and lesbian. Although we live in an in increasingly multicultural world, much of psychotherapy is still developed for and researched on the young and heterosexual. Let Ms. A remind us all of the clinical and research imperative to extend psychotherapy to the marginalized and oppressed in society.

The integrative therapist can share some credit for the salubrious outcome in this case, but Ms. A deserves the lion's share. She intentionally exposed herself to anxiety-provoking situations and topics. She was a bright, brave, and hard-working client who progressed from the contemplation stage to the action stage and ultimately to the maintenance stage.

Where the integrative therapist was probably most effective was in systematically tailoring the therapeutic relationship and treatment methods specifically to Ms. A. The treatment proceeded stepwise in accordance with the empirical research, the patient's preferences, and her other nondiagnostic characteristics. The therapist combined several treatment goals (action and insight), therapy methods (those traditionally associated with behavioral, cognitive, psychodynamic, experiential, and systemic approaches), healing resources (psychotherapy, self-help, and spirituality), and treatment formats (individual, couples, and family) in a seamless and responsive manner.

Would a psychotherapist endorsing a single, brand-name therapy have achieved such impressive and comprehensive changes in the same number of sessions as the integrative therapist? We immodestly think not.

SUMMARY

Integrative psychotherapies are intellectually vibrant, clinically popular, and demonstrably effective. Integration converges with the evidence-based movement in emphasizing that different problems require different solutions and that these solutions increasingly can be selected on the basis of outcome research. Integrative therapies offer the evidence, flexibility, and responsiveness to meet the multifarious needs of individual patients and their unique contexts. For these reasons, integration will assuredly be a therapeutic mainstay of the 21st century.

Integration can take several different paths—theoretical integration, technical eclecticism, common factors, and assimilative integration—but it consistently searches for new ways of conceptualizing and conducting psychotherapy that go beyond the confines of single schools. Integration encourages practitioners and researchers to examine what other therapies have to offer, particularly when confronted with difficult cases and therapeutic failures. Rival therapy systems are increasingly viewed not as adversaries, but as welcome partners (Landsman, 1974); not as contradictory, but as complementary.

Integration is a meta-psychotherapy. It does not offer a model of psychopathology or a theory of personality, nor does it limit the mechanisms through which psychotherapy works. Instead, integration embraces the therapeutic value of many systems of psychotherapy and can be superimposed on whichever psychopathology model or therapy system a clinician endorses.

This chapter outlined our integrative therapy and its process of systematic treatment selection. This process applies empirical knowledge from multiple theoretical orientations on both diagnostic and nondiagnostic patient characteristics to the optimal choice of technical and relational methods. Such a therapy posits that many treatment methods and interpersonal stances have a valuable place in the repertoire of the contemporary psychotherapist. Their particular and differential place can be determined through outcome research, seasoned experience, and positioning the individual client at the center of the clinical enterprise. In the future, psychotherapy will be defined not by its brand names but by its effectiveness and applicability.

ANNOTATED BIBLIOGRAPHY AND WEB RESOURCES

Beutler, L. E., & Harwood, T. M. (2000). *Prescriptive psychotherapy: A practical guide to systematic treatment selection.* New York: Oxford University Press.
Translates the principles of systematic treatment selection into a treatment manual, which has been used in two randomized controlled trials of integrative psychotherapy. Includes methods of assessment, rating therapist compliance with the principles, and assessment of progress and outcome.

Beutler, L. E., & Groth-Marnat, G. (Eds.). (2003). *Integrated assessment of adult personality* (2nd ed.). New York: Guilford Press.
Identifies psychological assessment procedures and tests to evaluate the dimensions that predict psychotherapy outcome. Based on systematic treatment selection, this book reveals the relationships among patient variables and treatment effects and describes the computerized systems for helping the clinician develop treatment plans.

Castonguay, L. G., & Beutler, L. E. (Eds.). (2006). *Principles of therapeutic change that work.* New York: Oxford University Press.
Reports the results of a Society of Clinical Psychology (APA Division 12) and North American Society for Psychotherapy Task Force that identified research-informed principles that account for therapeutic change.

Norcross, J. C. (Ed.). (2002). *Psychotherapy relationships that work.* New York: Oxford University Press.
Compiles the empirical research on what works in the therapy relationship in two ways: effective elements of therapy relationships (what works in general) and effective methods of tailoring or customizing therapy to the individual patient (what works for particular patients).

Norcross, J. C., & Goldfried, M. R. (Eds.). (2005). *Handbook of psychotherapy integration* (2nd ed.). New York: Oxford University Press.
A state-of-the-art, comprehensive description of psychotherapy integration and its clinical practices by the leading proponents. Along with integrative therapies, the book addresses the concepts, history, training, research, and future of psychotherapy integration.

Prochaska, J. O., & Norcross, J. C. (2010). *Systems of psychotherapy: A transtheoretical analysis* (7th ed.). Pacific Grove, CA: Cengage-Brooks/Cole.
A systematic and balanced survey of 15 systems of psychotherapy from an integrative perspective. The comparative analysis demonstrates how much psychotherapy systems agree on the processes producing change while disagreeing on the content that needs to be changed.

Prochaska, J. O., Norcross, J. C., & DiClemente, C. C. (1995). *Changing for good.* New York: Avon.
The best and most accessible summary of the stages and the processes of change. Written in a self-help format for educated laypersons and professionals.

Society for the Exploration of Psychotherapy Integration: www.sepiweb.com/
The homepage of SEPI, the foremost integration organization, provides information on membership, conferences, the *Journal of Psychotherapy Integration,* and training opportunities.

Inner Life: Systematic Treatment: www.innerlife.com/
Online assessment and treatment matching based on the 30 years of research on systematic treatment. Generates an individualized yet comprehensive report to treatment plans.

Transtheoretical Model: www.uri.edu/research/cprc/
The homepage of the transtheoretical model features publications, measures, and research studies on the stages of change.

CASE READINGS AND VIDEOTAPES

Beutler, L. E. (2008). *Evidence-based treatment.* DVD. Washington, DC: American Psychological Association.
Dr. Beutler demonstrates his research-directed systematic treatment. He uses a presession assessment to tailor his approach to working with a young man suffering with depression who wants to be able to enjoy life again.

Beutler, L. E., Consoli, A. J., & Lane, G. (2005). Systematic treatment selection and prescriptive psychotherapy. In J. C. Norcross & M. R. Goldfried (Eds.), *Handbook of psychotherapy integration* (2nd ed., pp. 121–143). New York: Oxford University Press.
This chapter summarizes research and practice of systematic treatment selection and of prescriptive therapy. A case study illustrates the use of principles rather than models to guide treatment.

Beutler, L. E., Harwood, T. M., Bertoni, M., & Thomann, J. (2006). Systematic treatment selection and prescriptive therapy. In G. Stricker & J. Gold (Eds.), *A casebook of psychotherapy integration.* Washington, DC: American Psychological Association. [Revised and reprinted in D. Wedding & R. J. Corsini (Eds.), (2011). *Case studies in psychotherapy.* Belmont, CA: Brooks/Cole.]
This chapter describes the systematic treatment selection model for planning and integrating treatment.

Norcross, J. C. (2005). *Prescriptive eclectic psychotherapy.* DVD. Washington, DC: American Psychological Association.
Dr. Norcross demonstrates his adaptable, client-focused approach that tailors the therapy on the basis of the client's unique needs and situation. In this session, he works with a 33-year-old man whose substance use and marital infidelity have resulted in problems with his relationships and career.

Norcross, J. C. (Ed.). (1987). *Casebook of eclectic psychotherapy.* New York: Brunner/Mazel.

This edited volume presents 13 cases that concretely illustrate the practice of eclectic and integrative psychotherapy. Each case presents extensive transcripts, therapist remarks, and written patient impressions, followed by two invited commentaries on the case.

Norcross, J. C., Beutler, L. E., & Caldwell, R. (2002). Integrative conceptualization and treatment of depression. In M. A. Reinecke & M. R. Davison (Eds.), *Comparative treatments of depression*. New York: Springer.

This book reviews the major treatments for clinical depression; our chapter presents the integrative perspective and applies it to the case of Ms. Nancy T., who suffers from unipolar depression and a mixed personality disorder.

Norcross, J. C., & Caldwell, N. A. (2000). Prescriptive eclectic approach with Ms. Katrina. *Cognitive and Behavioral Practice, 7,* 514–519.

This article illustrates prescriptive eclecticism with Ms. Katrina, a complex and challenging woman, by demonstrating the process of customizing psychological treatments and therapeutic relationships to her specific needs as defined by diagnostic and nondiagnostic considerations.

Stricker, G., & Gold, J. (Eds.). (2006). *Casebook of psychotherapy integration*. Washington, DC: American Psychological Association.

Prominent practitioners describe their respective integrative psychotherapies and then demonstrate them in brief cases.

REFERENCES

Antonuccio, D. O. (1995). Psychotherapy for depression: No stronger medicine. *American Psychologist, 50,* 450–452.

Arnkoff, D. B., Glass, C. R., & Shapiro, S. J. (2002). Expectations and preferences. In J. C. Norcross (Ed.), *Psychotherapy relationships that work: Therapist contributions and responsiveness to patients* (pp. 315–334). New York: Oxford University Press.

Beutler, L. E. (1983). *Eclectic psychotherapy: A systematic approach*. New York: Pergamon.

Beutler, L. E. (in press). Making science matter in clinical practice. *Clinical Psychology: Science and Practice.*

Beutler, L. E., Clarkin, J., & Bongar, B. (2000). *Guidelines for the systematic treatment of the depressed patient*. New York: Oxford University Press.

Beutler, L. E., & Groth-Marnat, G. (Eds.). (2003). *Integrative assessment of adult personality* (2nd ed.). New York: Guilford Press.

Beutler, L. E., & Harwood, T. M. (2004). Virtual reality in psychotherapy training. *Journal of Clinical Psychology, 60,* 317–330.

Beutler, L. E., Harwood, T. M., Alimohamed, S., & Malik, M. (2002). Functional impairment and coping style: Patient moderators of therapeutic relationships. In J. C. Norcross (Ed.), *Psychotherapy relationships that work: Therapists' relational contributors to effective psychotherapy* (pp. 145–170). New York: Oxford University Press.

Castonguay, L. G., & Beutler, L. E. (Eds.). (2006). *Principles of therapeutic change that work*. New York: Oxford University Press.

DeRubeis, R. J., Hollon, S. D., Amsterdam, J. D., et al. (2005). Cognitive therapy vs medications in the treatment of moderate to severe depression. *Archives of General Psychiatry, 62,* 409–416.

Eysenck, H. J. (1970). A mish-mash of theories. *International Journal of Psychiatry, 9,* 140–146.

Frances, A., Clarkin, J., & Perry, S. (1984). *Differential therapeutics in psychiatry*. New York: Brunner/Mazel.

Frank, J. D. (1973). *Persuasion and healing* (2nd ed.). Baltimore: Johns Hopkins University.

French, T. M. (1933). Interrelations between psychoanalysis and the experimental work of Pavlov. *American Journal of Psychiatry, 89,* 1165–1203.

Garfield, S. L. (1980). *Psychotherapy: An eclectic approach*. New York: Wiley.

Goldfried, M. R. (1980). Toward the delineation of therapeutic change principles. *American Psychologist, 35,* 991–999.

Goldfried, M. R., Pachankis, J. E., & Bell, A. C. (2005). History of psychotherapy integration. In J. C. Norcross & M. R. Goldfried (Eds.), *Handbook of psychotherapy integration* (2nd ed., pp. 24–60). New York: Oxford University Press.

Goldstein, A. P., & Stein, N. (1976). *Prescriptive psychotherapies*. New York: Pergamon.

Grencavage, L. M., & Norcross, J. C. (1990). Where are the commonalities among the therapeutic common factors? *Professional Psychology: Research and Practice, 21,* 372–378.

Griner, D., & Smith, T. B. (2006). Culturally adapted mental health interventions: A meta-analytic review. *Psychotherapy, 43,* 531–548.

Halford, G. S., Baker, R., McCredden, J. E., & Bain, J. D. (2005). How many variables can humans process? *Psychological Science, 16,* 70–76.

Harwood, T. M., & Williams, O. B. (2003). Identifying treatment relevant assessment. In L. E. Beutler & G. Groth-Marnat (Eds.), *Integrated assessment of adult personality* (2nd ed.). New York: Guilford Press.

Hays, P. A. (1996). Culturally responsive assessment with diverse older clients. *Professional Psychology: Research and Practice, 27,* 188–193.

Hollanders, H., & McLeod, J. (1999). Theoretical orientation and reported practice: A survey of eclecticism among counsellors in Britain. *British Journal of Guidance & Counselling, 27,* 405–414.

Hoyt, M. F. (1995). *Brief therapy and managed care*. San Francisco: Jossey-Bass.

Jensen, J. P., Bergin, A. E., & Greaves, D. W. (1990). The meaning of eclecticism: New survey and analysis of components. *Professional Psychology: Research and Practice, 21,* 124–130.

Lambert, M. J. (Ed.). (2005). Enhancing psychotherapy outcome through feedback. *Journal of Clinical Psychology: In Session, 61(2).* (special issue)

Lampropoulos, G. K., & Dixon, D. N. (2007). Psychotherapy integration in internships and counseling psychology doctoral programs. *Journal of Psychotherapy Integration, 17,* 185–208.

Landsman, J. T. (1974). *Not an adversity but a welcome diversity.* Paper presented at the meeting of the American Psychological Association, New Orleans, Louisiana.

Lazarus, A. A. (1967). In support of technical eclecticism. *Psychological Reports, 21,* 415–416.

Lazarus, A. A. (1989). *The practice of multimodal therapy.* Baltimore: Johns Hopkins University.

Lazarus, A. A. (1993). Tailoring the therapeutic relationship, or being an authentic chameleon. *Psychotherapy, 30,* 404–407.

Liff, Z. A. (1992). Psychoanalysis and dynamic techniques. In D. K. Freedheim (Ed.), *History of psychotherapy* (pp. 571–586). Washington DC: American Psychological Association.

Lunde, D. T. (1974). Eclectic and integrated theory: Gordon Allport and others. In A. Burton (Ed.), *Operational theories of personality* (pp. 381–404). New York: Brunner/Mazel.

Marlatt, G. A., & Donovan, D. M. (Eds.). (2007). *Relapse prevention: Maintenance strategies in the treatment of addictive behaviors* (2nd ed.). New York: Guilford.

Messer, S. B. (1992). A critical examination of belief structures in integrative and eclectic psychotherapy. In J. C. Norcross & M. R. Goldfried (Eds.), *Handbook of psychotherapy integration* (pp. 130–168). New York: Basic Books.

Messer, S. B. (2001). Introduction to the special issue on assimilative integration. *Journal of Psychotherapy Integration, 11,* 1–4.

Norcross, J. C. (Ed.). (1986). *Handbook of eclectic psychotherapy.* New York: Brunner/Mazel.

Norcross, J. C. (Ed.). (1987). *Casebook of eclectic psychotherapy.* New York: Brunner/Mazel.

Norcross, J. C. (Ed.). (2002). *Psychotherapy relationships that work: Therapist contributions and responsiveness to patient needs.* New York: Oxford University Press.

Norcross, J. C. (2005). The psychotherapist's own psychotherapy: Educating and developing psychologists. *American Psychologist, 60,* 840–850.

Norcross, J. C. (2010). The therapeutic relationship. In B. L. Duncan et al. (Eds.), *Heart and soul of change* (2nd ed.). Washington, DC: American Psychological Association.

Norcross, J. C., & Beutler, L. E. (1997). Determining the therapeutic relationship of choice in brief therapy. In J. N. Butcher (Ed.), *Personality assessment in managed health care: A practitioner's guide* (pp. 42–60). New York: Oxford University Press.

Norcross, J. C., Beutler, L. E., & Caldwell, R. (2002). Integrative conceptualization and treatment of depression. In M. A. Reinecke & M. R. Davison (Eds.), *Comparative treatments of depression.* New York: Springer.

Norcross, J. C., Beutler, L. E., & Levant, R. F. (Eds.). (2006). *Evidence-based practices in mental health: Debate and dialogue on the fundamental questions.* Washington, DC: American Psychological Association.

Norcross, J. C., & Caldwell, N. A. (2000). Prescriptive eclectic approach with Ms. Katrina. *Cognitive and Behavioral Practice, 7,* 514–519.

Norcross, J. C., & Goldfried, M. R. (Eds.). (2005). *Handbook of psychotherapy integration* (2nd ed.). New York: Oxford University Press.

Norcross, J. C., & Halgin, R. P. (2005). In J. C. Norcross & M. R. Goldfried (Eds.), *Handbook of psychotherapy integration* (pp. 459–493). New York: Oxford University Press.

Norcross, J. C., Hedges, M., & Prochaska, J. O. (2002). The face of 2010: A Delphi poll on the future of psychotherapy. *Professional Psychology: Research and Practice, 33,* 316–322.

Norcross, J. C., Hogan, T. P., & Koocher, G. P. (2008). *Clinician's guide to evidence-based practice: Mental health and the addictions.* New York: Oxford University Press.

Norcross, J. C., Karpiak, C. P., & Lister, K. M. (2005). What's an integrationist? A study of self-identified integrative and (occasionally) eclectic psychologists. *Journal of Clinical Psychology, 61,* 1587–1594.

Norcross, J. C., Karpiak, C. P., & Santoro, S. O. (2005). Clinical psychologists across the years: The Division of Clinical Psychology from 1960 to 2003. *Journal of Clinical Psychology,* 1467–1483.

Norcross, J. C., & Napolitano, G. (1986). Defining our journal and ourselves. *International Journal of Eclectic Psychotherapy, 5,* 249–255.

Paniagua, F. A. (2005). *Assessing and treating culturally diverse clients: A practical guide* (3rd ed.). Thousand Oaks, CA: Sage.

Paul, G. L. (1967). Strategy of outcome research in psychotherapy. *Journal of Consulting Psychology, 31,* 109–118.

Pederson, P. B., Crethar, H. C., & Carlson, J. (2008). *Inclusive cultural empathy.* Washington, DC: American Psychological Association.

Pinsof, W. M. (1995). *Integrative IPCT: A synthesis of biological, individual, and family therapies.* New York: Basic Books.

Prochaska, J. O. (1979). *Systems of psychotherapy: A transtheoretical analysis.* Homewood, IL: Dorsey.

Prochaska, J. O., & DiClemente, C. C. (1983). Stages and processes of self-change of smoking: Toward an integrative model of change. *Journal of Consulting and Clinical Psychology, 51,* 390–395.

Prochaska, J. O., DiClemente, C. C., Velicer, W. F., & Rossi, J. S. (1993). Standardized, individualized, interactive, and personalized self-help programs for smoking cessation. *Health Psychology, 12,* 399–405.

Prochaska, J. O., & Norcross, J. C. (2002). Stages of change. In J. C. Norcross (Ed.), *Psychotherapy relationships that work* (pp. 303–313). New York: Oxford University Press.

Prochaska, J. O., & Norcross, J. C. (2010). *Systems of psychotherapy: A transtheoretical analysis* (7th ed.). Pacific Grove, CA: Brooks/Cole.

Prochaska, J. O., Norcross, J. C., & DiClemente, C. C. (1995). *Changing for good.* New York: Avon.

Rosen, C. S. (2000). Is the sequencing of change processes by stage consistent across health problems? A meta-analysis. *Health Psychology, 19,* 593–604.

Rosenzweig, S. (1936). Some implicit common factors in diverse methods in psychotherapy. *American Journal of Orthopsychiatry, 6,* 412–415.

Schultz-Ross, R. A. (1995). Ideological insularity as a defense against clinical complexity. *American Journal of Psychotherapy, 49,* 540–547.

Schottenbauer, M. A., Glass, C. R., & Arnkoff, D. B. (2005). In J. C. Norcross & M. R. Goldfried (Eds.), *Handbook of psychotherapy integration* (pp. 459–493). New York: Oxford University Press.

Stricker, G., & Gold, J. (Eds.). (2006). *Casebook of psychotherapy integration.* Washington, DC: American Psychological Association.

Swift, J. & Callahan, J. L. (2009). The impact of client treatment preferences on outcome: A meta-analysis. *Journal of Clinical Psychology, 65,* 368–381.

Thorne, F. C. (1957). Critique of recent developments in personality counseling theory. *Journal of Clinical Psychology, 13,* 234–244.

Thorne, F. C. (1967). The structure of integrative psychology. *Journal of Clinical Psychology, 23,* 3–11.

Tracey, T. J. G., Lichtenberg, J. W., Goodyear, R. K., Claiborn, C. D., & Wampold, B. E. (2003). Concept mapping of therapeutic common factors. *Psychotherapy Research, 13,* 401–413.

Wachtel, P. L. (1977). *Psychoanalysis and behavior therapy: Toward an integration.* New York: Basic Books.

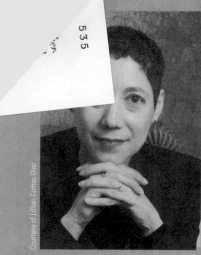

Courtesy of Lillian Comas-Díaz

Lillian Comas-Díaz

15 | MULTICULTURAL THEORIES OF PSYCHOTHERAPY

Lillian Comas–Díaz

OVERVIEW

Are the prevailing systems of psychotherapy relevant to culturally diverse individuals? Most therapeutic orientations recognize that individual differences must be respected and accepted. However, as a product of Western society, the dominant models of psychotherapy tend to be grounded in a monocultural perspective. As such, they support mainstream cultural values, neglecting multicultural worldviews. Unfortunately, a monocultural psychotherapy frequently promotes *ethnocentrism*. Ethnocentrism, the belief that one's worldview is inherently superior and desirable to others (Leininger, 1978), can compromise psychotherapy when therapists project their values and attitudes onto their culturally different clients. As a result, scholars and practitioners questioned the multicultural applicability of mainstream psychotherapy (Bernal, Bonilla, & Bellido, 1995; Sue, Bingham, Porche-Burke, & Vasquez, 1999). Multicultural psychotherapies emerged as a response to these concerns.

Proponents of multicultural psychotherapies advocate for cultural sensitivity—that is, awareness, respect, and appreciation for cultural diversity. Valuing diversity promotes a critical examination of established psychotherapeutic models and assumptions because definitions of health, illness, healing, normality, and abnormality are culturally embedded. Thus, multicultural psychotherapists examine their clients' as well as their own *worldviews*. The concept of worldview refers to people's systematized ideas and beliefs about the universe. When multicultural psychotherapists engage in self-examination, they explore their professional socialization and potential bias. They also examine the cultural applicability of their interventions and promote culturally relevant therapeutic strategies.

Monocultural, dominant psychotherapy tends to be decontextualized, ahistorical, and apolitical. When it fails to examine the historical and sociopolitical contexts, mainstream psychotherapy ignores the role of issues of power and privilege in people's lives. Multicultural psychotherapists consider power differences based on diversity characteristics such as ethnicity, race, gender, social class, sexual orientation, age, religion, national origin, ability/disability, language, place of residence, ideology, and membership in other marginalized groups. They believe that ethnocentric psychotherapy paradigms resist change because they preserve the status quo. To embrace change, multicultural psychotherapists promote empowerment and social justice. Instead of focusing on deficits, they affirm strengths. This emphasis on diversity leads multiculturalists to endorse interdisciplinary approaches. Indeed, *unity through diversity* is a multicultural maxim. Consequently, multicultural psychotherapists benefit from the contributions of sociology, anthropology, cultural/ethnic studies, humanities, arts, history, politics, law, philosophy, religion/spirituality, and many other disciplines. Accordingly, Multicultural psychotherapists also are represented in diverse theoretical schools including psychodynamic, cognitive–behavioral, rational–emotive, humanistic, Jungian, and various other combinations of dominant psychotherapies. Regardless of preferred theoretical approach, multicultural psychotherapists work to develop *cultural competence*. A basic concept in multicultural psychotherapies, cultural competence refers to the set of knowledge, behaviors, attitudes, skills, and policies that enables a practitioner to work effectively in a multicultural situation (Cross, Bazron, Dennis, & Isaacs, 1989).

Basic Concepts

The demographic changes in the United States signal the increasing number of culturally diverse individuals in need of psychotherapy. However, multiculturalism has not fully reached dominant psychotherapy. Accordingly, the lack of cultural relevance in dominant psychotherapies gave birth to multicultural psychotherapies. Simply put, multicultural psychotherapies infuse cultural competence into clinical practice. Regardless of theoretical orientation, most psychotherapists can incorporate a multicultural perspective into their practice. The term *multicultural* refers to the interaction between people across cultures. In the United States, multicultural refers to the interaction between culturally diverse individuals such as people of color, internationals, immigrants, temporary workers, and the dominant European American culture. Cultural misunderstandings and communication problems between psychotherapists and their clients interfere with treatment effectiveness. This observation illustrates how psychotherapists' ethnocentric worldviews interfere with psychotherapy's usefulness.

Worldviews

Harry Triandis (1995) classified worldviews according to how individuals define themselves and how they relate to others. Those cultures where individuals' identity is associated with their relationships to others are called collectivistic. In contrast, members who frequently view themselves independently from others are denominated individualistic (Triandis, 1995). Western societies tend to be identified as individualistic since their members define themselves primarily in terms of internal features such as traits, attitudes, abilities, and agencies. In other words, their ideal personal characteristics include being direct, assertive, competitive, self-assured, self-sufficient, and efficient. On the other hand, collectivistic members endorse relational values, prefer interdependence, encourage sharing resources, value harmony, tolerate the views of significant others, and prefer communication that minimizes conflicts (Triandis, 1995). Valuing connection, collectivistic persons frequently contextualize and have a holistic orientation. In reality, most people's worldviews can be placed within an individualist–collectivistic spectrum. For instance, many African Americans have a combined collectivistic and individualistic worldview.

The negotiation of client/therapist worldviews is crucial for effective psychotherapy. Regrettably, due to their individualistic worldview, mainstream psychotherapists tend to interpret multicultural clients' normative cultural behaviors as resistance, inferiority, and/or deviance (Young, 1990). For example, when collectivist members tolerate the limitations of significant others, individualist psychotherapists may misinterpret such behavior as poor judgment instead of viewing it as a culturally accepted norm. Moreover, individualistic psychotherapists can violate personal and family norms by asking collectivistic clients to reveal intimate personal information, soliciting the expression of emotion and affect, and requesting individuals to air family disputes, all before earning their clients' trust and establishing a positive therapeutic alliance (Varma, 1988). Since the notion of being understood is an important aspect in healing, effective psychotherapy depends on the therapist's understanding of his or her client's worldview. The development of cultural competence helps therapists to appreciate and manage diverse worldviews.

Cultural competence

Differences in therapists' and clients' worldviews frequently lead to communication problems, misdiagnosis, and/or client premature treatment termination. However, cultural competence enhances adherence to psychotherapy and completion of treatment. *Cultural competence* involves a set of congruent behaviors, attitudes, and policies that reflect an understanding of how cultural and sociopolitical influences shape individuals' worldviews and related health behaviors (Betancourt, Green, Carrillo, & Ananch-Firempong, 2003). Specifically, to become culturally competent you need to (1) become aware of your worldview; (2) examine your attitude toward cultural differences; (3) learn about different worldviews; and (4) develop multicultural skills (Sue et al, 1995). Likewise, culturally competent therapists develop the capacity to (1) value diversity; (2) manage the dynamics of difference; (3) acquire and incorporate cultural knowledge into their interventions and interactions; (4) increase their multicultural skills; (5) conduct self-reflection and assessment; and (6) adapt to diversity and to the cultural contexts of their clients. Since all therapeutic encounters are multicultural because everyone belongs to diverse cultures and subcultures, cultural competence enables psychotherapists to work effectively in most treatment situations. For the purpose of this chapter, *culture* is defined as individuals' total environment. It includes beliefs, values, practices, institutions, and psychological processes including language, cognition, and perception.

The American Psychological Association (APA) highlighted the importance of cultural competence by formulating a series of multicultural guidelines. The first set of principles, *Guidelines for Providers of Psychological Services to Ethnic, Linguistic, and Culturally Diverse Clients,* exhorted practitioners to (1) recognize cultural diversity; (2) understand the central role culture, ethnicity, and race play in culturally diverse individuals; (3) appreciate the significant impact of socioeconomic and political factors on mental health; and (4) help clients understand their cultural identification (APA, 1990). Afterward, APA (2003) published a second set of principles—*Guidelines on Multicultural Education, Training, Research, Practice and Organizational Change*—and encouraged psychologists to (1) recognize that we are cultural beings; (2) value cultural sensitivity and awareness; (3) use multicultural constructs in education; (4) conduct culture-centered and ethical psychological research with culturally diverse individuals; (5) use culturally appropriate skills in applied psychological practices; and (6) implement organizational change processes to support culturally informed organizational practices and policy (APA, 2003). The six specific multicultural guidelines are listed below:

Commitment to Cultural Awareness and Knowledge of Self and Others

1. "Psychologists are encouraged to recognize that, as cultural beings, they may hold attitudes and beliefs that can detrimentally influence their perceptions of and interactions with individuals who are ethnically and racially different from themselves."

2. "Psychologists are encouraged to recognize the importance of multicultural sensitivity/responsiveness, knowledge, and understanding about ethnically and racially different individuals."

Education

3. "As educators, psychologists are encouraged to employ the constructs of multiculturalism and diversity in psychological education."

Research

4. "Culturally sensitive psychological researchers are encouraged to recognize the importance of conducting culture-centered and ethical psychological research among persons from ethnic, linguistic, and racial minority backgrounds."

Practice

5. "Psychologists strive to apply culturally appropriate skills in clinical and other applied psychological practices."

Organizational Change and Policy Development

6. "Psychologists are encouraged to use organizational change processes to support culturally informed organizational (policy) development and practices." (APA, 2003, pp. 377–402)

The interested reader can access the complete document at: http://www.apa.org/pi/multiculturalguidelines/homepage.html.

All multicultural guidelines provide a context for multicultural psychotherapies. Nonetheless, three areas are of particular relevance to multicultural psychotherapies. These are the commitment to cultural awareness and knowledge of self and others, guidelines related to psychological practice, and organizational change and policy development. Multicultural psychotherapists respond to their Ethics Code (APA, 2002) regardless of purview of practice and setting.

The development of cultural competence is a lifelong process that requires acknowledging the need for ongoing learning. Cross and colleagues (1989) identified the development of cultural competence across the following spectrum: (1) cultural destructiveness is characterized by attitudes, policies, and practices that are destructive to cultures and to individuals within cultures (e.g., "English only" mandates); (2) cultural incapacity—individuals believe in the racial superiority of the dominant group and assume a paternalistic and ignorant position toward culturally diverse people; (3) cultural blindness—individuals believe that culture makes no difference and thus, the values of the dominant culture are universally applicable and beneficial; (4) cultural precompetence—individuals desire to provide an equitable and fair treatment with cultural sensitivity but do not know exactly how to proceed; (5) cultural competence—individuals value and respect cultural differences, engage in continuing self-assessment regarding culture, pay attention to the dynamics of difference, continue expanding their knowledge and resources, and endorse a variety of adaptations to belief systems, policies, and practices.

Multicultural psychotherapies' emphasis on context nurtured the emergence of cultural competence guidelines for organizations. Since many psychotherapists function within formal organizations, APA formulated multicultural guidelines for psychologists within organizations through its multicultural guideline number 6. Addressing this problem, Howard-Hamilton and colleagues (1998) outlined principles for those counselors working with multicultural clients. They exhorted therapists to (1) evaluate their institution's mission statement and policies to determine whether they include diversity issues; (2) assess policies with regard to diversity; (3) evaluate how people of color may perceive specific policies; (4) acknowledge within-group diversity; (5) be aware that diversity requires examination from both the individual and the institutional levels; and finally (6) recognize that multicultural sensitivity may mean advocating for culturally diverse people. Similarly, Wu and Martinez (2006) asked multicultural practitioners to help their organizations achieve cultural competence by (1) including community representation and input at all stages of implementation; (2) integrating all systems of the health care organization; (3) ensuring that changes made are manageable, measurable, and sustainable; (4) making the business case for implementation of cultural competency polices; (5) requiring commitment from leadership; and (6) helping to establish staff training on an ongoing basis.

Empowerment

In addition to promulgating cultural competence, multicultural psychotherapists challenged dominant approaches with conceptual, methodological, ethical, and sociopolitical concerns. Dominant psychotherapists' ignorance of the historical and sociopolitical contexts further disempowered marginalized individuals. This is detrimental for visible people of color, who, unlike majority group members, have a history of individual and collective oppression. A specific example of such disempowerment is dominant psychotherapists' inattention to racial microaggressions. *Racial microaggressions* refer to the assaults that individuals receive on a regular basis solely because of their race, color, and/or ethnicity (Pierce, 1995). Some illustrations of racial microaggressions include being harassed in public places, being ignored by clerks who favor White customers, being accused of being an "Affirmative Action baby" (racial favoritism), being targeted for racial profiling, and so forth. Unfortunately, racial microaggressions also occur in therapy and include therapists' cultural blindness, denial of racism, adherence to the myth of meritocracy (without acknowledging the roles of oppression and privilege), misdiagnosis, and pathologizing culturally diverse behaviors (Sue et. al., 2007). These therapists' behaviors promote disempowerment among culturally diverse clients.

Multicultural psychotherapists emphasize empowerment because many people of color tend to internalize their disempowerment as helplessness. Therapeutic empowerment helps clients increase their access to resources, develop options to exercise choice, improve self- and collective esteem, implement culturally relevant assertiveness, augment agency, affirm cultural strengths, overcome internalized oppression, and engage in transformative actions. Within their empowerment focus, multicultural psychotherapies frequently subscribe to the following assumptions: (1) Reality is constructed in a context; (2) experience is valuable knowledge; (3) learning/healing results from sharing multiple perspectives; and (4) learning/healing is anchored in meaningful and relevant contexts. Along these lines, several multicultural counselors espouse a liberation model, helping clients to critically analyze their situations, affirm ethnocultural strengths, promote personal transformation, and foster sociopolitical change.

Indeed, this emphasis on empowerment frequently leads psychotherapists to commit to social justice. The history of human rights violations against many minorities has resulted in a *cultural trauma*, a legacy of adversity, pain, and suffering among many minority group members. Duran and Ivey (2006) called this legacy a *soul wound*—the product of sociohistorical oppression, ungrieved losses, internalized oppression, and learned helplessness. Cultural trauma continues to afflict minorities through racism, sexism, elitism, heterosexism, ablism, xenophobia, ethnocentrism, and other types of oppression.

Group membership dynamics seem to reinforce oppression and privilege. For example, research has identified a human tendency to categorize individuals into in-group and out-group members (Allport, 1954). Membership in one group helps to shape our perceptions about our group as well as about other groups. When people belong to one group, they tend to prefer members of their own identity classification. Indeed, some studies have documented the existence of unconscious negative racial feelings and beliefs. By using cognitive psychology techniques (e.g., response latency as measure of bias), Dovidio and Gaertner (1998) demonstrated that individuals who in self-report measures appeared as nonprejudiced often have generally negative attitudes toward Blacks. Known as *aversive racism*, this phenomenon demonstrated that both liberal and conservative Whites discriminate against African Americans (and probably against other visible people of color) in situations that do not implicate racial prejudice as a basis for their actions (Whaley, 1998). Likewise, the expression of unintentional or symbolic racism can take subtle forms and thus is harder to identify. As a result, White individuals who grow up as members of a majority group may have either covertly or overtly racist attitudes (Brown, 1997). As an illustration, in-group favoritism—the informal networks that provide contacts, support, mentoring, rewards, and benefits to same-group members—tends to exclude people of color in predominantly White work environments (Rhodes & Williams, 2007).

Psychotherapy will be unsuccessful if clients feel that their therapist is unconsciously racist, ethnocentric, sexist, elitist, xenophobic, homophobic, or the like. To counteract bias, multicultural psychotherapists explore their beliefs, values, and attitudes toward their in-group members as well as their attitudes toward out-group members. That is, they become aware of and sensitive to their own attitudes toward others, as they may be unconscious of how culturally biased these attitudes may be. Besides becoming familiar with different worldviews, multicultural psychotherapists understand the stigmatizing effects of being a member of an oppressed group. More specifically, they recognize how minority members' history with the dominant society—such as African American slavery, concentration camps for Japanese Americans, the American Indian Holocaust, and the colonization of major Latino groups, including the forceful annexation of Mexican territories—can create cultural trauma and thus influence the worldview of people of color. An appreciation of such history requires awareness of how racism interacts with other types of discrimination such as sexism, classism, xenophobia, neocolonialism, and heterosexism.

To undertake this appreciation, therapists engage in cultural self-awareness. Therapists' cultural self-awareness includes learning about one's position in relation to societal power and privilege. Understanding power dynamics is an important part of appreciating the relationship between self and others. To achieve this goal, multicultural psychotherapists analyze the power differences between their life experiences and their client's. Different from most dominant therapies' analyses, a power analysis goes beyond the power differential inherent in the therapist/client dyad. Multicultural psychotherapists compare their client's cultural group's social status with their own. This comparison entails the identification and challenge of internalized privilege and oppression, since most individuals with power are unaware of its pervasive influence in their life. To increase awareness of power, Peggy McIntosh (1988) defined White privilege as unacknowledged systems that give power to European Americans and male individuals. She exhorted individuals to "unpack the invisible knapsack" by becoming aware of White privilege.

Examples of the invisible knapsack include those situations when European Americans and men can do the following:

1. Go shopping alone most of the time, pretty well assured that they will not be followed or harassed.

2. Turn on the television or open to the front page of the paper and see European American people widely represented.

3. Count on their skin color not to work against the appearance of financial reliability whenever they use checks, credit cards, or cash.

4. Rent or purchase housing in an area that they can afford and in which they would want to live.

5. Avoid the need to educate their children to be aware of systemic racism for their own daily physical protection.

6. Remain oblivious of the language and customs of persons of color who constitute the world's majority without feeling any penalty for such oblivion.

7. Exist with little fear about the consequences of ignoring the perspectives and powers of people of other races.

8. Confront a person of their own race if they ask to talk to the "person in charge."

9. Be confident that if a state trooper pulls them over, they haven't been singled out because of their race.

10. Take a job with an affirmative action employer without having their coworkers suspect that they got it because of their race.

You can review all of the examples of White privilege at www.case.edu/president/aaction/UnpackingTheKnapsack.pdf.

The illustrations of White privilege reflect the importance of recognizing the effects of institutionalized power disparities on people's lives because such disparities favor members of dominant groups while disenfranchising members of minority groups. The denial of the unacknowledged privilege protects the status quo.

To summarize, multicultural psychotherapies' underlying assumptions include the following:

•   Culture is complex and dynamic.

•   Reality is constructed and embedded in context.

•   Every encounter is multicultural.

•   Multicultural psychotherapies are relevant to all individuals.

•   Understanding nonverbal communication and behaviors is crucial to psychotherapy.

•   A Western worldview has dominated mainstream psychotherapy.

•   Psychotherapists engage in self-awareness.

•   Cultural competence is central to effective psychotherapy.

•   Healing entails empowering individuals and groups.

•   Healing is holistic and involves multiple perspectives.

Other Systems

Multiculturalism draws upon the benefits and perspectives of many disciplines, and multicultural psychotherapists acknowledge the contributions of diverse psychotherapeutic orientations. Although many multicultural therapists self-identify as adherents to one or another theoretical orientations, they also impart multicultural values into their specific therapeutic schools. Indeed, partly due to multiculturalism's criticisms, mainstream clinicians are revising psychotherapy's basic tenets with respect to their applicability to culturally diverse clients. Psychoanalysts, for instance, are including the experiences of culturally diverse individuals to incorporate their social, communal, and spiritual orientations into treatment. For example, Altman (1995) utilizes a modified psychoanalytic object relations framework, examining his clients' progress by their ability to use relationships to grow rather than by the insight that they gain.

Object relations theory focuses on the way in which significant interpersonal relationships are internalized and become central to the person's interactions with the world. Within this perspective, conflict and personality disturbance are viewed as arrest and or damage to the development of the child's sense of self and others. Object relations theory views damage to the development of relationships as a cause of conflict and personality disturbance.

In addition to the cultural adaptations of dominant psychotherapies, the specific influence of multicultural approaches is increasing. Research has reported inconsistent findings regarding the cultural sensitivity of mainstream psychological services. Although some studies found evidence-based practice (EBP) to be effective for a number of culturally diverse populations (CIEBP, 2008), other findings indicated that clients of color tend to drop out of cognitive–behavioral therapy (CBT) at a higher rate than their European American counterparts (Miranda, et al, 2005). Research findings suggest that to be effective, EBP needs to be culturally adapted to clients' contexts. These findings are consistent with the results of a study that showed African American clients who expressed positive expectations about seeking mental health services found treatment less positive than their European American counterparts after utilizing such services (Diala, et al., 2000).

Indeed, after reviewing the research on dominant psychotherapies' cultural adaptations, Whaley and Davis (2007) concluded that culture affects psychotherapeutic process more than it affects treatment outcome. Dominant psychotherapies' ethnocentrism could partly explain Whaley and King's conclusion. To illustrate, a major area of discontent among people of color is the United States' history of medical experimentation and additional abuses toward these populations. Such history has aggravated people of color's mistrust of the medical establishment. Called medical apartheid, this history ranges from the Tuskegee project, a research project where African American men with syphilis were given a placebo instead of medication (penicillin), despite the fact that a cure for syphilis was found during the course of the research and administered to White men, to the involuntary sterilization of Puerto Rican women when they came in for routine medical examinations (Comas-Díaz, 2008). As many culturally diverse individuals endorse a collectivistic orientation, they situate themselves in place and time. Therefore, personal and collective history is an important element in the lives of people of color.

HISTORY

Precursors

Interest in the "other" dates from the beginning of time. At times, such attention has been in the form of concern, awareness, and even fascination. Diverse religious and spiritual traditions assigned an important role to the other. For instance, in Judaism the other is associated with sacred because *otherness* means *holy* in Hebrew. In Christianity, the concept of the "necessary other" facilitates the recovery of the divided self. Furthermore, a Buddhist view on the other as enemy is that enemies are our best teachers because we learn the most from them. In accordance with spiritual traditions, multicultural psychotherapies aim to enhance the relationship between self and other.

Beginnings

Multicultural psychotherapies have interdisciplinary origins. Early theoretical influences include psychological anthropology, ethnopsychology, cultural anthropology, psycho-analytic anthropology, and folk healing. The interest in the other arrived in the mental health fields during the period between the 1940s and the 1960s. Anthropologists and psychoanalysts collaborated on studying the relationship between culture and psyche. Proponents of these movements applied psychoanalytic analyses to social and cultural phenomena. Some scholars examined cross-cultural mental health; some studied the effects of oppression on ethnic minorities' mental health; still others questioned the universal application of psychoanalytic concepts, such as the Oedipus complex.

Members of the Cultural School of Psychoanalysis argued that culture shapes behavior because individuals are contextualized and embedded in social interactions that varied across cultural contexts and historical periods (Seeley, 2000). Although the anthro-pological psychoanalytic orientations enriched the culture and behavior discourse, they failed to develop cultural theories that could be applied to psychotherapy (Seeley, 2000).

Psychological and psychiatric anthropologists studied the effects of culture on men-tal health and gave birth to transcultural psychiatry. Similar to *culturalism*—the psycho-therapeutic use of culture-specific folk healing—transcultural psychiatry and psychology advocated for the use of community and indigenous resources (clergy, teachers, folk healers, and other ethnic minority individuals) for mental health treatment.

The minority empowerment movements furthered the development of multicultural psychotherapies. These movements examined the power/oppression dynamics between dominant group members and minorities. Known as identity politics, women's rights, Black Power, Chicano/Brown power, and Gay, Lesbian, and Bisexual movements high-lighted the civil rights and needs of marginalized groups. Adherents of these movements raised consciousness and worked toward empowering marginalized groups in order to redress social and political inequities.

The desire to understand the effects of oppression on mental health led some clini-cians to examine the psychology of colonization. Frantz Fanon (1967) articulated the principles of the psychology of colonization in terms of the economic and emotional dependence of the colonized on the colonizer. He used the concepts of imperialism, dominance, and exploitation to examine the relationship between the colonizer and the colonized. The process of colonization echoed in the United States as the first president of color of the American Psychological Association, Kenneth B. Clark, identified the condition of Americans of color as colonization (Comas-Díaz, 2007).

A major influence on multicultural psychotherapies is the "education for the oppressed" model. Paulo Freire (1973) identified dominant models of education as instruments of oppression that reinforce and maintain the status quo and social inequi-ties. He coined the term *conscientization*, or *critical consciousness*, as a process of per-sonal and social liberation. Education for the oppressed teaches individuals to become aware of their circumstances and change them through a dialectical conversation with their world. Since oppression robs its victims of their critical thinking, the development of *conscientization* involves asking critical questions such as "What? Why? How? For whom? Against whom? By whom? In favor of whom? In favor of what? To what end?" (Freire & Macedo, 2000). Answering these questions helps clients to examine "what matters" and uncovers clients' existential reasons for being, purpose, and position in life. Critical consciousness helps oppressed individuals to author their own reality.

Re-evaluation counseling (RC) is another influence in the emergence of multicul-tural psychotherapies. RC is an empowering co-counseling approach where two or more individuals take turns listening to each other without interruption in order to recover from the effects of racism, classism, sexism, and other types of oppression (Roby, 1998).

Harvey Jackins developed RC based on his belief that everyone has tremendous intellectual and loving potential but that these qualities have become blocked as a result of accumulated distress. Recovery involves a natural discharge process through which the "counselor" encourages the "client" to discharge emotions (catharsis). Afterward, the "client" becomes the "counselor" and listens to the client. RC proponents are committed to ending racism at the individual, collective, and societal levels. For more information, visit www.rc.org.

The struggle against colonization and oppression challenged women's subservient position. As daughters of empowerment movements, feminist therapists embrace diversity as a foundation for practice. Such an empowerment position influenced the development of multicultural psychotherapies. Feminist clinicians believe dominant psychotherapists act as agents of the status quo; in contrast, feminist psychotherapy attempts to empower all people, women as well as men, and promote equality at individual, interpersonal, institutional, national, and international levels. Feminist therapy and multicultural therapies equally influence each other. For instance, women of color challenged feminist therapists to become culturally sensitive. As a result, cultural feminist therapy and Women of Color's feminist therapy were born. While cultural feminist therapists use the empathic relationship to increase women's connection to others' subjectivity, interdependence, and other female values (Worrell & Remer, 2003), Women of Color's feminist therapists address the interaction between racism, sexism, classism, heterosexism, ethnocentrism, ablism, and other forms of oppressions.

Ethnic Family Therapy

Like feminist therapy, family therapy has benefited from an interaction with multiculturalism. With its history of recognizing ethnicity and culture into its theory and practice (McGoldrick, Giordano & Pierce, 1982), family therapy witnessed the emergence of ethnic family therapy. Ethnic family therapists attempt to (1) know their own culture, (2) avoid ethnocentric attitudes and behaviors, (3) achieve an insider status, (4) use intermediaries, and (5) have selective disclosure (McGoldrick, et al., 1982). An illustration of ethnic family therapy is Boyd-Franklin's (2003) multisystemic approach for *Black Families in Therapy*. Just as family therapy uses genograms to show the relationships between family members (McGoldrick, Gerson, & Shellenberger, 1999), ethnic family therapists use cultural genograms (Hardy & Laszloffy, 1995). I discuss cultural genograms in more detail later in the chapter.

Several professional and academic organizations have supported the development of multicultural psychotherapies. For example, the American Psychological Association has a recent history of examining the needs of minority populations. Several of its societies, such as the Society of Psychology of Women, the Society for the Psychological Study of Ethnic Minority Psychology, and the Society for the Psychological Study of Gay, Lesbian, Bisexual, and Transgender Issues are examples. In particular, the Society for the Psychological Study of Ethnic Minority Psychology has promoted the need for multiculturalism in all aspects of psychology, especially in professional psychology. The society's official journal, *Cultural Diversity and Ethnic Minority Psychology,* is an important vehicle for dissemination of scholarly and professional work on multicultural psychology.

Counseling psychologists have demonstrated a commitment to multicultural issues and they have recognized the importance of multiculturalism in publications such as the *Journal of Multicultural Counseling and Development*. Feminist psychologists find an outlet for their writing in journals such as *Psychology of Women Quarterly*, the official journal of the American Psychological Association Society of Psychology of Women. Additionally, the Association of Women in Psychology publishes its official journal, *Women & Therapy*.

The ethnic minority psychological associations—the Asian American Psychological Association, the Association of Black Psychologists, the National Hispanic Psychological Association, and the Society of Indian Psychologists—have been powerful advocates for the mental health needs of people of color. Other organizations include the Council of National Psychological Associations for the Advancement of Ethnic Minority Issues (CNPAEMI). This coalition is composed of the APA Society for the Psychological Study of Ethnic Minority Issues, the Asian American Psychological Association, the Association of Black Psychologists, the National Hispanic Psychological Association, and the Society of Indian Psychologists. This group advocates for the delivery of effective psychological services to people of color. Additionally, the Society for the Study of Culture and Psychiatry is an interdisciplinary and international society devoted to furthering research, clinical care, and education in cultural *aspects* of mental health and illness (www.psychiatryandculture.org/cms/).

Current Status

The collectivistic concept of unity through diversity achieved preeminence during the 21st century. Multiculturalism promotes empowerment, change, and a transformative dialogue on oppression and privilege. The creation of the American Psychological Association Office of Ethnic Minority Affairs advanced the role of multiculturalism in psychological theory and practice. This office provided a forum for ethnic minority psychologists to voice their concerns about the lack of cultural relevance in psychological practice. Afterward, the establishment of the American Psychological Association's Society for the Psychological Study of Ethnic Minority Issues cemented the position of multicultural psychotherapies.

Currently, multicultural psychotherapists practice following three models: (1) cultural adaptation of dominant psychotherapy, (2) ethnic psychotherapies, and (3) holistic approaches. Frequently, psychotherapists combine these frameworks.

Psychotherapy can be culturally adapted through the development of generic cross-cultural skills or through the incorporation of culture specific skills (Lo & Fung, 2003). The generic term *cultural competence* refers to knowledge and skills required to work effectively in any cross-cultural clinical encounter. Psychotherapists working within the culture-specific skills level assimilate ethnic dimensions into mainstream psychotherapy. As an example of culture specificity, Bernal, Bonilla, and Bellido (1995) recommended the inclusion of eight cultural dimensions—language, persons, metaphors, content, concepts, goals, method, and context—into mainstream psychotherapy. Within this framework, therapists use culturally appropriate language to fit a client's worldview and life circumstances. The dimension of *persons* refers to the therapeutic relationship. *Metaphors* relate to concepts shared by members of a cultural group. The dimension of *content* refers to the therapist's cultural knowledge (e.g., Does the client feel understood by the therapist?). *Concepts* examine whether the treatment concepts are culturally consonant with the client's context. The dimension of *goals* examines whether clinical objectives are congruent with clients' adaptive cultural values. *Methods* pertain to the cultural adaptation and validation of methods and instruments. Finally, Bernal and his associates defined *context* as clients' environment, including history and sociopolitical circumstances.

In another example of culture specificity, Ricardo Muñoz (Muñoz & Mendelson, 2005) suggested culturally adapting cognitive behavioral treatments (CBT) through (1) involvement of culturally diverse people in the development of interventions; (2) inclusion of collectivistic values; (3) attention to religion/spirituality, (4) relevance of acculturation; and (5) acknowledgment of the effects of oppression on mental health. Notwithstanding CBT's evidence-based foundation, there is a dearth of empirical studies on the cultural validity of empirically supported treatments (Hall, 2001). Consequently, multicultural practitioners identified the need for culture-specific psychotherapy with an evidence base to address the day-to-day realities of people of color. As a response, the American Psychological Association Presidential Task Force included in its definition of evidence-based practice in psychology the integration of patients' characteristics, culture, and preferences with clinical expertise and research (APA, 2006).

Pamela Hays (2001) provided an example of a successful incorporation of cultural elements into therapy, highlighting cultural complexities in the conceptualization of identity. Her ADDRESSING framework recognizes the interacting cultural influences of age, developmental and acquired disabilities, religion, ethnicity, socioeconomic status, sexual orientation, indigenous heritage, national origin, and gender. Another culturally adapted psychotherapy, culturally sensitive psychotherapy (CSP), targets specific ethnocultural groups so that one group may benefit more from a specific intervention than from interventions designed for another (Hall, 2001). Furthermore, ethnocultural psychotherapy integrates cultural variables in treatment through the examination of worldviews, cultural transitions, relationships, and context (Comas-Diaz & Jacobsen, 2004).

Notwithstanding psychotherapy's cultural adaptation, several multiculturalists advocated for the use of ethnic psychotherapies in order to reaffirm their ethnocultural roots. As ethnic psychotherapies provide continuity, they may help clients repair their fractured identities. Ethnic and indigenous psychotherapies appeal to culturally diverse individuals because they are grounded in a cultural context and thus are responsive to clients' life experiences. They offer a culturally relevant framework that validates racial and ethnic meanings. Moreover, ethnic psychotherapies are based on a philosophical spiritual foundation that promotes connective, ancestral, and sacred affiliations in healing. As a result, they impart hope to sufferers, particularly when dominant approaches fail. Ethnic psychotherapies empower at both individual and collective levels. Some of the ethnic psychotherapies include folk healing, network therapy, narratives, the psychology of liberation, and holistic approaches based on Eastern philosophical traditions.

A historical antecedent of multicultural psychotherapies, folk healing is a form of indigenous psychotherapy. Folk healing re-establishes clients' sense of cultural belonging and historical continuity, promotes self-healing, and nurtures a balance between the sufferer, family, community, and cosmos (Comas-Diaz, 2006). Folk healers utilize mechanisms similar to those that mainstream psychotherapists use; the main difference is folk healers' spiritual belief systems. That is, folk healing fosters empowerment, encourages liberation, and promotes spiritual development. APA multicultural guideline number 5 encourages psychologists to strive to learn about non-Western healing traditions that could be appropriately integrated into psychotherapy. When appropriate, this guideline encourages psychologists to acknowledge and enlist the assistance of recognized helpers (community leaders, change agents) and traditional healers in treatment.

Carolyn Attneave developed network therapy as an extended family treatment and group intervention (Speck & Attneave, 1973). Based on a Native American healing approach, network therapy recreates the entire social context of a clan's network in order to activate and mobilize a person's family, kin, and relationships in the healing process. Network therapy is a community-based form of healing.

Another communal ethnic psychotherapy is the psychology of liberation. Based on Latin American theology of liberation, the psychotherapy of liberation emerged as a response to sociopolitical oppression. Its architect—Ignacio Martin-Baro (in Blanco, 1998)—was both a psychologist and a priest. Likewise, psychology of liberation resonates with African American psychology based on Black liberation theology and Africanist traditions. Such a spiritual basis affirms ethnocultural strengths through indigenous traditions and practices. Liberation practitioners attempt to work with people in context through strategies that enhance awareness of oppression and of the ideologies and structural inequality that have kept them subjugated and oppressed. Similar to Paulo Freire's critical consciousness, liberation therapists collaborate with the oppressed in developing critical analysis and engaging in transformative actions.

Ethnic psychotherapists frequently use narratives as a form of treatment. Therefore, stories are context-rich communications full of cultural nuances and meanings. Indeed, telling a story is a collectivistic way of relating. A reaction to Latin American political oppression, *testimonio* chronicles traumatic experiences and how these have affected the individual, family, and community (Cienfuegos & Monelli, 1982). Another healing narrative, *cuento* therapy, has been empirically proven to be an effective treatment for Puerto Rican children (Costantino, Malgady, & Rogler, 1997). Furthermore, *dichos* (sayings) are a form of flash psychotherapy that consists of Spanish proverbs or idiomatic expressions that capture folk wisdom (Comas-Diaz, 2006).

PERSONALITY

Theory of Personality

Multicultural psychotherapists recognize the development of identity within several contexts. As mind inhabits the body, personality develops within multiple contexts. Multicultural clinicians acknowledge multiple perspectives; hence, they adhere to diverse theories of personality and follow theories that are consistent with their preferred theoretical orientation. However, multicultural psychotherapies' unique contribution to the theory of personality is the formulation of cultural identity development theories.

Cultural Identity Development

Multicultural psychotherapists view the self as an internal representation of culture. For instance, being a member of an oppressed minority group influences identity development. People of color's identity formation involves both personal identity and cultural racial/ethnic group identity. Minority identity developmental theories illuminate people of color's worldviews. The minority identity development theories offer a lens for understanding how individuals process and perceive the world. Indeed, the ethnic and racial identity stage affects beliefs, emotions, behaviors, attitudes, expectations, and interpersonal style. As a result, these stages influence how individuals present to treatment and even how they select their psychotherapist.

The diverse models of minority identity development propose that members of racial and ethnic minority groups initially value the dominant group and devalue their own group, then move to value their own group while devaluing the dominant group, and in a final stage integrate appreciation for both groups (Atkinson, Morten, & Sue, 1998). More specifically, minority identity development stages include (1) conformity—individuals internalize racism and choose values, lifestyles, and role models from the dominant group; (2) dissonance—individuals begin to question and suspect the dominant group's cultural values; (3) resistance-immersion—individuals endorse minority-held views and reject the dominant culture's values; (4) introspection—individuals establish their racial/ethnic identity without following all cultural norms, beginning to question how certain values fit with their personal identity; and (5) synergistic—individuals experience a sense of self-fulfillment toward their racial/ethnic/cultural identity without having to categorically accept their minority group's values. Moreover, a key milestone in people of color's racial identity development is overcoming internalized racism and becoming critically conscientized.

Racial identity development potentially interacts with client and therapist ethnic match. Consider the case of Jose, a bilingual, bicultural teacher. Jose's racial ethnic identity placed him at the dissonance stage (characterized by suspicion of Whites). When referred to a mental health center, Jose refused to see a European American therapist. He asked to see a counselor who "spoke his language and understood" his culture. When Dr. Delgado was assigned to see Jose, the therapist said, "I'm sorry, I don't speak Spanish." Jose's answer: "That's okay, I just didn't want to see a White therapist." Jose's experience illustrates the relevance of understanding racial identity developmental stages.

Racial identity development models extend to members of the dominant society. A White American identity developmental theory suggests that European Americans develop a specific cultural identity due to their status as members of the dominant majority group. According to Janet Helms (1990), White American cultural racial identity occurs in specific stages: (1) contact—individuals are aware of minorities but do not perceive themselves as racial beings; (2) deintegration—they acknowledge prejudice and discrimination; (3) reintegration—they engage in blaming the victim and in reverse discrimination; (4) pseudoindependence—they become interested in understanding cultural differences; and (5) autonomy—they learn about cultural differences and accept, respect, and appreciate both minority and majority group members. Similar identity developmental stages have been proposed for biracial individuals (Poston, 1990). These are as follows: (1) personal identity; (2) choice of group categorization; (3) enmeshment/denial; (4) appreciation; and (5) integration.

Multicultural psychotherapies also contributed to the formulation of gays' and lesbians' minority identity development. Gay and lesbian identity developmental stages include (1) confusion—individuals question their sexual orientation; (2) comparison—individuals accept the possibility that they may belong to a sexual minority; (3) tolerance—recognition that one is gay or lesbian; (4) acceptance—individuals increase contacts with other gays and lesbians; (5) pride—people prefer to be gay or lesbian; and (6) synthesis—people find peace with their own sexual orientation and reach out to supportive heterosexuals (Cass, 2002).

Feminist identity developmental theory also emerged from the minority identity developmental models. The feminist identity development theory articulates the premise that women struggle and continuously work through their reactions to the prejudice and discrimination they encounter to achieve a positive feminist identity. According to Downing and Roush (1985), feminist identity develops in the following stages: (1) passive acceptance, (2) revelation, (3) embeddedness–emanation, (4) synthesis, and (5) active commitment.

PSYCHOTHERAPY

Theory of Psychotherapy

Multicultural psychotherapists do not subscribe to a unifying theory of psychotherapy; instead, they endorse multiple perspectives. However, at the center of their theoretical approach, multicultural psychotherapists attempt to answer the question, "How can a therapist understand the life of a culturally different client?" Multiculturalists view the cultivation of the therapeutic alliance as a crucial aspect in healing and critically important to understanding clients. For this reason, the therapeutic alliance guides the multicultural psychotherapy process.

Cultural Self-Awareness

Multicultural therapeutic encounters are full of conscious and/or unconscious messages about the client's and the therapist's feelings and attitudes about their cultural backgrounds. Indeed, the perception of cultural differences evokes feelings of being excluded, being compared, and being relatively powerless (Pinderhughes, 1989). To address these issues, multicultural psychotherapists engage in cultural self-awareness. They initiate the self-awareness by identifying the dominant culture's values in which they communicate and practice. Psychotherapists can explore these issues through the following questions (adapted from Pinderhughes, 1989):

- What is my cultural heritage?
- What was the culture of my parents and ancestors?
- With what cultural group(s) do I identify?
- What is the cultural meaning of my name?
- What is my worldview?
- What aspects of my worldview (values, beliefs, opinions, and attitudes) do I hold that are congruent with the dominant culture's worldview? Which are incongruent?
- How did I decide to become a psychotherapist? How was I professionally socialized? What professional socialization do I maintain? What do I believe to be the relationship between culture and psychotherapy/counseling?
- What abilities, expectations, and limitations do I have that might influence my relations with culturally diverse individuals?

Other potential questions include:

- How do my clients answer some of the questions above?
- Are there differences between my answers and those of my culturally diverse clients?
- How do I feel about these differences?
- How do I feel about the similarities?

To further their cultural self-awareness, psychotherapists can use Bennett's (2004) multicultural sensitivity development model. Bennett divided multicultural sensitivity development into ethnocentric and ethnorelative stages. The ethnocentric stages include (1) denial—individuals deny the existence of cultural differences and avoid personal contact with culturally diverse people; (2) defense—individuals recognize other cultures but denigrate them; and (3) minimization—individuals view their own culture as universal, and although they recognize cultural differences, they minimize them, believing that other cultures are just like theirs. The ethnorelative stages of developing multicultural sensitivity are (4) acceptance—individuals recognize and value cultural differences without judging them; (5) adaptation—individuals develop multicultural skills—that is, they learn to shift perspectives and move in and out of alternative worldviews; and finally (6) integration—individuals' sense of self expands to include diverse worldviews.

The development of multicultural sensitivity facilitates appreciation of diverse worldviews and the emergence of a positive therapeutic alliance. Indeed, a successful therapeutic relationship rests on the recognition of the self in the other.

Process of Psychotherapy

The Therapeutic Relationship

Most psychotherapists recognize that a positive alliance increases psychotherapy's effectiveness. Moreover, research has repeatedly demonstrated the importance of the therapeutic relationship as a curative factor. However, the development of a therapeutic alliance requires cultural congruence between clients' and therapists' worldviews. When both therapist and client share worldviews, the development of a positive alliance is enhanced. Conversely, different worldviews may obstruct the development of the therapeutic alliance and may require adjustments. For example, Kakar (1985) modified his psychoanalytic approach when working with East Indians by being active and didactic. In addition, he emphasized feeling and expressing pity, interest, and warmth.

Culture affects how clients perceive therapists. For example, cultural attitudes toward authority and healing figures shape clients' expectations about their therapists. If Eastern collectivistic clients perceive therapists as wise teachers, then they will adopt the role of students. The ideal therapist role varies from culture to culture. Hence, psychotherapists need to understand culturally diverse expectations. For example, therapists who have an egalitarian and nondirective style may not work well with clients who prefer hierarchical and directive relationships and specific instructions about what to do to change (Koss-Chioino & Vargas, 1992).

Similarly, Atkinson, Thompson, and Grant (1993) identified eight intersecting therapist roles that depend on clients' acculturation to the mainstream society. They asserted that low-acculturated clients expect therapists to behave as *advisor, advocate,* and/or *facilitator of indigenous support systems.* As an illustration, the use of modeling, selective self-disclosure, and didactic strategies seems culturally relevant for low-acculturated immigrant clients. More acculturated clients may expect their clinician to act as a consultant, change agent, counselor, and/or psychotherapist.

However, in reality, culturally diverse clients have complex expectations of their therapists. Besides acculturation, clients' expectations are shaped by interpersonal needs, developmental stages, ethnic identity, spirituality, and numerous other factors. Even though clients' expectations range from a collaborative to a hierarchical therapeutic style, these expectations are not mutually exclusive. For instance, regardless of clients' level of acculturation, psychotherapists tend to respond according to their clients' needs. In other words, therapists move from one role to another or simultaneously engage in several helping roles.

Along these lines, an empirical investigation found that although clients of color expected to get relief from their problems, they also expected to work in therapy to overcome their contribution to their distress (Comas-Diaz, Geller, Melgoza, & Baker, 1982). Even though they expected their therapist to be active, give advice, teach, and guide them, they also believed that psychotherapists would help them to grow emotionally in a process that at times would be painful. Concisely put, clients of color exhibited psychological mindedness and viewed psychotherapy as a process to work though their issues.

Cultural Empathy

Clients of color expect psychotherapists to demonstrate cultural credibility. Credibility refers to the client's perception of the psychotherapist as a trustworthy and effective helper. For example, many American Indians expect psychotherapists to exemplify empathy, genuineness, availability, respect, warmth, congruence, and connectedness. Certainly, a therapist's credibility and trust foster a positive therapeutic alliance. To achieve this goal, multicultural psychotherapists aim to develop empathy for the "other." Empathy is an interpersonal concept referring to a clinician's capacity to attend to the emotional experience of clients.

In dominant psychotherapy, empathy has somatic, cognitive, and affective components. The somatic aspect of empathy refers to nonverbal communication and body language. Therapists develop cognitive empathy for culturally diverse clients by becoming empathic witnesses. As empathic witnesses, psychotherapists study clients' culture and reaffirm clients' experience and reality. Empathy's affective component involves emotional connectedness, a capacity to take in and contain the feelings of the client. Succinctly put, affective empathy is similar to the subjective experience of *being* like the other. Therapists who can only empathize at a cognitive level keep their identity separate from their client's. This "separation" hinders the therapist's development of affective empathy for culturally different clients. Such empathic failure is associated with the difficulty of being "like the other." Indeed, the development of affective empathy is critical in multicultural psychotherapy because we tend to empathize with people who remind us of ourselves and, conversely, have difficulty empathizing with those who are culturally different from us.

Besides cognitive and affective empathy, therapists need to develop cultural empathy. Cultural empathy is a learned ability to obtain an understanding of the experience of culturally diverse individuals informed by cultural knowledge and interpretation (Ridley & Lingle, 1996). Therefore, cultural empathy promotes therapists' cultural responsiveness through the integration of perceptual, cognitive, affective, and communication skills. Cultural empathy involves a process using a cultural framework as a guide for understanding the client and recognizing cultural differences between self and other (Ridley & Lingle, 1996). Interestingly, research has suggested that practitioners reduce their stereotypic and ethnocentric attitudes if they are able to take the perspective of others (Galinsky & Moskowitz, 2000). Thus, cultural empathy entails an attunement to the other—a combined cultural, cognitive, emotional, affective, and behavioral connection to the culturally different person.

In short, cultural empathy is the ability to place yourself in the other's culture. As such, it facilitates the recognition of self in the culturally diverse other. Multicultural psychotherapists develop cultural empathy by engaging in self-reflection, unpacking their invisible knapsacks, exploring their own worldviews, challenging ethnocentrism, developing openness and respect for cultural differences, and understanding power dynamics.

Ethnocultural Transference and Countertransference

The therapeutic relationship is a fertile ground for the projection of conscious and unconscious feelings, and every therapeutic encounter promulgates the projection of conscious and/or unconscious messages about the client's and the therapist's cultures. The examination of transference (clients' projection of feelings from previous relationships onto their therapists) and countertransference (therapists' reaction to clients' transference) helps to manage these processes. Although the examination of transference reactions can be an important part of psychotherapy, most dominant psychotherapists ignore transferential cultural issues. Instead, they adhere to the universalistic perspective that endorses a culture-blind and race-neutral position of human relations (Pinderhughes, 1989). Simply put, many clinicians ignore ethnic, cultural, and racial aspects of transference and countertransference. Multicultural psychotherapists examine transferential reactions through the initiation of a dialogue on cultural differences and similarities. They specifically ask clients: "How do you feel about my being from a different culture from yours?" or, "How do you feel about our being from similar cultures?" This line of questioning fosters a discussion of ethnocultural transference and countertransference.

Ethnocultural transference and countertransference play a significant role in the therapeutic relationship because providers and clients tend to bring their imprinting of ethnic, cultural, and racial experiences into psychotherapy. Ethnocultural reactions can provide a blueprint for the relationship between self and others.

Comas-Díaz and Jacobsen (1991) described several types of ethnocultural transference and countertransference within intra- and inter-ethnic dyads. Some of the inter-ethnic transferential reactions include the following: (1) overcompliance and friendliness (observed when there is a societal power differential in the client/therapist dyad); (2) denial (when the client avoids disclosing issues pertinent to ethnicity and/or culture);

(3) mistrust, suspiciousness, and hostility ("What are this therapist's real motivations for working with me?"); and (4) ambivalence (clients in an inter-ethnic psychotherapy may struggle with negative feelings toward their therapist while simultaneously developing an attachment to him or her).

Intraethnic transference may transform a client's image of the therapist into one of several predictable roles: (1) the omniscient/omnipotent therapist (fantasy of the reunion with the perfect parent, promoted by the ethnic similarity); (2) the traitor (client exhibits resentment and envy at therapist's successes—equated with betrayal of his/her ethnoculture); (3) the auto-racist (client does not want to work with a therapist of his or her own ethnocultural group due to projection of the strong negative feelings onto the ethnoculturally similar therapist); and (4) the ambivalent (clients may feel at once comfortable with their shared ethnocultural background but at the same time they may fear too much psychological closeness).

Some inter-ethnic dyad countertransferential reactions include: (1) denial of cultural differences ("We are all the same"); (2) the clinical anthropologist's syndrome (excessive curiosity about clients' ethnocultural backgrounds at the expense of their psychological needs); (3) guilt (about societal and political realities that dictate a lower status for people of color); (4) pity (a derivative of guilt or an expression of political impotence within the therapeutic hour); (5) aggression; and (6) ambivalence (ambivalence toward the client's culture may originate from ambivalence toward a therapist's own ethnoculture).

Within the intra-ethnic dyad, some of the countertransferential manifestations include: (1) overidentification; (2) *us and them* mentality (shared victimization due to racial discrimination may contribute to therapist's ascribing the clients' problems as being solely due to membership in a minority group); (3) distancing; (4) survivor's guilt (therapists may have the personal experience of escaping the harsh socioeconomic circumstances of low-income ethnic minorities, leaving family and friends in the process, and generating guilt. Survivor's guilt can impede professional growth and may lead to denying their clients' psychological problems.); (5) cultural myopia (inability to see clearly due to ethnocultural factors that obscure therapy); (6) ambivalence (working through the therapist's own ethnocultural ambivalence); and (7) anger (being too ethnoculturally close to a client may uncover painful, unresolved intrapsychic issues).

Identifying the cultural parameters of transference and countertransference is central for multicultural psychotherapists. They recognize that ethnic, cultural, gender, and racial factors often lead to a more rapid unfolding of core problems in psychotherapy.

Mechanisms of Psychotherapy

Multicultural psychotherapists utilize whatever tools and techniques they learned in graduate school and those endorsed by their theoretical orientations and professional organizations. However, these techniques are not applied automatically and thoughtlessly; they also think carefully and hard to use psychotherapeutic mechanisms congruent with their clients' worldviews. For instance, many individualistic group members prefer a verbal therapy that works through and promotes change by externalizing, or moving from the unconscious to the conscious. Conversely, a significant number of collectivistic members require a holistic healing approach that acknowledges nonverbal communication and promotes change by internalizing, or moving from the conscious to the unconscious (Tamura & Lau, 1992). Therefore, many multicultural psychotherapists integrate holism into their practices. Most of these practices are based on non-Western philosophical and spiritual traditions. In addition to verbal therapy, many clients of color require a mind, body, and spirit approach. For example, Cane (2000) successfully used mind, body, and spirit self-healing practices complemented with a liberation method.

Also known as *contemplative* practices (see chapter 13), holistic approaches such as meditation, yoga, breath work, creative visualization, and indigenous healing are gaining popularity among mainstream psychotherapists. With their holistic emphasis, many multicultural psychotherapists promote spiritual development. Spirituality—a sense of connection to self, others, community, history, and context—is an important aspect in the lives of many people of color. Spirituality provides a worldview, a way of life, and a meaning-making process. Within this context, multicultural psychotherapists help individuals to overcome adversity and find meaning in their existence. Many people of color require liberation approaches in order to recover from historical and contemporary cultural and racial trauma.

Multicultural psychotherapists foster creativity as part of a holistic approach and they encourage clients to use art, folklore, ethnic practices, and other creative cultural forms. The therapeutic use of creativity enhances resilience and *cultural consciousness*— the affirmation, redemption, and celebration of one's ethnicity and culture (Comas-Diaz, 2007). For example, many psychotherapists use clients' oral traditions in healing because people of color frequently answer questions by telling a story. This communication style is consistent with an inferential reasoning based on contextual, interpersonal, and historical factors. In other words, telling a story is a creative way of constructing reality in both linear and nonlinear ways, and the patient's narrative combines both analytical and gestalt elements. Asking clients "What happened to you?" offers a cultural holding environment in which the therapist can become an emphatic witness. It is not surprising that storytelling has been found to be effective in cross-cultural psychotherapy (Semmler & Williams, 2000).

Moreover, due to their experiences of disconnection and trauma, people of color use creativity to cope with past trauma and create meaning and purpose in their lives. Examples of such resilient creativity include flamenco music (originated by Gypsy or Roma people), spoken word (New York Puerto Rican and African American urban spoken poetry), people of color's memoirs and narratives, and other narrative performances. For example, Southeast Indian novelist Chitra Banerjee Divakaruni began to write creatively after immigrating to the United States and confronting her first racist incident (personal communication, May 1, 2002).

Using photos for storytelling enhances self-esteem among visible people of color (Falicov, 1998) and addresses issues of skin color and race. Many oppressed people of color have used creativity as a means of resistance, recovery, redemption, and identity reformulation.

It is clear that creative activities promote healing, and songs, chants, music, and dance induce emotional states in patients that affect the way the immune system responds to illness (Lyon, 1993). Holistic healers understand this process very well. They use metaphors to help their clients manipulate sensory, emotional, and cognitive information to alter their perceptions of illness. For example, empirical studies revealed that folk healers who encouraged their patients to publicly perform their dreams in poetry, song, and dance were significantly more effective in healing as opposed to therapists who encouraged their patients to talk about their dreams in private (Joralemon, 1986).

There is an intimate relationship between multiculturalism and creativity, and research has demonstrated that exposure to diverse cultures enhances creativity. Leung, Maddux, Galinsky, and Chiu (2008) empirically showed that the relationship between multicultural experiences and creativity is stronger when people are open to new experiences and when the creative context emphasizes flexibility. In summary, multicultural psychotherapists use holistic approaches in addition to more traditional psychotherapy mechanisms used in mainstream healing approaches. Out of this amalgamation, with its specific emphasis on cultural strengths, healing emerges.

Ethnopsychopharmacology

All clients come to therapy expecting amelioration of symptoms and some relief from their distress. Medications such as antidepressants are often the quickest way to offer at least temporary relief from pain; consequently, psychotherapists need to work in tandem with physicians, prescribing psychologists, advanced practice nurses, and other health care providers to help patients access the medications they need.

Regrettably, ethnocentrism has resulted in culturally diverse clients' mistrust of psychopharmacology. This problem is compounded by the fact that different racial and ethnic minority groups may respond differently to medication than European American individuals (Rey, 2006). Notwithstanding the empirical evidence of the relevance of ethnicity in assessing likely pharmacological response to psychotropic medications (Ruiz, 2000), ignorance of the ways in which different ethnic groups respond to different medications has contributed to misdiagnosis and mistreatment. Ethnopharmacology is the field that specializes in the relationship between ethnicity and responses to medications. For example, African Americans with affective disorders are often misdiagnosed and thus mistreated with antipsychotic medications (Lawson, 1996; Strickland, Ranganeth, & Lin, 1991). Similarly, due to the fact that many health care providers do not understand or appreciate the different metabolic rates associated with different ethnic groups, many Asians and Latinos are treated inappropriately with psychotropic medications (Ruiz, 2000). Consequently, many people of color have deepened their mistrust of mental health establishments, especially with regard to the prescription of psychotropic medications. These individuals fear, sometimes correctly, that psychotherapists' ignorance of ethnic variations in drug metabolization reflects cultural unawareness, incompetence, and/or indifference.

The field of ethnopsychopharmacology emerged out of the need to address the specific mental health needs of culturally diverse people. Ethnopsychopharmacologists take special care in assessing potential gender and ethnic interactions when prescribing medications. Additionally, they are knowledgeable of the interface of multiculturalism and psychopharmacology (Rey, 2006). For example, it is common for Latinos to share medications with family members and significant others. This practice reflects the cultural value of familism, where family interdependence naturally and predictably results in the sharing of resources. Additionally they may self-medicate and combine medications with herbal remedies. Therefore, multicultural psychotherapists are alert to the need to educate clients about the dangers of self-medication, sharing medications with relatives, use of medications obtained over the counter from outside the United States, and combining herbal remedies with psychotropic medications.

Besides exploring the biological characteristics that affect response to medications, multicultural clinicians examine their clients' lifestyles. For example, the diets of some people of color contain foods (i.e., Mexican Americans' consumption of cheese) that are incompatible with certain kinds of psychotropic medications (MAOIs), but this problem can't be assessed unless the clinician knows something about the dietary habits of his or her client. In addition, multicultural psychotherapists collaborate with psychopharmacologists who are knowledgeable of ethnicity medication interactions.

APPLICATIONS

Who Can We Help?

Paraphrasing Murray and Kluckhohn's (1953) words, every multicultural therapist is "like all other therapists, like some other therapists, and like no other therapist." In other words, multiculturalists share similarities with all therapists (by virtue of being therapists), with some therapists (by belonging to a particular theoretical orientation), and with no other therapists (due to their unique personal and cultural experiences). Multicultural clinicians engage in diverse therapy formats, including individual, family, and group. Additionally, some use community interventions, such as network therapy. In this section, I present specific examples of clinical interventions prevalent in multicultural psychotherapies.

Multicultural psychotherapies apply to everyone because they emphasize a person-in-context model. As such, multicultural practitioners attempt to use culturally appropriate assessment and treatment modalities. However, multicultural psychotherapies are particularly helpful when individuals present to treatment with identity issues, relationships problems, cultural adaptation, ethnic and racial stressors, and conflicts of diverse nature.

Treatment

A multicultural assessment is a process-oriented tool that leads to culturally appropriate treatment. Some examples of multicultural assessment include the explanatory model of distress, cultural formulation, the use of a cultural genogram, and ethnocultural assessment.

Explanatory Model of Distress

Clients' worldviews and life experiences affect how they present their problems to their psychotherapists, the meaning they attribute to their distress, their help-seeking behavior, their level of social support, and their perseverance in treatment (Anderson, 1995). The explanatory model is a culture-centered assessment based on an anthropological method developed to address these issues. In other words, an explanatory model elicits clients' perspectives of their illness, experience, and healing (Kleinman, 1980). Multicultural psychotherapists use the explanatory model to unfold clients' treatment expectations by asking the following questions (Kleinman, 1980):

- What do you call your problem (illness)?
- What do you think your problem (illness) does?
- What do you think the natural course of your illness is?
- What do you fear?
- Why do you think this illness or problem has occurred?
- How do you think the distress should be treated?
- How do want me to help you?
- Who do you turn to for help?
- Who should be involved in decision-making?

Cultural Formulation and Analysis

The cultural formulation is a clinical tool for assessment and treatment included in the American Psychiatric Association's (2000) *Diagnostic and Statistical Manual* (DSM-IV). The cultural formulation is a process-oriented approach that places diagnosis in a cultural context. Although the cultural formulation is a medical model that emphasizes pathology, its application increases psychotherapists' cultural awareness. The cultural formulation examines (1) individuals' cultural identity; (2) cultural explanations for individual illnesses; (3) cultural factors related to the psychosocial environment and levels of functioning; (4) cultural elements of the therapist–client relationship; and (5) overall cultural assessment for diagnosis and treatment (APA, 2000).

The cultural formulation facilitates a cultural analysis. Like the explanatory model of distress, the cultural analysis uncovers the cultural knowledge people use to organize their behaviors and interpret their experiences (Spradley, 1990). Lo and Fung (2003) recommended a cultural analysis based on an object–relation treatment model, emphasizing the importance of self and relationships with others and with the world. The domains of the cultural analysis include self, relations, and treatment. According to Lo and Fung, the self domain captures cultural influences on the psychological aspects of the self that may be relevant in psychotherapy (i.e., affect, cognition, behavior, body, self-concept, plus individual goals and motivations). The relations domain relates to cultural influence on clients' relationships with family, groups, others, society, possessions, environment, spirituality, and time. The treatment domain accentuates therapy elements influenced by culture such as communication (both verbal and nonverbal), problem–solution models, and the therapeutic relationship.

Cultural Genogram

Psychotherapists use genograms to enhance their cultural self-awareness. A family therapy tool, genograms diagram a genealogical tree highlighting dynamics from a nuclear to an extended family perspective (McGoldrick, Gerson, & Shellenberger, 1999). Genograms are particularly useful when psychotherapists compare their genealogy to their clients' and examine similarities as well as differences. Many psychotherapists complete their own genogram during personal therapy or professional training. You can see how to complete a genogram at www.genopro.com/genogram_rules/default.htm.

Although the genogram is a well-known family therapy tool, few psychotherapists complete their cultural genograms, even when working with multicultural clients. Hardy and Laszloffy (1995) developed the cultural genogram as a tool to emphasize the role of culture and collective contexts in the lives of individuals and their families. Cultural genograms diagram the genealogical, developmental, historical, political, economical, sociological, ethnic, spiritual/religious, and racial influences in people's lives. The cultural genogram places individuals within their communal contexts.

Clinicians begin a cultural genogram with three or more generations of ancestors. If appropriate and if the information is unavailable, they invite clients to use their imaginations to summon up family information. To aid in this process, clients bring family photos to therapy sessions. This approach is useful when discussing racial differences and other types of physical characteristics. In preparing the cultural genogram, Hardly and Laszloffy recommended the use of color to designate different ethnic groups and mixed colors to identify mixed-race individuals. Likewise, clients can use their creativity—draw, paint, sculpt, and so forth—to prepare their cultural genogram. Cultural genograms share the symbols used in family genograms such as squares to designate males and circles for females.

The following factors can be used in completing a cultural genogram (adapted from Comas-Diaz and Ramos Grenier (1998) and Hardly and Laszloffy (1995)):

- Individual and family culture(s)
- Meaning of race
  - Identity and identification
  - Significance of skin color, body type, hair texture, phenotype
- Meaning of ethnicity
- National origin, collective history, wars, conflicts with other ethnic groups

- Languages spoken by client, family of origin, and current family
- Ethnocultural heritage
- Sexual orientation
  - Interaction of gender, ethnicity, race, class, and sexual orientation
- Family
  - Intact, blended, single parent, nuclear, extended, multigenerational, etc.
- Cultural meanings of family roles
  - Adoption and foster parenting
- Family of origin and multigenerational history
- Assessment of nonblood-related extended family members
- Family life cycle development and stages
- Family structure (nuclear, extended, traditional, intact, reconstituted)
- Gender and family roles
- Social class
- Educational level
- Financial history (e.g., Great Depression), culture of poverty, change in socioeconomic class
- Occupation, avocation
- Marriage
  - Common-law, civil law, religious, commitment ceremonies, same-sex unions, etc.
- Gender roles
  - Gender-specific trauma
  - Relations (intimate, friends, etc.)
  - Intra-ethnic, interethnic
- Migration
  - History of (im)migration and generations from (im)migrations
  - Patterns, reasons for migration
  - Refugee experience
  - Refugee trauma
  - Acculturation
  - Assimilation, separation, marginalization, integration
- Stress
  - Types of stress
  - Acculturative stress
  - Life stressors
  - Ecological stress (e.g., inner city living)
  - Stress management
- Spirituality and faith
- Spiritual assessment
- Use of contemplative practices
- History and politics

- Trauma
  - Political torture and repression
  - History of slavery, colonization, Holocaust, genocide, wars
  - History of human trafficking
  - Sexual and gender trauma
  - Rape, incest, molestation, harassment
- Meaning of differences
  - Individual, family, group, community

As learning about one's societal power is an important aspect of self-knowledge, multicultural assessments can be complemented with a *power differential analysis*. Such analysis requires going beyond the power differential inherent in the psychotherapist/client dyad. It should include an analysis of the client's cultural group's social status compared with the practitioner's. This comparison entails the identification and challenge of internalized privilege and oppression

Ethnocultural Assessment

A multicultural tool for both evaluation and treatment, the ethnocultural assessment explores diverse stages in the development of cultural identity. The stages of ethnocultural assessment include heritage, saga, niche, self-adjustment, and relationships (Comas-Diaz & Jacobsen, 2004). During the heritage stage, therapists explore clients' ethnocultural ancestry (including parents' genealogy), history, genetics, and sociopolitical contexts. Of particular relevance is the examination of cultural trauma. Exploring family saga entails examining the family, clan, and group story. During this stage, clinicians explore their clients' history of immigration and other significant transitions. The niche assessment stage entails the posttransition analysis. Special attention is given to clients' intellectual and emotional interpretation of their family saga. Therapists examine clients' individual adaptation separate from their family during the self-adjustment stage. Clients' coping styles, including cultural resilience, are assessed during this stage. The final stage of the ethnocultural assessment explores clients' significant affiliations, including the therapeutic relationship.

Evidence

Multicultural psychotherapists combine cultural knowledge with clinical skills and ecological understanding. Instead of endorsing cultural reductionism, they argue for research on the effectiveness of multicultural approaches to psychotherapy. That is, they advocate for research findings that are applicable to the lives of culturally diverse individuals and communities. Multicultural psychotherapies' evidence base is a reality-based perspective, one that moves from the "couch to the bench," and from the "clinic to the laboratory." Such an approach reflects the need for psychotherapy research to be culturally relevant and accountable to ethnic communities.

Some early psychotherapy research focused on ethnic similarity between psychotherapists and clients. Empirical findings suggested that clients working with psychotherapists of similar ethnic backgrounds and languages tend to remain in treatment longer than those whose therapists are not ethnically or linguistically similar. However, ethnic and linguistic match does not necessarily translate into mutual cultural identification (Hall, 2001), nor is it necessarily desirable for some clients. A review of the research on therapist/client ethnic matching revealed inconclusive results and low validity for ethnic matching (Karlsson, 2005). Nonetheless, research has indicated that clients of color in similar-race dyads participate more in their care than do those in race-dissimilar dyads (Cooper-Patrick et al., 1999). In contrast, an empirical study on the effects of ethnic matching on treatment satisfaction among migrant patients showed that these clients did not view ethnic matching as important and considered clinical competence, compassion, and sharing their worldview as far more important factors (Knipscheer & Kleber, 2004). In toto, however, the available research suggests that culturally competent therapists enhance their clients' satisfaction with treatment.

Much more research is needed on multicultural psychotherapies. Some of the questions that need to be answered include the following:

- What kinds of treatments work best with which kind of clients?
- What is the connection between a psychotherapist's cultural competence and his or her treatment outcomes?
- What is spirituality's effect on psychotherapy effectiveness?
- What are the effects of cultural resilience on physical and mental health?
- How does language (e.g., bilingualism, being a polyglot) influence psychotherapy process?
- How do creativity and multicultural experiences affect mental health?
- What are the gender, ethnobiological, and neurohomonal factors that influence clients' responses to psychotropic medications?
- What are the cultural and ethical contexts of therapists' self-disclosure?

The empirical exploration of these questions and others can reveal the effectiveness of multicultural psychotherapies.

Psychotherapy in a Multicultural World

The inclusion of a new section in each chapter of *Current Psychotherapies* on multicultural psychotherapy—and more significantly, the addition of an entire chapter devoted to the topic in the current edition—underscores the growing importance of multicultural issues for all psychotherapists. Students who are reading this chapter are encouraged to now go back and reread the multicultural sections of all of the other psychotherapy-specific chapters and to evaluate these sections, chapters, and therapies *vis-a-vis* what they have learned from reading the current chapter. To facilitate this process, students can examine the clinical insights provided by the application of multicultural psychotherapies in the following case illustration.

CASE EXAMPLE

Grace: " I don't know why I'm here."
Dr. Martin: "You are wondering why you are in therapy."
Grace: "Don't paraphrase me. I hate it when shrinks do that."
Dr. Martin: "It sounds like you have been in therapy before."
Grace: "Yes, and I despised it."
Dr. Martin: "What did you despise?"
Grace: "I was never understood."
Dr. Martin: "Help me understand you."
Grace: "It's simple: Just listen to me, look at me. What do you see?"
Dr. Martin: "An attractive young woman who needs help and doesn't know why she is here."

Grace:	"Now you are getting somewhere. Anything else?"
Dr. Martin:	"How do you see yourself"?
Grace:	"What do you mean?"
Dr. Martin:	"Let's start with where do you come from? Family, ethnic, racial, cultural background."
Grace:	"You are the first shrink who asked me that. Hum. Although I look White, I'm mixed race."

Background

Grace was the daughter of an African American man and a White European American woman. She grew up in an upper-middle class family—her father worked as a clinic administrator and her mother as a high school teacher. Both parents grew up Catholic and sent Grace to Catholic school. She excelled at academics until her senior year, when she experienced a traumatic loss. A drunk driver killed her boyfriend Adolph, who was on his way home after leaving his 17th birthday party.

"I created a macabre dance," Grace told Dr. Martin without crying.

Grace was referring to her birthday gift to Adolph—a choreographed piece that she created for him.

After the tragedy, Grace's grades plummeted. She saw three different therapists, all of whom she fired.

Grace's developmental history was unremarkable. Her health history indicated episodic sleep paralysis during times of severe stress. Based on her sleep laboratory study, Grace received medication (Tofranil 25 mg) to control her symptoms. However, she stopped treatment due to side effects from the medication she was taking. "I have a sleep paralysis episode every year on Adolph's birthday," Grace said.

Upon the completion of the explanatory model of distress, Grace told Dr. Martin: "This is the first time I feel a therapist listened to me." Dr. Martin cemented the emerging therapeutic alliance by teaching Grace relaxation techniques. Grace expressed some relief from her anxiety symptoms.

Assessment

Grace's responses to the explanatory model of distress revealed a fear of being cursed. Immediately after her birth, Grace's father lost his job. The "curse" continued until 2 years later when her parents had a second child.

"My sister, Mary, brought joy and luck," Grace said. "My parents won the lottery and used the money to pay for my father's graduate studies."

"What did your parents think about your 'curse'?" Dr. Martin asked Grace.

"My mother denied it, but Dad has always been distant from me."

As further evidence of her "curse," Grace connected her "macabre dance" with Adolph's death.

When asked about her views on her problem, Grace responded, "I'm a 25-year-old woman looking for myself."

Cultural genogram

Dr. Martin invited Grace to complete a cultural genogram. Grace began to gather information by talking with her relatives. She traced her maternal family to Germany back three generations. Dr. Martin asked her to bring photos of her relatives to therapy sessions. In response, Grace compiled a photo album and complemented it with drawings. She chose a pink color to identify her maternal ancestors and used lavender to assign her paternal side of the family. At this time, Grace did not choose a color to identify herself in the cultural genogram.

Grace had a dream about a town in Germany during the completion of her cultural genogram. She conducted research and discovered that part of her maternal family was from an area that Germany annexed from Denmark. She found a great aunt of German–Danish ancestry and began communicating with her through the Internet. Fortunately, her great aunt spoke enough English to communicate with Grace.

Grace became a genealogy fan and researched her paternal ancestry. She discovered that her father was a descendant of the free people of color in New Orleans. As the term implies, free people of color were not enslaved during the United States slavery period. Most of the free people of color were of mixed race and had similar rights to Whites. That is, they owned property, were educated, and participated in diverse occupations and professions. This legacy filled Grace with excitement and pride. "I'm the product of contradictions." The exploration of Grace's contrasts led to the examination of her cultural identity development. At the beginning of treatment, Grace appeared to be at the biracial identity appreciation stage. Her words during the first session with Dr. Martin, "Although I look White, I'm mixed race," denoted positive regard for her mixed-race identity. Interestingly, Grace's genealogy work signaled her movement toward an integrative stage where biracial identity began to coalesce. Grace selected a gold color to self-identify at the completion of her cultural genogram.

Treatment

Dr. Martin worked on Grace's complicated bereavement during the beginning stages of treatment. However, before deepening the treatment, Dr. Martin—a European American middle-aged married woman—engaged in cultural self-assessment. The process revealed an English and Italian ethnocultural heritage. Both maternal and paternal great-grandparents had been immigrants. Dr. Martin compared her ethnocultural heritage with Grace's. Like her client, she felt proud of being a product of the union of two ethnicities. Like her client, Dr. Martin had received a Catholic school education. Another connection between them was the loss of a significant person during adolescence; Dr. Martin's best friend died after an accident during her senior year in high school. These similarities seemed to facilitate Dr. Martin's development of empathy. Nonetheless, the therapist acknowledged not knowing what it was like to be a mixed-race woman.

Grief work helped Grace to accept Adolph's death. Her anxiety symptoms decreased. However, Adolph's next birthday/death anniversary found Grace with another sleep paralysis episode. Grace described it to Dr. Martin. "It's like someone is sitting on my chest and I can't move. Grandma says that when this happens, a witch is riding you."

Dr. Martin researched the topic of sleep paralysis and found that the condition is prevalent among some African Americans who suffer from anxiety (Paradis & Freidman, 2005). After reviewing the literature, Dr. Martin suggested that Grace consult her grandmother about the "riding witch." Grace, who was named after her paternal grandmother, reported that her grandmother believed Adolph to be the cause of her sleep affliction. When Dr. Martin asked her what she thought about this explanation, Grace replied that relationships don't end with death. Indeed, some people of color believe that relationships between significant others continue after death.

Dr. Martin used grief counseling to treat Grace's complicated bereavement. Although Grace was able to sleep better, she continued to experience sleep paralysis. Dr. Martin interpreted Grace's symptoms as survivor's guilt and treated Grace with cognitive behavioral techniques. After several months of treatment, Dr. Martin began to feel frustrated and angry toward Grace. She examined her countertransference and realized that she was comparing her own grief (around her friend's death) with Grace's experience of losing

Adolph. Dr. Martin consulted a colleague and worked through her own bereavement. Afterward, Dr. Martin suggested a guided imagery exercise to Grace. She asked Grace to remember the last time she saw Adolph. Grace used the relaxation techniques she learned in therapy to help her visualization.

"Adolph just turned into my father," Grace said during the exercise. "Was Adolph Black?" asked Dr. Martin. "Yes," Grace answered.

Dr. Martin realized that she had an ethnocultural countertransference involving a cultural denial: She had assumed that Adolph was White. The realization that Adolph was African American helped her to better understand Grace's circumstances around his death. Dr. Martin interpreted Grace's reaction to Adolph's death as a repetition of a pattern where Grace felt abandoned by significant others (like her father's reaction to her "curse"). Dr. Martin worked with Grace on this dynamic interpretation. She suggested another holistic guided visualization. In this exercise, Dr. Martin asked Grace to relax deeply and imagine a safe and serene place. Grace saw herself choreographing a new dance. While she danced, Grace envisioned herself getting healed. She named the piece the Dance of Life.

Grace did not experience sleep paralysis during Adolph's next birthday/death anniversary. She examined her relationships with significant others during the rest of psychotherapy. Grace improved her relationship with her father, and for the first time, she felt close to her sister Mary. Her grandmother died during the last phase of therapy. Grace experienced sadness, but she completed her bereavement. Afterward, Grace formed an advocacy group to raise community consciousness about drunk driving. Grace stayed in therapy for two and a half years. On her last therapy session, she said to Dr. Martin: "I found myself." She took a tissue from the Kleenex box. "I finally own my name. No longer a curse, I'm a Grace to my family, community, and to myself."

SUMMARY

The United States' population is becoming more culturally, racially, and ethnically diverse. The election of the first president of color of the United States is a sign of such diversity. Multiculturalism emerged as a product of sociopolitical and civil rights movements. Multicultural theories of psychotherapy came to light out of people of color's concerns and later expanded to embrace diversity regarding gender, sexual orientation, class, religion, spirituality, age, ability, and disability.

Originally considered a transforming force in psychology, multiculturalism is at the vanguard of psychotherapy. To illustrate, multicultural theories constitute a shift in psychological paradigm. They provide conceptual and practical methods designed to enhance all types of clinical interventions. Multicultural psychotherapies facilitate adaptation and growth because they address the management of diverse and complex environments. With their emphasis on context, multicultural theories enhance our ability to cope with change and thus foster transformation and evolution.

Multicultural psychotherapies promote the development of cultural competence as a lifelong process. Fostering flexibility, they facilitate the incorporation of pluralistic and holistic approaches into practice. Multicultural theories accommodate the current resurgence of ancient healing traditions and promote their integration into mainstream psychotherapy.

As every human encounter is multicultural in nature, multicultural psychotherapies are relevant to all individuals (Sue & Sue, 2008). They offer tools for the effective management of differences, similarities, and power disparities. Finally, multicultural theories facilitate our adjustment to the globalization of our society. They offer a compass for the multicultural journey upon which all of us embark.

ANNOTATED BIBLIOGRAPHY AND WEB RESOURCES

Fadiman, A. (1997). *The spirit catches you and you fall down: A Hmong child, her American doctors and the collision of two cultures.* New York: Noonday Press (Farrar, Straus & Giroux).
A true story of cultural misunderstanding within the healing profession. It illustrates the utility of the explanatory model of distress.

Hoffman, E. (1989). *Lost in translation: A life in a new language.* New York: Penguin Books.
A superb memoir of an immigrant woman who struggles with cultural change and eventually becomes a psychotherapist.

Pinderhughes, E. (1989). *Understanding race, ethnicity and power: The key to efficacy in clinical practice.* New York: Free Press.
This classic text articulates the relationship between race, ethnicity, and power in clinical work.

Ridley, C. R. (1995). *Overcoming unintentional racism in counseling and therapy: A practitioner's guide to intentional intervention.* Thousand Oaks: Sage.
An eye opener, this book offers practical guidelines for clinicians to overcome prejudice and racism.

Web resources

American Psychological Association Guidelines for Providers of Psychological Services to Ethnic, Linguistic and Culturally Diverse populations, www.apa.org/pi/oema/resources/policy/provider-guidelines.aspx

Genograms, www.genopro.com/genogram_rules/default.htm

Psychological Treatment of Ethnic Minority Populations (Council of National Psychological Associations, 2003), www.apa.org/pi/oema/resources/brochures/treatment-minority.pdf

CASE READING

Comas-Diaz, L. (2006). Latino healing: The integration of ethnic psychology into psychotherapy. *Psychotherapy: Theory, Research, Practice, Training, 46*(4), 436–453. [One of these cases is reprinted in D. Wedding & R. J. Corsini (Eds.), (2011). *Case studies in psychotherapy.* Belmont, CA: Brooks/Cole.]

This article illustrates the integration of ethnic psychology into mainstream psychotherapy and includes examples of Latino psychology such as *cuento, dichos* and spirituality.

REFERENCES

Allport, G. W. (1954). *The nature of prejudice.* Cambridge, MA: Addison-Wesley.

Altman, N. (1995). *The analyst in the inner city: Race, class and culture through a psychoanalytic lens.* New York: Analytic Press.

American Psychiatric Association. (2000). *Diagnostic and statistical manual of mental disorders, 4th Edition,* Text Revision. Washington, DC: Author.

American Psychological Association. (1990). *Guidelines for providers of psychological services to ethnic, linguistic, and culturally diverse populations.* Washington, DC: Office of Ethnic Minority Affairs, American Psychological Association.

American Psychological Association (2003). Ethical principles of psychologists and code of conduct. Available from www.apa.org/ETHICS/code2002.html.

American Psychological Association. (2003). Guidelines on multicultural education, training, research, practice, and organizational change for psychologists. *American Psychologist, 58,* 377–402.

American Psychological Association Presidential Task Force on Evidence-Based Practice. (2006). Evidence-based practice in psychology. *American Psychologist, 6*(4), 271–285.

Anderson, N. (1995). Behavioral and sociological perspectives on ethnicity and health: Introduction to the special issue. *Health Psychology, 14,* 589–591.

Atkinson, D.R. Morten, G. & Sue, D.W. (Eds). (1998). *Counseling American minorities* (5th edition). Boston: McGraw-Hill.

Atkinson, D. R., Thompson, C. E., & Grant, S. K. (1993). A three-dimensional model for counseling racial/ethnic minorities. *Counseling Psychologist, 21,* 257–277.

Bennett, M. J. (2004). From ethnocentrism to ethnorelativism. In J. S. Wurzel (Ed.), *Toward multiculturalism: A reader in multicultural education* (pp. 62–77). Newton, MA: Intercultural Resource Corporation.

Bernal, G., Bonilla, J., & Bellido, C. (1995). Ecological validity and cultural sensitivity for outcome research: Issues for cultural adaptation and development of psychosocial treatments with Hispanics. *Journal of Abnormal Child Psychology, 23*(1), 67–82.

Betancourt, J. R., Green, A. R., Carrillo, J. E., & Ananch-Firempong, O. (2003). Defining cultural competence: A practical framework for addressing racial/ethnic disparities in health and health care. *Public Health Reports, 118,* 293–302.

Blanco, A. (1998). *Psicología de la liberación de Ignacio Martín-Baró.* Madrid, Spain: Editorial Trotta.

Boyd-Franklin, N. (2003). *Black families in therapy: Understanding the African American experience* (2nd ed.). New York: Guilford.

Brown, L. S. (1997). The private practice of subversion: Psychology as Tikkun Olam. *American Psychologist, 52,* 449–462.

Cane, P. (2000). *Trauma, healing and transformation: Awakening a new heart with body mind spirit practices.* Watsonville, CA: Capacitar.

Cass, V. (2002). Gay and lesbian identity development model. In Ritter, K. & Terndrup, A. I. (Eds.), *Handbook of affirmative psychotherapy with lesbians and gay men* (pp. 90–107). New York: Guilford Press.

CIEBP. (2008, March 13–14). *Culturally informed evidence-based practice: Translating research and policy for the real world.* Bethesda, MD: Capacitar.

Cienfuegos, A. J., & Moneli, C. (1983). The testimony of political repression as a therapeutic instrument. *American Journal of Orthopsychiatry, 53,* 43–51.

Comas-Diaz, L. (2006). Latino healing: The integration of ethnic psychology into psychotherapy. *Psychotherapy: Theory, Research, Practice & Training, 43*(4), 436–453.

Comas-Diaz, L. (2007). Ethnopolitical psychology: Healing and transformation. In E. Aldarondo (Ed.), *Promoting social justice in mental health practice* (pp. 91–118). Mahwah, NJ: Lawrence Earlbaum Associates.

Comas-Diaz, L. (2008). *Spirita*: Reclaiming womanist sacredness in feminism. *Psychology of Women Quarterly, 32,* 13–21.

Comas-Diaz, L., Geller, J., Melgoza, B., & Baker, R. (1982, August). *Ethnic minority patients' expectations of treatment and of their therapists.* Presentation made at the American Psychological Association Annual Meeting. Los Angeles: CA.

Comas-Díaz, L., & Jacobsen, F. M. (1991). Ethnocultural transference and countertransference in the therapeutic dyad. *American Journal of Orthopsychiatry, 61*(3), 392–402.

Comas-Diaz, L., & Jacobsen, F. M. (2004). Ethnocultural psychotherapy. In E. Craighead & C. Nemeroff (Eds.), *The Corsini encyclopedia of psychology and behavioral science* (pp. 338–339). New York: Wiley.

Comas-Diaz & Ramos Grenier, J. (1998). Migration and acculturation. In J. Sandoval, C. L. Frisby, K. F. Geisinger, J. D. Scheuneman, & J. Ramos-Grenier, (Eds.), *Test interpretations and diversity: Achieving equity in assessment.* (pp. 213–239). Washington, DC: American Psychological Association.

Cooper-Patrick, L., Gallo, J., Gonzales, J. J., Vu, H. T., Powe, N. E., Nelson, C., & Ford, D. (1999). Race, gender and partnership in the patient–physician relationship. *Journal of the American Medical Association, 282,* 583–589.

Costantino, G., Malgady, R., & Rogler, L. (1986). *Cuento* therapy: A culturally sensitive modality for Puerto Rican

children. *Journal of Consulting and Clinical Psychology, 54,* 639–645.

Cross, T., Bazron, B., Dennis, K., & Isaacs, M. (1989). *Towards a culturally competent system of care: A monograph on effective services for minority children who are severely emotionally disturbed* (pp. 13–17). Washington, DC: CASPP Technical Assistance Center, Georgetown University Child Development Center.

Dala, C., Muntaner, C., Walrath, C., Nickerson, K., LaVeist, T., & Leaf, P. (2000). Racial differences in attitudes toward professional mental health care in the use of services. *American Journal of Orthopsychiatry, 70*(4), 455–456.

Dovidio, J. F., & Gaertner, S. L. (1998). On the nature of contemporary prejudice: The causes, consequences and challenges of aversive racism. In J. L. Eberhardt & S. T. Fiske (Eds.), *Confronting racism: the problem and the response* (pp. 3–32). Thousand Oaks, CA: Sage.

Downing, N., & Roush, K. (1985). From passive acceptance to active commitment: A model of feminist identity development for women. *The Counseling Psychologist, 13*(4), 695–709.

Duran, E., & Ivey, A. E. (2006). *Healing the soul wound: Counseling with American Indians and other Native People.* New York: Teachers College.

Falicov, C. J. (1998). *Latino families in therapy: A guide to multicultural practice.* New York: Guilford.

Fanon, F. (1967). *Black skin, White masks.* New York: Grove.

Freire, P. (1973). *Education for critical consciousness.* New York: Seabury.

Freire, P., & Macedo, D. (2000). *The Paulo Freire reader.* New York: Continuum.

Galinsky, A. D., & Moskowitz, G. B. (2000). Perspective-taking: Decreasing stereotype expression, stereotype accessibility, and in-group favoritism. *Journal of Personality & Social Psychology, 78,* 708–724.

Hall, G. C. N. (2001). Psychotherapy research with ethnic minorities: Empirical, ethical, and conceptual issues. *Journal of Consulting and Clinical Psychology, 69,* 502–510.

Hardy, K. V. & Laszloffy, T. (1995). The cultural genogram: Key to training culturally competent family therapists. *Journal of Marital and Family Therapy, 21*(3), 227–237.

Hays, P. (2001). *Addressing cultural complexities in practice: Assessment, diagnosis and therapy.* Washington, DC: American Psychological Association.

Helms, J. E. (1990). *Black and White racial identity: Theory, research and practice.* Westport, CT: Greenwood.

Howard-Hamilton, M. F., Phelps, R. E., & Torres, V. (1998). *Meeting the needs of all students and staff members: The challenge of diversity. New directions for student services.* San Francisco: Jossey-Bass.

Jo-alemon, D. (1986). The performing patient in ritual healing. *Social Science and Medicine, 23,* 841–845.

Kakar, S. (1985). Psychoanalysis and non-Western cultures. *International Review of Psychoanalysis, 12,* 441–448.

Karlsson, R. (2005). Ethnic matching between therapist and patient in psychotherapy: An overview of findings, together with methodological and conceptual issues. *Cultural Diversity and Ethnic Minority Psychology, 11*(2), 113–129.

Kleinman, A. (1980). *Patients and healers in the context of culture: An exploration of the borderland between anthropology, medicine, and psychiatry.* Berkeley: University of California Press.

Knipscheer, J. W., & Kleber, R. J. (2004). A need for ethnic similarity in the therapist–patient interaction? Mediterranean migrants in Dutch mental health care. *Journal of Clinical Psychology, 60*(6), 543–554.

Koss-Chioino, J., & Vargas, L. (1992). Through the cultural looking glass: A model for understanding culturally responsive psychotherapies. In L. A. Vargas & J. D. Koss-Chioino (Eds.), *Working with culture: Psychotherapeutic interventions with ethnic minorities, children and adolescents* (pp. 1–22). San Francisco: Jossey-Bass.

Lawson, W. B. (1996). Clinical issues in pharmacotherapy of African Americans. *Psychopharmacological Bulletin, 32*, 275–281.

Leininger, M. (1978). Changing foci in American nursing education: Primary and transcultural nursing care. *Journal of Advanced Nursing, 3*(2), 155–166.

Leung, A. K-y., Maddux, W., Galinsky, A., Chiu, C-y. (2008). Multicultural experience enhances creativity: The when and how. *American Psychologist, 63*(3), 169–181.

Lo, H.-T., & Fung, K. P. (2003). Culturally competent psychotherapy. *Canadian Journal of Psychiatry, 48*(3), 161–170.

Lyon, M. (1993). Psychoneuroimmonology: The problem of the situatedness of illness and the conceptualization of healing. *Culture, Medicine and Psychiatry, 17*, 77–97.

McGoldrick, M., Gerson, R., & Shellenberger, S. (1999). *Genograms: Assessment and Intervention.* New York: W. W. Norton.

McGoldrick, M. Giordano, J. & Pierce, J.K (Eds.) (1982). *Ethnicity and family therapy.* New York: Guilford.

McIntosh, P. (1988). *White privilege and male privilege: A personal account of coming to see correspondences through work in women's studies.* Available from the Wellesley College Center for Research on Women, Wellesley MA 02181.

Melfi, C. A., Croghan, T. W., Hanna, M. P., & Robinson, R. (2000). Racial variation in antidepressant treatment in a Medicare population. *Journal of Clinical Psychiatry, 61*(1), 16–21.

Miranda, J., Bernal, G., Lau, A., Kohn, L., Hwang, W.-C., & La Framboise, T. (2005). State of the science on psychosocial interventions for ethnic minorities. *Annual Review of Clinical Psychology, 1*, 113–142.

Muñoz, R. F., & Mendelson, T. (2005). Toward evidence-based interventions for diverse populations: The San Francisco General Hospital Prevention and Treatment Manuals. *Journal of Clinical and Consulting Psychology, 73*(5), 790–799.

Murray, H.A. & Kluckhohn, C (1953). *Personality in nature, society and culture.* Cambridge, MA: Harvard University Press.

Paradis, C., & Freidman, S. (2005). Sleep paralysis in African Americans with panic disorder. *Transcultural Psychiatry, 42*(1), 123–134.

Pierce, C. M. (1995). Stress analogs of racism and sexism: Terrorism, torture and disaster. In C. V. Willie, P. P. Reiker, & B. S. Brown (Eds.), *Mental health, racism and sexism* (pp. 277–293). Pittsburgh: University of Pittsburgh Press.

Pinderhughes, E. (1989). *Understanding race, ethnicity and power: The key to efficacy in clinical practice.* New York: Free Press.

Poston, W. C. (1990). The biracial identity development model: A needed addition. *Journal of Counseling and Development, 69*(2), 152–155.

Rey, J. (2006). The interface of multiculturalism and psychopharmacology. *Journal of Pharmacy Practice, 19*(6), 379–385.

Rhodes, D. L., & Williams, J. C. (2007). Legal perspectives on employment discrimination. In F. J. Crosby, M. S. Stockdale, & S. A. Ropp (Eds.), *Sex discrimination in the workplace* (pp. 235–270). Malden, MA: Blackwell.

Ridley, C., & Lingle, D. W. (1996). Cultural empathy in multicultural counseling: A multidimensional process model. In P. B. Pedersen, J. G. Draguns, W. J. Lonner, & J. E. Trimble (Eds.), *Counseling across cultures* (4th edition, pp. 21–46). Thousand Oaks, CA: Sage.

Roby, P. (1998). Creating a just world: Leadership for the twenty-first century. *Social Problems, 45*(1), 1–20.

Ruiz, P. (Ed.). (2000). *Ethnicity and psychopharmacology.* Washington, DC: American Psychiatric Press.

Seeley, K. M. (2000). *Cultural psychotherapy: Working with culture in the clinical encounter.* Northvale, NJ: Jason Aronson.

Semmler, P. L., & Williams, C. B. (2000). Narrative therapy: A storied context for multicultural counseling. *Journal of Multicultural Counseling and Development, 28*, 51–62.

Speck R. V., & Attneave, C. L. (1973). *Family networks.* New York: Pantheon Books.

Spradley, J. P. (1990). *Participant observation.* New York: Holt, Rinehart and Winston.

Strickland, T., L., Ranganeth, V., & Lin, K-M., (1991). Psychopharmacologic considerations in the treatment of Black American populations. *Psychopharmacology Bulletin, 27*, 441–448.

Sue, D.W. & Sue, D. (2008). *Counseling the culturally diverse: Theory and practice.* 5th edition. New York: Wiley.

Sue, D. W., Bingham, R. P., Porche-Burke, L., & Vasquez, M. (1999). The diversification of psychology: A multicultural revolution. *American Psychologist, 54*(12), 1061–1069.

Sue, D., Capodilupo, C. M., Torino, G. C., Bucceri, J. M., Holder, A. M., Nadal, K. L., & Esquilin, M. (2007). Racial micoraggressions in everyday life: Implications for clinical practice. *American Psychologist, 62*(4), 271–286.

Thompson, C. (1950). *Psychoanalysis: Evolution and development.* New York: Da Capo

Triandis, H. (1995). *Individualism and collectivism.* Boulder, CO: Westview.

*Varma, V. K. (1988). Culture, personality and psychotherapy. *International Journal of Social Psychiatry, 43*(2), 142–149.

Whaley, A. (1998). Racism in the provision of mental health services: A social–cognitive analysis. *American Journal of Orthopsychiatry, 68*, 47–57.

Whaley, A. L., & , King K. E. (2007). Cultural competence and evidence-based practice in mental health services: A complementary perspective. *American Psychologist, 62*(6), 563–574.

Worrell, J., & Remer, P. (2003). *Feminist perspectives in therapy* (2nd ed.). New York: Wiley.

Wu, E., & Martinez, M. (2006, October). Taking cultural competence from theory to action. *The Commonwealth Fund Publication No. 964.* www.commonwealthfund.org/Content/Publications/Fund-Reports/2006/Oct/Taking-Cultural-Competency-from-Theory-to-Action.aspx. Retrieved January 19, 2009.

Young, M. I. (1990). *Justice and the politics of difference.* Princeton, NJ: Princeton University Press.

16 CONTEMPORARY CHALLENGES AND CONTROVERSIES

Kenneth S. Pope and Danny Wedding

The other chapters in this book show psychotherapy's fascinating diversity. Therapists come from a variety of disciplines—psychology, psychiatry, social work, and counseling, to name just a few—and apply different principles from different perspectives in their work with people who come to them for help.

Yet for all the diversity, every therapist who shows up for work in a private office, clinic, community center, hospital, or elsewhere faces an array of contemporary challenges and controversies. This chapter takes a look at nine of them:

1. The mental health workforce
2. Physicians, medications, and psychotherapy
3. Empirically supported therapies
4. Phones, computers, and the Internet
5. Therapists' sexual involvement with patients, nonsexual physical touch, and sexual feelings
6. Nonsexual multiple relationships and boundary issues
7. Accessibility and people with disabilities
8. Detainee interrogations
9. Cultures

THE MENTAL HEALTH WORKFORCE

You and your partner have just moved to a new state. After a week, your partner tells you, "I've been feeling a little depressed and anxious since we moved. It's not one of those things I can pull myself out of. I think I need some help. We don't know anyone here, so there's no one we trust to ask for a recommendation, but I've looked in the phone book and here are the people who are available: a counselor, a life coach, a marriage and family therapist, a psychiatrist, a psychologist, and a social worker. The phone book doesn't give anything more than the title. Which do you think I should choose?" How do you respond to your partner?

Defining the mental health workforce with any precision presents complex challenges, especially in light of the fact that many therapists work part-time and many identify with more than one mental health profession (for example, a therapist may be both a social worker *and* a marriage and family therapist). However, we know that for every 100,000 U.S. citizens, there are about 6.5 psychiatric nurses, 11.4 school psychologists, 13.7 psychiatrists, 16.7 marriage and family therapists, 31.1 psychologists, 35.3 social workers, and 49.4 counselors (Robiner, 2006). Mental health services are also delivered by other health professionals, including rehabilitation counselors, pastoral counselors, substance abuse counselors, and general practice physicians and nurses (Wedding, DeLeon, & Olson, 2006). Whatever their professional identification, the majority of these individuals practice *technical eclecticism* (described in Chapter 14) and use a variety of methods, most of which are derived from the therapies described in *Current Psychotherapies*.

In recent years, psychologists and social workers have come closer to achieving the status of medical therapists, especially in the areas of insurance reimbursement, participation in federal health programs, and admission to psychoanalytic training. In many states, psychologists also have gained hospital admitting privileges, and some states enacted laws requiring hospitals that offer psychology services to allow psychologists to directly admit their patients. Other groups that practice counseling or psychotherapy are making rapid strides toward achieving those privileges now available to psychologists and social workers.

The accreditation standards of the Joint Commission on Accreditation of Healthcare Organizations (JCAHO) influence the hiring practices and staffing decisions made by administrators of hospitals, community mental health centers, and other settings where psychotherapy services are delivered. These administrators, confronted with fiscal limitations and budget constraints, are acutely aware that there is tremendous variation in the base salaries expected by therapists who may have different professional backgrounds but who deliver essentially comparable services.

Nearly all states classify psychotherapy as a legitimate part of medical practice without any requirement that its use be restricted to psychiatrists. However, psychiatrists now devote the majority of their time to medication management, and far fewer psychiatrists are being trained to provide psychotherapy to their patients (Luhrmann, 2000; Moran, 2009). This trend results in part from the fact that approximately half of new psychiatrists licensed in the United States are International Medical Graduates (IMGs), and these physicians are more likely to be trained in biological psychiatry. Bernard Beitman and other psychiatrists have decried the abdication of psychotherapy training by psychiatry residency programs and have developed time-limited, modular approaches to training that can be adapted to fit psychiatry residency curricula (Beitman & Yue, 1999).

In 2009, psychologists, psychiatric nurse practitioners, and social workers in all 50 states were required to be licensed or certified, and professional counselors had to be licensed or certified in almost all states. A growing number of states also require marriage/family and substance abuse counselors to be licensed or certified.

Licensing is more meaningful than certification because *licensure* restricts the practice of a profession, whereas *certification* restricts the use of a profession's name. These distinctions are difficult to apply to psychotherapy because it is virtually impossible to restrict the practice of a profession that includes such a varied range of activities. Certain professional activities may be state regulated, however. Psychological testing may be restricted to psychologists, for example, and the authority to prescribe medication may be granted only to physicians, dentists, and other health care practitioners such as advanced practice nurses, nurse practitioners, physicians' assistants, optometrists, and podiatrists. Regulatory authority is usually invested in a state board appointed by the governor and composed of professionals and members of the public. Frequently, state boards will use *reciprocity* to license professionals who hold a license to practice in other states.

It is difficult to decide who should have the right to practice psychotherapy because there are few unambiguous practice guidelines to define what is appropriate professional care for patients with mental and emotional disorders. A psychoanalyst and a behavior therapist may provide dramatically different treatment for a patient with an anxiety disorder, for example. Yet both will claim—and genuinely believe—that their mode of treatment is appropriate, and both will expect payment for their services.

PHYSICIANS, MEDICATIONS, AND PSYCHOTHERAPY

You are a psychologist practicing in a small town. You and a psychiatrist, who is also in solo practice, provide the town's only mental health services. Over the years, you have noticed that whenever one of your therapy patients needs to be evaluated for medications and you refer him or her to the psychiatrist, the patient soon stops seeing you. It's one of those small towns where there are few secrets, so you discover that the psychiatrist encourages your patients to discontinue seeing you so that they can consolidate their care and receive both medication and psychotherapy from the same person, even though many of them are subsequently treated only with medication. Rosa Gonzales, for example, had been seeing you in connection with her work-related depression. Her employer was exploitive, abusive, and disrespectful. She'd been working on developing the confidence and courage to change jobs. However, once she went to the psychiatrist for a medication consult, she stopped coming to therapy. When you happen to see her in the grocery store several months later, she looks at the floor and comments, "The medications made me feel better and the job doesn't seem so bad now." What are your reactions to your experiences with the psychiatrist? And how do you think you'd respond to your former patient's comment?

No therapist works in isolation. All therapists must cope with frequently changing rules about the allocation and delivery of clinical services. The patterns that reflect which people receive—and which people fail to receive—clinical services, in what forms, for what problems, and from whom continue to evolve. Therapists must decide how they want to respond to these shifting patterns and what role, if any, they want to play in changing them.

What are the major trends? Many studies document that treatment consisting solely of psychotherapy is becoming less common. Wang, Demler, Olfson, Pincus, Wells, and Kessler (2006), for example, found that a

mental-health-specialty-only profile, representing possible use of psychotherapy alone, had been the most popular profile in the NCS [National Comorbidity Survey] but declined significantly in the past decade. This finding is consistent with a significant decrease in psychotherapy visits during the 1990s. . . . It could reflect new restrictions on the number of psychotherapy sessions, increased patient cost sharing, and reduced provider reimbursements for psychotherapy visits imposed by many third-party payers. . . . It could also reflect changes in the popularity of therapeutic modalities, particularly patients' growing preferences for psychotropic medications. (p. 1195)

Those findings echo an earlier study by Olfson, Marcus, Druss, Elinson, Tanielian, and Pincus (2002) that found that

Significant growth occurred in the number of Americans who received treatment for depression during the past decade, and at the same time the treatments they received underwent a profound transformation. Antidepressant medications became established as a mainstay, psychotherapy sessions became less common and fewer among those receiving treatment, and physicians assumed a more prominent role. (pp. 206–207)

These data suggest that people seeking help for problems such as depression are turning more to physicians and less to psychologists. Olfson and his colleagues reported that

there was a significant increase in the proportion of patients whose treatment of depression involved visits to a physician. . . . By 1997, more than 8 (87.3%) of 10 patients who received outpatient treatment of depression were treated by a physician, compared with 68.9% in 1987. Conversely, the percentage who received treatment from psychologists declined (29.3% vs. 19.1%). Treatment of depression by social workers remained little changed and relatively uncommon. (p. 206)

Interestingly, this shift to seeking help from physicians, particularly primary care physicians, involves obtaining not only medications but also psychotherapy from those primary care physicians. Wang and his colleagues note that

The general medical-only profile experienced the largest growth over the past decade and is now the most common profile. This increased use of general medical providers without specialists may be because primary care physicians now act as "gatekeepers" for nearly one-half of patients. . . . The development and heavy promotion of new antidepressants and other psychotropic medications with improved safety profiles have further spurred care of mental disorders exclusively in general medical settings. . . . There has also been a growing tendency for some primary care physicians to deliver psychotherapies themselves. (Wang et al., 2006, p. 1194)

Although some mental health practitioners may be concerned about competition with physicians, there is a growing national trend toward collaborative practice and integrated care (Bluestein & Cubic, 2009; Ruddy, Borresen, & Gunn, 2008). This model involves co-location of mental health practitioners with physicians and nurses, joint training, and shared continuing education opportunities. The model facilitates respect between different professional groups and supports the "curbside consults" and "hallway hand-offs" that are so critical to continuity of care (Wedding & Mengel, 2004).

Several studies also suggest a shift away from longer-term psychotherapies. Olfson, Marcus, Druss, and Pincus (2002) examined changes that occurred between 1987 and 1997. In 1987, about 16% of the outpatients had more than 20 sessions of psychotherapy. Ten years later, only about 10% had more than 20 sessions. In both years, about one third of the patients reported only one or two therapy sessions. In 1987, about 48% of the therapy sessions were conducted by physicians, about 32% by psychologists, about 7% by social workers, and about 23% by others. By 1997, the percentage of physicians conducting therapy sessions had increased to about 65%, psychologist-led therapy sessions had increased to around 35%, social worker-led therapy had almost doubled to 13%, and sessions conducted by others had decreased to around 15%.

In some cases, the focus on medication may mean that patients receive little monitoring or other help of any kind. A study of 84,514 adult and pediatric patients found that "during the first 4 weeks of treatment with antidepressants, only 55.0% of the patients saw a healthcare provider for any purpose, and only 17.7% saw a provider for mental healthcare" (Stettin, Yao, Verbrugge, & Aubert, 2006, p. 453).

The increased use of medications to treat psychological disorders was one factor that led psychologists to seek prescription privileges. The issue soon erupted in controversy, with thoughtful arguments made on each side. Would prescription privileges enable psychologists to provide a more comprehensive array of clinical services to clients? Would psychologists' ability to prescribe enable them to provide services in geographic areas of critical need that lacked psychiatrists? Would psychologists betray their professional identity and values, shifting toward a medical model in which medication is often an initial intervention? If psychologists were not going to add a year or two to their doctoral training, what part of their current curriculum and training would have to be abandoned to make room for training in psychopharmacology? Those interested in reviewing the proposed standards and reading a broader and more detailed discussion of the arguments for and against psychologists' prescription privileges should review publications by the American Psychological Association (2007a), Ax, Bigelow, Harowski, Meredith, Nussbuam, and Taylor (2008), Fagan, Ax, Liss, Resnick, & Moody (2007), and Rae, Jensen-Doss, Bowden, Mendoza, and Banda (2008).

As this chapter is written, only New Mexico, Louisiana, and the U.S. Territory of Guam have laws providing limited prescription privileges to psychologists with special training, and slightly more than 1,500 psychologists have completed Level 3 Clinical Pharmacotherapy training (Ax, Fagan, & Resnick, 2009). The New Mexico law authorizing prescription privileges for psychologists is online at the New Mexico Board of Psychologist Examiners Web site (www.rld.state.nm.us/Psychology/ruleslaw.html). The Louisiana law authorizing prescription privileges for psychologists is online at the Louisiana State Board of Examiners of Psychologists Web site (www.lsbep.org). Hawaii passed legislation authorizing prescription privileges for psychologists, but the governor vetoed the bill.

EMPIRICALLY SUPPORTED THERAPIES

It is your first week as executive director of a community mental health clinic. The clinic offers individual therapy, group therapy, and family therapy, as well as a suicide hotline and a walk-in crisis clinic. At the end of the week, the Board of Directors informs you that because they want to be sure that money is spent wisely and effectively, they have adopted a new policy for you to implement: The clinic will offer only services that have been empirically supported through well-designed scientific research. If research has not demonstrated that an intervention is both safe and effective, it is prohibited. Would you agree with this policy? If required to implement it, what steps would you take?

The push to put therapy on sound scientific footing led to the concept of *empirically supported therapies* (ESTs). Proponents of ESTs believed that each form of therapy needs to be tested in carefully controlled experimental research. The results would show which therapies actually worked and which, though well intended, did nothing to help the patient or, worse, were harmful.

Eager to stop wasting money on worthless interventions, managed care companies and other third-party payment sources rushed to embrace the concept. ESTs held the promise of allowing insurance companies to restrict payments to those therapies that well-designed experiments had demonstrated to be the most effective and efficient.

The concept of empirically supported therapy, appealing to so many in theory, has turned out to be difficult and controversial to put into practice. Drew Westen and Rebekah Bradley (2005) note that

> evidence-based practice is a construct (i.e., an idea, abstraction, or theoretical entity) and thus must be operationalized (i.e., turned into some concrete form that comes to define it). The way it is operationalized is not incidental to whether its net effects turn out to be positive, negative, or mixed. (p. 226; see also Westen, Novotny, & Thompson-Brenner, 2004)

One challenge is that a therapy cannot be described simply as "effective" any more than a psychological test can be described simply as "valid" or "reliable." The validity and reliability of psychological tests do not exist in the abstract. They must be established for a specific purpose (e.g., identifying malingering), for a specific setting (e.g., forensic), and for a specific population (e.g., adults who can read and write English at a seventh-grade or more advanced level). Gordon Paul acknowledged this complexity in 1967 when many were searching for therapies that were "effective." Paul wrote that both therapists and researchers must confront the question "What treatment, by whom, is most effective for this individual with that specific problem, and under which set of circumstances?" (p. 111).

David Barlow reviewed research showing the importance of these complex sets of variables. He notes, for example, that studies show "that therapist variables such as experience contribute to successful outcome. . . . But this research on therapist variables occurs in the context of considering, first and foremost, the presenting pathology of the patient" (2004, p. 874). He concludes that

> there are three overriding principles in evaluating the robustness of [psychotherapies]. . . . First, it is important to match the psychological intervention to the psychological or physical disorder or problem. . . . Second, it is important to match the treatment to patient and therapist characteristics. . . . Finally, the evaluation of treatments must be considered in the context of the actual settings in which the treatments are provided. (p. 874)

Another challenge is that it is difficult to define with precision exactly what variables are significant in a specific situation. Imagine, for example, that a series of experiments had evaluated the effectiveness and efficiency of different treatments for a specific psychological syndrome, perhaps one of those found in DSM-IV. As Robert Sternberg points out,

> If every client was a textbook-pure case of a particular syndrome, then it might be possible to comfortably generalize the results of many and even most . . . [random assignment studies] . . . to clinical settings. [But] the degree of fidelity is, at best, variable. . . . [E]cological validity is a matter of degree, and as the universe of therapy situations to which one wishes to generalize expands, one has to be increasingly cautious in interpreting the results of RAS designs. Will the treatment work in other cultures? Will it work for people with comorbid diagnoses? Will it work for people on a particular combination of drugs? How will it work for people who are highly resistant to psychotherapy? In the end, one must ask just how general the results of any given study or set of studies can be. (2006, p. 269)

The daunting complexity of the research needed to investigate a particular psychological therapy adequately stands in stark contrast with the sheer number of available therapies. Kazdin (2008b; see also 2008a), for example, notes that there are more than 550 psychological interventions for children and adolescents but that only a relatively small minority have been subjected to research.

Trying to determine whether a set of studies can be validly generalized to other individuals, other cultures, and other situations is difficult enough, but Alan Kazdin (2006) takes the challenge to a deeper level: In light of the kinds of measures used in most therapy research, do we have logical, empirical, or other scientific proof that the individuals in the research studies themselves are being helped? A fundamental scientific and clinical question, according to Kazdin, "is whether our findings 'generalize' to patient functioning. Stated more empirically, what exactly is the evidence that EBTs [Evidence Based Therapies] help patients? I believe it is possible to delineate an EBT . . . that improves the life of no one" (p. 46). Furthermore, he says,

> In most therapy studies, measures are not linked to specific referents in everyday life and are arbitrary metrics. Fancy data transformations, creation of new metrics, and

statistical razzle-dazzle can be very useful (and worked with my dissertation committee, even if only for the first hour of my six-hour root-canal-like oral defense). However, these statistical strategies do not alter the arbitrariness of the metric, and in the case of psychotherapy research, they say little to nothing about whether patients have changed in ways that make a difference. (p. 46)

Carol Goodheart (2006) identified a challenge on yet another level:

Psychotherapy is first and foremost a human endeavor. It is messy. It is not solely a scientific endeavor, nor can it be reduced meaningfully to a technical mechanistic enterprise. . . . Psychotherapy is a fluid, mutual, interactive process. Each participant shapes and is shaped by the other. They are masters of tact and timing, of when to push and when to be patient. They know the spectrum of disruptions that can occur in a working alliance and are versatile and empathetic in their reparative responses. They are creative in finding paths to understanding, in matching an intervention to a need. (pp. 42–42)

Despite such challenges, the APA 2005 Presidential Task Force on Evidence-Based Practice reached an optimistic conclusion about evidence-based practice, defining it as

the integration of the best available research with clinical expertise in the context of patient characteristics, culture, and preferences. . . . Many strategies for working with patients have emerged and been refined through the kinds of trial and error and clinical hypothesis generation and testing that constitute the most scientific aspect of clinical practice. Yet clinical hypothesis testing has its limits, hence the need to integrate clinical expertise with the best available research.

Perhaps the central message of this task force report—and one of the most heartening aspects of the process that led to it—is the consensus achieved among a diverse group of scientists, clinicians, and scientist–clinicians from multiple perspectives that [evidence-based psychology practice] requires an appreciation of the value of multiple sources of scientific evidence. In a given clinical circumstance, psychologists of good faith and good judgment may disagree about how best to weigh different forms of evidence; over time, we presume that systematic and broad empirical inquiry—in the laboratory and in the clinic—will point the way toward best practice in integrating best evidence. What this document reflects, however, is a reassertion of what psychologists have known for a century: The scientific method is a way of thinking and observing systematically, and it is the best tool we have for learning about what works for whom. (p. 282)

Despite the widespread optimism and enthusiasm among some, controversies remain. Goodheart and Kazdin (2006), for example, in their introduction to the APA-published book *Evidence-Based Psychotherapy: Where Practice and Research Meet,* wrote:

It is not clear whether the EBP movement is good for clients. . . . There is agreement on the interest and priority of improving client care. There is disagreement on the extent to which conclusions from research ought to be applied to and constrain clinical practice and the extent to which practitioners can genuinely identify client needs and apply the best or more appropriate combination of treatments based on that evaluation. (pp. 7–8)

The debate about evidence-based practice is not limited to the mental health professions; the absence of clear guidelines characterizes much of medical practice. The United States government has attempted to deal with this lack of uniform standards by establishing the Agency for Healthcare Research and Quality (AHRQ). This agency and a number of professional organizations have developed explicit treatment guidelines for behavioral problems such as depression and anxiety, but the use of practice guidelines in mental health remains controversial. Proponents of practice guidelines argue that they bring much-needed standardization to a field that has suffered greatly from extensive but unnecessary variance in practice (largely as the result of a lack of standardized training in the mental health professions). Critics of the guidelines, on the other hand, argue that every clinical case is unique and adamantly reject any attempt to apply standardized treatment protocols, algorithms, or "cookbooks." Moreover, Terrence Shaneyfelt and Robert Centor (2009) argue that "too many current guidelines have become marketing and opinion-based pieces, delivering directive rather than assistive statements" and that "Most current articles called 'guidelines' are actually expert consensus reports" (p. 868). They wrote:

> The overreliance on expert opinion in guidelines is problematic. All guideline committees begin with implicit biases and values, which affects the recommendations they make. However, bias may occur subconsciously and, therefore, go unrecognized. Converting data into recommendations requires subjective judgments; the value structure of the panel members molds those judgments. (p. 868)

In a similar vein, John Kraemer and Laurence Gostin (2009) caution against the "politization of professional practice guidelines."

Anyone interested in reviewing the large number of existing guidelines for treating behavioral disorders should visit the *AHRQ Guideline Clearinghouse* (www.guidelines.gov).

The other chapters in this book illustrate the great diversity of approaches to psychotherapy. In light of that diversity, and the diversity of human nature itself, perhaps it should not be surprising that there is no general agreement about the definition, methodology, or value of evidence-based psychotherapy. Diverse views and a lack of general agreement among therapists about basic definitions, methodology, and the like have deep historical roots. APA president Carl Rogers set in motion an organized effort to define psychotherapy when he appointed David Shakow to chair a special committee. The APA convention of 1947 adopted the Shakow committee report, which led to the Boulder Conference in 1949. The Boulder Conference recorder summarized the result of this massive effort to define psychotherapy in a memorable passage: Psychotherapy is "an undefined technique which is applied to unspecified problems with a nonpredictable outcome. For this technique we recommend rigorous training" (Lehner, 1952, p. 547).

PHONES, COMPUTERS, AND THE INTERNET

You have established a busy practice, and you schedule eight 1-hour sessions each day. You use your computer both for billing and for record keeping, and all of your client files are maintained on your office computer. You also use e-mail extensively as a way to follow up and check on your patients. Because so much of your work depends on access to your computer, it is especially frustrating when your hard drive crashes, and you realize that you have not backed up your files in months. When you frantically call a local computer repair company, you are told that your data can probably be recovered but that a technician will need access to your computer for an entire day. You can bring your computer into the shop for repair, or the technician can visit your clinic to do the work on site. A colleague is on vacation, and you will be able to use her office to see your patients, so you tell the computer repair company to send somebody out the next day. What ethical dilemmas does this vignette present? Is it reasonable to expect a therapist to cancel eight patients in order to simply sit and watch someone work on her computer for 8 hours? Is it sufficient to simply "check in" on the technician between patients?

Scenario One

The digital age makes it possible for psychotherapy to occur without therapist and patient ever meeting face to face or even being in the same country. Consider this scenario:

Someone seeking therapy begins the search on the Internet, examining a number of therapists' Web sites. One site offers just what the prospective patient is looking for. The site provides a list of available times for initial sessions, one of which is convenient. The soon-to-be patient reads a series of passages describing the nature and ground rules of the therapy, the exceptions to confidentiality, the responsibilities of both therapist and patient, and so on. After reading each passage, the individual indicates "agree" or "disagree" as part of the informed-consent process.

Once the basics are covered, the soon-to-be patient answers a series of open-ended questions about personal history, demographics, health status, the reasons for seeking therapy, and so on. The therapist offers an initial session at half price—therapist and prospective patient will get to know a little about each other and decide whether they both want to work together. The prospective patient must pay the fee in advance, by credit card, to reserve the time for the initial session.

Therapist and patient meet on the Internet once a week for 45-minute sessions for a total of 12 weeks. They focus on the patient's depression, which they trace to the patient's unsatisfying career. They discuss the barriers—both internal and external—that have kept the patient from finding a new line of work. When the patient decides it is time to end the therapy after 3 months, the depression is no longer constant and debilitating. The patient has started to implement a plan to change careers.

Scenario Two

The therapist and patient in this scenario live more than 300 miles from each other. They communicate only by computer. The words of both therapist and patient appear on their computer monitors.

The patient in this scenario is particularly appreciative of this mode of therapy. Not only was she able to find a therapist whose skills and personal approach were what she was looking for—the kind of therapist who was simply not available in her own small, remote community—but this patient is in the advanced stages of a neuromuscular disease that makes it very difficult for her to leave home. No longer able to speak, she communicates with others via assistive technology on her computer that enables her to control the computer using a "sip and puff" switch. Her words are displayed on a monitor.

Technologies enabling therapist and client to work together without meeting each other face to face, without living in the same state or even in the same country, and without either of them leaving home have brought many benefits. Patients, especially those living in small or remote communities, are more likely to find a therapist with particular qualities, values, approaches, skills, or experience. Therapists specializing in a very rare disorder can reach patients with this disorder living across a wide range of states, provinces, and other locales. Many patients—for example, those in the final stages of terminal diseases; those whose physical conditions limit their mobility, and those with highly contagious diseases—can choose among a great variety of therapeutic approaches, even though any attempted travel outside their home is arduous, painful, risky, and perhaps impossible. Some patients whose fears, anxieties, or conditions (such as agoraphobia) might discourage them from trying more traditional modes of therapy may find that therapy by computer or telephone seems safe as an initial intervention. Therapists whose physical condition makes it impractical for them to travel to and from a job site or to spend extended time in an office can work from home, hospital, or hospice.

Scenario Three

These forms of long-distance therapy have also brought challenges and controversy. For example, imagine a scenario in which a therapist begins work traditionally, working with the client in an office setting. However, the company for which the client works transfers the client to another state. Both client and therapist believe that it would be in the client's interest to continue working with the same therapist rather than starting over in the new state with a new therapist. Therapist and client continue to work for the next 2 years, holding sessions by phone and computer. However, the client becomes profoundly depressed and confesses to the therapist that he has been sexually abusing children in his new neighborhood. Then the client becomes acutely suicidal and takes his life. The client's family subsequently sues the therapist for malpractice.

During the extended litigation, a number of issues arise:

- Was the therapist practicing without a license in the state to which the client had moved? If a therapist and patient are in different jurisdictions during therapy sessions, must the therapist maintain appropriate licensing status in both jurisdictions? If a therapist lives in Missouri and is licensed only in Missouri, what authority, if any, does the state licensing board in Missouri have over the therapist's work via telephone or Internet with a client living in Illinois? What authority, if any, does the licensing board in Illinois have to regulate the work of the therapist who lives in Missouri? Does it make any difference if the patient and therapist live only minutes apart, but on different sides of the Mississippi river?

- What are the standards of care regarding basic competence when therapy is conducted by telephone or Internet? What education, training, or supervised experience in telephone therapy or Internet therapy establishes that therapists are not working outside their areas of competence?

- Do the laws regarding privacy, confidentiality, privilege, mandatory reporting (of child abuse or elder abuse, for example), and duty to protect third parties that prevail in the state where the therapist lives apply, or do such laws of the state in which the client lives apply, or do both sets of laws apply? What happens if the laws in the therapist's state conflict with the laws in the client's state? For example, what if the laws in one state require that certain information be kept confidential, whereas the laws of the other state require that the information be reported?

- What information about telephone therapy or Internet therapy must a therapist be sure that a client understands and consents to as part of the process of informed consent and informed refusal?

- Under what conditions is telephone therapy or Internet therapy covered—or not covered—under different professional liability policies?

One useful source of guidance in considering these issues is Gerry Koocher and Elizabeth Morray's (2000) article "Regulation of Telepsychology: A Survey of State Attorneys General." In closing their review, Koocher and Morray offer seven maxims:

1. Before engaging in the remote delivery of mental health services via electronic means, practitioners should carefully assess their competence to offer the particular services and should consider the limitations of efficacy and effectiveness that may be a function of remote delivery.

2. Practitioners should consult with their professional liability insurance carrier to ascertain whether the planned services will be covered. Ideally, a written confirmation from a representative of the carrier should be obtained.

3. Practitioners are advised to seek consultation from colleagues and to provide all clients with clear, written guidelines regarding planned emergency practices (e.g., suicide risk situations).

4. Because no uniform standards of practice exist at this time, thoughtful written plans that reflect careful consultation with colleagues may suffice to document thoughtful professionalism in the event of an adverse incident.

5. A careful statement on limitations of confidentiality should be developed and provided to clients at the start of the professional relationship. The statement should inform clients of the standard limitations on confidentiality (e.g., child abuse reporting mandates), any state-specific requirements, and cautions about privacy problems with broadcast conversations (e.g., overheard wireless phone conversations or captured Internet transmissions).

6. Clinicians should thoroughly inform clients of what they can expect in terms of services offered, unavailable services (e.g., emergency or psychopharmacology coverage), access to the practitioner, emergency coverage, and similar issues.

7. If third parties are billed for services offered via electronic means, practitioners must clearly indicate that fact on billing forms. If a third-party payer who is unsupportive of electronic service delivery is wrongly led to believe that the services took place in person rather than online, fraud charges may ultimately be filed.

Formal guidelines relevant to therapy provided by telephone or Internet, as well as discussion of the other topics included in this chapter, can be found on the Web page *Ethics Codes & Practice Guidelines for Assessment, Therapy, Counseling, & Forensic Practice* (http://kspope.com/ethcodes/index.php), which provides links to more than 100 formal sets of guidelines and codes, including the National Board for Certified Counselors' "The Practice of Internet Counseling" and the APA's "American Psychological Association: Statement on Services by Telephone, Teleconferencing, & Internet."

The continuing evolution of the digital revolution has great potential for transforming the relationship between clinicians and patients. In "Take Two Aspirin and Tweet Me in the Morning: How Twitter, Facebook, and Other Social Media Are Reshaping Health Care," Carleen Hawn (2009) describes the ways in which "new media tools like weblogs, instant messaging platforms, video chat, and social networks are reengineering the way doctors and patients interact" (p. 361).

Digital technology has created changes and challenges for therapists in another area of practice: the storage and transmission of records. Even though the widely hailed "paperless office" has not come to pass for most therapists, many therapists use computers to handle clinical data. Some may use computers to administer, score, or interpret psychological tests and other assessment instruments. Many use computers for recording information about their clients and notes on psychotherapy sessions. Spreadsheets and specialized software handle billing, track accounts receivable, and provide documentation to insurance companies and other third-party payment sources.

How can therapists make sure that this confidential information is restricted to those authorized to see it? It may seem a reasonably easy challenge, but therapists and patients have been stunned by instances in which supposedly secure information fell into the wrong hands. Here are some of the things that can happen:

• A desktop or laptop computer containing confidential patient information is stolen from an office.

• A car is vandalized, and a laptop stored in the trunk is stolen.

• Someone hacks into a computer that is connected to the Internet and steals the information stored on the computer's hard drive.

- A virus, worm, Trojan, or other malware infects a computer and sends confidential files to a hacker, uploads confidential files to a Web site where anyone can read them, and sends confidential files to everyone listed in the computer's address book. This includes all the Internet discussion groups to which the therapist belongs and all addresses in the computer's memory.

- A hacker makes subtle and undetected changes in a therapist's files (such as adding numbers randomly to billing records or changing the dates in the records of therapy sessions).

- Someone sits down at an unattended computer that is not password-protected or whose password is easy to find (in the desk drawer, under the keyboard, or on a Post-it note nearby) or easy to guess (the person's name, the word "password") and reads, downloads, or transmits confidential data to unauthorized sources.

- Someone reads a monitor—and obtains confidential information—by standing near the monitor or sitting next to a laptop user in an airport, on a flight, or in some other public setting.

- A therapist and client discuss extremely sensitive information, unaware that because one of them is using a cordless phone, the conversation can be overheard by someone using a cordless phone close by.

- A therapist e-mails a message containing confidential information to a colleague who is authorized to have it, but accidentally uses the wrong e-mail address.

- A therapist e-mails a message containing confidential information to a colleague who is authorized to have it, but the recipient shares his or her computer with someone else who opens the e-mail message.

- A therapist faxes confidential information, but the recipient's fax machine is shared with others.

- A therapist keeps clinical and financial records on a computer, unaware that spyware has been installed on the computer.

- A therapist faxes confidential information but, by mistake, punches in the wrong fax number.

- A therapist sells a computer, forgetting that confidential information, thought "erased" from the hard drive, is still recoverable because a more thorough form of "scrubbing" the hard drive was not used.

Computers and other electronic devices for storing information and communicating with others offer obvious benefits. However, the mental health community has been slow to recognize their potential pitfalls and the need for creativity and care in their use. Therapists have extensive education, training, and supervised experience in working with people. For most of us in this field, however, working with computers and other digital devices is not our strong suit. When we use digital devices to handle the most sensitive and private information about our clients, we must remember to live up to an ancient precept: First, do no harm.

Therapists—and all students learning to be therapists—should also realize that most clients will "Google" their therapist's name either before or immediately after the first session. This can be particularly problematic when a therapist's Facebook page or a similar social networking site (e.g., a dating service) contains highly personal information that one would not want to have shared with one's clients. Admissions committees for professional training programs are currently grappling with the issue of whether or not highly personal information (e.g., nude photos) obtained from an Internet search is appropriate data to be shared with other members of the committee and used in making decisions about admission to professional training programs.

THERAPISTS' SEXUAL INVOLVEMENT WITH PATIENTS, NONSEXUAL PHYSICAL TOUCH, AND SEXUAL FEELINGS

You are a therapist in a hospital and mental health center seeing your last client of the day. She is dressed in a short skirt and t-shirt, and she has for several sessions hinted at some secret that she is too embarrassed to talk about. You find her very attractive and enjoy spending time with her. She begins by saying that she had an intense dream that may have given her the courage to work on her secret in therapy. She tells you the dream in detail. It is an erotic dream, and you find yourself becoming intensely aroused. She says that all the graphic sexual activity in the dream is related to her secret, which is that she has always been ashamed that her breasts were so small and that she had wanted to ask you if you thought so. She immediately pulls her t-shirt off. What do you think you would do if you were this therapist? What, if anything, would you tell your supervisor about it? What, if anything, would you write in the client's chart? If you imagine the same scenario adapted to a male patient who is concerned about the size of his penis and suddenly pulls down his pants, are your responses to these questions different in any way?

Sex is the focus of one of the most ancient rules of working with patients, is a cause of discomfort and confusion for many therapists, and is a contemporary challenge for the profession.

Therapist–Patient Sexual Involvement

No circumstances or rationale justify sexual involvement with a patient. This basic rule has ancient roots. Annette Brodsky's (1989) research led to her discovery that the prohibition is older than the Hippocratic Oath, which included it. In fact, she found that this prohibition was set forth centuries earlier in the Nigerian Code of the Healing Arts.

The prohibition continues to be fundamental to the profession for many reasons, including the issue of harm to patients. In the landmark 1976 case of *Roy v. Hartogs*, for example, New York Supreme Court Presiding Justice Markowitz wrote, "Thus from [Freud] to the modern practitioner we have common agreement of the harmful effects of sensual intimacies between patient and therapist" (*Roy v. Hartogs*, 1976, p. 590).

Studies of the effects of therapist–patient sexual involvement have looked at both patients who never returned to therapy and those who worked with a subsequent therapist; have compared those who engaged in sex with a therapist with matched groups of those who engaged in sex with a nontherapist physician and of those who did not engage in sex with a health care professional; and have evaluated the effects of sexual involvement between patients and therapists using an array of measures including standardized psychological tests, clinical interview by subsequent therapists and by independent clinicians, behavioral observation, and self-report (Pope, 1994). Reading first-person accounts of therapist–patient sexual involvement—its course of development and its aftermath—can deepen the understanding provided by research-based findings. Client accounts include those by Bates and Brodsky (1989), Freeman and Roy (1976), Noel and Waterson (1992), Plaisil (1985), and Walker and Young (1986).

The effects of therapist–patient sexual involvement on clients often seem to cluster into 10 very general areas: (1) ambivalence, (2) guilt, (3) emptiness and isolation, (4) sexual confusion, (5) impaired ability to trust, (6) confused roles and boundaries, (7) emotional liability, (8) suppressed rage, (9) increased suicidal risk, and (10) cognitive dysfunction, frequently in the areas of concentration and memory and often involving flashbacks, intrusive thoughts, unbidden images, and nightmares (Pope, 1988, 1994; Pope & Vasquez, 2007).

In light of the harm associated with sexual boundary violations, almost half the states have determined that the civil legislation and case law prohibiting sex with patients were insufficient and have added criminal penalties that can be applied in some situations.

Despite the harm that therapist–patient sexual involvement can cause to patients, despite the longstanding professional prohibition, and despite civil and even criminal penalties, a small minority of therapists sexually exploit their patients. A study of the combined data from the first eight national, anonymous self-report surveys that appeared in peer-reviewed journals found that 4.4% of the 5,148 therapists surveyed reported having engaged in sex with at least one patient (Pope & Vasquez, 2007).

Statistical analysis found no significant differences among the three professions surveyed in these studies: Social workers, psychiatrists, and psychologists report becoming sexually involved with their patients at roughly the same rates.

These studies do, however, reveal significant gender differences. Male therapists reported engaging in sex with their patients at much higher rates (6.8%) than did female therapists (1.6%). By far the most common pairing is a male therapist with a female patient, accounting for about 88–95% of the instances of therapist–patient sex in large-scale peer-reviewed studies that report gender data.

Gender is a significant factor in a variety of other sexual dual or multiple relationships and boundary issues (e.g., supervisor–supervisee, professor–student)—even when the base rates of gender in each role are taken into account—and in other nonsexual dual or multiple relationship situations. An early national study of sex between therapists and patients, supervisors and supervisees, and professors and their students noted that

> When sexual contact occurs in the context of psychology training or psychotherapy, the predominant pattern is quite clear and simple: An older higher status man becomes sexually active with a younger, subordinate woman. In each of the higher status professional roles (teacher, supervisor, administrator, therapist), a much higher percentage of men than women engage in sex with those students or clients for whom they have assumed professional responsibility. In the lower status role of student, a far greater proportion of women than men are sexually active with their teachers, administrators, and clinical supervisors. (Pope, Levenson, & Schover, 1979, p. 687; see also Pope, 1994 Pope & Vasquez, 2007)

Therapists usually become sexually involved with their patients through a variety of common scenarios. Pope and Bouhoutsos (1986, p. 4) presented 10 of the scenarios that seem to occur most often (see Table 15.1).

Nonsexual Physical Touch

It is important to distinguish therapist–patient sexual involvement from two very different phenomena. First, nonsexual physical touch is clearly different from sexual involvement. Pope, Sonne, and Holroyd (1993) documented the ways in which nonsexual physical touch within therapy had acquired a "guilt by association" with sexual touch. Their review of the research and other professional literature found no harm from nonsexual touch per se, although context, culture, and meaning should always be considered before touching a patient. When consistent with the patient's clinical needs and the therapist's approach, nonsexual touch can be comforting, reassuring, grounding, caring, and an important part of the healing process. When discordant with clinical needs, context, competence, or consent, even the most well-intentioned nonsexual

TABLE 16.1   **Ten Common Scenarios**

Scenario	Description
Role Trading	Therapist becomes the "patient" and the wants and needs of the therapist become the focus
Sex Therapy	Therapist fraudulently presents therapist–patient sex as valid treatment for sexual or related difficulties
As If . . .	Therapist treats positive transference as if it were not the result of the therapeutic situation
Svengali	Therapist creates and exploits the dependence of the patient
Drugs	Therapist uses cocaine, alcohol, or other drugs as part of the seduction
Rape	Therapist uses physical force, threats, and/or intimidation
True Love	Therapist uses rationalizations that attempt to discount the clinical/professional nature of the professional relationship and its duties
It Just Got Out of Hand	Therapist fails to treat the emotional closeness that develops in therapy with sufficient attention, care, and respect
Time Out	Therapist fails to acknowledge and take account of the fact that the therapeutic relationship does not cease to exist between scheduled sessions or outside the therapist's office
Hold Me	Therapist exploits patient's desire for nonerotic physical contact and [patient's] possible confusion between erotic and nonerotic contact

physical contact may be experienced as aggressive, frightening, intimidating, demeaning, arrogant, unwanted, insensitive, threatening, or intrusive.

Sexual Attraction to Patients

Like nonsexual touch, sexual feelings about patients seem to have acquired a guilt by association with therapist–patient sex. National studies indicate that *simply experiencing sexual attraction to a client*—without acting on it and without necessarily even feeling tempted to act on it—makes a majority of both social workers and psychologists feel guilty, anxious, and confused (see Pope & Vasquez, 2007). Although a large majority of therapists report feeling sexually attracted to one or more clients, and most also report discomfort with the feelings, these studies also suggest that adequate training in this area is relatively rare. A majority reported no training in the area, and only around 10% of social workers and psychologists reported adequate training in their graduate programs and internships. Gerry Koocher, the 2006 president of the American Psychological Association, asked, "How can the extant population of psychotherapists be expected to adequately address [these issues] if we pay so little attention to training in these matters?" (1994, p. viii).

Pope, Sonne, and Greene (2006) discuss the seemingly taboo nature of sexual feelings about clients as reflecting one of several basic myths about therapists that interfere with training and effective therapy. The myth is

that *good* therapists (those who don't sexually exploit their patients) never have sexual feelings about their patients, don't become sexually aroused during therapy sessions, don't vicariously enjoy the (sometimes) guilty pleasures of their patients' sexual experiences, don't have sexual fantasies or dreams about their patients. (p. 28)

Because of the widespread discomfort with sexual feelings about clients and the inadequacy of training in this area, it is not surprising that many professional books do not focus on this topic.

In light of the multitude of books in the areas of human sexuality, sexual dynamics, sex therapies, unethical therapist–patient sexual contact, management of the therapist's or patient's sexual behaviors, and so on, it is curious that sexual attraction to patients per se has not served as the primary focus of a wide range of texts. The professor, supervisor, or librarian seeking books that turn their *primary* attention to exploring the therapist's *feelings* in this regard would be hard pressed to assemble a selection from which to choose an appropriate course text. If someone unfamiliar with psychotherapy were to judge the prevalence and significance of therapists' sexual feelings on the basis of the books that focus exclusively on that topic, he or she might conclude that the phenomenon is neither widespread nor important. (Pope, Sonne, & Holroyd, 1993, p. 23)

There may be a circular process at work here: The discomfort about sexual feelings may have fostered a relative absence of books and a lack of adequate training in this area. The relative dearth of books and training may have, in turn, led to further discomfort with the topic.

NONSEXUAL MULTIPLE RELATIONSHIPS AND BOUNDARY ISSUES

You are a social worker providing weekly psychotherapy sessions to an extremely rich and successful CEO, Ms. Chin. Your client is struggling with how to implement her decision to acquire a medium-sized company. When she makes the public announcement that she is buying the company, should she immediately announce the planned lay-offs at the new company or should she take time to try to cushion the blow? It is about this time that you decide to buy some stock in her company. Ms. Chin is so appreciative of your help in sorting through her difficult issues that she asks you if you will attend a special event at her home, a celebration of her installation as the new president of the company. You accept the invitation and, during the all-day celebration, wind up playing tennis with her and some of her friends in the business community, leading to new referrals to your practice and to a weekly tennis game on the courts of her estate. As your practice and the value of your stock holdings grow, you reflect on your choices. Your buying the stock harmed no one, did not disclose confidential information, was not based on illegally obtained information, and, as you think about it, was something you had planned to do all along, even before you heard that Ms. Chen's investment group would be buying a new company. Your weekly visits to Ms. Chen's estate allow you to see her in another setting and interacting with other people—and this provides invaluable information that helps you understand and treat your client. The visits enable you to bond with your client more deeply and in more varied ways, strengthening your working relationship with her and giving you a better basis for your therapy. It is all very proper, and everyone benefits. As you imagine yourself as the therapist in this vignette, do you have any second thoughts?

Sound judgments about nonsexual boundaries always depend on context.

Nonsexual boundary crossings can enrich therapy, serve the treatment plan, and strengthen the therapist–client working relationship. They can also undermine the therapy, sever the therapist–patient alliance, and cause immediate or long-term harm to the client. Choices about whether to cross a boundary confront us daily, are often subtle and complex, and can sometimes influence whether therapy progresses, stalls, or ends. (Pope & Keith-Spiegel, 2008, p. 638)

In the 1980s and the early and mid-1990s, the full, often daunting complexity of boundary issues made itself known to the profession through clinical experimentation, research, articles challenging virtually every aspect of the status quo, and open discussion from diverse points of view. A vigorous, wide-ranging, and healthy controversy over therapists' nonsexual multiple relationships and other boundary excursions blossomed. Was it good practice for a therapist to enter into dual professional roles with a client, serving both as a client's therapist and as that client's employer? What about multiple social roles? Is it helpful, hurtful, or completely irrelevant for a therapist to provide therapy to a close friend, spouse, or stepchild? Are there any potential benefits or risks to social outings with a client (meeting for dinner, going to a movie, playing golf, or heading off for a weekend of sightseeing), so long as there is no sexual or romantic involvement? Are financial relationships (say, the therapist borrowing a large sum from a client to buy a new house or car, or inviting a client to invest in the therapist's new business venture) compatible with the therapeutic relationship? What about lending a client money to help pay the rent or buy food and medications, or driving a patient home after a session because she doesn't have a car and can't afford cab fare? Under what circumstances should a therapist accept bartered services or products as payment for therapy sessions?

The 15 years or so from the early 1980s to the mid-1990s saw these and other questions about multiple relationships and boundaries discussed—and often argued—from virtually every point of view, every discipline, and every theoretical orientation. In 1981, for example, Samuel Roll and Leverett Millen presented "A Guide to Violating an Injunction in Psychotherapy: On Seeing Acquaintances as Patients." In her 1988 article on "Dual Role Relationships," ethicist Karen Kitchener provided systematic guidance to readers on the kinds of "counselor–client relationships that are likely to lead to harm and those that are not likely to be harmful" (p. 217). According to Kitchener, the kinds of dual relationships that were most likely to be problematic were those in which there were "(1) incompatibility of expectations between roles; (2) diverging obligations associated with different roles, which increases the potential for loss of objectivity; and (3) increased power and prestige between professionals and consumers, which increases the potential for exploitation" (p. 217). Similarly, in the 1985 edition of their widely used textbook *Ethics in Psychology: Professional Standards and Cases,* Patricia Keith-Spiegel and Gerald Koocher discussed ways in which boundary crossings may be unavoidable in good clinical practice and presented ways to think through the ethical implications of specific dual relationships or other boundary issues. Patrusksa Clarkson, who wrote "In Recognition of Dual Relationships," discussed the "mythical, single relationship" and wrote that "it is impossible for most psychotherapists to avoid all situations in which conflicting interests or multiple roles might exist"(1994, p. 32).

Vincent Rinella and Alvin Gerstein argued that "the underlying moral and ethical rationale for prohibiting dual relationships (DRs) is no longer tenable" (1994, p. 225). Similarly, Robert Ryder and Jeri Hepworth (1990) set forth thoughtful arguments that the AAMFT ethics code should not prohibit dual relationships. Jeanne Adleman and Susan Barrett (1990) took a fresh and creative look, from a feminist perspective, at how to make careful decisions about dual relationships and boundary issues. Laura Brown (1989; see also 1994) examined the implications of boundary decisions from another perspective in "Beyond Thou Shalt Not: Thinking about Ethics in the Lesbian Therapy Community." Ellen Bader (1994) urged that the focus on the duality of roles be replaced by an examination of whether each instance did or did not involve exploitation.

Elisabeth Horst (1989) and Amy Stockman (1990) were among those who explored issues of dual relationships and boundaries in rural settings. Melanie Geyer (1994) examined some of the decision-making principles that had evolved for evaluating multiple relationships and boundary issues in rural settings and adapted them for some of the unique challenges faced by Christian counselors (and counselors for whom other religious faiths are a focus of practice). *Ethics & Behavior* was one of many journals in the 1980s and early 1990s that spotlighted the richness of creative thinking in this area. In 1994, it published a special section in which nine prominent authorities debated sharp disagreements about the issue of boundaries in therapy and explored their contrasting approaches.

The care with which these diverse articles and books in the 1980s and first half of the 1990s examined a diverse array of contextual issues such as the nature of the community (e.g., rural or small town) and the therapist's theoretical orientation, in thinking through whether a specific multiple relationship or boundary crossing was likely to be healing or hurtful, helped develop a more complex appreciation for both the potential benefits and the risks in this area. In 1989, a survey (return rate = 49%) of 1,600 psychiatrists, 1,600 psychologists, and 1,600 social workers found that therapists' behaviors and beliefs about a wide range of dual relationships and other boundary issues tended to be significantly associated with factors such as

1. Therapist's gender
2. Therapist's profession (psychiatrist, psychologist, social worker)
3. Therapist's age
4. Therapist's experience
5. Therapist's marital status
6. Therapist's region of residence
7. Client's gender
8. Practice setting (such as solo or group private practice or outpatient clinic)
9. Practice locale (size of the community)
10. Therapist's theoretical orientation (Borys & Pope, 1989; see also Baer & Murdock, 1995; Gutheil & Brodsky, 2008; Lamb & Catanzaro, 1998; Lamb, Catanzaro, & Moorman, 2004)

Research Leading to a Call for a Change in the APA Ethics Code

The first ethics code of the American Psychological Association was empirically based. APA members responded to a survey asking them what ethical dilemmas they encountered in their day-to-day work. A replication of that survey, performed 50 years after the original, led to a call for a change in the APA ethics code regarding dual relationships.

The second most often reported ethical dilemma that psychologists reported was in the area of blurred, dual, or conflictual relationships. These responses from such a wide range of psychologists led the investigators, Pope and Vetter (1992), to include in their report a call for changes to the APA ethics code in the areas of dual relationships, multiple relationships, and boundary issues so that the ethics code would, for example,

1. define dual relationships more carefully and specify clearly conditions under which they might be therapeutically indicated or acceptable;
2. address clearly and realistically the situations of those who practice in small towns, rural communities, remote locales, and similar contexts (emphasizing that neither

the current code in place at the time nor the draft revision under consideration at that time fully acknowledged or adequately addressed such contexts); and

3.   distinguish between dual relationships and accidental or incidental extratherapeutic contacts (e.g., running into a patient at the grocery market or unexpectedly seeing a client at a party) . . . [in order] to address realistically the awkward entanglements into which even the most careful therapist can fall.

The following section from the *American Psychologist* report of the study presents the relevant findings, examples, specific suggestions for changes, and reasoning.

Blurred, Dual, or Conflictual Relationships

The second most frequently described incidents involved maintaining clear, reasonable, and therapeutic boundaries around the professional relationship with a client. In some cases, respondents were troubled by such instances as serving as both "therapist and supervisor for hours for [patient/supervisee's] MFCC [marriage, family, and child counselor] license" or when "an agency hires one of its own clients." In other cases, respondents found dual relationships to be useful "to provide role modeling, nurturing and a giving quality to therapy"; one respondent, for example, believed that providing therapy to couples with whom he has social relationships and who are members of his small church makes sense because he is "able to see how these people interact in group context." In still other cases, respondents reported that it was sometimes difficult to know what constitutes a dual relationship or conflict of interest; for example, "I have employees/supervisees who were former clients and wonder if this is a dual relationship." Similarly, another respondent felt a conflict between his own romantic attraction to a patient's mother and responsibilities to the child who had developed a positive relationship with him:

> I was conducting therapy with a child and soon became aware that there was a mutual attraction between myself and the child's mother. The strategies I had used and my rapport with the child had been positive. Nonetheless, I felt it necessary to refer to avoid a dual relationship (at the cost of the gains that had been made).

Taken as a whole, the incidents suggest, first, that the ethical principles need to define dual relationships more carefully and to note with clarity if and when they are ever therapeutically indicated or acceptable. For example, a statement such as "Minimal or remote relationships are unlikely to violate this standard" ("Draft," 1991, p. 32) may be too vague and ambiguous to be helpful. A psychologist's relationship to a very casual acquaintance whom she or he meets for lunch a few times a year, to an accountant who only does very routine work in filling out her or his tax forms once a year (all such business being conducted by mail), to her or his employer's husband (who has no involvement in the business and with whom the psychologist never socializes), and to a travel agent (who books perhaps one or two flights a year for the psychologist) may constitute relatively minimal or remote relationships. However, will a formal code's assurance that minimal or remote relationships are unlikely to violate the standard provide a clear, practical, valid, and useful basis for ethical deliberation to the psychologist who serves as therapist to all four individuals? Research and the professional literature focusing on nonsexual dual relationships underscores the importance and implications of decisions to enter into or refrain from such activities (e.g., Borys & Pope, 1989; Ethics Committee, 1988; Keith-Spiegel & Koocher, 1985; Pope & Vasquez, 2007; Stromberg et al., 1988).

Second, the principles must address clearly and realistically the situations of those who practice in small towns, rural communities, and other remote locales. Neither the current code nor the current draft revision explicitly acknowledges and adequately addresses such geographic contexts. Forty-one of the dual relationship incidents involved such locales. Many respondents implicitly or explicitly complained that the principles seem to ignore the special conditions in small, self-contained communities. For example,

> I live and maintain a . . . private practice in a rural area. I am also a member of a spiritual community based here. There are very few other therapists in the immediate vicinity who work with transformational, holistic, and feminist principles in the context of good clinical training that "conventional" people can also feel confidence in. Clients often come to me because they know me already, because they are not satisfied with the other services available, or because they want to work with someone who understands their spiritual practice and can incorporate its principles and practices into the process of transformation, healing, and change. The stricture against dual relationships helps me to maintain a high degree of sensitivity to the ethics (and potentials for abuse or confusion) of such situations, but doesn't give me any help in working with the actual circumstances of my practice. I hope revised principles will address these concerns!

Third, the principles need to distinguish between dual relationships and accidental or incidental extratherapeutic contacts (e.g., running into a patient at the grocery market or unexpectedly seeing a client at a party) and to address realistically the awkward entanglements into which even the most careful therapist can fall. For example, a therapist sought to file a formal complaint against some very noisy tenants of a neighboring house. When he did so, he was surprised to discover "that his patient was the owner–landlord." As another example, a respondent reported,

> Six months ago a patient I had been working with for 3 years became romantically involved with my best and longest friend. I could write no less than a book on the complications of this fact! I have been getting legal and therapeutic consultations all along, and continue to do so. Currently they are living together and I referred the patient (who was furious that I did this and felt abandoned). I worked with the other psychologist for several months to provide a bridge for the patient. I told my friend soon after I found out that I would have to suspend our contact. I'm currently trying to figure out if we can ever resume our friendship and under what conditions.

The latter example is one of many that demonstrate the extreme lengths to which most psychologists are willing to go to ensure the welfare of their patients. Although it is impossible to anticipate every pattern of multiple relationship or to account for all the vicissitudes and complexities of life, psychologists need and deserve formal principles that provide lucid, useful, and practical guidance as an aid to professional judgment. (Pope & Vetter, 1992, pp. 400–401)

It is worth emphasizing that the complexity of both therapy itself and specifically of boundary issues can never obscure, erode, or minimize the clinician's inescapable responsibility to maintain boundaries that protect and serve the patient's safety and the goals of therapy. Robert Simon and Daniel Shuman (2007) wrote:

It is always the therapist's responsibility to maintain appropriate boundaries, no matter how difficult or boundary testing the patient may be. . . . The conduct of psychotherapy is an impossible task because there are no perfect therapists and no perfect therapies. Knowing one's boundaries, however, makes the impossible task easier. (p. 212; see also Appelbaum & Gutheil, 2007; Gutheil & Brodsky, 2008)

Some Helpful Guidelines

The topic of multiple relationships and boundary issues is complex and rich with multiple points of view from diverse perspectives. Fortunately for therapists and counselors, there is no shortage of well-informed, thoughtful, practical guides to this area. For those in search of decision-making help as they think through the various issues, here are six highly respected and widely used sets of guidelines:

1. Gottlieb's 1993 guide in "Avoiding Exploitive Dual Relationships: A Decision-Making Model" (*Note:* This set of guidelines is on the Web at http://kspope.com/dual/index.php.)

2. Faulkner and Faulkner's 1997 guide for practice in rural settings in "Managing multiple relationships in rural communities: Neutrality and boundary violations"

3. Lamb and Catanzaro's 1998 model in "Sexual and Nonsexual Boundary Violations Involving Psychologists, Clients, Supervisees, and Students: Implications for Professional Practice"

4. Younggren's 2002 model in "Ethical Decision-Making and Dual Relationships" (*Note:* This set of guidelines is on the web at http://kspope.com/dual/index.php; see also Younggren & Gottlieb, 2004.)

5. Campbell and Gordon's 2003 five-step approach for considering multiple relationships in rural communities in "Acknowledging the Inevitable: Understanding Multiple Relationships in Rural Practice"

6. Sonne's 2006 "Nonsexual Multiple Relationships: A Practical Decision-Making Model for Clinicians" (*Note:* This set of guidelines is on the web at http://kspope.com/dual/index.php.)

For those seeking guidance in internship settings, Burian and Slimp (2000) wrote a helpful article titled "Social Dual-Role Relationships during Internship: A Decision-making Model" (see also Slimp & Burian, 1994).

Finally, published articles, standards, research studies, some of the widely used guides mentioned above, and other resources in the area of multiple relationships and other boundary issues are online at http://kspope.com/dual/index.php.

On Not Overlooking How Difficult This Topic Tends to Be for Us

In closing this section, it's worth noting what a vexing challenge this area is for mental health practitioners. Part of the problem is the difficulty of psychotherapy itself. We can never go on automatic pilot, never let the formal standards and guidelines do our thinking for us, and never let the general principles obscure the uniqueness of every therapeutic encounter.

Awareness of the ethics codes is crucial to competence in the area of ethics, but the formal standards are not a substitute for an active, deliberative, and creative approach to fulfilling our ethical responsibilities. They prompt, guide, and inform our ethical consideration; they do not preclude or serve as a substitute for it. There is no way that the codes and principles can be effectively followed or applied in a rote, thoughtless manner. Each new client, whatever his or her similarities to previous clients, is a unique individual. Each situation also is unique and is likely to change significantly over time. The explicit codes and principles may designate many possible approaches as clearly unethical. They may identify with greater or lesser degrees of clarity the types of ethical concerns that are likely to be especially significant, but they cannot tell us how these concerns will manifest themselves in a particular clinical situation. They may set forth essential tasks that we must fulfill, but they cannot tell us how we can accomplish these tasks with a unique client facing unique problems. . . . There is no legitimate way to avoid these struggles. (Pope & Vasquez, 1998)

But another part of the difficulty is the topic itself, how often we jump to conclusions, rely on stereotypes, or fail to consider carefully what is actually occurring rather than what seems to be happening. Former APA president Gerry Koocher (2006) provides a vivid example of how others tend to react when he tells them about crossing time boundaries (i.e., letting a session run far beyond its schedule), financial boundaries (i.e., not charging), and other boundaries with one of his clients.

On occasion I tell my students and professional audiences that I once spent an entire psychotherapy session holding hands with a 26-year-old woman together in a quiet darkened room. That disclosure usually elicits more than a few gasps and grimaces. When I add that I could not bring myself to end the session after 50 minutes and stayed with the young woman holding hands for another half hour, and when I add the fact that I never billed for the extra time, eyes roll.

Then, I explain that the young woman had cystic fibrosis with severe pulmonary disease and panic-inducing air hunger. She had to struggle through three breaths on an oxygen line before she could speak a sentence. I had come into her room, sat down by her bedside, and asked how I might help her. She grabbed my hand and said, "Don't let go." When the time came for another appointment, I called a nurse to take my place. By this point in my story most listeners, who had felt critical of or offended by the "hand holding," have moved from an assumption of sexualized impropriety to one of empathy and compassion. The real message of the anecdote, however, lies in the fact that I never learned this behavior in a classroom. No description of such an intervention exists in any treatment manual or tome on empirically based psychotherapy. (p. xxii)

Setting appropriate boundaries and limits presents vexing dilemmas for all therapists. Consider the following situations and discuss how you would respond:

- Several of your clients ask to follow you on Twitter and to be listed as a friend on Facebook.

- A longtime client dies, and her sister asks you to say a few words at your client's funeral.

- Your client, a travel agent, offers you a free upgrade to first class when you are only paying for an economy-class seat.

(continued)

(continued)

- A patient you have seen for many years commits suicide, and the patient's sister—a trial attorney who has been paying the bills for therapy for many years—asks to have a private session to "get closure on David's death."

- A client reveals that she is in fact "Maria," a woman you have been flirting with on an Internet dating site for the past 2 months.

- A state trooper—who also happens to be one of your clients—stops you for speeding, but tells you he is only going to give you a warning ticket because you've helped him so much in therapy.

ACCESSIBILITY AND PEOPLE WITH DISABILITIES

You are a therapist with a thriving practice in a large city. You see clients in a large suite atop a high-rise office building, with a magnificent view of the city. There is a new client who will be showing up that evening for an initial session. The office building closes and locks its doors at 5 p.m. each day, but both heating in winter and air conditioning in summer remain on until 10 p.m., and at the top of the front steps is a call-box system allowing people outside to call the phone in any of the offices to ask to be buzzed in. The new client never shows up at your office. It is only the next day that you learn that the client is blind. Finding the front door locked, he was unable to locate a way to enter the building. There were no instructions in Braille or any other indications of how to gain access to the building that would be perceived by someone who was blind or had any form of severely impaired vision. As you consider this situation, the phone rings. It is someone whose initial appointment is scheduled to begin 5 minutes from now. She is calling with her cell phone. She is outside your building but does not know how to enter. She uses a wheelchair for mobility and is unable to use the front steps that lead up to your building's front door. What are your feelings as you imagine yourself the therapist in this vignette? What do you think you would say to these two people? What, if anything, do you wish you had done differently?

This vignette illustrates two of the many ways in which psychotherapists and their offices may be blocked off from people with disabilities. These physical barriers may shut out many people. Psychologist Martha Banks noted that

> Approximately one-fifth of U.S. citizens have disabilities. The percentage is slightly higher among women and girls (21.3%) than among men and boys (19.8%). Among women, Native American women and African American women have the highest percentages of disabilities. . . . As a result of limited access to funds, more than one-third of women with work disabilities and more than 40% of those with severe work disabilities are living in poverty . . . (2003, p. xxiii)

Individual therapists and the profession as a whole face the challenge of identifying the barriers that screen out people with disabilities or that make it unnecessarily difficult for them to become therapists or to find appropriate therapeutic services. Think back to the classrooms, lecture halls, and therapy offices you have seen. Would a person using a wheelchair or walker find reasonable access to those places? Would a person who is blind or has severe visual impairment experience unnecessary hardships in navigating those buildings? For additional information and strategies to identify and address issues of physical access, see Pope (2005), Chapter 4, in *How to Survive and Thrive as a Therapist: Information, Ideas, and Resources for Psychologists* (Pope & Vasquez, 2005), and the Web site *Accessibility & Disability Information & Resources in Psychology Training & Practice* at http://kpope.com.

In addition to the challenge of identifying and addressing physical barriers is the challenge of providing adequate training. A survey of American Psychological Association members by Irene Leigh and her colleagues found reports of problems resulting from lack of adequate training.

"A deaf woman [was] diagnosed as having schizophrenia by a mental health agency because she flailed her arms around; she was signing." Another respondent indicated that a child with hearing impairment had been misdiagnosed with mental retardation. With regard to test interpretation, a respondent reported that a provider administered a short version of the Minnesota Multiphasic Personality Inventory and did not take into consideration how disability might affect some responses such as "I have difficulty standing or walking." Other examples . . . included providers not using an interpreter and provider refusal to treat persons with disabilities. (Leigh, Powers, Vash, & Nettles, 2004)

Similarly, in "Impact of Professional Training on Case Conceptualization of Clients with a Disability," Nancy Kemp and Brent Mallinckrodt (1996) reported the results of their study:

Therapists gave different priorities to treatment themes depending on whether the client had a disability and whether they, the therapists, had received any training in disability issues. Untrained therapists were more likely to focus on extraneous issues and less likely to focus on appropriate themes for a sexual abuse survivor with a disability" (p. 378).

Among the findings were that "even a small amount of training on issues of disability may be associated with significantly less bias in case conceptualization and treatment planning" (p. 383).

Unfortunately, studies of how therapists are trained suggest that we have a long way to go in meeting these challenges. In "ADA Accommodation of Therapists with Disabilities in Clinical Training," Hendrika Kemp and her colleagues noted that

Despite the obvious need . . . disability is not a standard part of clinical training. . . . We found that of the 618 internship sites recently listed on the APPIC web-site, only 81 listed a disabilities rotation. . . . The picture is even bleaker when we examine how training sites accommodate clinicians with disabilities. (Kemp, Chen, Erickson, & Friesen, 2003)

DETAINEE INTERROGATIONS

Scenario One

You are a therapist in independent practice. Several government officials arrive at your office to explain that one of your clients has been placed in a high-security center for questioning. The Department of Homeland Security has reason to believe that your client has knowledge of a terrorist network planning a massive attack. An interrogation team hopes to obtain enough information from your client, who has so far refused to discuss the topic, in time to prevent the attack. Emphasizing that lives are at stake and there is not a moment to waste, the officials ask for your client's evaluation and treatment records so that they can be faxed immediately to the interrogation team. They ask you to accompany them to the holding center so that the interrogation team can consult with you about the strategies most likely to gain the client's trust and persuade him to cooperate. They also ask you to talk with your client because he trusts you. When you hesitate, they stress that the attack may be only a matter of hours away, that surely you would not want to be the one person who could have prevented the attack and whose delay or refusal to help resulted in widespread death and destruction.

What ethical issues does this scenario raise? What reasons would you give for cooperating fully, cooperating in some ways but not in others, or refusing to cooperate with the government officials?

Scenario Two

You are a military psychologist transferred to a detention center holding those suspected of being enemy combatants, unlawful combatants, and others who pose a threat to national security. You are ordered to use interviews and other appropriate methods to prepare psychological profiles of several detainees so that they may be interrogated effectively.

What ethical issues, if any, does this scenario present? Would you have concerns about any aspects of your participation?

Should psychologists, psychiatrists, and other mental health care specialists participate in the planning or implementation of detainee interrogations? Does this kind of work compromise the profession's ethical values, or do the special skills, training, and values of health care professionals help to ensure that interrogations are safe, effective, and ethical? Are the consequences of undertaking this work foreseeable and clear, or are there unexpected complications and unintended consequences?

Such questions confronted the professions with a striking urgency when, in the aftermath of 9/11, reports began to surface that some interrogators were using methods characterized as enhanced or extreme. Professional organizations created formal policies endorsing or prohibiting members' participation in detainee interrogations.

In 2005, the president of the American Psychological Association appointed a Presidential Task Force on Psychological Ethics and National Security [PENS]. The PENS Task Force Report (APA, 2005) did not prohibit psychologists from involvement in detainee interrogations but specified various limits. For example, psychologists could use medical records in some ways but not others for detainee interrogations:

> Psychologists who serve in the role of supporting an interrogation do not use health care related information from an individual's medical record to the detriment of the individual's safety and well-being. While information from a medical record may be helpful or necessary to ensure that an interrogation process remains safe, psychologists do not use such information to the detriment of an individual's safety and well-being. (APA, 2005, p. 4)

The PENS Report left several issues open because members were unable to reach consensus. For example, although it permitted psychologists not to disclose what they are doing or why, there was no agreement about prohibiting how far a psychologist could go in disguising his or her role in interrogations:

> While all members of the Task Force agreed that full disclosure of the nature and purpose of a psychologist's work is not ethically required or appropriate in every circumstance, members differed on the degree to which psychologists may ethically dissemble their activities from individuals whom they engage directly. (APA, 2005, p. 9)

The American Psychological Association took the position that psychologists were playing a key role in detainee interrogations because the interrogations were inherently a psychological process requiring psychological expertise. The "Statement of the

American Psychological Association on Psychology and Interrogations Submitted to the United States Senate Select Committee on Intelligence" stated:

> Conducting an interrogation is inherently a psychological endeavor. . . . Psychology is central to this process because an understanding of an individual's belief systems, desires, motivations, culture and religion likely will be essential in assessing how best to form a connection and facilitate educing accurate, reliable and actionable intelligence. Psychologists have expertise in human behavior, motivations and relationships. . . . Psychologists have valuable contributions to make toward . . . protecting our nation's security through interrogation processes. (APA, 2007b)

Psychologists' special expertise sets them apart, according to the American Psychological Association, from psychiatrists and other physicians. The Director of the APA Ethics Office wrote: "This difference, which stems from psychologists' unique competencies, represents an important distinction between what role psychologists and physicians may take in interrogations" (Behnke, 2006, p. 66).

Adopting a starkly different policy, the American Psychiatric Association's Board of Trustees and the Assembly of District Branches approved a clear prohibition:

> No psychiatrist should participate directly in the interrogation of persons held in custody by military or civilian investigative or law enforcement authorities, whether in the United States or elsewhere. Direct participation includes being present in the interrogation room, asking or suggesting questions, or advising authorities on the use of specific techniques of interrogation with particular detainees (American Psychiatric Association, 2006).

Similarly, the American Medical Association prohibited participation in detainee interrogations to such a degree that they banned even monitoring an interrogation with an intent to intervene (Moran, 2006; Ray, 2006).

Why did the American Psychiatric Association and the American Medical Association adopt an approach to involvement in detainee interrogations that differed so sharply from the American Psychological Association's policy? As noted earlier, the American Psychological Association presented the difference as one of "unique competencies." The American Psychiatric Association however, viewed the difference as one of ethical values. Discussing psychiatrists' "core values," American Psychiatric Association president Steven Sharfstein (2006) wrote:

> I told the generals that psychiatrists will not participate in the interrogation of persons held in custody. Psychologists, by contrast, had issued a position statement allowing consultations in interrogations. If you were ever wondering what makes us different from psychologists, here it is. This is a paramount challenge to our ethics and our Hippocratic training. Judging from the record of the actual treatment of detainees, it is the thinnest of thin lines that separates such consultation from involvement in facilitating deception and cruel and degrading treatment. Innocent people being released from Guantanamo—people who never were our enemies and had no useful information in the War on Terror—are returning to their homes and families bearing terrible internal scars. Our profession is lost if we play any role in inflicting these wounds. (p. 1713)

The American Psychiatric Association's stance distancing itself from the detainee interrogations at Guantanamo and prohibiting members from participation, in contrast to the American Psychological Association's emphasis on its unique competencies in interrogation and the value of its contributions to the interrogations, led the Pentagon to adopt a new policy in 2006 that focused solely on psychologists, rather than including psychiatrists, for help in developing strategies for interrogating detainees. *The New York Times* reported:

> Pentagon officials said Tuesday they would try to use only psychologists, not psychiatrists, to help interrogators devise strategies to get information from detainees at places like Guantánamo Bay, Cuba. The new policy follows by little more than two weeks an overwhelming vote by the American Psychiatric Association discouraging its members from participating in those efforts. Stephen Behnke, director of ethics for the counterpart group for psychologists, the American Psychological Association, said psychologists knew not to participate in activities that harmed detainees. But he also said the group believed that helping military interrogators made a valuable contribution . . . (Lewis, 2006)

What were the effects of psychologists' participation in detainee interrogations? The American Psychological Association emphasized important benefits such as psychologists' knowing "not to participate in activities that harmed detainees" and their "valuable contributions" toward "protecting our nation's security through interrogation processes." In 2007, the president of the American Psychological Association wrote: "The Association's position is rooted in our belief that having psychologists consult with interrogation teams makes an important contribution toward keeping interrogations safe and ethical."

It is worth noting, however, that some reports suggested that the effects of psychologists' involvement were not all positive. Eban (2007; see also Goodman, 2007), for example, documented ways in which "psychologists weren't merely complicit in America's aggressive new interrogation regime. Psychologists, working in secrecy, had actually designed the tactics and trained interrogators in them . . ." According to the Associated Press, "Military psychologists were enlisted to help develop more aggressive interrogation methods, including snarling dogs, forced nudity and long periods of standing, against terrorism suspects, according to a Senate investigation." Mayer (2008) reported: "[General] Dunlavey soon drafted military psychologists to play direct roles in breaking detainees down. The psychologists were both treating the detainees clinically and advising interrogators on how to manipulate them and exploit their phobias . . ." After publishing a series of investigative reports, the *Boston Globe* (2008) stated: "From the moment US military and civilian officials began detaining and interrogating Guantanamo Bay prisoners with methods that the Red Cross has called tantamount to torture, they have had the assistance of psychologists."

The sharp disagreements over interpretations of the effects of psychologists' participation in detainee interrogations is exemplified by the contrasting reactions to a set of government documents obtained by the American Civil Liberties Union (ACLU). The ACLU released the documents under the heading: "Newly Unredacted Report Confirms Psychologists Supported Illegal Interrogations in Iraq and Afghanistan." The ACLU disagreed with the view that the Director of the APA Ethics Office had expressed:

> We do not, however, agree with your conclusion that documents recently obtained by the ACLU through its Freedom of Information Act Litigation demonstrate that the APA's 'policy of engagement served the intended purpose'. . . . Rather, we are deeply concerned by the fact that, viewed in context, these documents warrant the opposite conclusion. (Romero, 2008)

APA's controversial policies attracted sharp criticism. The editor of *British Medical Journal* wrote that APA's approach was shocking (Goddlee, 2009). Amnesty International, Physicians for Human Rights, and 11 other organizations (2009) sent an open letter to APA describing necessary steps to acknowledge and confront "the terrible stain on . . . American psychology."

Here is an excerpt:

> Any meaningful approach to this issue must start by acknowledging the fact that psychologists were absolutely integral. . . . When the Bush administration decided to engage in torture, they turned to psychologists. . . . American Psychological Association] leadership has much work ahead to begin to repair the harm they have caused to the profession, the country, former and current detainees and their families.

The American Psychological Association has not yet reached a final or complete resolution of the complex and difficult issues underlying psychologists' participation in detainee interrogations. In 2008, the APA membership formally approved a petition that prohibited psychologists from working in some settings. APA's press release stated:

> The petition resolution stating that psychologists may not work in settings where "persons are held outside of, or in violation of, either International Law (e.g., the UN Convention Against Torture and the Geneva Conventions) or the US Constitution (where appropriate), unless they are working directly for the persons being detained or for an independent third party working to protect human rights" was approved by a vote of the APA membership. (APA, 2008a)

APA had previously stated that this new resolution would not be enforceable. Prior to the vote, the APA Office of Public Affairs had issued a fact sheet in the form of a Q & A: "Petition on Psychologists' Work Settings: Questions and Answers." APA's response to the question "If adopted would the petition be enforceable by APA?" included the following clarification: "As explained above, the petition would not become part of the APA Ethics Code nor be enforceable as are prohibitions set forth in the Ethics Code" (APA 2008b).

Working our way through these difficult issues, to which there are no easy answers, will require a careful review of the available documents, evidence, and arguments; critical thinking coupled with a willingness to consider contrary views; and open discussion. Some works presenting basic information, reviews, and/or analysis include APA (2005, 2007b, 2008a, 2008b), Levine (2007), Pope & Gutheil (2009a, 2009b), and Soldz (2009). A comprehensive online archive of more than 320 citations of articles, chapters, and books representing the full range of views of the controversy over psychologists, psychiatrists, and other health care professionals participating in the planning or implementation of detainee interrogations is available at http://kspope.com/interrogation/index.php.

CULTURES

You are a marriage and family counselor who works in a large mental health clinic. One client immigrated to the United States from another country and has learned enough English to communicate adequately during therapy. During the fourth session, the client says, "As you know, I come from another culture and I was wondering: Do you think that your own culture and the culture of this clinic have any effects on me and my therapy? For example, I notice that all the therapists and administrators in this clinic seem to be of the same race, while the people who clean the building and take care of the grounds all seem to be of a different race. Why do you think that is and do you think it has any effects on what happens between us in my therapy?"

How do you think you would respond to the client? What are your thoughts about how a therapist's culture and a mental health organization's culture might affect individual clients and the therapeutic process? How would you design a research study to explore the possible effects of culture on therapy, therapists, and clients? What hypotheses would you advance? When you imagined this situation, what country did you imagine the client emigrated from? What race was the client? The therapist? The cleaning staff? Why did these particular images come to mind?

The United States is a diverse nation enriched by the presence of many different cultures. However, cultural differences between therapist and client can sometimes pose significant challenges to everyone involved. One of the most obvious challenges occurs when the cultures speak different languages. In "Language Barriers to Health Care in the United States," Glen Flores (2006) writes,

> Some 49.6 million Americans (18.7 percent of U.S. residents) speak a language other than English at home; 22.3 million (8.4 percent) have limited English proficiency, speaking English less than "very well," according to self-ratings. Between 1990 and 2000, the number of Americans who spoke a language other than English at home grew by 15.1 million (a 47 percent increase), and the number with limited English proficiency grew by 7.3 million (a 53 percent increase . . .). The numbers are particularly high in some places: in 2000, 40 percent of Californians and 75 percent of Miami residents spoke a language other than English at home, and 20 percent of Californians and 47 percent of Miami residents had limited English proficiency. (pp. 229–230)

Even when therapist and patient both speak the same language (Spanish or Chinese, for example), each language may have many dialects that can prevent clear communication. And furthermore, "variations in language barriers experienced by immigrant groups are often reflective of differences in the local migration histories and socioeconomic status of these groups" (Kretsedemas, 2005, p. 109).

In addition to language challenges are the challenges imposed when the research studies that inform our understanding overlook potentially significant cultural and other group differences. For example, Beverly Greene (1997) notes:

> A preponderance of the empirical research on or with lesbians and gay men has been conducted with overwhelmingly white, middle-class respondents. . . . Similarly, research on members of ethnic minority groups rarely acknowledges differences in sexual orientation among group members. Hence there has been little exploration of the complex interaction between sexual orientation and ethnic identity development, nor have the realistic social tasks and stressors that are a component of gay and lesbian identity formation in conjunction with ethnic identity formation been taken into account. Discussion of the vicissitudes of racism and ethnic identity in intra- and interracial couples of the same gender and their effects on these couples' relationships has also been neglected in the narrow focus on heterosexual relationships found in the literature on ethnic minority clients. There has been an equally narrow focus on predominantly white couples in the gay and lesbian literature. (pp. 216–217)

Research that does take into account cultural complexity suggests that culture may sometimes play a significant role in the development of psychological disorders. Jeanne Miranda (2006) wrote,

> Rates of depression and substance abuse disorders are low among Mexican Americans born in Mexico (Vega et al., 1998), and immigrant Mexican American women have a lifetime rate of depression of 8%, similar to the rates of nonimmigrant Mexicans (Vega et al., 1998). However, after 13 years in the United States, rates of depression for those women who immigrated to the U.S. rise precipitously. U.S.-born women of Mexican heritage experience lifetime rates of depression similar to those of the White population in the United States, nearly twice the rate of immigrants. These findings are mirrored in other indicators of health. . . . Despite high rates of

poverty, Mexican American immigrant women have low rates of physical and mental health problems (Vega et al., 1998), Chinese American immigrant women have a lifetime rate of major depression near 7%, approximately half that of White women (Takeuchi et al., 1998). These results suggest that some aspects of culture protect against depression. (pp. 115–116.)

Shankar Vedantam (2005) provides other examples of how culture and other group differences may influence mental health:

- Patients with schizophrenia, a disease characterized by hallucinations and disorganized thinking, recover sooner and function better in poor countries with strong extended family ties than in the United States, two long-running studies by the World Health Organization have shown.

- People of Mexican descent born in the United States have twice the risk of disorders such as depression and anxiety, and four times the risk of drug abuse, compared with recent immigrants from Mexico. This finding is part of a growing body of literature that indicates that the newly arrived are more resilient to mental disorders, and that assimilation is associated with higher rates of psychiatric diagnoses.

- Black and Hispanic patients are more than three times as likely to be diagnosed with schizophrenia as White patients—even though studies indicate that the rate of the disorder is the same in all groups.

- White women in the United States are three times as likely to commit suicide as Black and Hispanic women—a difference that experts attribute in part to the relative strengths of different social networks.

- A host of small studies suggest that the effects of psychiatric drugs vary widely across different ethnic groups. There are even differences in the effect with dummy pills.

It is crucial to remember that even though any names and descriptions we might use to identify cultures, groups, and similar characteristics relevant to a client may help us understand the client's words, experiences, and behavior, they are *not* a substitute for learning directly from and about this unique individual. Individual differences within a group may overwhelm between-group differences, and an individual within a group may not reflect group characteristics. Any attempt to view, describe, or understand a person as the sum of a fixed set of descriptors oversimplifies in ways that are misleading. The descriptors themselves may not be as clear as some of the research seems to assume. As Connie Chan (1997) puts it,

> Although identity is a fluid concept in psychological and sociological terms, we tend to speak of identities in fixed terms. In particular, those aspects of identity that characterize observable physical characteristics, such as race or gender, are perceived as unchanging ascribed identities. Examples of these would include identifications such as *Chinese woman,* or *Korean American woman,* or even broader terms such as *woman of color,* which are ways of grouping together individuals who are not of the hegemonic "white" race in the United States. We base these constructions of identity upon physical appearance and an individual's declaration of identity. However, even these seemingly clear distinctions are not definitive. For example, I, as a woman of Asian racial background, may declare myself a woman of color because I see myself as belonging to a group of ethnic/racial minorities. However, my (biological) sister could insist that she is not a woman of color because she does not feel an affiliation with our group goals, even though she is a person of Chinese ancestry. Does her nonaffiliation take her out of the group of people of color? Or does she remain in regardless of her own self-identification because of her obvious physical characteristics? Generally, in the context of identities based upon racial and physical characteristics,

ascribed identities will, rightly or wrongly, continue to be attributed to individuals by others. It is left up to individuals themselves to assert their identities and demonstrate to others that they are or are *not* what they might appear to be upon first notice. (pp. 240–241; see also Wyatt, 1997)

It is also crucial that therapists be aware not only of the client's culture but also of the therapist's own culture and how it influences the therapist's values, frameworks, theoretical orientation, understanding, and decisions. An exceptional book, *The Spirit Catches You and You Fall Down: A Hmong Child, Her American Doctors, and the Collision of Two Cultures* (Fadiman, 1997) documents in vivid detail the efforts of health care professionals at a California hospital and a refugee family from Laos to help a Hmong child whom the health care professionals had determined was experiencing epileptic seizures. Despite the great expertise and dedication of the girl's physicians, the failure to take culture into account had disastrous consequences. Medical anthropologist Arthur Kleinman is quoted in the book:

As powerful an influence as the culture of the Hmong patient and her family is on this case, the culture of biomedicine is equally powerful. If you can't see that your own culture has its own set of interests, emotions, and biases, how can you expect to deal successfully with someone else's culture? (p. 261)

Kleinman addresses the effects of culture, such as the culture of biomedicine, in more detail in an article (2004) in the *New England Journal of Medicine:*

The culture of biomedicine is also responsible for some of the uncertainty surrounding depression. Symptoms that represent a depressive disorder for the practitioner (say, sadness and hopelessness in a patient dying from cancer) may not denote a medical problem to the patient, his or her family, or their clergy, for whom depression may be a sign of the moral experience of suffering. What is seen by a particular social network as a normal emotional response—say, grief lasting for years—may count as a depressive disorder for the psychiatrist, since the *Diagnostic and Statistical Manual of Mental Disorders,* 4th edition (DSM-IV), defines normal bereavement as lasting for two months. In this area, the professional culture, driven by the political economy of the pharmaceutical industry, may represent the leading edge of a worldwide shift in norms.

Yet many people with clinical depression—at least 50 percent among immigrants and minority groups in the United States—still receive neither a diagnosis nor treatment from a biomedical practitioner. Lack of access to appropriate services is a major reason for this failure, but cultural causes of misdiagnosis also contribute. Culture confounds diagnosis and management by influencing not only the experience of depression, but also the seeking of help, patient–practitioner communication, and professional practice. Culture also affects the interaction of risk factors with social supports and protective psychological factors that contribute to depression in the first place. Culture may even turn out to create distinctive environments for gene expression and physiological reaction, resulting in a local biology of depression: research already shows that persons from various ethnic backgrounds metabolize antidepressant drugs in distinct ways. (pp. 951–952)

Melba Vasquez (2007; see also Comas-Diaz, 2006; Sue & Sue, 2007; Sue et al., 2006) provides an evidence-based analysis of the ways in which cultural differences can affect the therapeutic alliance specifically and therapy more generally. Lillian Comas-Dias explores the relationship between culture and psychotherapy more fully in Chapter 15 of this book.

The same question arises here as with the other challenges and controversies noted in this chapter: Are we addressing these issues adequately in our training programs? Research conducted by Nancy Hansen and her colleagues (2006) suggests that we may need to pay more attention to issues of culture in our graduate programs, practica, internships, and other educational settings to develop competencies in this area and the ability to follow through. Hansen and colleagues' "Do We Practice What We Preach?" provides the results of a survey that found that "Overall and for 86% of the individual items, participants did not practice what they preached" (p. 66) in terms of what they endorsed as the need for multicultural competencies. Hansen and her colleagues concluded that

> psychotherapists need to recognize their vulnerability to not following through with what they know to be competent practice, and they need, in advance, to problem solve creative solutions. It would be helpful to identify your personal barriers in this regard: Are you anxious about raising certain issues with racially/ethnically different clients? Are you uncertain about how best to intervene? Do you fear you will "get in over your head" exploring these issues? What will it take to work through (or around) these barriers to become more racially/ethnically responsive in your psychotherapy work? (Hansen, et al. 2006, p. 72)

Taking seriously the reality that *every* therapist is influenced by culture and *every* client is influenced by culture saves us from the misleading stereotype that multicultural counseling is something you need to know about only if you happen to find yourself working with someone from a different country, say, or someone of a different ethnicity who speaks a different language. As Pedersen, Draguns, Lonner, and Trimble (1989, p. 1) remind us in *Counseling Across Cultures:* "Multicultural counseling is not an exotic topic that applies to remote regions, but is the heart and core of good counseling with any client."

REFERENCES

Adleman, J., & Barrett, S. E. (1990). Overlapping relationships: Importance of the feminist ethical perspective. In H. Lermamn & N. Portman (Eds.), *Feminist ethics in psychotherapy* (pp. 87–91). New York: Springer.

American Psychiatric Association (2006, May). Psychiatric participation in interrogation of detainees: position statement. Retrieved March 27, 2009, from http://archive.psych.org/edu/other_res/lib_archives/archives/200601.pdf

American Psychological Association, Presidential Task Force on Evidence-Based Practice. (2006). Evidenced-based practice in psychology. *American Psychologist, 61,* 271–285.

American Psychological Association. (2005, June). Report of the American Psychological Association Presidential Task Force on Psychological Ethics and National Security. Retrieved March 27, 2009, from http://www.apa.org/releases/PENSTaskForceReportFinal.pdf

American Psychological Association. (2007a). *Recommended postdoctoral education and training program in psychopharmacology for prescriptive authority* (Rev.). Washington, DC: Author.

American Psychological Association. (2007b, September 21). Statement of the American Psychological Association on

Psychology and Interrogations submitted to the United States Senate Select Committee on Intelligence. Retrieved March 27, 2009, from http://www.apa.org/ethics/statement092107.html

American Psychological Association. (2008a, September 17). *APA members approve petition resolution on detainee settings.* (APA Press Release). Retrieved March 28, 2009, from http://www.apa.org/releases/petition0908.html

American Psychological Association. (2008b, July 28). *Petition on psychologists' work settings: questions and answers.* Retrieved March 28, 2009, from http://www.apa.org/governance/resolutions/qa-work-settings.html

Amnesty International, Physicians for Human Rights, and 11 other organizations. Open letter in response to the American Psychological Association Board. June 29, 2009. http://bit.ly/Y2bFj. Accessed November 19, 2009

Appelbaum, P. S., & Gutheil, T. G. (2007). *Clinical handbook of psychiatry and the law* (4th ed.). New York: Lippincott Williams & Wilkins.

Ax, R. K., Bigelow, B. J., Harowski, K., Meredith, J. M., Nussbaum, D., & Taylor, R. R. (2008). Prescriptive authority for psychologists: Serving underserved health care consumers. *Psychological Services, 5*(2), 184–197.

Ax, R. K., Fagan, T. J., & Resnick, R. J. (2009). Predoctoral prescriptive authority training: The rationale and a combined model. *Psychological Services, 6*(1), 85–95.

Bader, E. (1994). Dual relationships: Legal and ethical trends. *Transactional Analysis Journal, 24*(1), 64–66.

Baer, B. E., & Murdock, N. L. (1995). Nonerotic dual relationships between therapists and clients: The effects of sex, theoretical orientation, and interpersonal boundaries. *Ethics & Behavior, 5,* 131–145.

Banks, M. E. (2003). Preface. In M. E. Banks & E. Kaschak (Eds.), *Women with visible and invisible disabilities: Multiple intersections, multiple issues, multiple therapists* (pp. xxi–xxxix). New York: Haworth Press.

Barlow, D. H. (2004). Psychological treatments. *American Psychologist, 59*(9), 869–878.

Bates, C. M., & Brodsky, A. M. (1989). *Sex in the therapy hour: A case of professional incest.* New York: Guilford Press.

Behnke, S. (2006). Ethics and interrogations: Comparing and contrasting the American Psychological, American Medical and American Psychiatric Association positions. *Monitor on Psychology, 37*(7), 66.

Beitman, B., & Yue, M. D. (1999). *Learning psychotherapy.* New York: Norton.

Bluestein, D., & Cubic, B. A. (2009). Psychologists and primary care physicians: A training model for creating collaborative relationships. *Journal of Clinical Psychology in Medical Settings, 16,* 101–112.

Borys, D. S., & Pope, K. S. (1989). Dual relationships between therapist and client: A national study of psychologists, psychiatrists, and social workers. *Professional Psychology: Research and Practice, 20,* 283–293; also available at http://kspope.com

Boston Globe. (2008, August 30). Boston Globe Editorial: Psychologists and torture. *Boston Globe.* Retrieved March 28, 2009, from http://tinyurl.com/5qhtf2

Brehm, S. (2007, January 9). American Psychological Association news release of letter from the APA president to the editor of *The Washington Monthly.* Retrieved March 28, 2009, from http://www.apa.org/releases/washingtonmonthly.pdf

Brodsky, A. M. (1989). Sex between patient and therapist: Psychology's data and response. In G. O. Gabbard (Ed.), *Sexual exploitation in professional relationships* (pp. 15–25). Washington, DC: American Psychiatric Press.

Brown, L. S. (1989). Beyond thou shalt not: Thinking about ethics in the Lesbian therapy community. *Women and Therapy, 8,* 13–25.

Brown, L. S. (1994). *Subversive dialogues.* New York: Basic Books.

Burian, B. K., & Slimp, A. O. (2000). Social dual-role relationships during internship: A decision-making model. *Professional Psychology: Research & Practice, 31,* 332–338.

Campbell, C., & Gordon, M. (2003). Acknowledging the inevitable: Understanding multiple relationships in rural practice. *Professional Psychology: Research and Practice, 34,* 430–434.

Chan, C. S. (1997). Don't ask, don't tell, don't know: The formation of a homosexual identity and sexual expression among Asian American lesbians. In B. Greene (Ed.), *Ethnic and cultural diversity among lesbians and gay men* (pp. 240–248). Thousand Oaks, CA: Sage.

Clarkson, P. (1994). In recognition of dual relationships. *Transactional Analysis Journal, 24*(1), 32–38.

Comas-Diaz, L. (2006). Cultural variation in the therapeutic relationship. In C. D. Goodheart, A. E. Kazdin, & R. J. Sternberg (Eds.), *Evidence-based psychotherapy: Where practice and research meet* (pp. 81–105). Washington, DC: American Psychological Association.

Eban, K. (2007, July 17). Rorschach and awe. *Vanity Fair.* Retrieved March 28, 2009, from http://tinyurl.com/2zkg9p

Fadiman, A. (1997). *The spirit catches you and you fall down: A Hmong child, her American doctors, and the collision of two cultures.* New York: Farrar, Straus and Giroux.

Fagan, T. J., Ax, R. K., Liss, M., Resnick, R. J., & Moody, W. (2007). Prescriptive authority and preferences for training. *Professional Psychology: Research and Practice, 38*(1), 104–111.

Faulkner, K. K., & Faulkner, T. A. (1997). Managing multiple relationships in rural communities: Neutrality and boundary violations. *Clinical Psychology: Science and Practice, 4*(3), 225–234.

Flores, G. (2006). Language barriers to health care in the United States. *New England Journal of Medicine, 355*(3), 229–231.

Freeman, L., & Roy, J. (1976). *Betrayal.* New York: Stein and Day.

Geyer, M. C. (1994). Dual role relationships and Christian counseling. *Journal of Psychology & Theology, 22*(3), 187–195.

Godlee F. (2009). Rules of conscience. *British Medical Journal.* 2009;338:b1972. http://www.bmj.com/cgi/content/full/338/may14_1/b1972. Accessed November 19, 2009.

Goodheart, C. D. (2006). Evidence, endeavor, and expertise in psychological practice. In C. D. Goodheart, A. E. Kazdin, & R. J. Sternberg (Eds.), *Evidence-based psychotherapy: Where practice and research meet* (pp. 37–61). Washington, DC: American Psychological Association.

Goodheart, C. D., & Kazdin, A. E. (2006). Introduction. In C. D. Goodheart, A. E. Kazdin, & R. J. Sternberg (Eds.), *Evidence-based psychotherapy: Where practice and research meet* (pp. 3–10). Washington, DC: American Psychological Association.

Goodman, A. (2007, June 8). Psychologists implicated in torture. *Seattle Post-Intelligencer.* Retrieved March 28, 2009, from http://seattlepi.nwsource.com/opinion/318745_amy07.html

Gottlieb, M. C. (1993). Avoiding exploitive dual relationships: A decision-making model. *Psychotherapy: Theory, Research, Practice, Training, 30*(1), 41–48; also available at http://kspope.com

Greene, B. G. (Ed.). (1997). *Ethnic and cultural diversity among lesbians and gay men.* Thousand Oaks, CA: Sage.

Gutheil, T. G., & Brodsky, A. (2008). *Preventing boundary violations in clinical practice.* New York: Guilford.

Hansen, N. D., Randazzo, K. V., Schwartz, A., Marshall, M., Kalis, D., Frazier, R., Burke, C., Kershner-Rice, K., & Norvig, G. (2006). Do we practice what we preach? An exploratory survey of multicultural psychotherapy competencies. *Professional Psychology: Research and Practice, 37*(1), 66–74.

Hawn, C. (2009). Take two aspirin and tweet me in the morning: How Twitter, Facebook, and other social media are reshaping health care. *Health Affairs, 28*(2), 361–368.

Horst, E. A. (1989). Dual relationships between psychologists and clients in rural and urban areas. *Journal of Rural Community Psychology, 10*(2), 15–24.

Kazdin, A. E. (2006). Arbitrary metrics: Implications for identifying evidence-based treatments. *American Psychologist, 61*(1), 42–49.

Kazdin, A. E. (2008a). Evidence-based treatments and delivery of psychological services: Shifting our emphases to increase impact. *Psychological Services, 5*(3), 201–215.

Kazdin, A. E. (2008b). Evidence-based treatment and practice: New opportunities to bridge clinical research and practice, enhance the knowledge base, and improve patient care. *American Psychologist, 63*(3), 146–159.

Keith-Spiegel, P., & Koocher, G. P. (1985). *Ethics in psychology: Professional standards and cases.* New York: Crown/ Random House.

Kemp, H. V., Chen, J. S., Erickson, G. N., & Friesen, N. L. (2003). ADA accommodation of therapists with disabilities in clinical training. *Women & Therapy, 26*(1–2), 155–168.

Kemp, N. T., & Mallinckrodt, B. (1996). Impact of professional training on case conceptualization of clients with a disability. *Professional Psychology: Research and Practice, 27*(4), 378–385.

Kitchener, K. S. (1988). Dual role relationships: What makes them so problematic? *Journal of Counseling & Development, 67*(4), 217–221.

Kleinman, A. (2004). Culture and depression. *New England Journal of Medicine, 351*(10), 951–953.

Koocher, G. P. (1994). Foreword. In K. S. Pope, *Sexual involvement with therapists: Patient assessment, subsequent therapy, forensics* (pp. vii–ix). Washington, DC: American Psychological Association.

Koocher, G. P. (2006). Foreword to the second edition: Things my teachers never mentioned. In K. S. Pope, J. L. Sonne, & B. Greene. *What therapists don't talk about and why: Understanding taboos that hurt us and our clients* (2nd ed.) (pp. xxi–xxiv). Washington, DC: American Psychological Association.

Koocher, G. P., & Morray, E. (2000). Regulation of telepsychology: A survey of state attorneys general. *Professional Psychology: Research and Practice, 31*(5), 503–508.

Kraemer, J. D., & Gostin, L. O. (2009). Science, politics, and values: The politicization of professional practice guidelines. *Journal of the American Medical Association, 301*(6), 665–667.

Kretsedemas, P. (2005). Language barriers & perceptions of bias. *Journal of Sociology & Social Welfare, 32*(4), 109–123.

Lamb, D. H., & Catanzaro, S. J. (1998). Sexual and nonsexual boundary violations involving psychologists, clients, supervisees, and students: Implications for professional practice. *Professional Psychology: Research and Practice, 29*, 498–503.

Lamb, D. H., Catanzaro, S. J., & Moorman, A. S. (2004). A preliminary look at how psychologists identify, evaluate, and proceed when faced with possible multiple relationship dilemmas. *Professional Psychology: Research and Practice, 35*(3), 248–254.

Lehner, G. F. J. (1952). Defining psychotherapy. *American Psychologist, 7*, 547.

Leigh, I. W., Powers, L., Vash, C., & Nettles, R. (2004). Survey of psychological services to clients with disabilities: The need for awareness. *Rehabilitation Psychology, 49*(1), 48–54.

Levine, A. (2007, January–February). Collective unconscionable: How psychologists, the most liberal of professionals, abetted torture. *Washington Monthly.* Retrieved March 28, 2009, from http://www.washingtonmonthly.com/features/2007/0701.levine.html

Lewis, A. (2006, June 7). Psychologists preferred for detainees. *New York Times.* Retrieved November 18, 2009, from http://tinyurl.com/2gfjdz

Luhrmann, T. M. (2000). *Of two minds: The growing disorder in American psychiatry.* New York: Knopf.

Mayer, J. (2008). *The dark side.* New York: Doubleday.

Miranda, J. (2006). Improving services and outreach for women with depression. In C. M. Mazure & G. P. Keita (Eds.), *Understanding depression in women: Applying empirical research to practice and policy* (pp. 113–135). Washington, DC: American Psychological Association.

Moran M. (2006). American Medical Association interrogation policy similar to American Psychiatric Association's position. *Psychiatric News, 41*(13), 1–5. Retrieved March 27, 2009, from http://pn.psychiatryonline.org/cgi/content/full/41/13/1

Moran, M. (2009). Psychiatrists lament decline of key treatment modality. *Psychiatric News, 44*(13), 8. Retrieved July 7, 2009, from http://pn.psychiatryonline.org/cgi/content/full/44/13/8

Noel, B., & Waterson, K. (1992). *You must be dreaming.* New York: Poseidon.

Olfson, M., Marcus, S. C., Druss, B., Elinson, L., Tanielian, T., & Pincus, H. A. (2002). National trends in the outpatient treatment of depression. *Journal of the American Medical Association, 287*(2), 203–209.

Olfson, M., Marcus, S. C., Druss, B., & Pincus, H. A. (2002). National trends in the use of outpatient psychotherapy. *American Journal of Psychiatry, 159*(11), 1914–1920.

Paul, G. L. (1967). Strategy of outcome research in psychotherapy. *Journal of Consulting Psychology, 31*(2), 109–118.

Pedersen, P. D., Draguns, J. G., Lonner, W. J., & Trimble, E. J. (1989). Introduction and overview. In P. D. Pedersen, J. G. Draguns, W. J. Lonner, & E. J. Trimble (Eds.), *Counseling across cultures* (3rd ed., pp. 1–2). Honolulu: University of Hawaii Press.

Plaisil, E. (1985). *Therapist.* New York: St. Martin's/Marek.

Pope, K. S. (1988). How clients are harmed by sexual contact with mental health professionals. *Journal of Counseling and Development, 67,* 222–226.

Pope, K. S. (1994). *Sexual involvement with therapists: Patient assessment, subsequent therapy, forensics.* Washington, DC: American Psychological Association.

Pope, K. S. (2005). Disability and accessibility in psychology: Three major barriers. *Ethics & Behavior, 15*(2), 103–106; also available at http://kspope.com

Pope, K. S., & Bouhoutsos, J. C. (1986). *Sexual intimacies between therapists and patients.* New York: Praeger/Greenwood.

Pope K. S. & Gutheil T. G. (2009). Contrasting ethical policies of physicians and psychologists concerning interrogation of detainees. *British Medical Journal. 338,* b1653. Accessed November 19, 2009, from http://www.bmj.com/cgi/section_pdf/338/apr30_2/b1653.pdf

Pope K. S. & Gutheil T. G. (2009). Psychologists abandon the Nuremberg ethic: concerns for detainee interrogations. *International Journal of Law & Psychiatry, 32, 4,* 161–166. Accessed November 19, 2009 from http://kspope.com/nuremberg.php

Pope, K. S., & Keith-Spiegel, P. (2008). A practical approach to boundaries in psychotherapy: Making decisions, bypassing blunders, and mending fences. *Journal of Clinical Psychology: In Session, 64*(5), 638–652.

Pope, K. S., & Vasquez, M. J. T. (1998). *Ethics in psychotherapy and counseling.* San Francisco: Jossey-Bass.

Pope, K. S., & Vasquez, M. J. T. (2005). *How to survive and thrive as a therapist: Information, ideas, and resources for psychologists in practice.* Washington, DC: American Psychological Association.

Pope, K. S., & Vasquez, M. J. T. (2007). *Ethics in psychotherapy and counseling: A practical guide* (3rd ed.). San Francisco: Jossey-Bass.

Pope, K. S., & Vetter, V. A. (1992). Ethical dilemmas encountered by members of the American Psychological Association: A national survey. *American Psychologist, 47,* 397–411; also available at http://kspope.com

Pope, K. S., Levenson, H., & Schover, L. R. (1979). Sexual intimacy in psychology training: Results and implications of a national survey. *American Psychologist, 34,* 682–689; also available at http://kspope.com

Pope, K. S., Sonne, J. L., & Holroyd, J. (1993). *Sexual feelings in psychotherapy: Explorations for therapists and therapists-in-training.* Washington, DC: American Psychological Association.

Pope, K. S., Sonne, J. L., & Greene, B. (2006). *What therapists don't talk about and why: Understanding taboos that hurt us and our clients.* Washington, DC: American Psychological Association.

Rae, W. A., Jensen-Doss, A., Bowden, R., Mendoza, M., & Banda, T. (2008). Prescription privileges for psychologists:

Opinions of pediatric psychologists and pediatricians. *Journal of Pediatric Psychology, 33*(2), 176–184.

Ray, P. (2006, June 12). *New AMA ethical policy opposes direct physician participation in interrogation.* American Medical Association news release. Retrieved March 27, 2009, from http://www.ama-assn.org/ama/pub/category/16446.html

Rinella, V. J., & Gerstein, A. I. (1994). The development of dual relationships: Power and professional responsibility. *International Journal of Law and Psychiatry, 17*(3), 225–237.

Robiner, W. N. (2006). The mental health professions: Workforce supply and demand, issues, and challenges. *Clinical Psychology Review, 26*(5), 600–625.

Roll, S., & Millen, L. (1981). A guide to violating an injunction in psychotherapy: On seeing acquaintances as patients. *Psychotherapy: Theory, Research & Practice, 18*(2), 179–187.

Romero, A. D. (2008, June 18). Letter from the American Civil Liberties Executive Director to Dr. Stephen Behnke, Director, Ethics Office, American Psychological Association. Retrieved March 28, 2009, from http://tinyurl.com/6o5grc

Roy v. Hartogs. (1976). 381 N.Y.S. 2d 587; 85 Misc.2d 891.

Ruddy, N. B., Borresen, D. A., & Gunn Jr., W. B. (2008). *The collaborative psychotherapist: Creating reciprocal relationships with medical professionals.* Washington, DC: American Psychological Association.

Ryder, R., & Hepworth, J. (1990). AAMFT ethical code: "Dual relationships." *Journal of Marital & Family Therapy, 16*(2), 127–132.

Shaneyfelt, T. M., & Centor, R. M. (2009). Reassessment of clinical practice guidelines. *Journal of the American Medical Association, 301*(8), 868–869.

Simon, R. I., & Shuman, D. W. (2007). *Clinician's manual of psychiatry & law.* Washington, DC: American Psychiatric Press.

Slimp, A. O., & Burian, B. K. (1994). Multiple role relationships during internship: Consequences and recommendations. *Professional Psychology: Research and Practice, 25*(1), 39–45.

Soldz, S. (2009). Closing eyes to atrocities: U.S. psychologists, detainee interrogations, and the response of the American Psychological Association. In R. Goodman & M. J. Roseman (Eds.). *Interrogations, forced feedings, and the role of health professionals: New perspectives on international human rights, humanitarian law and ethics* (Harvard Law School Human Rights Program series) (pp. 103–142). Cambridge, MA: Harvard University Press. Retrieved March 28, 2009, from http://tinyurl.com/cc9yw4

Sonne, J. L. (2006). Nonsexual multiple relationships: A practical decision-making model for clinicians. Retrieved November 19, 2009 from http://kspope.com/dual/index.php

Sternberg, R. J. (2006). Evidence-based practice: Gold standard, gold plated, or fool's gold? In C. D. Goodheart,

A. E. Kazdin, & R. J. Sternberg (Eds.), *Evidence-based psychotherapy: Where practice and research meet* (pp. 261–271). Washington, DC: American Psychological Association.

Stettin, G. D., Yao, J., Verbrugge, R. R., & Aubert, R. E. (2006, August). Frequency of follow-up care for adult and pediatric patients during initiation of antidepressant therapy. *American Journal of Managed Care, 12,* 453–461.

Stockman, A. F. (1990). Dual relationships in rural mental health practice: An ethical dilemma. *Journal of Rural Community Psychology, 11*(2), 31–45.

Stromberg, C. D., Haggarty, D. J., Leibenluft, R. F., McMillian, M. H., Mishkin, B., Rubin, B. L., & Trilling, H. R. (1988). *The psychologist's legal handbook.* Washington, DC: Council for the National Register of Health Service Providers in Psychology.

Sue, D. W., & Sue, D. (2007). *Counseling the culturally diverse: Theory and practice* (5th ed.). New York: Wiley.

Sue, S., Zane, N., Levant, R. F., Silverstein, L. B., Brown, L. S., Olkin, R., & Taliafero, G. (2006). How well do both evidence-based practices and treatment as usual satisfactorily address the various dimensions of diversity? In J. Norcross, L. Beutler, & R. Levant (Eds.), *Evidence-based practices in mental health: Debate and dialogue on the fundamental questions.* (pp. 329–374). Washington, DC: American Psychological Association: Washington.

Vasquez, M. J. T. (2007). Cultural difference and the therapeutic alliance: An evidence-based analysis. *American Psychologist, 62*(8), 878–885.

Vedantam, S. (2005, June 26). Patients' diversity is often discounted: Alternatives to mainstream medical treatment call for recognizing ethnic, social differences. *Washington Post,* p. A1.

Walker, E., & Young, T. D. (1986). *A killing cure.* New York: Holt.

Wang, P. S., Demler, O., Olfson, M., Pincus, H. A., Wells, K. B., & Kessler, R. C. (2006). Changing profiles of service sectors used for mental health care in the United States. *American Journal of Psychiatry, 163*(8), 1187–1198.

Wedding, D., DeLeon, P. H., & Olson, R. P. (2006). Mental health care in the United States. In P. Olson (Ed.), *Mental health systems compared* (pp. 185–230). Springfield, IL: Charles C Thomas.

Wedding, D., & Mengel, M. (2004). Models of integrated care in primary care settings. In L. Haas (Ed.), *Handbook of psychology in primary care* (pp. 47–62). New York: Oxford University Press.

Westen, D., & Bradley, R. (2005). Empirically supported complexity: Rethinking evidence-based practice in psychotherapy. *Current Directions in Psychological Science, 14,* 266–271.

Westen, D., Novotny, C. M., & Thompson-Brenner, H. (2004). The empirical status of empirically supported psychotherapies: Assumptions, findings, and reporting in controlled clinical trials. *Psychological Bulletin, 130,* 631–663.

Wyatt, G. E. (1997). *Stolen women: Reclaiming our sexuality, taking back our lives.* New York: Wiley.

Younggren, J. (2002). *Ethical decision-making and dual relationships.* Retrieved August 22, 2006, from http://kspope.com

Younggren, J. N., & Gottlieb, M. C. (2004). Managing risk when contemplating multiple relationships. *Professional Psychology: Research and Practice, 35*(3), 255–260.

GLOSSARY

The following abbreviations are used to indicate primary associations: (AD) Adlerian Psychotherapy; (AP) Analytical Psychotherapy; (BT) Behavior Therapy; (CC) Client-Centered Therapy; (CN) Contemplative Psychotherapy; (CT) Cognitive Therapy; (EX) Existential Therapy; (FT) Family Therapy; (GT) Gestalt Therapy; (INT) Integrative Therapy; (IPT) Interpersonal Psychotherapy; (MC) Multicultural Psychotherapy; (PA) Psychoanalysis; (REBT) Rational Emotive Behavior Therapy.

Abreaction (PA) The reliving or recovery of painful, repressed emotional experiences in psychotherapy, accompanied by a discharge of affect or intense feelings. *See also* Catharsis.

Acceptance and Commitment Therapy (BT) A form of behavior therapy developed by Steven Hayes that focuses on experiential avoidance and cognitive fusion as key determinants of psychopathology and commitment as one component of therapeutic success.

Active Imagination (AP) A form of reflection through which people activate and follow their imaginative reveries in a purposive way.

Activity Scheduling (CT, BT) Setting up routine activity in order to offset inertia.

Actualizing Tendency (CC) An innate human predisposition toward growth and fulfilling one's potential.

Agape Unconditional love for humanity (literally, "love between friends").

Aggression (GT) The basic biological movement of energy extending out from the organism to the environment. Aggression is required for assimilation, love, assertion, creativity, hunger, humor, discrimination, warmth, etc.

Agoraphobia An excessive fear of open spaces and/or leaving one's own home.

Aha! (GT) Awareness of a situation in which a number of separate elements come together to form a meaningful whole; sudden insight into the solution to a problem or the structure of a situation.

Albert Ellis Institute (REBT) An organization founded by Albert Ellis in 1959. There was considerable controversy in psychotherapy circles in 2005 when the Institute removed Albert Ellis from the Board.

Albert Ellis Foundation (REBT) An organization established in 2006 to support the work and legacy of Albert Ellis.

Anal Phase (PA) Freud's second phase of psychosexual development, extending roughly from 18 months to 3 years of age, in which most libidinal pleasure is derived from retaining and expelling feces.

Anima (AP) A feminine archetypal image that serves as a bridge to the unconscious in both men and women, but is most often expressed as the feminine part of a man. *See also* Animus.

Animus (AP) A masculine archetypal image that serves as a bridge to the unconscious in both men and women, but is most often expressed as the masculine part of a woman. *See also* Anima.

Anorectic A person engaging in self-starving behavior.

Antisuggestion (AD) *See* Paradoxical Intervention.

Aphasia An organic speech deficit involving difficulty understanding or using language.

Applied Behavior Analysis (BT) A form of behavior therapy, closely tied to Skinner's philosophy of radical behaviorism, that stresses observable behavior rather than private events and uses single-subject experimental design to determine the relationship between behavior and its antecedents and consequences.

Arbitrary Inference (CT) Drawing conclusions without supporting evidence or despite evidence to the contrary.

Archetype (AP) An innate universal pattern or organizing principle similar to an instinct. It has no specific form but can be seen through archetypal images observable in the common motifs present in myths, fairy tales, legends, and dreams across cultures and times. Examples include the Earth Mother, the Wise Old Man, the Hero's Quest, the Shadow, and the Trickster.

Armamentarium The complete range of psychotherapeutic methods and techniques used by a therapist.

Assertion Training (BT) A treatment procedure designed to teach clients to openly and effectively express both positive and negative feelings.

Assimilation (GT) The process of breaking something into component parts so that these parts can be accepted and made part of the person, rejected, or modified into suitable form.

Assimilative Integration (INT) An approach to psychotherapy integration that entails a firm grounding in one system of psychotherapy, but with a willingness to selectively incorporate (assimilate) practices and views from other systems.

Attachment Theory (FT, IPT) A theory developed by John Bowlby, who proposed that all humans have an innate tendency to develop strong affectional bonds and that threat to these bonds resulted in psychopathology.

Authentic Mode (EX) A way of being described by Heidegger in which one understands and appreciates the fragility of being while acknowledging responsibility for one's own life. Also referred to as the *Ontological Mode*.

Autoeroticism (PA) Obtaining gratification from self-stimulating a sensual area of the body.

Automatic Thought (CT) A personal notion or idea triggered by particular stimuli that lead to an emotional response.

Autonomy A personality dimension based on needs to be independent, to be self-determining, and to attain one's goals.

Auxiliary A person who aids a therapist or client in enacting a particular scene.

Aversive Racism (MC) A theory proposed by Gaertner & Dovidio that maintains that Whites can sincerely endorse egalitarian values while at the same time being racist and harboring unacknowledged negative attitudes toward racial/ethnic out-groups.

Awfulizing (REBT) Seeing something inconvenient or obnoxious as awful, horrible, or terrible.

Basic Encounter (CC) One member of a group's responding with empathy to another member's being genuine and real.

Basic Mistake (AD) Myth used to organize and shape one's life. Examples include overgeneralizations, a desperate need for security, misperceptions of life's demands, denial of one's worth, and faulty values.

Behavioral Experiment (CT, REBT) Testing distorted beliefs or fears scientifically in a real-life situation (e.g., having a shy person initiate a conversation to see what actually happens).

Behavioral Medicine (BT) Applying learning theory techniques to prevent or treat physical problems (e.g., pain reduction, weight loss).

Behavioral Rehearsal (CT, BT) Practicing an emotionally charged event and one's response to it prior to its actual occurrence.

Belonging (AD, BT) An innate need, drive, and source of human behavior. It leads people to seek relationship and involvement with other human beings.

Boundary (FT) A barrier between parts of a system, as in a family, in which rules establish who may participate and in what manner.

Catastrophizing (REBT, CT) Exaggerating the consequences of an unfortunate event.

Catharsis The expression and discharge of repressed emotions; sometimes used as a synonym for *abreaction*.

Cathexis (PA) Investment of mental or emotional (libidinal) energy into a person, object, or idea.

Circular Causality (FT) The feedback model of a network of interacting loops that views any causal event as the effect of a prior cause, as in family interactions.

Circular Questioning (FT) An interviewing technique directed at eliciting differences in perceptions about events or relationships from different family members, especially regarding those points in the family life cycle when significant coalition shifts occur.

Classical Conditioning (BT) A form of learning in which existing responses are attached to new stimuli by pairing those stimuli with those that naturally elicit the response; also referred to as *respondent conditioning*.

Closed System (FT) A self-contained system that has impermeable boundaries and thus is resistant to new information and change.

Cognitive Behavior Modification (BT) A recent extension of behavior therapy that treats thoughts and cognition as behaviors amenable to behavioral procedures. Cognitive behavior modification is most closely associated with the work of Aaron Beck, Albert Ellis, and Donald Meichenbaum.

Cognitive Distortion (CT) Pervasive and systematic errors in reasoning.

Cognitive Restructuring (AD, BT, REBT) An active attempt to alter maladaptive thought patterns and replace them with more adaptive cognitions.

Cognitive Shift (CT) A systematic and biased interpretation of life experiences.

Cognitive Triad (CT) Negative views of the self, the world, and the future that characterize depression.

Cognitive Vulnerability (CT) Individual ways of thinking that predispose one to particular psychological distress.

Collaborative Empiricism (CT) A strategy of seeing the patient as a scientist capable of objective interpretation.

Collective Unconscious (AP) The part of the unconscious that is universal in humans, in contrast to the personal unconscious belonging to individual experience. The contents of the collective unconscious come into consciousness through archetypal images or basic motifs common to all people. *See also* Personal Unconscious.

Common Factors Approach (INT) An approach that seeks to determine and apply the core ingredients different therapies share, predicated on the assumption that commonalities across therapies account for more of the variance in therapeutic success than do unique factors. Common factors include the therapeutic alliance, catharsis, acquisition of new behaviors, and positive expectations.

Complex (AP) An energy-filled cluster of emotions and ideas circling a specific subject. A complex has an archetypal core but expresses aspects of the personal unconscious. Jung's discovery and explanation of the complex lent validity to Freud's belief in the personal unconscious.

Conditional Assumption (CT) An erroneous "if then" interpretation of events that leads to an erroneous conclusion (e.g., "*If* one person dislikes me, *then* I am not likable").

Confluence (GT) A state in which the contact boundary becomes so thin, flexible, and permeable that the distinction between self and environment is lost. In confluence, one does not experience self as distinct but merges self into the beliefs, attitudes, and feelings of others. Confluence can be healthy or unhealthy.

Congruence (CC) Agreement between the feelings and attitudes a therapist is experiencing and his or her professional demeanor; one of Rogers's necessary and sufficient conditions for therapeutic change. *See also* Genuineness.

Conscientization (MC) An educational concept, also known as critical consciousness, that was developed by Paulo Freire. Conscientization involves learning to perceive the social, political, and economic contradictions associated with oppression.

Consensus Trance (CN) View of the normal waking state as dreamlike, lacking real awareness, and shared consensually by most people.

Conjoint Session (FT) Psychotherapy in which two or more patients are treated together.

Constructivism (FT) The view that emphasizes the subjective ways in which each individual creates a perception of reality.

Contact (GT) Basic unit of relationship involving an experience of the boundary between "me" and "not me"; feeling a connection with the "not-me" while maintaining a separation from it.

Convenient Fiction A philosophy of science phase signifying concepts that are imaginary and unreal, but that may be helpful in conceptualization.

Conviction Conclusion based on personal experience and perceptions, usually biased because each person's perspective is unique.

Core Conditions (CC) According to Carl Rogers, the core conditions for growth in therapy are congruence, unconditional positive regard, and empathy. Other theorists such as Albert Ellis have argued that these three conditions are neither necessary nor sufficient for therapeutic growth.

Core Conflictual Relationship Theme Method (PA) A supportive-expressive psychotherapy method used to examine the inner workings of a patient's relationship patterns; an operational version of transference. Each CCRT pattern has three elements: wish, response of others, and response of self.

Counterconditioning (BT) Replacing a particular behavior by conditioning a new response incompatible with the maladaptive behavior. Counterconditioning is one of the explanations for the effectiveness of systematic desensitization.

Countertransference (PA, AP) The activation of unconscious wishes and fantasies on the part of the therapist toward the patient. It can either be elicited by and indicative of the patient's projections or come from the therapist's tendency to respond to patients as though they were significant others in the life, history, or fantasy of the therapist.

Courage (AD) Willingness to take risks without being sure of the consequences; necessary for effective living.

Cultural Competency (MC) The set of knowledge, behaviors, attitudes, skills, and policies that enables a practitioner to work effectively in a multicultural situation. Cultural competence requires congruent behaviors, attitudes, and policies that reflect an understanding of how cultural and sociopolitical influences shape individuals' worldviews and related health behaviors.

Cultural Genogram (MC) A therapeutic tool that emphasizes the role of culture and context in the lives of individuals and their families.

Cybernetic Epistemology (FT) A framework for conceptualizing and analyzing what is being observed in terms of the flow of information through a system.

Cybernetic System (FT) The study of methods of feedback control within a system.

Decatastrophizing (CT, REBT) A "what if" technique designed to explore actual rather than feared events and consequences.

Decentering (CT) Moving the supposed focus of attention away from oneself.

Deconstructionism A theory of literary criticism that challenges many of the prevailing assumptions of psychotherapy. Therapists influenced by deconstructionism attempt to "deconstruct" the ideological biases and traditional assumptions that shape the practice of psychotherapy. Like postmodernism, deconstructionism rejects all claims of ultimate truth.

Defense Mechanism (PA) Method mobilized by the ego in response to its danger signal of anxiety as protection from inner and outer threat. Examples include repression, denial, and projection.

Deflection (GT) A means of blunting the impact of contact and awareness by not giving or receiving feelings or thoughts directly. Vagueness, verbosity, and understatement are forms of deflection.

Dehypnosis (CN) Awakening from a hypnotic trance, especially the enculturated consensus trance shared by most people. This involves disidentifying from mental phenomena such as thoughts and fantasies rather than assuming them to be "real."

Demandingness (REBT) The belief of some clients that they must get what they want in life and that it is a terrible tragedy if this does not occur.

Dementia Praecox An obsolete term for schizophrenia.

Denial (PA) A basic defense through which aspects of experienced reality are treated as if they did not exist; often directed against personal existential death anxieties.

Dereflection (CN) Directing one's attention away from the self.

Determinism The assumption that every mental event is causally tied to earlier psychological experience.

Dialectical Behavior Therapy (BT) A therapy developed by Marsha Linehan for use with patients with borderline personality disorders. DBT balances the need to change with acceptance of the way things are; this is the central dialectic of psychotherapy. Mindfulness is a central component of DBT.

Dialogue (EXT, GT) Genuine, equal, and honest communication between two people; the "I—Thou" relationship.

Dichotomous Thinking (CT, REBT) Categorizing experiences or people in black-and-white or extreme terms only (e.g., all good vs. all bad), with no middle ground.

Dichotomy (GT) A split in which a field is experienced as comprising competing and unrelated forces that cannot be meaningfully integrated into a whole.

Differentiation of Self (FT) Psychological separation by a family member, increasing resistance to being overwhelmed by the emotional reactivity of the family.

Discriminative Stimulus (BT) A stimulus signifying that reinforcement will (or will not) occur.

Disengaged Family (FT) A family whose members are psychologically isolated from one another because of overly rigid boundaries between the participants.

Disorientation Inability to correctly identify time and place (e.g., dates and locations).

Disturbances at the Boundary (GT) A disturbance in the ongoing movement between connection and withdrawal. Blocking connection results in *isolation*; blocking withdrawal results in *confluence*.

Double The auxiliary role that involves playing the protagonist's inner self or what the protagonist might be feeling or thinking but not expressing outwardly. *See also* Auxiliary.

Double Bind (FT) Conflict created in a person who receives contradictory messages in an important relationship but is forbidden to leave or escape from the relationship or to comment on the discrepancy.

Drama Therapy Use of theater techniques to gain self-awareness or increase self-expression in groups.

Dramaturgical Metaphor Framing situations as if they were scenes in a play, which helps to include and more effectively describe vividly the range of psychosocial phenomena that are difficult to describe in more prosaic or abstract terms.

Dual-Instinct Theory (PA) The notion that humans operate primarily in terms of pervasive and innate drives toward both love and aggression. *See also* Eros, Thanatos.

Dyadic (FT) Pertaining to a relationship between two persons.

Dynamics (PA) Interactions, usually conflicted, between one's basic drives or id and the ego's defenses. *See also* Psychodynamics.

Dysarthria Speech deficit involving difficulty with the mechanical production of language.

Early Recollection (AD) Salient memory of a single incident from childhood; used as a projective technique by Adlerian therapists.

Eclecticism The practice of drawing from multiple and diverse sources in formulating client problems and devising treatment plans. Multimodal therapists are technical eclectics (e.g., they employ multiple methods without necessarily endorsing the theoretical positions from which they were derived).

Early Maladaptive Schemas (CT) Broad, pervasive themes regarding oneself and one's relationship with others, developed during childhood and elaborated throughout one's lifetime; dysfunctional to a significant degree.

Effectiveness Study Less well-controlled studies that do not typically use treatment manuals or specific training for the therapists involved in the study. Effectiveness research tends to be conducted in community settings under conditions that approximate day-to-day clinical practice. Contrast with *Efficacy Study*.

Efficacy Study A controlled study that typically uses random assignment of patients to treatments, treatment manuals, carefully trained therapists, and rigorous assessment of outcome by impartial evaluators. This is the type of research typically conducted in universities. Contrast with *Effectiveness Study*.

Ego (PA) The central controlling core of the personality mediating between the *id* (primitive, instinctive needs) and the *superego* (civilized, moralistic elements of the mind).

Eigenwelt (EX) One level of the ways each individual relates to the world. *Eigenwelt* literally means "own world" and refers to the way each of us relates to self.

Electra Complex (PA) Erotic attraction of the female child for her father, with accompanying hostility for her mother; the female equivalent of the Oedipus complex. *See also* Oedipus Complex.

Elegant Solution (REBT) Solution that helps clients make a profound philosophical change that goes beyond mere symptom removal.

Emotional Cognition (PA) The means by which, both consciously and unconsciously, we perceive and process emotionally charged information and meaning in the service of adaptation.

Emotive Techniques (REBT) Therapy techniques that are vigorous, vivid, and dramatic.

Empathic Understanding (CC) The ability to appreciate a person's phenomenological position and to accompany the person's progress in therapy; one of the necessary conditions for therapeutic change.

Empathy (CC) Accurately and deeply feeling someone else's expressed emotions, concerns, or situation.

Empirically Supported Treatments Therapies that have been shown to be effective in scientific studies that meet rigid criteria (e.g., randomized clinical trials). For a treatment to be empirically supported, patients receiving the treatment must have been shown to be better off than patients who receive no treatment, and outcomes must be at least equal to those obtained by alternative therapies that have been documented to be beneficial.

Empty Chair (GT) A chair whose inhabitant is imagined by a client, with all the client's projected attitudes. The imaginary occupant might be a significant person in the client's life, a figure from a dream, a part of the client's body or mind, or even the therapist. The chair is usually used along with role reversal, and the term "shuttling" is used to describe the client's moving back and forth between the chairs as the two parts engage in an encounter. *See also* Encounter, Role Reversal.

Enactment Showing (rather than verbalizing) a situation that deserves to be explored.

Encounter (GT) A dialogue between two persons, or two aspects of the same person, either in reality or with one part played by someone else.

Encounter Group A small number of people who meet (sometimes only once, sometimes on a weekly basis for a specified time) to truly know and accept themselves and others.

Enmeshed Family (FT) Family in which individual members are overly involved in each other's lives, making individual autonomy impossible.

Eros (PA) The life instinct, fueled by libidinal energy and opposed by Thanatos, the death instinct. *See also* Libido, Thanatos.

Epistemology The study of the origin, nature, methods, and limits of knowledge.

Ethicality (CN) Internally based emphasis on moral or principled behavior.

Ethnocentrism (MC) The belief that one's worldview is inherently superior and desirable to others.

Existential Isolation (EX) Fundamental and inevitable separation of each individual from others and the world; it can be reduced but never completely eliminated.

Existentialism (EX) A philosophical movement that stresses the importance of actual existence, one's responsibility for and determination of one's own psychological existence, authenticity in human relations, the primacy of the here and now, and the use of experience in the search for knowledge.

Existential Neurosis (EX) Feelings of emptiness, worthlessness, despair, and anxiety resulting from inauthenticity, abdication of responsibility, failure to make choices, and a lack of direction or purpose in life.

Experiencing (CC) Sensing or awareness of self and the world, whether narrowly and rigidly or openly and flexibly. Experience is unique for each person.

Experiential Family Therapist (FT) A therapist who reveals himself or herself as a real person and uses that self in interacting with families.

Extinction (BT) In classical conditioning, the result of repeated presentation of a conditioned stimulus without the unconditioned stimulus and the resulting gradual diminution of the conditioned response. In operant conditioning, extinction (no response) occurs when reinforcement is withheld following performance of a previously reinforced response.

Facilitator An individual who aids a group in going the direction they choose and accomplishing their chosen goals without doing harm to any member.

Factors of Enlightenment (CN) Seven mental qualities identified by Buddhist psychology as important for psychological well-being and maturation: mindfulness, effort, investigation, rapture, concentration, calm, and equanimity.

Family Constellation (AD) The number, sequencing, and characteristics of the members of a family. The family constellation is an important determinant of life-style.

Family Sculpting (FT, PD) A nonverbal technique to be used by individual family members for physically arranging other family members in space to represent the arranger's symbolic view of family relationships.

Feedback The process by which a system makes adjustments in itself; can be negative (reestablishing equilibrium) or positive (leading to change).

Field Theory (GT) A theory about the nature of reality and our relationship to reality in which our experiences are understood within a specific context. A field is composed of mutually interdependent elements, and changes in the field influence how a person experiences reality. No one can transcend embeddedness in a field, and therefore no one can have an objective perspective on reality.

First-Order Change (FT) Change within a system that does not alter the basic organization of the system itself.

Formative Tendency (CC) An overall inclination toward greater order, complexity, and interrelatedness common to all nature, including human beings.

Free Association (PA) A basic technique of psychoanalysis in which analysands are asked to report, without structure or censure, whatever thoughts come to mind.

Functionally Specific States (CN) States of consciousness in which particular abilities such as introspection are increased, while others are reduced.

Fusion (EXT, FT) In existential therapy, the giving up of oneself to become part of another person or a group; a particular attempt to reduce one's sense of isolation. In family therapy, a blurring of boundaries between family members with the resultant loss of a separate sense of self by each member.

Future Projection Demonstration of what one sees going on in life at some specified time in the future.

Gemeinschaftsgefühl (AD) A combination of concern for others and appreciation of one's role in a larger social order; usually translated as "social interest."

Generalization (BT) The occurrence of behavior in situations that resemble but are different from the stimulus environment in which the behavior was learned.

Genital Stage (PA) The final stage in psychosexual development, also termed the oedipal phase, in which heterosexual relations are achieved. Its roots are formed at ages 5 to 6, and it is said to be the basis for the mature personality.

Genogram (FT, MC) A schematic diagram of a family's relationship system that is used to trace recurring family patterns over generations.

Genuineness (CC) The characteristic of being real and true to oneself; lack of pretense, social facade, or refusal to allow certain aspects of one's self into awareness. See *congruence*.

Gestalt (GT) A word with no literal English translation, referring to a perceptual whole or a unified configuration of experience.

Givens of Human Existence (EX) Psychiatrist Irvin Yalom defines these as death, freedom, isolation, and meaninglessness. The courage with which we meet the givens of human existence defines our life.

Graded-Task Assignment (CT, BT) Starting with a simple activity and increasing the level of complexity or difficulty in a step-by-step fashion.

Guided Discovery A series of questions to assist the client to uncover relevant information out of his or her current awareness, examine his or her interpretations of events and discover alternative meanings.

Hidden Agenda The actual goal of an interaction between people (as in a game), which is different from what superficially appears to be the goal.

Higher States (CN) States of consciousness containing normal mental capacities plus additional, heightened ones.

Holism (AD) Studying individuals in their entirety, including how they proceed through life, rather than trying to separate out certain aspects or parts, such as studying the mind apart from the body.

Homeostasis A balanced and steady state of equilibrium.

Homework (REBT, BT) Specific activities to be done between therapy sessions.

Hot Cognition (CT) A powerful and highly meaningful idea that produces strong emotional reactions.

Hysteria An early term for conversion reaction, a disorder in which psychological disturbance takes a physical form (e.g., paralysis in the absence of organic disturbance). Many of Freud's theories grew out of his experience in treating hysterical patients.

Id (PA) The reservoir of the biological, instinctual drives with innate and developmental components. *See also* Ego, Superego.

Identification (PA) A mental mechanism, used unconsciously in normal interactions and as a psychic defense, through which one person absorbs and takes on the traits, values, and defenses of another person.

Identified Patient (FT) The person who seeks treatment or for whom treatment is sought.

Inauthentic Mode (EX) Heidegger believed the inauthentic mode of being was characterized by mindless responding and a failure to take responsibility for becoming one's true self.

Inclusion (GT) Putting oneself as completely as possible into another's experience without judging or evaluating, while still maintaining a separate sense of self.

Individual Psychology (AD) An approach to understanding human behavior that sees each person as a unique, whole entity who is constantly becoming rather than being and one whose development can only be understood within a social context.

Individuation (AP) The process by which an individual becomes an indivisible and integrated whole person responsibly embodying his or her individual strengths and limitations.

Inferiority Complex (AD) An exaggeration of feelings of inadequacy and insecurity resulting in defensiveness and neurotic behavior. It is usually, but not always, abnormal.

Inferiority Feeling (AD) Seeing oneself as inadequate or incompetent in comparison with others, with one's ideal self, or with personal values; considered universal and normal. *Contrast with* Inferiority Complex.

Integration Organized and harmonious relationships among personality components.

Intensive Group (CC) A small number of people who come together for a brief but condensed period (e.g., a weekend) to engage in special interpersonal experiences that are designed to expand awareness of self and others.

Interlocking Pathologies (FT) Multiple forms of dysfunction within a family that are interdependent in the way they are expressed and maintained.

Interlocking Triangles (FT) Basic units of family relationships consisting of a series of three-person sets of interactions (e.g., father—mother—child; grandparent—parent—child).

Internal Frame of Reference (CC) A view or perception of both the world and self as seen by the individual, as distinguished from the viewpoint of an observer, psychotherapist, or other person.

Interpersonal Problem Areas (IPT) Grief, interpersonal disputes, role transitions, and interpersonal deficits. These four problem areas serve as the triggers for depressive episodes.

Intrapsychic Within the mind or psyche of the individual.

Introject (FT) Internalized object from one's past that affects current relationships.

Introjection (PA, GT) In psychoanalysis, an unconscious process of identifying with other persons, real or imagined, by incorporating attributes of these others into oneself. In Gestalt therapy, accepting information or values from the outside without evaluation; not necessarily psychologically unhealthy.

Irrational Belief (REBT) Unreasonable conviction that produces emotional upset (for example, insisting that the world should or must be different from what it actually is).

Isolation (GT) A state in which the contact boundary is so thick, rigid, and impermeable that the psychological connection between self and environment is lost, and the person does not allow access from or to the outside. Isolation can be healthy or unhealthy. *Contrast with* Withdrawal.

Latency Period (PA) A relatively inactive period of psychosexual development said to begin around age 6 and end around age 11.

Leaning Tower of Pisa Approach (FT) A variation of paradoxical intention in which a therapist intentionally makes a problem worse until it falls of its own weight and is thereby resolved.

Libido (PA) The basic driving force of personality in Freud's system. It includes sexual energy but is not restricted to it.

Life-style (AD) One's characteristic way of living and pursuing long-term goals.

Life Tasks (AD) The basic challenges and obligations of life: society, work, and sex. The additional tasks of spiritual growth and self-identity are included by Rudolf Dreikurs and Harold Mosak.

Linear Causality (FT) The view that one event causes the other, not vice versa.

Locus of Evaluation (CC) The place of a judgment's origin, its source; whether the appraisal of an experience comes more from within the individual (internal) or from outside sources (external).

Logotherapy (EX) A therapeutic approach developed by Viktor Frankl emphasizing value and meaning as prerequisites for mental health and personal growth.

Lucid Dreaming (CN) A sleep state in which people know they are dreaming.

Magnification (CT) Exaggerating something's significance.

Manual-Based Treatments (BT) The use of standardized, manual-based treatments is advocated by most proponents of evidence-based treatment because manuals increase the likelihood of treatment fidelity. Critics of manualized treatment argue that the use of manuals represents a Procrustean approach that ignores individual differences in patients and problems.

Marital Schism (FT) A disturbed family arrangement characterized by disharmony, undermining of the spouse, and frequent threats of divorce. *See also* Marital Skew.

Marital Skew (FT) A disturbed family arrangement in which one person dominates to an extreme degree, and in which the marriage is maintained through the distortion of reality. *See also* Marital Schism.

Maya (CN) An illusory and encompassing distortion of one's perception and experience that is not recognized as such.

Mediational Stimulus-Response Model (BT) A behavioral model that posits internal events, such as thoughts and images, as links between perceiving a stimulus and making a response.

Medical Model (IPT) An approach that is used to allow depressed individuals to adopt a "sick role" and understand that it is a treatable medical problem like diabetes.

Meditation (CN) Practices designed to train attention and bring various mental processes under greater voluntary control.

Microaggressions (MC) Psychological assaults that individuals receive on a regular basis solely because of their race, color, or ethnicity.

Mindfulness (CN) Clear objective awareness of experience.

Mindfulness-Based Cognitive Therapy (CT) An approach to cognitive therapy that uses acceptance and meditation strategies to promote resiliency and prevent recurrences of depressive episodes.

Minimization (CT) Making an event far less important than it actually is.

Mirror Person who imitates a client's behavior and demeanor so that the client can more clearly see him- or herself in action.

Morita (CN) A Japanese therapy for treating anxiety by redirecting one's attention away from the self.

Mitwelt (EX) The way in which each individual relates to the world, socially and through being with others; the age we live in, our age, our own times, the present generation, our contemporaries.

Mode (CT) Network of cognitive, affective, motivational, and behavioral schemas that composes personality and interprets ongoing situations.

Monadic (FT) Based on the characteristics or traits of a single person.

Monodrama (PD, GT) One client's playing both parts in a scene by alternating between them.

Multigenerational Transmission Process (FT) The passing on of psychological problems over generations as a result of immature persons marrying others with similar low levels of separateness from their families.

Multiple Psychotherapy (AD) A technique in which several therapists simultaneously treat a single patient.

Musturbation (REBT) A term coined by Albert Ellis to characterize the behavior of clients who are absolutistic and inflexible in their thinking, maintaining that they *must* not fail, *must* be exceptional, *must* be successful, and so on.

Mystification (FT) The deliberate distortion of another person's experience by misinterpreting or mislabeling it.

Naikan (CN) Japanese therapy using intensive reflection on past relationships to increase social and interpersonal contributions.

Narcissism (PA) Self-absorption, self-concern, and self-love arising from psychic energy directed at the self; the term currently is used to include tension regulation, self-image, and self-esteem.

Narrative Therapy (FT) An approach to family therapy built on the belief that reality is constructed, organized, and maintained through the stories we create. Associated with Australian therapist Michael White and others.

Negative Feedback (FT) The flow of output information back into a system to correct too great a deviation from normal and return the system to its steady state.

Negative Reinforcement (BT) Any behavior that increases the probability of a response by terminating or withdrawing an unpleasant stimulus. Negative reinforcement increases the likelihood of future occurrence of the behavior it follows.

Neurosis (PA) A term first used by Freud to include all but the most severe psychological syndromes; currently narrowly defined as an emotional disorder in which psychic functioning is relatively intact and contact with reality is sound.

Neurotic Anxiety (EX) A state of fear or apprehension out of proportion to an actual threat. Neurotic anxiety is destructive or paralyzing and cannot be used constructively. *Compare with* Normal Anxiety.

Nondirective Attitude (CC) Valuing the client's inherent capacity for and right to self-determination.

Normal Anxiety (EX) A sense of apprehension appropriate to a given threatening situation, which can be faced, dealt with, and used creatively. *Compare with* Neurotic Anxiety.

Object Relations Theory (PA, FT) The view that the basic human motive is the search for satisfying object (person) relationships. Associated with the writings of W. Ronald Fairbairn.

Oedipus Complex (PA) Erotic attraction of the male child for his mother, accompanied by hostility toward the father. *See also* Electra Complex.

Ontological (EX) Concerned with the science of being or existence.

Open System (FT) A system with relatively permeable boundaries permitting the exchange of information with its environment.

Operant Conditioning (BT) A type of learning in which responses are modified by their consequences. Reinforcement increases the likelihood of future occurrences of the reinforced response; punishment and extinction decrease the likelihood of future occurrences of the responses they follow.

Oral Phase (PA) The earliest phase of psychosexual development, extending from birth to approximately 18 months, in which most libidinal gratification occurs through biting, sucking, and oral contact.

Organ Inferiority (AD) Perceived or actual congenital defects in organ systems believed by Alfred Adler to result in compensatory striving to overcome these deficits.

Organismic Valuing Process (CC) Making individual judgments or assessments of the desirability of an action or choice on the basis of one's own sensory evidence and life experience.

Overgeneralization (CT, REBT) Constructing a general rule from isolated incidents and applying it too broadly.

Panacea A remedy for all diseases and difficulties; a cure-all.

Paradigm A set of assumptions limiting an area to be investigated scientifically and specifying the methods used to collect and interpret the forthcoming data.

Paradigm Shift A significant and widespread change in the concepts, values, perceptions, and practices that define a community or a structured activity (e.g., psychotherapy).

Paradoxical Intervention (FT) A therapeutic technique whereby the patient is directed to continue the symptomatic behavior. To comply is to admit voluntary control over the symptom; to rebel is to give up the symptom.

Paradoxical Theory of Change. (GT) A theory of change that is based on a paradox: The more one tries to be who one is not, the more one stays the same; the more one tries to stay the same in a changing world, the more one changes relative to the world. When a person knows and accepts himself or herself, maximum growth can occur. When one rejects oneself, e.g., by forcing oneself beyond one's support, growth is hindered by internal conflict.

Paraphilias Unusual or atypical sexual behaviors that are thought to have clinical relevance. The major paraphilias include exhibitionism, fetishism, frotteurism, pedophilia, sexual masochism, sexual sadism, transvestic fetishism, and voyeurism.

Persona (AP) A mask or way of appearing that is appropriate to a specific role or social setting. It both shields an individual and reveals suitable aspects of the personality, but is often at variance with the personality as a whole.

Personal Unconscious (AP) An individual unconscious layer of the personality containing undeveloped parts of the personality, repressed ideas, experiences, emotions, and subliminal perceptions. *See also* Collective Unconscious.

Personalization (CT) Taking personal responsibility for negative events without supporting evidence of personal involvement.

Phallic Phase (PA) A psychosexual phase in boys of ages 3 to 5 in which penile experiences and fantasies of thrusting and exhibiting are predominant. The comparable phase in girls is termed the vaginal phase. *See also* Vaginal Phase.

Phases of Dynamic Psychotherapy (PA) Opening; working through; termination.

Phenomenology (AD, EXT, GT) A method of exploration that primarily uses human experience as the source of data and attempts to include all human experience without bias (external observation, emotions, thoughts, and so on). Subjects are taught to distinguish between current experience and the biases brought to the situation. Phenomenology is the basic method of most existentialists.

Placebo In medicine, placebos are inert substances given to patients in place of bona fide medications. In psychotherapy, placebos are most often sham treatments used in research to control for the nonspecific effects of attention.

Pleasure Principle (PA) The basic human tendency to avoid pain and seek pleasure, especially salient in the first years of life. *Contrast with* Reality Principle.

Positive Feedback (FT) The flow of output information back into the system in order to amplify deviation from a steady state, thus leading to instability and change.

Positive Reinforcement (BT) Any stimulus that follows a behavior and increases the likelihood of the occurrence of the behavior that it follows.

Postmodern Therapies (GT) Any approach to therapy that recognizes the validity and assumptions of multiple realities while rejecting the primacy of the worldview of the therapist. Postmodern therapies stress the importance of culture in determining reality and emphasize the influence of language and power relationships in shaping and defining psychopathology.

Primary Process Thinking (PA) Nonlogical thinking such as is found in dreams, creativity, and the operation of the unconscious. Freud believed primary process thinking characterized the operations of the Id. Contrast with *Secondary Process Thinking*.

Principled Nondirectiveness (CC) An unwaivering attitude of respect adopted by the client centered therapist to provide an optimal environment in which clients can change. Ususally contrasted with instrumental nondirectiveness in which the therapist's empathic responding is goal directed.

Projection (PA, AP) Attributing to others unacceptable personal thoughts, feelings, or behaviors.

Projective Identification (PA) An interactional form of projection, used both normally and as a defense, through which one person places into another person his or her inner state and defenses.

Protagonist In psychodrama, the term used for the client whose situation is being explored, who is also usually the main player in the role-playing process.

Pseudohostility (FT) Superficial bickering that allows one to avoid dealing with deeper, more genuine, and more intimate feelings.

Pseudomutuality (FT) A facade of family harmony that gives the appearance of an open and satisfying relationship that does not truly exist.

Psychodynamic Diagnostic Manual (PA) A psychodynamic alternative to the *Diagnostic and Statistical Manual (or DSM)*. The *Psychodynamic Diagnostic Manual* is based on a psychoanalytic model of human functioning and addresses the subjective experiences associated with various diagnoses.

Psychodrama A method of psychotherapy developed by J. L. Moreno in the mid-1930s in which clients role-play their problems.

Psychodynamics (PA) A term similar to dynamics that refers to mental interactions and conflict, usually formulated in terms of ego, id, and superego. *See also* Dynamics.

Psychodynamic Psychotherapy (PA) A general term for a variety of therapies that evolved from psychoanalysis. Dynamic psychotherapists generally see their clients once or twice each week and the client is sitting up.

Psychological Masquerade Apparent psychological symptoms actually caused by physical or organic conditions.

Punishment (BT) An aversive event likely to terminate any behavior that it follows.

Randomized controlled trial (IPT; BT) A prospective experiment in which investigators randomly assign patients to one or more treatment groups; considered the gold standard in evidence-based therapy. Most widely used in interpersonal psychotherapy and behavior therapy. (Also known as **randomized clinical trial**.)

Rapture(CN) Somatically experienced ecstasy that accompanies clear awareness in advanced meditation.

Reality An individual's private world, but more generally, a group of perceptions or "facts" with substantial consensus about their meaning.

Reality Principle (PA) The guiding principle of the ego, which permits postponement of gratification to meet the demands of the environment or secure greater pleasure at a later time. *Contrast with* Pleasure Principle.

Reattribution (CT) Assigning alternative causes to events; reinterpreting one's symptoms.

Redundancy Principle (FT) Repetitive behavioral sequences between participants, as within a family.

Re-evaluation Counseling (MC) An empowering co-counseling approach in which two or more individuals take turns listening to each other without interruption in order to recover from the effects of racism, classism, sexism, and other types of oppression.

Reframing (FT) Relabeling behavior by putting it into a new, more positive perspective.

Regression (PA) Variously defined as an active or passive slipping back to more immature levels of defense or functioning, or seeking gratification from earlier phases of development.

Reinforcement (BT) The presentation of a reward or the removal of an aversive stimulus following a response. Reinforcement always increases the future probability of the reinforced response.

Replay (PD, BT) A psychodramatic technique, often used in behavior therapy and other approaches, in which the client repeats a previous scene. It is often applied in the mastery of interpersonal skills.

Repression (PA) A major defense mechanism in which distressing thoughts are barred from conscious expression.

Resistance (PA, GT) In psychoanalysis, any obstacle, pathological or nonpathological, to the progress of an analysis or therapy, usually involving a modification of a ground rule of treatment and based on unconscious sources within both patient and analyst (i.e., interactionally determined). In Gestalt therapy, the reluctance of people to know, show, or own aspects of themselves. Resistance can be healthy or unhealthy.

Respondent Conditioning (BT) *See* Classical Conditioning.

Retroflection (GT) A contact boundary disturbance in which a person substitutes self for the environment and does to self what he or she originally did or tried to do to others. Retroflection is the chief mechanism of isolation and is not necessarily unhealthy.

Role Playing Acting the part of oneself or someone else under therapeutic guidance. (Originally used in psychodrama, the term has now come to be used also as a way of problem exploration in many other therapies, as well as in education and business.)

Role Reversal In psychodrama, the dropping of the point of view of one's own role and taking on the attitudes and physical position and perspective of the other person in an interaction. A plays B and B plays A. Or sometimes, if the actual other person isn't present, A takes the role of whoever he imagines B to be, using an empty chair, thus opening his mind to a deeper level of empathy. *See also* Empty Chair.

Samadhi (CN) Yogic state of consciousness marked by deep calm and concentration.

Scapegoating (FT) Casting a person in a role that unfairly exposes him or her to criticism, blame, or punishment.

Schema (CT) Strategy or way of thinking comprising core beliefs and basic assumptions about how the world operates.

Schema Therapy (CT) A strategy developed by Jeffrey Young that elaborates on classic cognitive therapy by incorporating techniques drawn from psychodynamic theory and other systems. Schema therapy specifically focuses on childhood experiences believed to be associated with anxiety and depression.

Secondary Process Thinking (PA) Linear, logical, and verbal thinking, associated with the operations of the ego. Contrast with *Primary Process Thinking*.

Second-Order Change (FT) Fundamental change in a system's organization and function.

Selective Abstraction (CT) Basing a conclusion on a detail taken out of context and ignoring other information.

Self-Actualization A basic human drive toward growth, completeness, and fulfillment.

Self-Concept One's own definition of who one is, including one's attributes, emotions, abilities, character, faults, and so on.

Self-Instructional Training (BT) A technique, described most completely by Donald Meichenbaum, for replacing self-defeating thoughts with self-enhancing cognitions.

Self Psychology (PA) A psychoanalytic approach associated with the work and writings of Heinz Kohut. Self psychology stresses empathy, mirroring, and support for positive esteem.

Self-Regard (CC) That aspect of the self-concept that develops from the esteem or respect accorded oneself.

Sensate Focus (BT) A series of exercises used in sex therapy designed to reintroduce clients to receiving and giving sensual pleasure.

Shadow (AP) Unconscious, unaccepted, or unrecognized parts of the personality that are most often, but not always, negative.

Sharing The third phase of a psychodramatic enactment in which other group members in the audience and even auxiliaries share how that role playing may have touched on similar or related events in their own lives—in contrast to giving advice, interpretations, or analysis.

Social Interest (AD) The feeling of being part of a social whole; the need and willingness to contribute to the general social good. *See also* Gemeinschaftsgefühl.

Social Learning Theory (BT) A system that combines operant and classical conditioning with cognitive mediational processes (e.g., vicarious learning and symbolic activity) to account for the development, maintenance, and modification of behavior.

Sociometry A method in which groups give feedback about their interpersonal preferences (e.g., attraction or repulsion).

Sociotrophy (CT) A personality dimension characterized by dependency on interpersonal relationships and needs for closeness and nurturance.

Socratic Dialogue (CT) A series of questions designed to arrive at logical answers to and conclusions about a hypothesis.

Splitting (PA, GT) In psychoanalysis, a primitive defense through which persons are classified as all-good or all-bad individuals, making it impossible to have a full and balanced picture of other people. In Gestalt therapy, a situation in which a person splits off part of him- or herself as a polar opposite. The individual is aware of one pole and oblivious to the other. For example, an individual may split into competent and incompetent selves and vacillate between these roles. A split is one form of a dichotomy.

Spontaneity A frame of mind enabling one to address situations afresh, often with a significant measure of improvisation.

Stages of Change (INT) A model developed by Prochaska and DiClemente and used to match therapeutic approaches to a client's readiness to change. The model posits five stages: Precontemplation, contemplation, preparation, and action. See Table 1 in chapter 14.

Stimulus Control (BT) Arranging the environment in such a way that a given response is either more likely or less likely to occur (e.g., buying only one pack of cigarettes per day in order to decrease the likelihood of smoking).

Strategic Intervention Therapy (FT) An approach to family therapy employing specific strategies, plans, and tactics to force changes in behavior.

Structuralism (FT) An approach to family therapy, associated with Salvador Minuchin, that emphasizes the importance of the nuclear family and seeks to change pathological alliances and splits in the family.

Structuralist (FT) A therapist who emphasizes changing or realigning a family's organizational structure to improve its transactional patterns.

Structural Theory or Hypothesis (PA) Freud's second model of the mind. The model postulates three agencies of the mind—ego, superego, and id—each with conscious and unconscious components. *See also* Id, Ego, *and* Superego.

Stuck-Togetherness (FT) A situation observed in schizophrenic families in which roles and boundaries are blurred and no family member has an identity distinct from the family.

Subjective Reasoning (CT) Believing that feelings are the same as, or equivalent to, facts.

Subsystem (FT) An organized component within an overall system, such as a family.

Superego (PA) A structure of the mind, developed from innate tendencies and early parental interactions and identifications, that embraces moral and other standards and regulates psychic tensions, self-image, self-esteem, and drive-discharge. *See also* Ego, Id.

Support (GT) To provide the psychological, physiological, social, or material aid needed to initiate, terminate, regulate, and maintain contact or withdrawal as needed by the person or the environment. People are self-supporting to the degree that they are the chief agents in initiating, terminating, regulating, and maintaining contact/withdrawal and do so based on self-identification.

Surplus Reality Psychological experiences involving other than physical reality (e.g., spiritual events, a relationship with a significant deceased other).

Survival An innate need, drive, and source of human behavior. It leads human beings to seek health, nutrition, and protection from physical danger.

Symbiosis (FT) A relationship in which two people, often a mother and her child, become so intertwined that it is impossible to find a boundary between them.

Symbolization (CC) A process of allowing a life event or experience into one's consciousness or awareness and interpreting it in terms of the self-concept; it may be straightforward, distorted, or prohibited altogether.

Symptom—Context Method (PA) A way to decode the meanings of symptoms; used in supportive–expressive psychotherapy for both research and therapy purposes.

Syncretism (INT) A pejorative term referring to the uncritical and unsystematic combination of various therapeutic approaches.

Synthesis Making a whole from elements or parts; constructing the overall meaning of a situation from many different aspects of it.

System A complete unit made up of interconnected and interdependent parts operating in a stable way over time.

Systematic Desensitization (BT) A step-by-step procedure for replacing anxiety with relaxation while gradually increasing exposure to an anxiety-producing situation or object.

Systematic Eclecticism (INT) An approach advocated by Norcross and Beutler (chapter 14) in which the various approaches to eclecticism (e.g., technical eclecticism, theoretical integration, common factors, and assimilative integration) are blended to meet the unique needs of each individual patient. Also referred to as *systematic treatment selection (STS)*.

Technical Eclecticism (INT) An integrative approach in which therapists use multiple procedures drawn from various therapeutic systems without particular concern about the theories from which they came.

Thanatos (PA) An instinct toward death and self-destruction posited by Freud to oppose and balance Eros, the life instinct.

Theoretical Integration (INT) The integration of two or more therapies with an emphasis on integrating the underlying theories associated with each therapeutic system.

Therapeutic Alliance The partnership between therapist and client that develops as the two work together to reach the goals of therapy.

Third-Party Payer Financial intermediary that controls payment to therapists. In therapy, third-party payers are usually insurance companies or government agencies.

Third Wave of Behavior Therapy (BT) The first wave of behavior therapy focused on modifying overt behavior. The second wave addressed cognitions (e.g., cognitive behavior therapy). The third wave addresses mindfulness and self-awareness and includes dialectical behavior therapy (DBT) and acceptance and commitment therapy (ACT).

Token Economy (BT) A program that provides people with short-term reinforcement for specific behaviors by allotting tokens (poker chips or points) that are accumulated and later exchanged for privileges or desired objects.

Topographic Theory (PA) Freud's first model of the mind in which access to awareness of contents and functions was the defining criterion. The model had interactional elements but was eventually replaced by Freud's structural model. *See also* Unconscious.

Trait Theory The belief in stable and enduring personality characteristics.

Transference (PA, AP) The therapy situation in which the patient responds to the therapist as though he or she were a significant figure in the patient's past, usually a parent. *See also* Countertransference.

Triadic (FT) Pertaining to a relationship involving the interaction of three or more persons.

Trust (CC) Basic faith in oneself and others as being growth-directed and positively oriented.

Two-chair Technique (GT) An affective, experiential procedure in which the client engages in dialogue with another person (or with another part of the self) symbolically represented by an empty chair. The client may assume different roles by switching from one chair to the other.

Umwelt (EX) A way of relating to the world through its biological and physical aspects; one's relationship with nature and the surrounding world.

Unconditional Positive Regard (CC) A nonpossessive caring and acceptance of the client as a human being, irrespective of the therapist's own values. One of Rogers's necessary and sufficient conditions for therapeutic change.

Unconscious (PA, AP) A division of the psyche; the repository of psychological material of which the individual is unaware.

Vaginal Phase (PA) The phase in girls that corresponds to boys' phallic phase, ages 3 to 5, during which vaginal sensations and incorporative imagery predominate.

Vicarious Learning (BT) Learning through observation and imitation; a synonym for *modeling*.

Voluntary Simplicity (CN) Self-motivated choice to live more simply and to de-emphasize material goods.

Warming Up The process of becoming more spontaneous, often associated with a relaxation of self-consciousness and anxiety, a higher level of trust, and an increasing degree of involvement in the task at hand.

Warmth (CC) Positive and real feelings of acceptance toward another person.

Will to Power (AD) Individual striving for superiority and dominance in order to overcome feelings of inadequacy and inferiority.

Withdrawal (GT) Temporary withdrawing from contact while maintaining a permeable contact boundary. Withdrawal can be healthy or unhealthy. *Contrast with* Isolation.

Work (GT) The process of exploring by phenomenological focusing in order to increase awareness. One can work in any setting and can focus on any theme (here-and-now contact, life problems, developmental themes, spiritual concerns, creativity and emotional expansion, dreams, belief systems, etc.)

Worldview (MC) Those ideas and beliefs, shaped by one's culture, that influence the way an individual interprets the world and interacts with it. Associated with the writings of Harry Triandis.

Yoga (CN) Disciplines dealing with ethics, lifestyle, body postures, breath control, intellectual study, and meditation.

Zeitgeist The spirit of the times; the prevailing cultural climate.

NAME INDEX

SUBJECT INDEX